Clinical Diagnosis and Management of Hearing Loss

Clinical Diagnosis and Management of Hearing Loss

Edited by Freya Brown

hayle medical

New York

Hayle Medical,
750 Third Avenue, 9th Floor,
New York, NY 10017, USA

Visit us on the World Wide Web at:
www.haylemedical.com

ISBN: 978-1-64647-517-9

Cataloging-in-Publication Data

Clinical diagnosis and management of hearing loss / edited by Freya Brown.
p. cm.
Includes bibliographical references and index.
ISBN 978-1-64647-517-9
1. Deafness. 2. Deafness--Etiology. 3. Deafness--Prevention. 4. Deafness--Treatment. 5. Ear--Diseases.
6. Hearing disorders. I. Brown, Freya.
RF290 .H43 2023
617.8--dc23

Table of Contents

Preface

The main aim of this book is to educate learners and enhance their research focus by presenting diverse topics covering this vast field. This is an advanced book which compiles significant studies by distinguished experts in the area of analysis. This book addresses successive solutions to the challenges arising in the area of application, along with it; the book provides scope for future developments.

Hearing loss refers to the partial or complete inability to hear. This condition affects people of all ages and may be inherited or acquired after birth. Mixed hearing loss, conductive hearing loss and sensorineural hearing loss are the three types of hearing loss. It has various signs and symptoms such as difficulty in hearing consonants, muffling of speech and other sounds, withdrawal from conversations, and difficulty in understanding words. Hearing loss can range from mild to moderate to severe. It makes hearing high pitched sounds or conversational speech difficult, and can affect one or both ears. The causes of hearing loss include a variety of factors such as aging, certain infections, some toxins or medications, genetics, trauma to the ear, exposure to noise, and birth complications. Medical treatments, hearing aids, cochlear implants and other options are used to treat and manage hearing loss. This book contains a detailed explanation of the various diagnostic and therapeutic techniques associated with hearing loss. It will help new researchers by foregrounding their knowledge on this medical condition.

It was a great honour to edit this book, though there were challenges, as it involved a lot of communication and networking between me and the editorial team. However, the end result was this all-inclusive book covering diverse themes in the field.

Finally, it is important to acknowledge the efforts of the contributors for their excellent chapters, through which a wide variety of issues have been addressed. I would also like to thank my colleagues for their valuable feedback during the making of this book.

Editor

1

The Effect of Endolymphatic Hydrops and Mannitol Dehydration Treatment on Guinea Pigs

Shu-Qi Wang[1,2†], Chen-Long Li[1,2,3†], Jing-Qi Xu[1,2], Li-Li Chen[1,2,3], You-Zhou Xie[1,2,3], Pei-Dong Dai[1,2], Liu-Jie Ren[1,2,3], Wen-Juan Yao[4,5*] and Tian-Yu Zhang[1,2,3*]*

[1] Department of Facial Plastic Reconstruction Surgery, Eye and ENT Hospital of Fudan University, Shanghai, China, [2] ENT Institute, Eye and ENT Hospital of Fudan University, Shanghai, China, [3] Hearing Medicine Key Laboratory, National Health Commission of China, Shanghai, China, [4] School of Mechanics and Engineering Science, Shanghai University, Shanghai, China, [5] Shanghai Institute of Applied Mathematics and Mechanics, Shanghai, China

***Correspondence:**
Liu-Jie Ren
renliujie@fudan.edu.cn
Wen-Juan Yao
wjyao@shu.edu.cn
Tian-Yu Zhang
ty.zhang2006@aliyun.com

† These authors have contributed equally to this work

Background: Endolymphatic hydrops (EH) is considered as the pathological correlate of Menière's disease (MD) and cause of hearing loss. The mechanism of EH, remaining unrevealed, poses challenges for formalized clinical trials.

Objective: This study aims to investigate the development of hearing loss, as well as the effect of dehydration treatment on EH animal models.

Methods: In this study, different severity EH animal models were created. The laser Doppler vibrometer (LDV) and auditory brainstem responses (ABR) were used to study the effects of EH and the dehydration effects of mannitol. The LDV was used to measure the vibration of the round window membrane (RWM) reflecting the changes in inner ear impedance. ABR was used to evaluate the hearing changes. Furthermore, tissue section and scanning electron microscopy (SEM) observations were used to analyze the anatomical change to the cochlea and outer hair cells.

Results: The RWM vibrations decreased with the severity of EH, indicating an increase in the cochlear impedance. The dehydration therapy lowered the impedance to restore acoustic transduction in EH 10- and 20-day animal models. Simultaneously, the ABR thresholds increased in EH models and were restored after dehydration. Moreover, a difference in the hearing was found between ABR and LDV results in severe EH animal models, and the dehydration therapy was less effective, indicating a sensorineural hearing loss (SNHL).

Conclusion: Endolymphatic hydrops causes hearing loss by increasing the cochlear impedance in all tested groups, and mannitol dehydration is an effective therapy to restore hearing. However, SNHL occurs for the EH 30-day animal models, limiting the effectiveness of dehydration. Our results suggest the use of dehydrating agents in the early stage of EH.

Keywords: endolymphatic hydrops, dehydration therapy, Ménière's disease, laser Doppler vibrometry, cochlear impedance

HIGHLIGHTS

- This study investigated the development of hearing loss on guinea pig EH models, as well as the effect of dehydration treatment. By combining analogical observations and objective measurement of hearing loss (ABR and LDV measurement of RWM vibration). The highlights of this study are:

1. EH induced hearing loss progressed with the development of EH, it starts at low frequencies, and later involves medium to high frequencies.
2. EH increases the cochlear impedance, causing conductive dysfunction. This dysfunction can be cured by dehydration treatment in early stage. But irreversible sensorineural component becomes significant for long-time EH.
3. Early dehydration treatment is suggested for reserving hearing.

- This study gives an overview of the development of hearing loss in EH, and partly revealed the mechanical basis and biological influences of EH. Moreover, the investigation of dehydration treatment may provide a reference for clinical practice.

INTRODUCTION

Menière's disease (MD) is an inner ear disorder named after Prosper Menière (Atkinson, 1961), who in 1861 described patients with episodic vertigo accompanied by fluctuating hearing, tinnitus, and aural fullness in the affected ear. Later, the correlation between MD and endolymphatic hydrops (EH) was found by Hallpike and Cairns (1938) and Yamakawa (1938). As the presence of histopathological EH was reported postmortem, the essential relationship between EH and MD were being questioned until Merchant's study found that EH and MD are associated with 100% of cases when the current definition of MD is strictly applied (Merchant et al., 2005; Gluth, 2020). Recently, the development of gadolinium chelate (GdC)-enhanced MRI demonstrated EH *in vivo* and further confirmed EH is a common pathological feature of inner ear diseases characterized by low-frequency hearing loss, including MD (Naganawa et al., 2014; Zou et al., 2020).

The physiological mechanisms of Méniere are still poorly understood, yet causative relationships between EH and disordered auditory physiology in MD have been supported by much clinical and experimental evidence. It is widely believed that the dysregulation of endolymph volume may lead to EH and cause a chain reaction. Since morphological changes such as the collapse of stereocilia of outer hair cells (Albers et al., 1987) or losing synapses in inner hair cells (Valenzuela et al., 2020) fail to explain the correlation of EH and hearing loss, potential explanations have mainly focused on the mechanical impact caused by high endolymphatic pressure on endolymph components (Oberman et al., 2017) and the function of the lymphatic sac (Swinburne et al., 2018). Among those theories, the mechanical mechanism of high pressure in the endolymphatic duct explains the clinical hearing symptoms in early and mid-stage Méniere's disease (Ichimiya and Ichimiya, 2019), prompting the dehydration therapy for patients with MD. The effectiveness of dehydration therapy has not been strictly evaluated (Quaranta et al., 2019), and a recent meta-analysis further concluded that it was unclear whether diuretics were effective (Nevoux et al., 2018), even though patients have stated subjective perception improvements (Ward et al., 2019). Whether hyperosmolar agents, such as glycerol, urea, or mannitol, can improve patient hearing and act as a diagnostic tool are still under debate (Thomsen and Vesterhauge, 1979; Angelborg et al., 1982; Van de Water et al., 1986; Sterkers et al., 1987; Magliulo et al., 2001). This apparent contradiction raises the question of why patients report relief of symptoms while most of the available studies query the effectiveness of dehydration.

As the hearing ability can be predicted by the mechanical transfer of acoustic vibration and the round window is considered as an accurate proxy for cochlear fluid displacement (Ryan et al., 2020), we propose using peak-to-peak displacement of round window membrane (RWM) to analyze the change in intra-cochlear pressure under the effects of dehydration agents on EH animal models. We chose RWM as the reflection of the inner ear transfer function because it can estimate the cochlear input impedance as a whole, so it is free from the influence of the inertia of the perilymph inside the helicontrema, thus the compliance of it can better describe the total pressure inside the cochlea (Marquardt and Hensel, 2013). As the laser Doppler vibrometer (LDV) is an established optical technique to analyze the vibration of the ossicular chain, RWM, and tympanic membranes (Zhang and Gan, 2013), we used LDV to measure the dynamic behavior of RWM to evaluate cochlear impedance and sound transmission. To better illustrate the effectiveness of dehydration therapy, we created a series of different severity EH models using guinea pigs to simulate various stages of MD, then treated with mannitol. By measuring the auditory brainstem response (ABR), the linear displacement of RWM, and observing the changes in the organ of Corti, we assessed the influence of high endolymphatic pressure and the dehydration effects of mannitol on EH models.

MATERIALS AND METHODS

Animals and Research Program

Healthy albino guinea pigs (male, weighed 250–300 g), with a positive Preyer reflex and free of tympanic membrane perforation or otitis media, were used in this study. Pre-recruiting ABR measurements (click stimuli) were conducted to exclude animals with abnormal hearing function.

Guinea pigs were classified into 10-day EH, 20-day EH, 30-day EH, and blank control groups equally (12 individuals in the blank control group and 18 animals in the EH group). For the EH group, ABR (tone burst stimuli) was conducted to evaluate the auditory responses of one-third (6 animals) of the animals, and LDV measurement was used for the other two-thirds (12 animals). For all EH groups (10, 20, and 30 days), the ABR measurements were conducted both before and after dehydration with mannitol. Bilateral ears were used in all measurements.

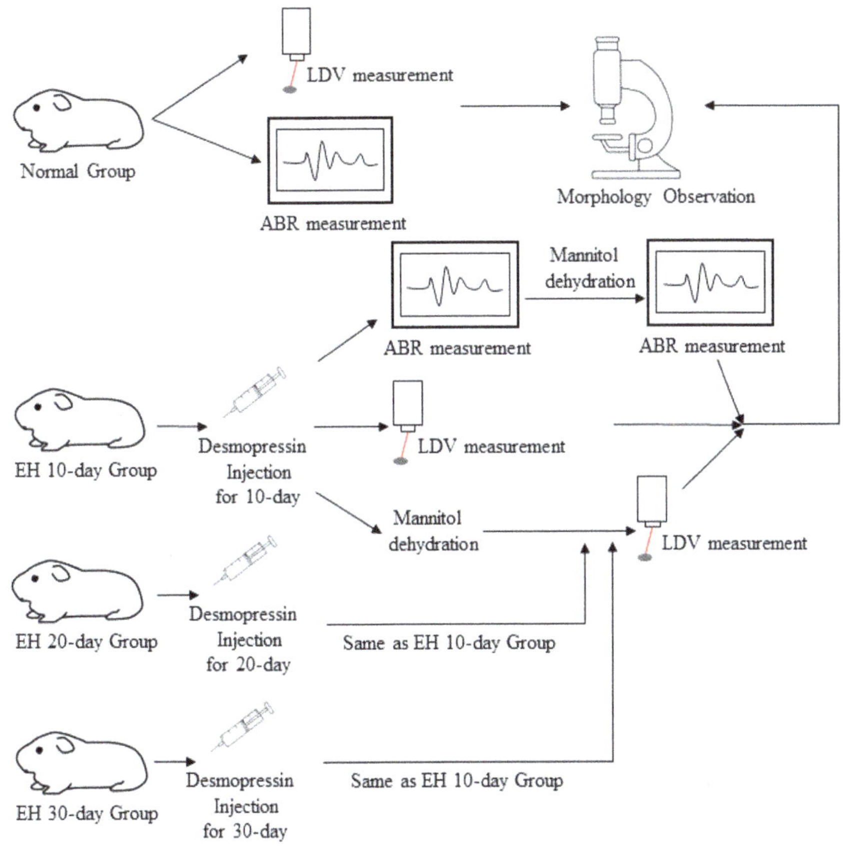

FIGURE 1 | The experimental design.

For the LDV measurements, the twelve animals in each EH group were divided into two subgroups, one for direct LDV measurement and the other for vibrometry after mannitol treatment. An operation is necessary for LDV measurement, making it hard to keep the animals healthy if further mannitol treatments are followed, which may influence the effect of dehydration. The ABR and LDV results were also obtained as baselines by the blank control groups. **Figure 1** and **Table 1** give a flowchart and roadmap of the experimental program.

After the measurements, the animals were sacrificed using an overdose of anesthetic. The cochleas were sectioned and stored in 10% polymerized formaldehyde or 2.5% glutaraldehyde for further histography.

The research program follows the principles of the guidelines for care and use of laboratory animals and was approved by the Ethics Committee of the Eye and ENT Hospital of Fudan University.

Endolymphatic Hydrops Model and Mannitol Treatment

As several studies report the importance of the endolymphatic sac and further confirm its function of regulating endolymph (Baluk et al., 2007; Swinburne et al., 2018), we used desmopressin without combining surgery to create our EH models.

The EH guinea pig model was conducted by intraperitoneal injection of desmopressin acetate (T5144, CAS: 62288-83-9, TargetMol, United States), once a day, at a dose of 8 μg/kg weight. The dose of desmopressin reported to induce EH models was variable, but there was evidence supporting increasing dosage and injection days can provide a more severe EH status in animal models at a low dose level (Takeda et al., 2000; Katagiri et al., 2014). The dose of 4–6 μg/kg weight has been widely used for EH guinea pigs modeling (Degerman et al., 2019; Jiang et al., 2019). Considering the potential for long-time medication tolerance, we increased the dose of desmopressin for our animal models (Takeda et al., 2000). To create an EH model with different levels of severity, the duration of model creation was 10, 20, and 30 days for the 10-, 20-, and 30-day EH groups, respectively.

Different kinds of hyperosmolar dehydration agents, such as glycerol, urea, isosorbide, sodium bicarbonate, and mannitol, were used to discuss their influence on the inner ears (Baldwin et al., 1992; Yazawa et al., 1998). Given the report of the rebound phenomenon of glycerol (Takeda et al., 1999) and the recent discovery of aquaporin-3 (also termed as aquaglyceroporin) in the labyrinthine membrane (Agre et al., 2002; Beitz et al., 2003), we chose mannitol as the dehydration agent applied in this study. The percentage of mannitol used in research varies from 10 to 40% (Larsen et al., 1982; Baldwin et al., 1992; Yazawa et al., 1998; Morawski et al., 2003; Le and Blakley, 2017). A high

TABLE 1 | A flowchart of the experimental procedure.

Groups	Experimental procedure		
Blank control (12 animals)	ABR (6 animals, N = 12)		
	LDV (6 animals, N = 12)		
EH 10-day (18 animals)	1st ABR (6 animals, N = 12)	Mannitol dehydration	2nd ABR (6 animals, N = 12)
	LDV (6 animals, N = 12)	–	–
	–	Mannitol dehydration	LDV (6 animals, N = 12)
EH 20-day (18 animals)	same as EH 10-day group		
EH 30-day (18 animals)	same as EH 10-day group		

dose of mannitol would cause a lethal effect, while a low dose may not ensure sufficient dehydration. In our experiment, the dehydration treatment was fulfilled by the intravenous injection of an 18% mannitol-saline solution at a safer dose of 0.5 g/kg. The dose and concentration were chosen by experience. During the dehydration process, the infusion rate was set slow, and the measurement started approximately an hour after the full dose of mannitol was given.

Auditory Brainstem Responses Measurement

Before the ABR measurement, the animals were anesthetized with an intramuscular injection of ketamine hydrochloride (40 mg/kg) and xylazine hydrochloride (10 mg/kg).

The ABR measurements were conducted in a soundproof, electromagnetically shielded room. The measurements were conducted using the RZ6/BioSigRZ system (Tucker-Davis Technologies, Alachua, FL, United States). Electrodes were inserted into the skin, one electrode at the vertex for signal recording and two electrodes at the bilateral mastoids as reference and ground. Repeated tone bursts (5 ms duration, 0.5 ms rise-fall time, Blackman envelope) were presented by a closed-field speaker at a rate of 21 stimuli/s. The test frequency points are 2, 4, 8, 16, 24, and 32 kHz. The sound-intensity level ranges from 20 to 90 dB sound pressure level (SPL) at an interval of 5 dB. ABR responses were recorded and averaged after 1,024 stimuli. The threshold for each frequency point was determined typically by the ABR I, III, and V waves.

Laser Doppler Vibrometer Measurement

The vibration of the RWM was measured to evaluate the hearing function of normal, EH-modeled, and mannitol-treated guinea pigs. The feasibility of using RWM vibration as a measure of auditory function has been previously proven (Zhang et al., 2019).

The guinea pig was anesthetized using an intramuscular injection of ketamine hydrochloride (40 mg/kg) and xylazine hydrochloride (10 mg/kg). For the duration of the surgery, the animal was placed on a heating blanket to maintain its body temperature. Bilateral auricles were partially removed, and the dorsal auditory bulla was opened to sufficiently expose the RWM (**Figure 2A**). A reflective tape (0.2×0.2 mm^2, < 0.01 mg Polytec, Germany) was carefully placed on the center of the RWM. The tympanic membrane and the ossicular chain were kept intact.

Figure 2B illustrates the setup of the LDV system. The experiment was conducted in a soundproof chamber with < 30 dB SPL noise floor. The animal was placed on a platform. An insert earphone (ER-4PT, Etymotic, United States) was inserted into the ear canal, coupled with a tiny sound pressure probe (ER-7C, Etymotic, United States). Pure tones at 85 dB SPL in the frequency range of 0.5–10 kHz (5 points/octave) were produced by the earphones, driven by a power amplifier (Type 2718, B&K, Denmark) connected with a signal generator (NI 9263, National Instruments, United States). The tip of the pressure probe was positioned approximately 2 mm from the tympanic membrane to accurately monitor the input sound pressure.

An LDV (CLV 2534-4, Polytec, Germany) was adopted to measure the vibration of the RWM. The measuring laser beam generated by the device was controlled so that the measuring angle was greater than 70°. The RWM velocity (sensitivity: 2 mm/s/V) and input sound pressure (sensitivity: 20 Pa/V) were simultaneously recorded using a four-channel data acquisition card (NI9234, sampling rate: 51.2 kHz, National Instruments, United States). Two channels were used. An in-house MATLAB code was developed for measurement control, data acquisition, and analysis. The FFT algorithm was used to obtain the velocity amplitude and sound pressure.

Histological Section

For histology, specimens (stored in 10% polymerized formaldehyde at 4°C) were decalcified in 10% ethylenediaminetetraacetic acid (EDTA), dehydrated with 15 and 30% sucrose solution, and coated with Optimum Cutting Temperature (OCT) compound. Then the cochlea was frozen and sectioned in the plane parallel to the modiolus (section thickness: 8 μm), followed by hematoxylin and eosin (H&E) stain.

For scanning electron microscopy (SEM), during specimen collection, the apical of the cochlea and RWM were opened, poured, and fixed with 2.5% glutaraldehyde at 4°C for 48 h. Then the membranous labyrinth was fully exposed. All other tissues were removed, leaving only the basement membrane, fixed in osmium tetroxide solution, and treated with tannic acid. Finally, the specimens were dehydrated with alcohol, dried, sprinkled with gold, and observed by a scanning electron microscope (SU8010, HITACHI, Toyko, Japan).

Data Processing

For sections, since the EH model is induced by desmopressin, the SAM ratio is not suitable for our case. We provided changes in the angle formed by Reissner's membrane and basilar membrane (BM) to reflect the severity of EH and response to mannitol. For LDV measured data, the RWM velocity amplitude was converted to peak-to-peak displacement according to the mathematical

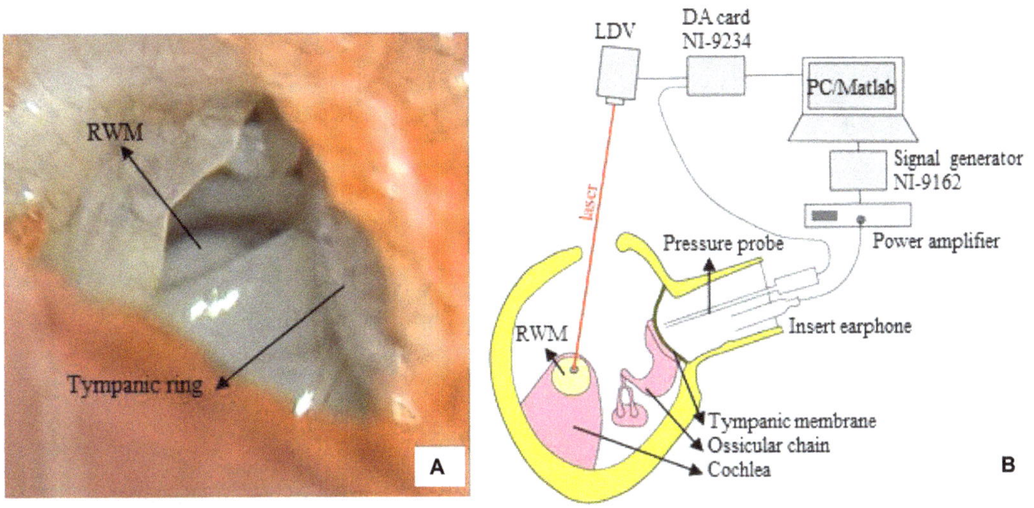

FIGURE 2 | The LDV measurement. **(A)** The surgical exposure was photographed *via* a dissecting microscope. The tympanic ring and round window membrane (RWM), with a radius of 0.5–0.6 mm, are seen from the opened middle ear cavity (right ear of tested guinea pig). **(B)** A sketch of the measurement system. The RWM velocity was measured *via* a compact LDV, and the signal was acquired by an AD card (NI-9234) and analyzed by an in-house MATLAB program.

relation: $U\text{peak-to-peak} = V/(\pi \cdot f)$ (where Upeak–to–peak is the peak-to-peak displacement, V is the velocity amplitude, and f is the frequency). Then the displacement is normalized by the sound pressure near the tympanic membrane. To statistically analyze the displacement and ABR threshold, the mean and standard deviation (SD) were calculated for each group. Two-tailed Student t-tests were used for data comparison, and p-values of < 0.05 were considered as a significant difference.

RESULTS

Observation of Tissue Sections of the Cochlea in Ears With Endolymphatic Hydrops

Figure 3 presents the H&E stained section of the cochlea for the EH groups and the blank controlled group (more section samples are presented in **Supplementary Appendix**). Turn 2 was shown. In the control group (**Figure 3A**), the Reissner's membrane (RM) did not deform so that the membrane and the BM formed a sharp angle. However, the RM bulged toward the scala vestibula (SV) in the EH groups (**Figures 3B–D**). The tissue of RM deformation became more significant with the duration of EH, indicating an increase in EH severity. These observations, consistent with the previous reports (Katagiri et al., 2014), verified our EH models.

Figures 3E–G shows turn 2 of the cochleae after dehydration. Compared with the non-dehydration results, a significant volumetric change in the scala media (SM) was shown, and in the EH 10- and 20-day groups, the RM nearly relocated to its normal location, indicating the effectiveness of mannitol treatment. Slight foldings and distortions of the RM were observed (**Figures 3E–G** and **Supplementary Figure 1**). Additionally, some cases showed the deformation of the organ of Corti (**Figures 3F,G**). The mean and SD of the angle between RM and BM were calculated and shown in **Table 2** (sections were used to calculate the mean of the angle, thus forming the sample number of 8).

Effect of Endolymphatic Hydrops and Dehydration Treatment on Auditory Brainstem Responses Measurement

Auditory brainstem response thresholds of all groups are presented in **Figure 4**. **Figure 4A** plots the ABR thresholds in the EH groups of different severity, together with the result of the control group as a baseline. In the EH 10-day group, the mean thresholds increased by approximately 10 dB, mainly at low frequencies (2, 4, and 8 kHz). In the EH 20-day group, high-frequency thresholds also increased significantly (by 10–15 dB at 16, 24, and 32 kHz, $p < 0.05$), but low-frequency thresholds were still more prominent (with an increase of 20–30 dB at 2–8 kHz, $p < 0.05$). In the EH 30-day group, the ABR thresholds increased over a broad frequency range (by approximately 30 dB at 2–32 kHz, $p < 0.05$).

The mannitol dehydration treatment effect on ABR thresholds is shown in **Figures 4B–D**, with each sub-figure corresponding to EH 10-, 20-, and 30-day groups, respectively. Compared with non-dehydration status, the ABR thresholds at the low-frequency range of EH 10-day had remarkable improvements (9.1 dB SPL at 2 kHz, 5.0 dB SPL at 4 kHz, and 5.4 dB SPL at 8 kHz; **Figure 4B**, $p < 0.05$) and almost went back to normal. In the EH 20-day group, significant improvements of approximately 10 dB ($p < 0.05$) were observed in all frequencies. The improved thresholds were still notably higher than that of the normal baseline (refer to **Figure 4C**). In the EH 30-day group, the ABR thresholds were not changed after mannitol injection (except for a slight improvement at 2 kHz), indicating the ineffectiveness of dehydration treatment (refer to **Figure 4D**).

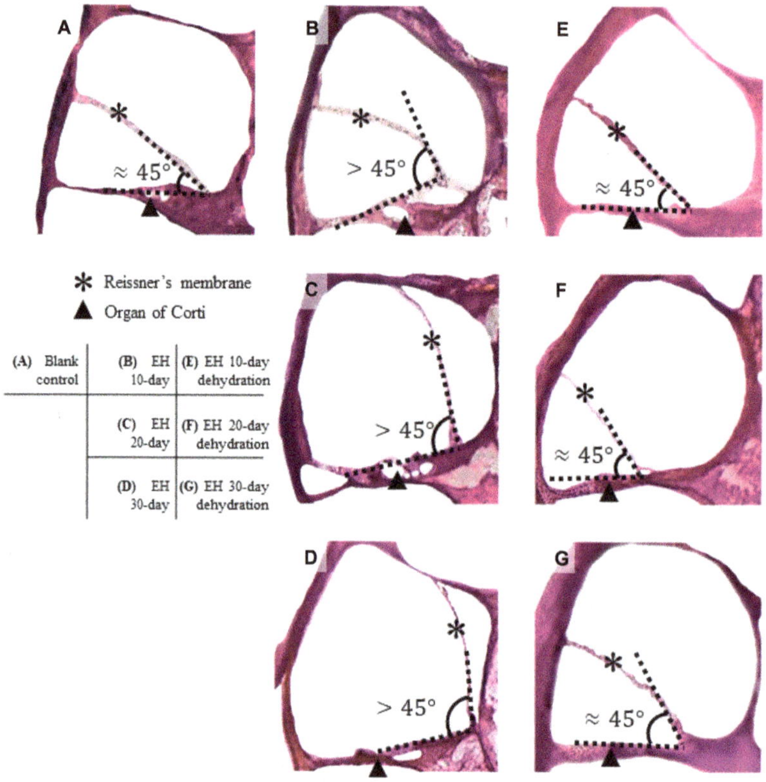

FIGURE 3 | Section of cochlear turn 2 of normal, EH-modeled, and dehydration-treated guinea pigs. In the control group **(A)**, the Reissner's membrane (RM) and the organ of Corti are in the normal position, and the RM and BM form a sharp angle (approximately 45°). In the EH groups **(B–D)**, the RM are bent, and the deformation becomes remarkable as the EH goes severe. **(E–G)** The dehydration effect where the RM is partly restored. Some distortion of the RM and the organ of Corti are shown.

Effect of Endolymphatic Hydrops and Dehydration Treatment on Round Window Membrane Vibration

Figure 5A shows the mean peak-to-peak displacement and SD of RWM in the control and EH 10-, 20-, and 30-day groups. For the normal baseline, the displacements generally decrease as frequency increases in the range of 0.5–10 kHz. The most reduction occurred at 1–5 kHz and the plateau had been reached at above 7 kHz, which coincide with the reported data (Zhang et al., 2019). In the EH 10-day group, there existed a slight reduction (approximately 10 dB) in RWM displacement at 0.5–4 kHz (11.3 dB at 0.5 kHz). For the EH 20-day group, the RWM displacement significantly decreased at the frequency range of 0.5–10 kHz (at approximately 15 dB). In the EH 30-day group, a further reduction of 15–20 dB was observed.

After dehydration treatment, the RWM vibration is shown in **Figures 5B–D**. In the EH 10-day group, the peak-to-peak displacement of RWM nearly went back to its normal range and was slightly higher than normal at 4–10 kHz (less than 4 dB, $p < 0.05$). In the EH 20-day group, the peak-to-peak displacements also showed a great improvement. However, at the range of 0.5–1 kHz, the recovery exhibited a mild reduction, compared with the normal curve (**Figure 5C**). In the EH 30-day group, the improvements were 3–8 dB, which was still 10–15 dB worse than the normal cases, suggesting the limited effect of dehydration therapy (**Figure 5D**).

Observation of Outer Hair Cells of the Cochlea in Ears With Endolymphatic Hydrops

Figure 6 shows the SEM observations of outer hair cells (OHC) in the EH 10-, 20-, and 30-day groups. Turns 2 and 3 were presented. In the EH 10-day group, the stereocilia of outer hair cells in turn 2 (**Figure 6A**) have already exhibited slight swelling and lodging, and accidental loss of stereocilia has been noticed. However, the OHC remains intact at turn

TABLE 2 | The angle between RM and BM of turn 2 in each group ($N = 8$).

Angle between RM and BM	Mean	*SD*
Normal	41.9°	3.3
EH 10-day	59.7°	4.9
EH 20-day	77.8°	7.3
EH 30-day	90.7°	8.1
EH 10-day Mannitol Tx	50.0°	5.1
EH 20-day Mannitol Tx	54.4°	3.5
EH 30-day Mannitol Tx	57.6°	4.5

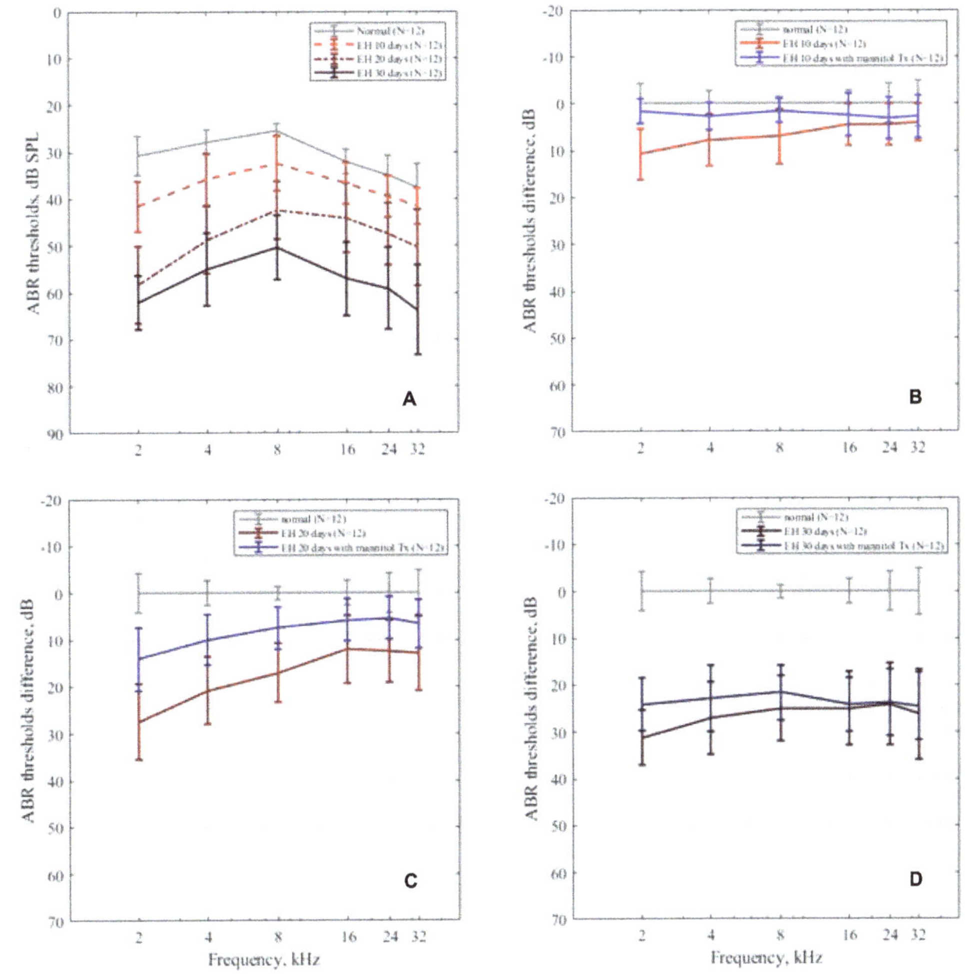

FIGURE 4 | The ABR thresholds change. **(A)** The ABR thresholds in the control, EH 10-, 20-, and 30-day groups, presenting with mean and SD; as the degree of EH became more severe, the thresholds increased. **(B–D)** The ABR threshold differences between the EH groups and the dehydration groups of 10, 20, and 30 days, compared with the control group.

3 (**Figure 6B**). In the EH 20-day group, the damage of stereocilia of OHC in turn 2 (**Figure 6C**) is very obvious, and the lodging and collapse of stereocilia have started to show up in turn 3 (**Figure 6D**). The changes in OHC were most prominent in the EH 30-day groups. The injury to OHC was more severe compared with the EH 20-day group in both turns (**Figures 6E,F**), and collapse of cilia and swelling inner hair cells (IHC) have started to appear (**Figures 6E,F**). Those finding indicating sensation dysfunction in severe EH may be the explanation of poor response to mannitol in the EH 30-day group.

DISCUSSION

The Hearing Loss in Endolymphatic Hydrops Animal Models

Animal models are commonly used in identifying and characterizing the pathophysiology of EH. Current existing animal models can resemble the dilation of SM and low-frequency hearing loss. It is widely accepted that the EH animal models, created through surgical operation, medication application, or their combination, can reproduce the chronic phase of MD (Seo and Brown, 2020).

The EH surgical model was created *via* ablation of the endolymphatic duct and endolymphatic sac by electrocauterization. It produces reliable EH models, but the permanent surgical damage and irreversible hearing loss limit its feasibility in studying the curative effect (Horner, 1991). The EH medication models are created with injections of low-dose vasopressin (VP), desmopressin, or aldosterone. In hydropic cochleae confirmed by X-ray micro-tomography (micro-CT), desmopressin influences all frequency ranges of the cochlea but is more prominent at low frequencies (Takeda et al., 2000; Chihara et al., 2013; Katagiri et al., 2014).

A similar phenomenon was observed in our EH model experiments. The ABR results showed that the hearing loss started at low frequencies (the EH 10-day group) and progressed

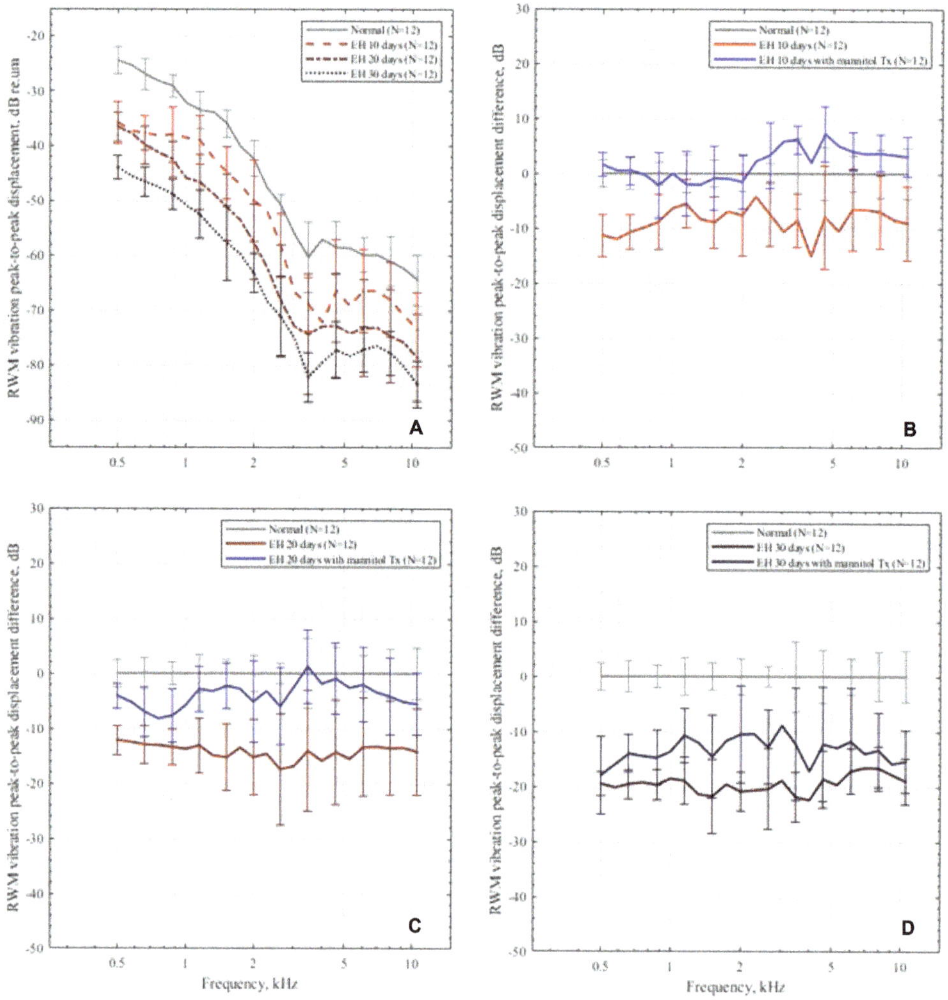

FIGURE 5 | The RWM peak-to-peak displacements in the dB scale. **(A)** The RWM peak-to-peak displacement in the control group and the EH 10-, 20-, and 30-day groups, presenting with mean and SD. The displacements are normalized by sound pressure in the ear canal. **(B–D)** The RWM peak-to-peak displacement differences in the 10-, 20-, and 30-day EH groups before and after dehydration treatment, compared with the normal baseline.

to higher frequencies (the EH 20- and 30-day groups, refer to **Figure 4A**). Note that the large variations in our ABR results may be caused by individual differences in response and the vasopressin escape phenomenon (Ecelbarger et al., 1998).

The increasing hearing losses were also reflected by the reduction of RWM vibrations (refer to **Figure 5A**). A positive correlation was found between the reduction of the RWM vibration and the severity of EH. However, the vibration reductions were not frequency-sensitive compared with the ABR results. The RWM vibration, different from ABR thresholds, is an evaluation of the mechanical influence of EH. This may cause the inconsistency between ABR and LDV results.

The Effect of Dehydration Therapy on Endolymphatic Hydrops

In clinical trials, dehydration agents (e.g., mannitol, isosorbide, and glycerol) are commonly used in the diagnosis and treatment of MD (Kakigi et al., 2004), as their influences on hearing improvement have been confirmed by clinical trials and research (Filipo et al., 1997; Degerman et al., 2019). The impacts of dehydration agents in animal models have usually been analyzed by tissue section or micro-CT. Among those studies, common morphological changes such as folding of the distended RM and deformation of the organ of Corti have been observed and reported (Egami et al., 2016). In our study, those morphological changes were also noticed (**Figures 3F,G**).

Hearing restoration after dehydration treatment was also evaluated in this study. As shown in both ABR (**Figures 4B–D**) and RWM vibration (**Figures 5B–D**) results, the hearing loss was nearly fully recovered after dehydration in the EH 10-day group and partly recovered in the EH 20-day group. In the EH 30-day group, the hearing loss was sustained. Considering the remarkable OHC injury in the EH 30-day group (**Figures 6E,F**), at that time, the causes of hearing loss may

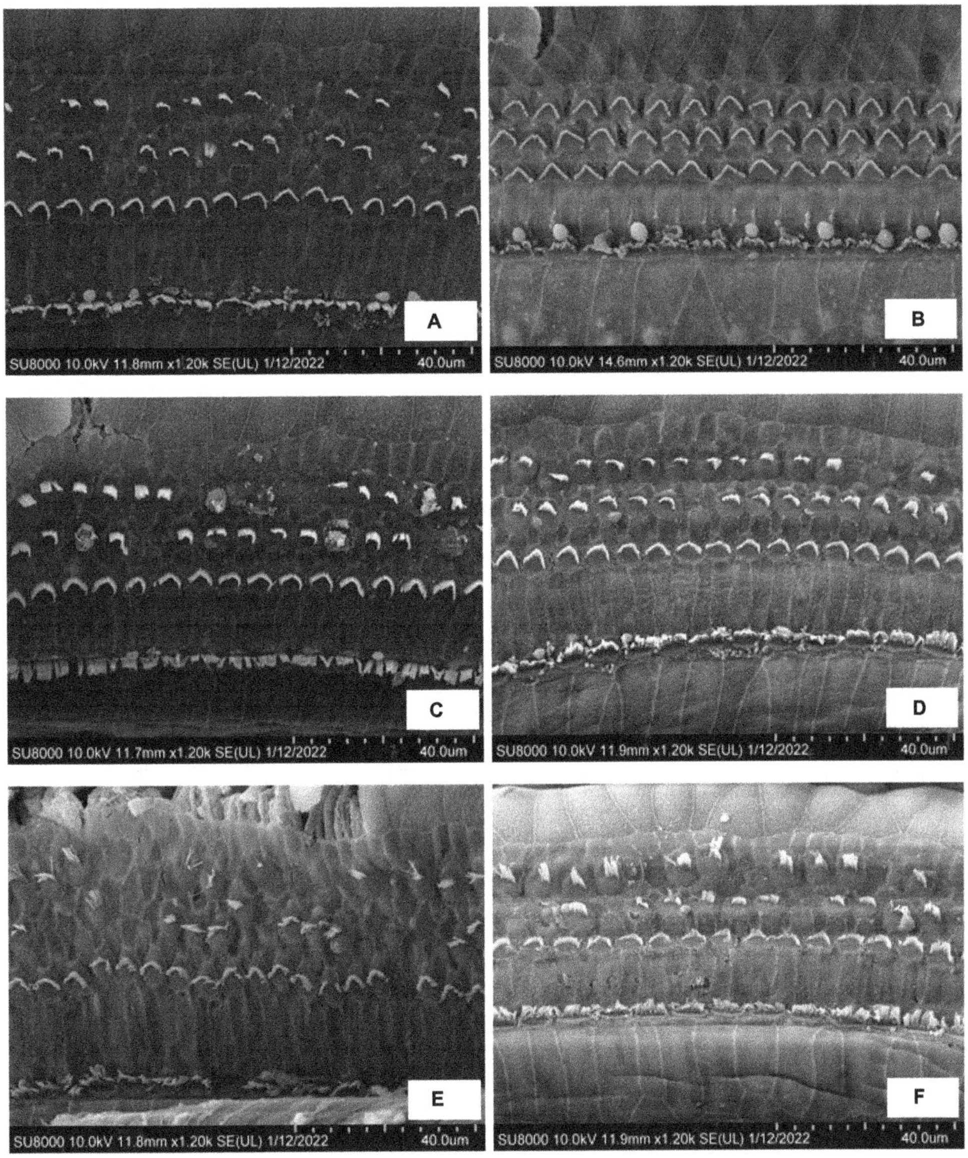

FIGURE 6 | The SEM observation of OHC in the EH 10-, 20-, and 30-day groups. **(A,C,E)** Turn 2 of the cochlea in the EH 10-, 20-, and 30-day groups. **(B,D,F)** Turn 3 of the cochlea in each group accordingly.

be transferred from conductive dysfunction to sensory impair, restoring of conductive function by dehydration is not enough to improve hearing.

Conductive and Sensorineural Hearing Loss

Typically, patients with MD experience fluctuating low-frequency hearing loss followed by medium- to high-frequency involvement. Gluth (2020) reviewed the hypothesis for MD development. The mechanical effect of high endolymphatic pressure affects cochlear conductive problems and damages the sensory hair cells, resulting in sensation dysfunction. The same damage to hair cell stereocilia in our study was also reported in many EH animal models (Momin et al., 2010; Jia et al., 2012; Ding et al., 2016).

Our results support this assumption. In the EH 10-day group, the injury stereocilia of OHC at turn 2 is minimal, and turn 3 is almost normal. The RWM vibration decreased by 7.6, 15.0, and 7.0 dB at 2,4, and 8 kHz, respectively (referring to normal range in **Figure 5B**), which were similar to ABR threshold changes (10.8, 7.9, and 7.1 dB at 2, 4, and 8 kHz, respectively, refer to **Figure 4B**). In the EH 20-day group, the hearing loss evaluated by RWM vibration was 15.2, 15.8, and 13.5 dB at 2, 4, and 8 kHz, respectively (**Figure 5C**), while the ABR threshold elevation was significantly higher (27.5, 20.8, and 17.1 dB at 2, 4, and 8 kHz, respectively, refer to **Figure 4C**). The gap was even more significant in the EH 30-day group. The ABR increases were

31.3, 27.1, and 25.0 dB, and the LDV results were 20.9, 22.4, and 16.6 dB at 2, 4, and 8 kHz, respectively (**Figures 4D, 5D**). For long-time EH models, the hearing loss evaluated by ABR was higher than that by RWM vibration, which is consistent with OHC stereocilia injury (**Figures 6C–F**).

The RWM vibration is a measurement of cochlear impedance, representing the conductive dysfunction component in acoustic transferring, while the ABR change is a sum of the conductive and sensation dysfunction. Therefore, the gap between ABR and RWM vibration may represent the SNHL. In our study, there is no gap in the EH 10-day animal models, indicating minimal SNHL at that time. However, the gap occurs in the EH 20- and 30-day groups, suggesting an increasing sensorineural component. Therefore, the dehydration treatment shows a significant curative effect in the EH 10- and 20-day groups (**Figures 3B, 4B**) while less effective in the EH 30-day group (**Figures 3C,D, 4C,D**).

Endolymphatic Hydrops-Induced Cochlear Damage

Besides the dislocations of RM in EH, the BM may also deform (Xenellis et al., 2004) as shown in **Figure 3**, caused by the pressure difference between SM and scale tympani. However, the BM deformation is quite small, and sectioning observations may not be solid evidence of BM deformation since slight deformation may also be caused during the sectioning. The BM deformation in EH has been numerically calculated using finite element analysis (Lee and Koike, 2017; Areias et al., 2021). The numerical analysis also predicts a low-frequency conductive hearing loss caused by BM deformation.

There are also assumptions that the EH-induced BM deformation may damage the sensory cells and cause SNHL. Lee and Kalinec (2016) measured the deformation of the organ of Corti in acute guinea pig EH models. They observed a significant decrease in the average area and height of the organ of Corti in the apical turn. They found that the lengths of OHC and Deiters' cells in the apical turn were significantly reduced. Lee suggested that the compression and deformation of the organ of Corti may decouple the tectorial membrane and stereocilia. However, *in vivo* observations need further solid evidence. Optical coherence tomography may be a promising technique (Liu et al., 2017; Badash et al., 2021).

Limitations of This Study

The first limitation of this study is the mismatch between the frequency range in ABR and LDV measurements. The LDV measurement range was 0.5–10 kHz. Frequencies beyond this interval had not been surveyed, so the paired frequencies in ABR thresholds and RWM vibrations were restricted to 2–8 kHz. Second, mannitol injection is used in the diagnosis of MD in clinical practice instead of treatment due to severe side effects. However, it does not affect the conclusion of this study.

CONCLUSION

This study investigated the development of hearing loss in guinea pig EH models as well as the effect of dehydration treatment. By combining analogical observations (frozen section) and objective measurements of hearing loss (ABR and LDV measurement of RWM vibration), we are able to obtain an overview of the development of hearing loss in EH, both mechanically and biologically. The main conclusions of this study are as follows:

1. EH-induced hearing loss progressed with the development of EH; it starts at low frequencies and later involves medium to high frequencies.
2. EH increases the cochlear impedance, causing conductive dysfunction. This dysfunction can be cured by dehydration treatment at an early stage. But the irreversible sensorineural component becomes significant for long-time EH.
3. Early dehydration treatment is suggested for preserving hearing.

AUTHOR CONTRIBUTIONS

S-QW: methodology, formal analysis, visualization, and writing—original draft. C-LL: methodology, formal analysis, visualization, and writing—review and editing. J-QX and L-LC: methodology. Y-ZX and P-DD: writing—review and editing. L-JR: conceptualization, software, writing—review and editing, supervision, and funding acquisition. W-JY: supervision and funding acquisition. T-YZ: conceptualization, supervision, and funding acquisition. All authors contributed to the article and approved the submitted version.

REFERENCES

Agre, P., King, L. S., Yasui, M., Guggino, W. B., Ottersen, O. P., Fujiyoshi, Y., et al. (2002). Aquaporin water channels–from atomic structure to clinical medicine. *J. Physiol.* 542, 3–16. doi: 10.1113/jphysiol.2002.020818

Albers, F. W., Veldman, J. E., and Huizing, E. H. (1987). Early hair cell loss in experimental hydrops. *Ann. Otol. Rhinol. Laryngol.* 96, 282–285. doi: 10.1177/000348948709600309

Angelborg, C., Klockhoff, I., Larsen, H. C., and Stahle, J. (1982). Hyperosmotic solutions and hearing Meniere's disease. *Am. J. Otol.* 3, 200–202.

Areias, B., Parente, M. P. L., Gentil, F., Caroça, C., Paço, J., and Natal Jorge, R. M. (2021). A finite element model to predict the consequences of endolymphatic hydrops in the basilar membrane. *Int. J. Numer. Method Biomed. Eng.* 2021:e3541. doi: 10.1002/cnm.3541

Atkinson, M. (1961). Meniere's original papers. Reprinted with an English translation together with commentaries and biographical sketch. *Acta Otolaryngol.* 162, 1–78.

Badash, I., Applegate, B. E., and Oghalai, J. S. (2021). In vivo cochlear imaging provides a tool to study endolymphatic hydrops. *J. Vestib. Res.* 31, 269–276. doi: 10.3233/VES-200718

Baldwin, D. L., Ohlsén, K. A., Miller, J. M., and Nuttall, A. L. (1992). Cochlear blood flow and microvascular resistance changes in response to hypertonic glycerol, urea, and mannitol infusions. *Ann. Otol. Rhinol. Laryngol.* 101, 168–175. doi: 10.1177/000348949210100212

Baluk, P., Fuxe, J., Hashizume, H., Romano, T., Lashnits, E., Butz, S., et al. (2007). Functionally specialized junctions between endothelial cells of lymphatic vessels. *J. Exp. Med.* 204, 2349–2362. doi: 10.1084/jem.20062596

Beitz, E., Zenner, H. P., and Schultz, J. E. (2003). Aquaporin-mediated fluid regulation in the inner ear. *Cell Mol. Neurobiol.* 23, 315–329. doi: 10.1023/a:1023636620721

Chihara, Y., Wong, C., Curthoys, I. S., and Brown, D. J. (2013). The effect of systemic administration of desmopressin on cochlear function in guinea pigs. *Acta Otolaryngol.* 133, 676–684. doi: 10.3109/00016489.2013.771282

Degerman, E., Zandt, R., Pålbrink, A., and Magnusson, M. (2019). Endolymphatic hydrops induced by different mechanisms responds differentially to spironolactone: a rationale for understanding the diversity of treatment responses in hydropic inner ear disease. *Acta Otolaryngol.* 139, 685–691. doi: 10.1080/00016489.2019.1616819

Ding, C. R., Xu, X. D., Wang, X. W., Jia, X. H., Cheng, X., Liu, X., et al. (2016). Effect of Endolymphatic hydrops on sound transmission in live guinea pigs measured with a laser doppler vibrometer. *Neural. Plast.* 2016, 1–12. doi: 10.1155/2016/8648297

Ecelbarger, C. A., Chou, C. L., Lee, A. J., DiGiovanni, S. R., Verbalis, J. G., and Knepper, M. A. (1998). Escape from vasopressin-induced antidiuresis: role of vasopressin resistance of the collecting duct. *Am. J. Physiol.* 274, F1161–F1166. doi: 10.1152/ajprenal.1998.274.6.F1161

Egami, N., Kakigi, A., Takeda, T., and Yamasoba, T. (2016). Dehydration effects of a V2 antagonist on endolymphatic hydrops in guinea pigs. *Hear. Res.* 332, 151–159. doi: 10.1016/j.heares.2015.12.017

Filipo, R., Barbara, M., Cordier, A., Mafera, B., Romeo, R., Attanasio, G., et al. (1997). Osmotic drugs in the treatment of cochlear disorders: a clinical and experimental study. *Acta Otolaryngol.* 117, 229–231. doi: 10.3109/00016489709117777

Gluth, M. B. (2020). On the relationship between menière's disease and endolymphatic hydrops. *Otol. Neurotol.* 41, 242–249. doi: 10.1097/MAO.0000000000002502

Hallpike, C. S., and Cairns, H. (1938). Observations on the pathology of ménieres syndrome: (section of otology). *Proc. R. Soc. Med.* 31, 1317–1336.

Horner, K. C. (1991). Old theme and new reflections: hearing impairment associated with endolymphatic hydrops. *Hear. Res.* 52, 147–156. doi: 10.1016/0378-5955(91)90194-e

Ichimiya, I., and Ichimiya, H. (2019). Complex tone stimulation may induce binaural diplacusis with low-tone hearing loss. *PLoS One.* 14:e0210939. doi: 10.1371/journal.pone.0210939

Jia, X. H., Liang, Q., Chi, Z. C., Dai, P. D., Zhang, T. Y., and Wang, T. F. (2012). [Morphological changes associated with low-tone hearing loss in guinea pig models of early endolymphatic hydrops]. *Sheng Li Xue Bao* 64, 48–54.

Jiang, L. Y., He, J. J., Chen, X. X., Sun, X. J., Wang, X. Z., Zhong, S., et al. (2019). Arginine vasopressin-aquaporin-2 pathway-mediated dehydration effects of electroacupuncture in guinea pig model of AVP-induced eendolymphatic hydrops. *Chin. J. Integr. Med.* 25, 763–769. doi: 10.1007/s11655-017-2411-2

Kakigi, A., Takeda, S., Takeda, T., Sawada, S., Azuma, H., Higashiyama, K., et al. (2004). Time course of dehydrating effects of isosorbide on experimentally induced endolymphatic hydrops in guinea pigs. *ORL J. Otorhinolaryngol. Relat. Spec.* 66, 291–296. doi: 10.1159/000081884

Katagiri, Y., Takumida, M., Hirakawa, K., and Anniko, M. (2014). Long-term administration of vasopressin can cause Méniere's disease in mice. *Acta Otolaryngol.* 134, 990–1004. doi: 10.3109/00016489.2014.902989

Larsen, H. C., Angelborg, C., and Hultcrantz, E. (1982). Cochlear blood flow related to hyperosmotic solution. *Arch. Otorhinolaryngol.* 234, 145–150. doi: 10.1007/BF00453621

Le, T. N., and Blakley, B. W. (2017). Mannitol and the blood-labyrinth barrier. *J. Otolaryngol. Head Neck Surg.* 46:66. doi: 10.1186/s40463-017-0245-8

Lee, S., and Koike, T. (2017). Simulation of the basilar membrane vibration of endolymphatic hydrops. *Procedia. IUTAM* 24, 64–71. doi: 10.1016/j.piutam.2017.08.043

Lee, S. H., and Kalinec, F. (2016). Measurement of the mechanical deformation of organ of corti in a model of acute endolymphatic hydrops. *Kor. J. Otorhinolaryngol. Head Neck Surg.* 59, 110–119. doi: 10.3342/kjorl-hns.2016.59.2.110

Liu, G. S., Kim, J., Applegate, B. E., and Oghalai, J. S. (2017). Computer-aided detection and quantification of endolymphatic hydrops within the mouse cochlea in vivo using optical coherence tomography. *J. Biomed. Opt.* 22:76002. doi: 10.1117/1.JBO.22.7.076002

Magliulo, G., Cianfrone, G., Triches, L., Altissimi, G., and D'Amico, R. (2001). Distortion-product otoacoustic emissions and glycerol testing in endolymphatic hydrops. *Laryngoscope* 111, 102–109. doi: 10.1097/00005537-200101000-00018

Marquardt, T., and Hensel, J. (2013). A simple electrical lumped-element model simulates intra-cochlear sound pressures and cochlear impedance below 2 kHz. *J. Acoust. Soc. Am.* 134, 3730–3738. doi: 10.1121/1.4824154

Merchant, S. N., Adams, J. C., and Nadol, J. B. Jr. (2005). Pathophysiology of Meniere's syndrome: are symptoms caused by endolymphatic hydrops? *Otol. Neurotol.* 26, 74–81. doi: 10.1097/00129492-200501000-00013

Momin, S. R., Melki, S. J., Alagramam, K. N., and Megerian, C. A. (2010). Spiral ganglion loss outpaces inner hair cell loss in endolymphatic hydrops. *Laryngoscope.* 120, 159–165. doi: 10.1002/lary.20673

Morawski, K., Telischi, F. F., Merchant, F., Abiy, L. W., Lisowska, G., and Namyslowski, G. (2003). Role of mannitol in reducing postischemic changes in distortion-product otoacoustic emissions (DPOAEs): a rabbit model. *Laryngoscope* 113, 1615–1622. doi: 10.1097/00005537-200309000-00039

Naganawa, S., Yamazaki, M., Kawai, H., Bokura, K., Iida, T., Sone, M., et al. (2014). MR imaging of Méniere's disease after combined intratympanic and intravenous injection of gadolinium using HYDROPS2. *Magn. Reson. Med. Sci.* 13, 133–137. doi: 10.2463/mrms.2013-0061

Nevoux, J., Barbara, M., Dornhoffer, J., Gibson, W., Kitahara, T., and Darrouzet, V. (2018). International consensus (ICON) on treatment of Méniere's disease. *Eur. Ann. Otorhinolaryngol. Head Neck Dis.* 135, S29–S32. doi: 10.1016/j.anorl.2017.12.006

Oberman, B. S., Patel, V. A., Cureoglu, S., and Isildak, H. (2017). The aetiopathologies of Méniere's disease: a contemporary review. *Acta Otorhinolaryngol. Ital.* 37, 250–263. doi: 10.14639/0392-100X-793

Quaranta, N., Picciotti, P., Porro, G., Sterlicchio, B., Danesi, G., Petrone, P., et al. (2019). Therapeutic strategies in the treatment of Menière's disease: the Italian experience. *Eur. Arch. Otorhinolaryngol.* 276, 1943–1950. doi: 10.1007/s00405-019-05423-7

Ryan, M., Lally, J., Adams, J. K., Higgins, S., Ahmed, M., Aden, J., et al. (2020). Mechanical energy dissipation through the ossicular chain and inner ear using laser doppler vibrometer measurement of round window velocity. *Otol. Neurotol.* 41, e387–e391. doi: 10.1097/MAO.0000000000002509

Seo, Y. J., and Brown, D. (2020). Experimental animal models for meniere's disease: a mini-review. *J. Audiol. Otol.* 24, 53–60. doi: 10.7874/jao.2020.00115

Sterkers, O., Leriche, P., Ferrary, E., and Paquelin, F. (1987). Effets du mannitol sur les liquides de l'oreille interne. Application au traitement des surdités [Effects of mannitol on the fluids of the internal ear. Use in the treatment of deafness]. *Ann. Otolaryngol. Chir. Cervicofac.* 104, 127–135.

Swinburne, I. A., Mosaliganti, K. R., Upadhyayula, S., Liu, T. L., Hildebrand, D. G. C., Tsai, T. Y., et al. (2018). Lamellar projections in the endolymphatic sac act as a relief valve to regulate inner ear pressure. *Elife* 7:e37131. doi: 10.7554/eLife.37131

Takeda, T., Takeda, S., Kitano, H., Okada, T., and Kakigi, A. (2000). Endolymphatic hydrops induced by chronic administration of vasopressin. *Hear Res.* 140, 1–6. doi: 10.1016/s0378-5955(99)00180-x

Takeda, T., Takeda, S., Saito, H., Hamada, M., and Sawada, S. (1999). The rebound phenomenon of glycerol-induced changes in the endolymphatic space. *Acta Otolaryngol.* 119, 341–344. doi: 10.1080/00016489950181369

Thomsen, J., and Vesterhauge, S. (1979). A critical evaluation of the glycerol test in Ménière's disease. *J. Otolaryngol.* 8, 145–150.

Valenzuela, C. V., Lee, C., Mispagel, A., Bhattacharyya, A., Lefler, S. M., Payne, S., et al. (2020). Is cochlear synapse loss an origin of low-frequency hearing loss associated with endolymphatic hydrops? *Hear Res.* 398:108099. doi: 10.1016/j.heares.2020.108099

Van de Water, S. M., Arenberg, I. K., and Balkany, T. J. (1986). Auditory dehydration testing: glycerol versus urea. *Am. J. Otol.* 7, 200–203.

Ward, B., Wettstein, V., Golding, J., Corallo, G., Nuti, D., Trabalzini, F., et al. (2019). Patient perceptions of effectiveness in treatments for menière's disease: a national survey in italy. *J. Int. Adv. Otol.* 15, 112–117. doi: 10.5152/iao.2019.5758

Xenellis, J. E., Linthicum, F. H. Jr., Webster, P., and Lopez, R. (2004). Basilar membrane displacement related to endolymphatic sac volume. *Laryngoscope* 114, 1953–1959. doi: 10.1097/01.mlg.0000147927.98766.e1

Yamakawa, K. (1938). Uber ide patholgische Veranderung bei einem Meniere-Kranken. *J. Otolaryngol. Soc. Japn.* 4, 2310–2312.

Yazawa, Y., Kitano, H., Suzuki, M., Tanaka, H., and Kitajima, K. (1998). Studies of cochlear blood flow in guinea pigs with endolymphatic hydrops. *ORL J. Otorhinolaryngol. Relat. Spec.* 60, 4–11. doi: 10.1159/000027554

Zhang, T. Y., Ren, L. J., Yang, L., Dai, P. D., Zhang, T. Y., and Liang, Q. (2019). Ethanol infiltration into the stapedio-vestibular joint reduces low-frequency vibration of the ossicular chain and round window membrane in the guinea pig. *Acta Otolaryngol.* 139, 403–408. doi: 10.1080/00016489.2019.1575521

Zhang, X., and Gan, R. Z. (2013). Dynamic properties of human round window membrane in auditory frequencies running head: dynamic properties of round window membrane. *Med. Eng. Phys.* 35, 310–318. doi: 10.1016/j.medengphy.2012.05.003

Zou, J., Wang, Z., Chen, Y., Zhang, G., Chen, L., and Lu, J. (2020). MRI detection of endolymphatic hydrops in Meniere's disease in 8 minutes using MIIRMR and a 20-channel coil after targeted gadolinium delivery. *World J. Otorhinolaryngol. Head Neck Surg.* 5, 180–187. doi: 10.1016/j.wjorl.2019.04.001

2

Autophagy Regulates the Survival of Hair Cells and Spiral Ganglion Neurons in Cases of Noise, Ototoxic Drug and Age-Induced Sensorineural Hearing Loss

Lingna Guo[1,2†], Wei Cao[2†], Yuguang Niu[3†], Shuangba He[4], Renjie Chai[1,5,6,7*] and Jianming Yang[2*]*

[1] State Key Laboratory of Bioelectronics, School of Life Sciences and Technology, Jiangsu Province High-Tech Key Laboratory for Bio-Medical Research, Southeast University, Nanjing, China, [2] Department of Otolaryngology Head and Neck Surgery, The Second Affiliated Hospital of Anhui Medical University, Hefei, China, [3] Department of Ambulatory Medicine, The First Medical Center of PLA General Hospital, Beijing, China, [4] Department of Otolaryngology Head and Neck Surgery, Nanjing Tongren Hospital, School of Medicine, Southeast University, Nanjing, China, [5] Co-Innovation Center of Neuroregeneration, Nantong University, Nantong, China, [6] Institute for Stem Cell and Regeneration, Chinese Academy of Sciences, Beijing, China, [7] Beijing Key Laboratory of Neural Regeneration and Repair, Capital Medical University, Beijing, China

Correspondence:
Shuangba He
hesb@njtrh.org
Renjie Chai
renjiec@seu.edu.cn
Jianming Yang
Jmyang88@163.com

† These authors have contributed equally to this work

Inner ear hair cells (HCs) and spiral ganglion neurons (SGNs) are the core components of the auditory system. However, they are vulnerable to genetic defects, noise exposure, ototoxic drugs and aging, and loss or damage of HCs and SGNs results in permanent hearing loss due to their limited capacity for spontaneous regeneration in mammals. Many efforts have been made to combat hearing loss including cochlear implants, HC regeneration, gene therapy, and antioxidant drugs. Here we review the role of autophagy in sensorineural hearing loss and the potential targets related to autophagy for the treatment of hearing loss.

Keywords: hearing loss, hair cells, spiral ganglion neurons, autophagy, mechanism

INTRODUCTION

According to the World Health Organization (WHO, 2021), about 5% of the world's population (or 430 million people) suffer from hearing impairment, and it is expected that the number of people with disabling hearing loss will be around 700 million by 2050. Hearing loss is not only a physical and financial burden in social life, but also causes psychological problems and psychiatric disorders, including cognitive decline and depression (Strawbridge et al., 2000; Steffens et al., 2006; Lin et al., 2013). Indeed, hearing loss has become a serious threat to global population health and economic development.

Genetic alterations, noise, ototoxic drugs, and aging can all contribute to hearing loss. Although the causes vary, the most common causes of deafness are damage or loss of hair cells (HCs) and degeneration of spiral ganglion neurons (SGNs). HCs are responsible for converting external sound signals into electrical signals that are transmitted to the brainstem through SGNs (Groves and Fekete, 2012). Recent studies have shown that these sensory cells cannot spontaneously regenerate in adult mammals (Stone et al., 1998; Brigande and Heller, 2009; Cox et al., 2014), so damage or loss of HCs and degeneration of SGNs can result in permanent deafness.

Cochlear implants offer strategies to mitigate hearing loss, but their effectiveness has been reported to be highly correlated with the remaining HCs and SGNs in the cochlea. Efforts have been made to protect HCs and SGNs against noise or ototoxic drugs-induced death, and N-acetylcysteine and neurotrophins have been shown to prevent HC death and SGN degeneration to some extent (Aladag et al., 2016; Chen et al., 2018; Wu et al., 2020). Recently, autophagy has been reported to play an antioxidative role in preventing sensorineural hearing loss (SNHL) (Ye et al., 2019a). In this review, we present the role of autophagy in hearing loss induced by noise exposure, ototoxic drugs and aging, and describe the molecules and signaling pathways involved in autophagy in the inner ear.

THE MECHANISM AND PROCESS OF AUTOPHAGY

Autophagy is a highly conserved degradation system in eukaryotic cells that maintains cellular homeostasis, and autophagy can be induced by nutrient deficiency and reactive oxygen species (ROS) accumulation (Mizushima, 2007; Eskelinen, 2019). Through the autophagy pathway, damaged cytoplasmic components are absorbed and transferred to lysosomes, where they are degraded and recycled. There are three main types of autophagy, the most common form being macroautophagy, which is the form generally being referred to by the term "autophagy." In this process, bilayer organelles called autophagosomes carry cytoplasmic products to lysosomes for degradation (Mizushima, 2007; Mizushima and Komatsu, 2011). This dynamic process generally comprises the following four steps: first is the initiation of autophagy through the envelopment of the cytosolic contents within phagophores; second is the formation of the autophagosome, which is a double-membrane vesicle; third is the fusion of autophagosomes with lysosomes to form autolysosomes; and fourth is the degradation of the contents of the autolysosomes (Feng et al., 2014). The second form is microautophagy, in which the cytoplasmic contents enter the lysosome through direct invagination or through deformation of the lysosomal membrane (Li et al., 2012). The third form is molecular chaperone-mediated autophagy, which is a highly specific process in which proteins containing a KFERQ motif are recognized and transported to the lysosomal membrane (Kaushik and Cuervo, 2018; Yang et al., 2019).

The biogenesis of autophagy requires many autophagy-related (ATG) proteins. So far more than 30 ATGs have been shown to be involved in the initiation and maturation of autophagy (Klionsky et al., 2003; Xie and Klionsky, 2007; Mizushima et al., 2011; Wesselborg and Stork, 2015), and the ATGs that are required for autophagosome formation are divided into several functional units. The autophagy-related 2 (ATG1)–Unc51-like kinase (ULK) complex (ULK1) plays a vital role during the initiation stage, and because this complex is negatively regulated by mammalian target of rapamycin complex 1 (mTORC1) (Noda and Ohsumi, 1998; Kamada et al., 2010), the inactivation of mTORC1 by rapamycin stimulates autophagy. Alternatively, the activation of autophagy can also be regulated by AMP-activated protein kinase (AMPK) (Kim et al., 2011; Li and Chen, 2019). The phosphatidylinositol 3-kinase complex (PI3KC), which is activated by ULK1, participates in the formation of autophagic vesicle membranes. ATG9 is the only known transmembrane protein shown to be involved in the delivery of membrane particles to form autophagosomes (Noda et al., 2000; Webber and Tooze, 2010). During the maturation stage, two ubiquitin-like conjugation systems, the ATG5-ATG12 system and the LC3-PE system, play vital roles in the elongation of autophagosomes (Geng and Klionsky, 2008). After the autophagosome is encapsulated, the autophagosome and lysosome fuse to form the autolysosome through the function of proteins such as SNARE (Itakura et al., 2012).

THE PROTECTIVE EFFECT OF AUTOPHAGY AGAINST SNHL

Autophagy is responsible for normal cell survival and homeostasis. A variety of human conditions, such as neurodegenerative diseases, cancer, and inflammation, have been reported to be associated with dysregulated autophagic processes (Levine et al., 2011; White, 2012; Kochergin and Zakharova, 2016). In the inner ear, many studies have shown that autophagy played an important role in cell development, differentiation, and survival (Fujimoto et al., 2017; Magarinos et al., 2017), and recently there has been renewed interest in regulating autophagy to prevent SNHL.

Noise and ototoxic drugs increased the levels of oxidative stress in HCs, which contributed to cell death (Warchol, 2010; Tabuchi et al., 2011; Sheth et al., 2017; Wu et al., 2020), and in a mouse model that was exposed to noise, the level of autophagy was increased in HCs (Xu et al., 2021). It is worth noting that the oxidative stress level in response to noise was dose dependent, and moderate noise induced temporary threshold shifts and increased the level of autophagy in outer hair cells, while severe noise produced excess ROS that induced permanent threshold shifts (Yuan et al., 2015). Increasing autophagy with rapamycin can reduce the accumulation of ROS and prevent cell death from noise exposure. In contrast, blocking autophagy through the autophagy inhibitor 3-methyladenine (3-MA) or knocking down LC3 can increase the accumulation of ROS and promote cell death (Yuan et al., 2015). More recently, a study reported that treatment with FK506 (tacrolimus), a calcineurin inhibitor, increased autophagy and inhibited ROS and alleviated moderate noise-induced HC damage and hearing loss (He et al., 2021b).

Ototoxic drugs such as aminoglycoside antibiotics and cisplatin can also result in HC damage and hearing loss. He et al. (2017) found that autophagy activity was increased in neomycin or gentamicin-treated HCs and HEI-OC1 cells. Treatment with rapamycin increased autophagy activity and decreased ROS accumulation and apoptosis, while treatment with 3-MA or knockdown of ATG5 resulted in reduced autophagy activity and increased ROS levels and apoptosis. Other studies also showed that upregulation of autophagy alleviated cisplatin-induced ototoxicity in HCs (Fang and Xiao, 2014; Liu et al., 2019;Liang et al., 2021).

Presbycusis (age-related hearing loss) is a common sensory disorder associated with aging. The level of autophagy decreased with age, and the upregulation of autophagy can promote aging HC survival and slow the degeneration of auditory cells (Yuan et al., 2018; He et al., 2021a).

Autophagy also exerts a protective effect in SGNs against ototoxic drug-induced damage. Administration of kanamycin and furosemide induced HC loss and subsequent SGN degeneration by impairing autophagic flux and lysosomal biogenesis, and restoration of autophagy by promoting transcription factor EB (TFEB) translocation into the nucleus attenuated SGN degeneration (Ye et al., 2019b). In cisplatin-induced SGN damage, activation of autophagy by rapamycin alleviated SGN apoptosis and hearing loss, and inhibition of autophagy by 3-MA aggravated the degeneration of SGNs (Liu et al., 2021). Thus, autophagy has a protective effect against HC loss, SGN degeneration and subsequent hearing impairment.

THE PRO-APOPTOTIC EFFECT OF AUTOPHAGY IN SNHL

Autophagy has a dual function of pro-survival and pro-apoptotic, which has been demonstrated in many diseases, especially cancers, and the role of autophagy depends on the developmental stage and tumor type (Singh et al., 2018). Several reports have demonstrated the pro-apoptotic role of autophagy in SNHL. In a model of cisplatin-induced HC damage, exposure to 15 μM cisplatin for 48 h induced excessive autophagy, while co-treatment of cisplatin with meclofenamic acid, a highly selective inhibitor of fatmass and obesity-associated enzyme, inhibited the cisplatin-induced excessive autophagy in HEI-OC1 cells and reduced oxidative stress and cell apoptosis (Li et al., 2018). Another study indicated that pretreatment with U0126, an inhibitor of the ERK1/2 signaling pathway, can reduce the level of cisplatin-induced autophagy in HEI-OC1 cells and HCs and can reduce cisplatin-induced ROS and apoptosis (Wang et al., 2021). Interestingly, a study showed that in cisplatin-treated HEI-OC1 cells, autophagy promoted cell survival in the early phase (during the first 8 h) of cisplatin treatment, while autophagy induced cell death in the late phase (Youn et al., 2015).

MITOPHAGY IN SNHL

Autophagy is considered to be a non-selective process in the degradation of a large number of cytoplasmic components. However, recent studies have shown that there are many types of selective autophagy. Some types of selective autophagy have recently been found in the inner ear, for example, mitophagy and pexophagy. Defective, excessive, and aged mitochondria produce toxic byproducts, particularly ROS, and mitophagy is a specific autophagic process that selectively removes these redundant or damaged mitochondria in order to reduce ROS levels and to maintain the normal function of the mitochondria (Kroemer et al., 2007; Novak, 2012). Mitophagy has been linked to neurodegenerative diseases, cancer, and aging (Bernardini et al., 2017; Chu, 2019; Tran and Reddy, 2021). Recent studies have indicated potential associations between mitophagy and age-related hearing loss, and in the cochlea of aged mice, mitophagy was reduced along with decreased expression of mitophagy-related genes and proteins (Oh et al., 2020; Youn et al., 2020). Damaged mitochondria were increased in HCs and SGNs in aged mice, and activation of mitophagy alleviated cellular senescence by promoting mitochondrial protein degradation (Kim et al., 2021). The same phenomenon was observed in carbonyl cyanide m-chlorophenyl hydrazone-induced cytotoxicity in HEI-OC1 cells and in the organ of Corti, and the protein level of mitochondrial cytochrome c oxidase subunit 4 was downregulated (Setz et al., 2018). However, in aminoglycoside-induced HC loss, neither neomycin nor gentamicin exposure had an impact on the level of mitophagy, thus suggesting a mitophagy-independent pathway of aminoglycoside ototoxicity (He et al., 2017; Setz et al., 2018).

PEXOPHAGY IN SNHL

Pexophagy is another selective autophagy pathway, in which peroxisomes are selectively degraded in vacuoles in response to environmental stimuli (Farre et al., 2009; Germain and Kim, 2020). It has been reported that pexophagy was related to inflammation induced by lipopolysaccharide exposure, and impaired pexophagy resulted in the accumulation of impaired peroxisomes and redox disequilibrium (Vasko et al., 2013). Pexophagy was associated with noise-induced HC damage, overexposure to noise led to an increased level of peroxisome in HCs and SGNs, and defective pexophagy led to noise-induced hearing loss (Delmaghani et al., 2015; Defourny et al., 2019). Pejvakin was a peroxisome-associated protein that directly recruited LC3B to promote pexophagy in order to protect cochlear HCs against noise-induced damage (Defourny et al., 2019).

PROTEINS THAT MODULATE AUTOPHAGY IN SNHL

A number of molecules have been reported to respond to cell damage by regulating autophagy. TFEB is a major regulator of autophagy and lysosomal biogenesis, and phosphorylated TFEB is inactive and remains in the cytoplasm, while dephosphorylated TFEB is translocated to the nucleus where it promotes the transcription of its target genes (Martina et al., 2012; Settembre et al., 2012). In kanamycin-induced degenerated SGNs, TFEB remained in the cytoplasm and the autophagic flux was impaired, while the mTOR inhibitor temsirolimus (CCI-779) promoted the translocation of TFEB to the nucleus thus restoring autophagic flux and ameliorating SGN degeneration (Ye et al., 2019b). Phosphatase and tensin homolog (PTEN)-induced putative kinase 1 (PINK1) also shown a protective effect against

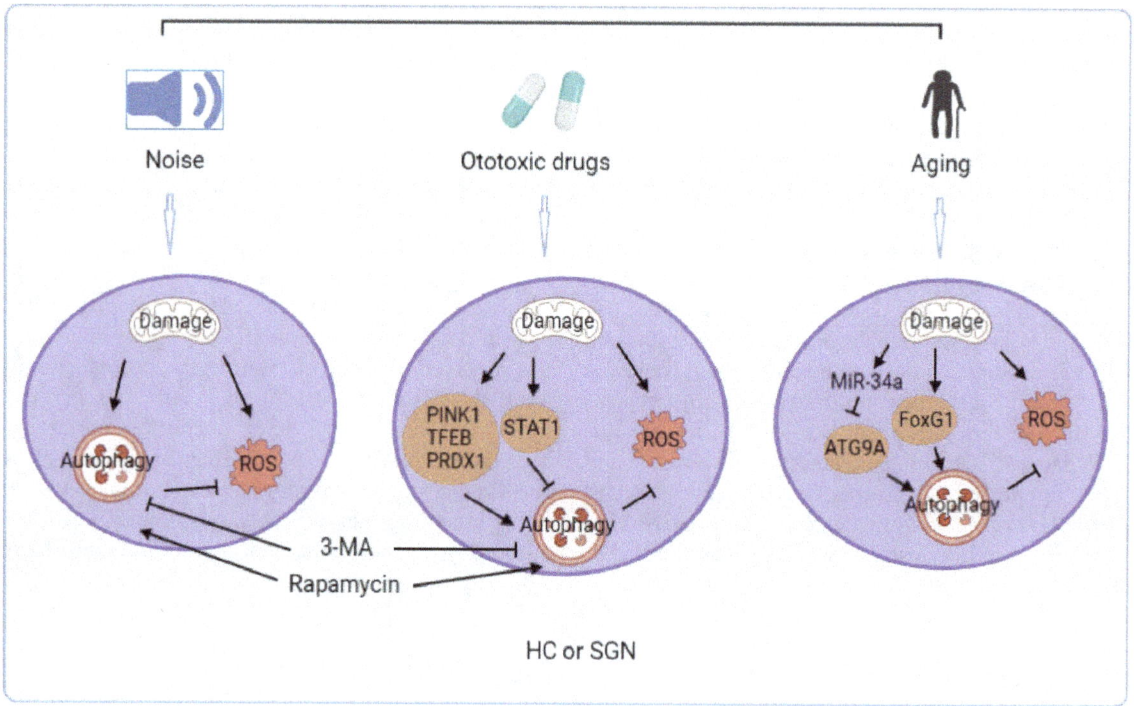

FIGURE 1 | Summary diagram of the role of autophagy in noise, ototoxic drug, and age-induced sensorineural hearing loss. (The picture is created in BioRender.com).

gentamicin and cisplatin-induced ototoxicity. PINK1 promoted autophagy and inhibited the P53 pathway in gentamicin-induced HC damage (Yang et al., 2018b), while in response to cisplatin-induced HC and SGN damage, PINK1 induced autophagy and inhibited the JNK signaling pathway (Yang et al., 2018a). Peroxiredoxin 1 (PRDX1) also played a protective role in cisplatin-induced SGN damage by activating autophagy through the activation of the PTEN-AKT signaling pathway (Liu et al., 2021). FoxG1 protected HC and delayed age-related hearing loss via autophagy making it be used as a strategy to delay age-related hearing loss (He et al., 2021a).

In addition, some proteins have detrimental effects regarding ototoxicity. For example, STAT1 is a regulator of cell death and has been reported to participate in cisplatin-induced HC damage. Knockdown of STAT1 by siRNA reduced cisplatin-induced ototoxicity (Kaur et al., 2011), and Levano et al. found that STAT1 played a role in modulating the autophagy pathway, with higher levels of autophagy seen in STAT1−/− explants in response to gentamicin and cisplatin (Levano and Bodmer, 2015). Thus, different molecules and pathways regulate the occurrence and development of SNHL in different contexts.

miRNAs RELATED TO AUTOPHAGY IN SNHL

miRNAs are a class of small endogenous RNAs with a length of about 21–23 nucleotides, and they play a variety of important regulatory roles in cells (Rupaimoole and Slack, 2017). miRNAs are potential therapeutic targets for treating cancer and other diseases, and miRNAs are also involved in SNHL (Chen et al., 2019). miR-34a was shown to be associated with age-related hearing loss in mice and humans (Pang et al., 2016, 2017), and miR-34a was activated with aging and overexpression of miR-34a significantly decreased the level of ATG9A thus inhibiting autophagic flux and inducing cell death (Pang et al., 2017). A considerable number of miRNAs have been found to be involved in autophagy cascades, such as miR-204, miR-216a, and miR-375 etc. (Su et al., 2015), but the roles of these miRNAs are poorly studied in relation to SNHL (**Figure 1**).

CONCLUSION

There is no doubt that autophagy plays an important role in SNHL. Although excessive autophagy can lead to cell death under some conditions, activation of autophagy protects HCs and SGNs against oxidative stress-induced death. It is important to be clear that the mechanisms of autophagy are complex and that different stimuli may lead to activation of different pathways. Though we have known that some proteins and miRNAs participate in the autophagic pathways involved in SNHL making them potential targets for treatment of SNHL, however, the specific signaling pathways they participate in remain unclear, let alone the known connections between these proteins and miRNAs. Furthermore, there are potential proteins and miRNAs whose functions in SNHL have not yet been identified. Future studies should thus further clarify the mechanism of autophagy in response to different stimuli in order to develop ways to regulate autophagy and thus protect HCs and SGNs. However, the application of autophagy as a treatment for deafness is still a long way off. Current research has been limited to cell lines, explants and animals, and few clinical trials have examined the role of autophagy. Given the complexity of mechanisms and functions of autophagy, the safest and most effective strategies must be studied in future research.

AUTHOR CONTRIBUTIONS

All authors listed have made a substantial, direct and intellectual contribution to the work, and approved it for publication.

ACKNOWLEDGMENTS

We are grateful to Matthew Hogg for revising the manuscript. We are thankful to the reviewers for their insightful comments.

REFERENCES

Aladag, I., Guven, M., and Songu, M. (2016). Prevention of gentamicin ototoxicity with N-acetylcysteine and vitamin A. *J. Laryngol. Otol.* 130, 440–446. doi: 10.1017/S0022215116000992

Bernardini, P., Lazarou, M., and Dewson, G. (2017). Parkin and mitophagy in cancer. *Oncogene* 36, 1315–1327. doi: 10.1038/onc.2016.302

Brigande, J. V., and Heller, S. (2009). Quo vadis, hair cell regeneration? *Nat. Neurosci.* 12, 679–685. doi: 10.1038/nn.2311

Chen, H. R., Wijesinghe, P., and Nunez, D. A. (2019). MicroRNAs in acquired sensorineural hearing loss. *J. Laryngol. Otol.* 133, 650–657. doi: 10.1017/S0022215119001439

Chen, Y., Xing, L. Xia, Chen, Z., Yin, S., and Wang, J. (2018). AAV-mediated NT-3 overexpression protects cochleae against noise-induced synaptopathy. *Gene Ther.* 25, 251–259. doi: 10.1038/s41434-018-0012-0

Chu, C. T. (2019). Mechanisms of selective autophagy and mitophagy: implications for neurodegenerative diseases. *Neurobiol. Dis.* 122, 23–34. doi: 10.1016/j.nbd.2018.07.015

Cox, B. C., Chai, R. J., Lenoir, A., Liu, Z. Y., Zhang, L. L., Nguyen, D. H., et al. (2014). Spontaneous hair cell regeneration in the neonatal mouse cochlea in vivo. *Development* 141, 816–829. doi: 10.1242/dev.109421

Defourny, J., Aghaie, A., Perfettini, I., Avan, P., Delmaghani, S., and Petit, C. (2019). Pejvakin-mediated pexophagy protects auditory hair cells against noise-induced damage. *Proc. Natl. Acad. Sci. U.S.A.* 116, 8010–8017. doi: 10.1073/pnas.1821844116

Delmaghani, S., Defourny, J., Aghaie, A., Beurg, M., Dulon, D., Thelen, N., et al. (2015). Hypervulnerability to sound exposure through impaired adaptive proliferation of peroxisomes. *Cell* 163, 894–906. doi: 10.1016/j.cell.2015.10.023

Eskelinen, E. L. (2019). Autophagy: supporting cellular and organismal homeostasis by self-eating. *Int. J. Biochem. Cell Biol.* 111, 1–10. doi: 10.1016/j.biocel.2019.03.010

Fang, B., and Xiao, H. J. (2014). Rapamycin alleviates cisplatin-induced ototoxicity in vivo. *Biochem. Biophys. Res. Commun.* 448, 443–447. doi: 10.1016/j.bbrc.2014.04.123

Farre, J. C., Krick, R., Subramani, S., and Thumm, M. (2009). Turnover of organelles by autophagy in yeast. *Curr. Opin. Cell Biol.* 21, 522–530. doi: 10.1016/j.ceb.2009.04.015

Feng, Y. C., He, D., Yao, Z. Y., and Klionsky, D. J. (2014). The machinery of macroautophagy. *Cell Res.* 24, 24–41. doi: 10.1038/cr.2013.168

Fujimoto, C., Iwasaki, S., Urata, S., Morishita, H., Sakamaki, Y., Fujioka, M., et al. (2017). Autophagy is essential for hearing in mice. *Cell Death Dis.* 8:e2780. doi: 10.1038/cddis.2017.194

Geng, J., and Klionsky, D. J. (2008). The Atg8 and Atg12 ubiquitin-like conjugation systems in macroautophagy. 'Protein modifications: beyond the usual suspects' review series. *EMBO Rep.* 9, 859–864. doi: 10.1038/embor.2008.163

Germain, K., and Kim, P. K. (2020). Pexophagy: a model for selective autophagy. *Int. J. Mol. Sci.* 21:578.

Groves, K., and Fekete, D. M. (2012). Shaping sound in space: the regulation of inner ear patterning. *Development* 139, 245–257. doi: 10.1242/dev.078257

He, Z. H., Guo, L. N., Shu, Y. L., Fang, Q. J., Zhou, H., Liu, Y. Z., et al. (2017). Autophagy protects auditory hair cells against neomycin-induced damage. *Autophagy* 13, 1884–1904. doi: 10.1080/15548627.2017.1359449

He, Z. H., Pan, S., Zheng, H. W., Fang, Q. J., Hill, K., and Sha, S. H. (2021b). Treatment with calcineurin inhibitor FK506 attenuates noise-induced hearing loss. *Front. Cell Dev. Biol.* 9:648461. doi: 10.3389/fcell.2021.648461

He, Z. H., Li, M., Fang, Q. J., Liao, F. L., Zou, S. Y., Wu, X., et al. (2021a). FOXG1 promotes aging inner ear hair cell survival through activation of the autophagy pathway. *Autophagy.* doi: 10.1080/15548627.2021.1916194 [Epub ahead of print].

Itakura, E., Kishi-Itakura, C., and Mizushima, N. (2012). The hairpin-type tail-anchored SNARE syntaxin 17 targets to autophagosomes for fusion with endosomes/lysosomes. *Cell* 151, 1256–1269. doi: 10.1016/j.cell.2012.11.001

Kamada, Y., Yoshino, K., Kondo, C., Kawamata, T., Oshiro, N., Yonezawa, K., et al. (2010). Tor directly controls the Atg1 kinase complex to regulate autophagy. *Mol. Cell. Biol.* 30, 1049–1058. doi: 10.1128/Mcb.01344-09

Kaur, T., Mukherjea, D., Sheehan, K., Jajoo, S., Rybak, L. P., and Ramkumar, V. (2011). Short interfering RNA against STAT1 attenuates cisplatin-induced ototoxicity in the rat by suppressing inflammation. *Cell Death Dis.* 2:e180.

Kaushik, S., and Cuervo, A. M. (2018). The coming of age of chaperone-mediated autophagy. *Nat. Rev. Mol. Cell Biol.* 19, 365–381. doi: 10.1038/s41580-018-0001-6

Kim, J., Kundu, M., Viollet, B., and Guan, K. L. (2011). AMPK and mTOR regulate autophagy through direct phosphorylation of Ulk1. *Nat. Cell Biol.* 13, 132–141. doi: 10.1038/ncb2152

Kim, Y. J., Choo, O. S., Lee, J. S., Jang, J. H., Woo, H. G., and Choung, Y. H. (2021). BCL2 interacting protein 3-like/NIX-mediated mitophagy plays an important role in the process of age-related hearing loss. *Neuroscience* 455, 39–51. doi: 10.1016/j.neuroscience.2020.12.005

Klionsky, D. J., Cregg, J. M., Dunn, W. A., Emr, S. D., Sakai, Y., . Sandoval, I. V., et al. (2003). A unified nomenclature for yeast autophagy-related genes. *Dev. Cell* 5, 539–545. doi: 10.1016/S1534-5807(03)00296-X

Kochergin, J. A., and Zakharova, M. N. (2016). The role of autophagy in neurodegenerative diseases. *Neurochem. J.* 10, 7–18. doi: 10.1134/S1819712416010098

Kroemer, G., Galluzzi, L., and Brenner, C. (2007). Mitochondrial membrane permeabilization in cell death. *Physiol. Rev.* 87, 99–163. doi: 10.1152/physrev.00013.2006

Levano, S., and Bodmer, D. (2015). Loss of STAT1 protects hair cells from ototoxicity through modulation of STAT3, c-Jun, Akt, and autophagy factors. *Cell Death Dis.* 6:e2019.

Levine, B., Mizushima, N., and Virgin, H. W. (2011). Autophagy in immunity and inflammation. *Nature* 469, 323–335. doi: 10.1038/nature09782

Li, H., Song, Y. D., He, Z. H., Chen, X. Y., Wu, X. M., Li, X. F., et al. (2018). Meclofenamic acid reduces reactive oxygen species accumulation and apoptosis, inhibits excessive autophagy, and protects hair cell-like HEI-OC1 cells from cisplatin-induced damage. *Front. Cell. Neurosci.* 12:139. doi: 10.3389/fncel.2018.00139

Li, J., and Chen, Y. Y. (2019). AMPK and autophagy. autophagy: biology and diseases. *Basic Sci.* 1206, 85–108. doi: 10.1007/978-981-15-0602-4_4

Li, W. W., Li, J., and Bao, J. K. (2012). Microautophagy: lesser-known self-eating. *Cell. Mol. Life Sci.* 69, 1125–1136. doi: 10.1007/s00018-011-0865-5

Liang, Z. R., Zhang, T., Zhan, T., Cheng, G., Zhang, W. J., Jia, H. Y., et al. (2021). Metformin alleviates cisplatin-induced ototoxicity by autophagy induction possibly via the AMPK/FOXO3a pathway. *J. Neurophysiol.* 125, 1202–1212. doi: 10.1152/jn.00417.2020

Lin, F. R., Yaffe, K., Xia, J., Xue, Q. L., Harris, T. B., Purchase-Helzner, E., et al. (2013). Hearing loss and cognitive decline in older adults. *JAMA Int. Med.* 173,

293–299.

Liu, T. Y., Zong, S. M., Luo, P., Qu, Y. J., Wen, Y. Y., Du, P. Y., et al. (2019). Enhancing autophagy by down-regulating GSK-3 beta alleviates cisplatin-induced ototoxicity in vivo and in vitro. *Toxicol. Lett.* 313, 11–18. doi: 10.1016/j.toxlet.2019.05.025

Liu, W. W., Xu, L., Wang, X., Zhang, D. G., Sun, G. Y., Wang, M., et al. (2021). PRDX1 activates autophagy via the PTEN-AKT signaling pathway to protect against cisplatin-induced spiral ganglion neuron damage. *Autophagy*. doi: 10.1080/15548627.2021.1905466 [Epub ahead of print].

Magarinos, M., Pulido, S., Aburto, M. R., Rodriguez, R. D., and Varela-Nieto, I. (2017). Autophagy in the vertebrate inner ear. *Front. Cell Dev. Biol.* 5:56. doi: 10.3389/fcell.2017.00056

Martina, J. A., Chen, Y., Gucek, M., and Puertollano, R. (2012). MTORC1 functions as a transcriptional regulator of autophagy by preventing nuclear transport of TFEB. *Autophagy* 8, 903–914. doi: 10.4161/auto.19653

Mizushima, N. (2007). Autophagy: process and function. *Genes Dev.* 21, 2861–2873. doi: 10.1101/gad.1599207

Mizushima, N., and Komatsu, M. (2011). Autophagy: renovation of cells and tissues. *Cell* 147, 728–741. doi: 10.1016/j.cell.2011.10.026

Mizushima, N., Yoshimori, T., and Ohsumi, Y. (2011). The role of Atg proteins in autophagosome formation. *Ann. Rev. Cell Dev. Biol.* 27, 107–132. doi: 10.1146/annurev-cellbio-092910-154005

Noda, T., and Ohsumi, Y. (1998). Tor, a phosphatidylinositol kinase homologue, controls autophagy in yeast. *J. Biol. Chem.* 273, 3963–3966. doi: 10.1074/jbc.273.7.3963

Noda, T., Kim, J., Huang, W. P., Baba, M., Tokunaga, C., Ohsumi, Y., et al. (2000). Apg9p/Cvt7p is an integral membrane protein required for transport vesicle formation in the Cvt and autophagy pathways. *J. Cell Biol.* 148, 465–479. doi: 10.1083/jcb.148.3.465

Novak, I. (2012). Mitophagy: a complex mechanism of mitochondrial removal. *Antioxid. Redox Signal.* 17, 794–802. doi: 10.1089/ars.2011.4407

Oh, J., Youn, C. K., Jun, Y., Jo, E. R., and Cho, S. I. (2020). Reduced mitophagy in the cochlea of aged C57BL/6J mice. *Exp. Gerontol.* 137:110946. doi: 10.1016/j.exger.2020.110946

Pang, J. Q., Xiong, H., Lin, P. L., Lai, L., Yang, H. D., Liu, Y. M., et al. (2017). Activation of miR-34a impairs autophagic flux and promotes cochlear cell death via repressing ATG9A: implications for age-related hearing loss. *Cell Death Dis.* 8:e3079.

Pang, J. Q., Xiong, H., Yang, H. D., Ou, Y. K., Xu, Y. D., Huang, Q. H., et al. (2016). Circulating miR-34a levels correlate with age-related hearing loss in mice and humans. *Exp. Gerontol.* 76, 58–67. doi: 10.1016/j.exger.2016.01.009

Rupaimoole, R., and Slack, F. J. (2017). MicroRNA therapeutics: towards a new era for the management of cancer and other diseases. *Nat. Rev. Drug Discov.* 16, 203–221. doi: 10.1038/nrd.2016.246

Settembre, C., Zoncu, R., Medina, D. L., Vetrini, F., Erdin, S., Erdin, S., et al. (2012). A lysosome-to-nucleus signalling mechanism senses and regulates the lysosome via mTOR and TFEB. *Embo J.* 31, 1095–1108. doi: 10.1038/emboj.2012.32

Setz, C., Benischke, A. S., Bento, A. C. P. F., Brand, Y., Levano, S., Paech, F., et al. (2018). Induction of mitophagy in the HEI-OC1 auditory cell line and activation of the Atg12/LC3 pathway in the organ of Corti. *Hear. Res.* 361, 52–65. doi: 10.1016/j.heares.2018.01.003

Sheth, S., Mukherjea, D., Rybak, L. P., and Ramkumar, V. (2017). Mechanisms of cisplatin-induced ototoxicity and otoprotection. *Front. Cell. Neurosci.* 11:338. doi: 10.3389/fncel.2017.00338

Singh, S. S., Vats, S., Chia, A. Y. Q., Tan, T. Z., Deng, S., Ong, M. S., et al. (2018). Dual role of autophagy in hallmarks of cancer. *Oncogene* 37, 1142–1158. doi: 10.1038/s41388-017-0046-6

Steffens, D. C., Otey, E., Alexopoulos, G. S., Butters, M. A., Cuthbert, B., Ganguli, M., et al. (2006). Perspectives on depression, mild cognitive impairment, and cognitive decline. *Arch. Gen. Psychiatry* 63, 130–138. doi: 10.1001/archpsyc.63.2.130

Stone, J. S., Oesterle, E. C., and Rubel, E. W. (1998). Recent insights into regeneration of auditory and vestibular hair cells. *Curr. Opin. Neurol.* 11, 17–24. doi: 10.1097/00019052-199802000-00004

Strawbridge, W. J., Wallhagen, M. I., Shema, S. J., and Kaplan, G. A. (2000). Negative consequences of hearing impairment in old age: a longitudinal analysis. *Gerontologist* 40, 320–326. doi: 10.1093/geront/40.3.320

Su, Z. Y., Yang, Z. Z., Xu, Y. Q., Chen, Y. B., and Yu, Q. (2015). MicroRNAs in apoptosis, autophagy and necroptosis. *Oncotarget* 6, 8474–8490. doi: 10.18632/oncotarget.3523

Tabuchi, K., Nishimura, B., Nakamagoe, M., Hayashi, K., Nakayama, M., and Hara, A. (2011). Ototoxicity: mechanisms of cochlear impairment and its prevention. *Curr. Med. Chem.* 18, 4866–4871. doi: 10.2174/092986711797535254

Tran, M., and Reddy, P. H. (2021). Defective autophagy and mitophagy in aging and Alzheimer's disease. *Front. Neurosci.* 14:612757. doi: 10.3389/fnins.2020.612757

Vasko, R., Ratliff, B. B., Bohr, S., Nadel, E., Chen, J., Xavier, S., et al. (2013). Endothelial peroxisomal dysfunction and impaired pexophagy promotes oxidative damage in lipopolysaccharide-induced acute kidney injury. *Antioxid. Redox Signal.* 19, 211–230. doi: 10.1089/ars.2012.4768

Wang, D., Shi, S. M., Zhang, Y. P., Guo, P., Wang, J. L., and Wang, W. Q. (2021). U0126 pretreatment inhibits cisplatin-induced apoptosis and autophagy in HEI-OC1 cells and cochlear hair cells. *Toxicol. Appl. Pharmacol.* 415:115447.

Warchol, M. E. (2010). Cellular mechanisms of aminoglycoside ototoxicity. *Curr. Opin. Otolaryngol. Head and Neck Surg.* 18, 454–458. doi: 10.1097/MOO.0b013e32833e05ec

Webber, L., and Tooze, S. A. (2010). New insights into the function of Atg9. *Febs Lett.* 584, 1319–1326. doi: 10.1016/j.febslet.2010.01.020

Wesselborg, S., and Stork, B. (2015). Autophagy signal transduction by ATG proteins: from hierarchies to networks. *Cell. Mol. Life Sci.* 72, 4721–4757. doi: 10.1007/s00018-015-2034-8

White, E. (2012). Deconvoluting the context-dependent role for autophagy in cancer. *Nat. Rev. Cancer* 12, 401–410. doi: 10.1038/nrc3262

WHO (2021). *Deafness and Hearing Loss*. Available online at: https://www.who.int/news-room/fact-sheets/detail/deafness-and-hearing-loss (accessed April 1, 2021).

Wu, F., Xiong, H., and Sha, S. H. (2020). Noise-induced loss of sensory hair cells is mediated by ROS/AMPK alpha pathway. *Redox Biol.* 29: 101406.

Xie, Z. P., and Klionsky, D. J. (2007). Autophagosome formation: core machinery and adaptations. *Nat. Cell Biol.* 9, 1102–1109. doi: 10.1038/ncb1007-1102

Xu, L., Cheng, Y. J., and Yan, W. Y. (2021). Up-regulation of autophagy and apoptosis of cochlear hair cells in mouse models for deafness. *Arch. Med. Sci.* 17, 535–541.

Yang, Q. Q., Zhou, Y. W., Yin, H. Y., Li, H. R., Zhou, M. J., Sun, G. Y., et al. (2018b). PINK1 protects against gentamicin-induced sensory hair cell damage: possible relation to induction of autophagy and inhibition of p53 signal pathway. *Front. Mol. Neurosci.* 11:403. doi: 10.3389/fnmol.2018.00403

Yang, Q. Q., Sun, G. Y., Yin, H. Y., Li, H. R., Cao, Z. X., Wang, J. H., et al. (2018a). PINK1 protects auditory hair cells and spiral ganglion neurons from cisplatin-induced ototoxicity via inducing autophagy and inhibiting JNK signaling pathway. *Free Radic. Biol. Med.* 120, 342–355. doi: 10.1016/j.freeradbiomed.2018.02.025

Yang, R., Wang, L., and Zhu, L. (2019). Chaperone mediated autophagy. autophagy: biology and diseases. *Basic Sci.* 1206, 435–452. doi: 10.1007/978-981-15-0602-4_20

Ye, B., Fan, C., Shen, Y. L., Wang, Q., Hu, H. X., and Xiang, M. L. (2019a). The antioxidative role of autophagy in hearing loss. *Front. Neurosci.* 12:1010. doi: 10.3389/fnins.2018.01010

Ye, B., Wang, Q., Hu, H. X., Shen, Y. L., Fan, C., Chen, P. H., et al. (2019b). Restoring autophagic flux attenuates cochlear spiral ganglion neuron degeneration by promoting TFEB nuclear translocation via inhibiting MTOR. *Autophagy* 15, 998–1016. doi: 10.1080/15548627.2019.1569926

Youn, C. K., Jun, Y., Jo, E. R., and Cho, S. I. (2020). Age related hearing loss in C57BL/6J mice is associated with mitophagy impairment in the central auditory system. *Int. J. Mol. Sci.* 21:7202.

Youn, C. K., Kim, J., Park, J. H., Do, N. Y., and Cho, S. I. (2015). Role of autophagy in cisplatin-induced ototoxicity. *Int. J. Pediatr. Otorhinolaryngol.* 79, 1814–1819. doi: 10.1016/j.ijporl.2015.08.012

Yuan, H., Wang, X. R., Hill, K., Chen, J., Lemasters, J., Yang, S. M., et al. (2015). Autophagy attenuates noise induced hearing loss by reducing oxidative stress. *Antioxid. Redox Signal.* 22, 1308–1324. doi: 10.1089/ars.2014.6004

Yuan, J., Zhao, X. Y., Hu, Y. J., Sun, H. Y., Gong, G. Q., Huang, X., et al. (2018). Autophagy regulates the degeneration of the auditory cortex through the AMPK-mTOR-ULK1 signaling pathway. *Int. J. Mol. Med.* 41, 2086–2098. doi: 10.3892/ijmm.2018.3393

3

An *in vivo* Biomarker to Characterize Ototoxic Compounds and Novel Protective Therapeutics

*Joseph A. Bellairs[1], Van A. Redila[1,2], Patricia Wu[2,3], Ling Tong[1,2], Alyssa Webster[4], Julian A. Simon[4], Edwin W. Rubel[1,2] and David W. Raible[1,2,3]**

[1] *Department of Otolaryngology-Head and Neck Surgery, University of Washington, Seattle, WA, United States,* [2] *Virginia Merrill Bloedel Hearing Research Center, University of Washington, Seattle, WA, United States,* [3] *Department of Biological Structure, University of Washington, Seattle, WA, United States,* [4] *Fred Hutchinson Cancer Research Center, Seattle, WA, United States*

***Correspondence:**
David W. Raible
draible@uw.edu

There are no approved therapeutics for the prevention of hearing loss and vestibular dysfunction from drugs like aminoglycoside antibiotics. While the mechanisms underlying aminoglycoside ototoxicity remain unresolved, there is considerable evidence that aminoglycosides enter inner ear mechanosensory hair cells through the mechanoelectrical transduction (MET) channel. Inhibition of MET-dependent uptake with small molecules or modified aminoglycosides is a promising otoprotective strategy. To better characterize mammalian ototoxicity and aid in the translation of emerging therapeutics, a biomarker is needed. In the present study we propose that neonatal mice systemically injected with the aminoglycosides G418 conjugated to Texas Red (G418-TR) can be used as a histologic biomarker to characterize *in vivo* aminoglycoside toxicity. We demonstrate that postnatal day 5 mice, like older mice with functional hearing, show uptake and retention of G418-TR in cochlear hair cells following systemic injection. When we compare G418-TR uptake in other tissues, we find that kidney proximal tubule cells show similar retention. Using ORC-13661, an investigational hearing protection drug, we demonstrate *in vivo* inhibition of aminoglycoside uptake in mammalian hair cells. This work establishes how systemically administered fluorescently labeled ototoxins in the neonatal mouse can reveal important details about ototoxic drugs and protective therapeutics.

Keywords: biomarker, ototoxicity, otoprotection, mouse model, aminoglycloside, hair cell

INTRODUCTION

Aminoglycosides are potent, broad-spectrum antibiotics that are clinically employed to treat mycobacterial infections (*Mycobacterium tuberculosis*), Gram-negative urinary and respiratory infections, and severe neonatal infections (Durante-Mangoni et al., 2009). Despite their wide antibacterial coverage, low cost, and stability at ambient temperatures, use of aminoglycosides in developed countries is generally limited by dose-dependent damage to the kidney (nephrotoxicity) and inner ear (ototoxicity) (Forge and Schacht, 2000; Rizzi and Hirose, 2007; Van Boeckel et al., 2014). Aminoglycoside nephrotoxicity can be monitored for with regular kidney function screening and injury can be minimized or even reversed with strategies like adjusting dose for kidney function, hydration, limiting therapy duration, and once-daily dosing (Hatala et al., 1996; Munckhof et al., 1996; Bailey et al., 1997; Guo and Nzerue, 2002). To date there are no reliable clinical strategies or therapeutics that are approved or used to prevent or minimize aminoglycoside ototoxicity.

Aminoglycoside ototoxicity targets the mechanosensory hair cells within the inner ear, which convert mechanical energy from sound waves into electrical impulses. These cells are also exceptionally vulnerable to a wide variety of genetic and environmental challenges, including excessive noise exposure and off-target effects from therapeutics such as antineoplastic agents in addition to aminoglycoside antibiotics (Forge and Schacht, 2000; Rizzi and Hirose, 2007). While aminoglycoside antibiotics have been known to cause disabling hearing loss and vestibular disfunction for decades (Rybak et al., 2008), the cellular mechanisms underlying this pathology remain under intensive study. Previous work has implicated a diverse array of cellular insults caused by aminoglycosides, including excessive free radical accumulation (Priuska and Schacht, 1995; Hirose et al., 1997), mitochondrial damage (Qian and Guan, 2009), plasma-membrane interactions (Marche et al., 1983), calcium dysregulation (Esterberg et al., 2014, 2016), and both caspase-dependent (Cheng et al., 2003; Coffin et al., 2013) and caspase-independent (Jiang et al., 2006) cell death pathways. The diverse range of cytotoxic effects attributed to aminoglycosides makes target selection and rational drug design for protective therapeutics challenging. As an alternative approach, previous studies employed drug and compound screens for phenotypic drug discovery using the zebrafish model. Zebrafish lateral line hair cells closely resemble mammalian hair cells, and importantly they demonstrate susceptibility to known ototoxins such as aminoglycosides and the anticancer therapeutic cisplatin (Pickett and Raible, 2019). Utilizing high-throughput chemical screens in zebrafish to assess for hair cell protection from aminoglycosides, several promising protective compounds have been discovered (Owens et al., 2008; Kenyon et al., 2021), optimized (Chowdhury et al., 2018), and advanced to clinical trials (Kitcher et al., 2019).

Despite recent successes, translation of preclinical otoprotective leads to mammals and ultimately human clinical trials remains an immense challenge. Indeed, across numerous biomedical fields a majority of drug discovery pipelines fail to traverse the preclinical and clinical divide (Seyhan, 2019). Many preclinical ototoxicity studies occur in zebrafish and/or mammalian neonatal explant models, and while these models faithfully recapitulate parts of the auditory system (e.g., hair cells), they lack the complex pharmacokinetics and pharmacodynamics of an *in vivo* mammalian model. *In vivo* mammalian studies assessing clinical outcomes such as hearing loss with pre- and post-treatment auditory brainstem response (ABR) thresholds are the gold standard, but these studies in mice and rats are resource-intensive and take weeks to months to complete. Translating *in vitro* exposure conditions to *in vivo* dosing regimens is also a complex endeavor when considering pharmacokinetics of multiple compounds and the assessment of efficacy is limited to the clinical endpoint of ABR threshold shifts. As such, *in vivo* studies are often reserved for only the most promising lead compounds, and even then, finding a safe and effective drug candidate can be likened to the Herculean task akin to finding a needle in a haystack.

A biomarker is a measured characteristic that is an indicator of a normal biologic process, a pathogenic process, or a response to an exposure or intervention (FDA-NIH Biomarker Working Group, 2016). For studies of ototoxicity, there is a clear need for rapid, low-cost predictive biomarkers that can determine the ability of interventions and therapeutics to inhibit the accumulation of ototoxins in mammalian hair cells *in vivo*. Previous studies have used a variety of preparations such as cochlear cultures from neonatal mice (Richardson and Russell, 1991) and derived cell lines such as HEI-OC1 cells (Kalinec et al., 2003), and more recent reports proposed circulating microRNAs (Lee et al., 2018) and proteins such as prestin (Naples et al., 2018) as specific markers of hair cell injury. However, the translational utility of these markers remain to be validated. Here, we propose utilizing *in vivo* hair cell uptake of fluorescently labeled aminoglycosides as a histologic biomarker for ototoxicity. Despite the variety of mechanisms described for aminoglycoside-induced ototoxicity, there is consensus that a fundamental property of susceptible cells is their uptake and retention of aminoglycosides. Previous studies demonstrated that proximal convoluted tubule (PCT) cells within the kidney and inner ear mechanosensory hair cells show aminoglycoside uptake and retention following *in vivo* systemic aminoglycoside administration, and there appears to be good correlation between aminoglycoside uptake and cell death (Imamura and Adams, 2003; Dai et al., 2006; Kim and Ricci, 2022).

We examine intracellular accumulation of the aminoglycoside geneticin (G418) conjugated to the fluorophore Texas red (TR) in neonatal (P5) mouse hair cells following systemic injection. Building off recent studies (Makabe et al., 2020; Qian et al., 2021), we performed experiments in neonatal mice because (I) neonatal mice can be readily obtained in large number and at low costs from a small number of breeding adults and (II) neonatal otic capsules are incompletely ossified, allowing for rapid tissue fixation and easy dissection of sensory epithelium. We demonstrate that neonates, like juvenile mice (P25-30) with mature hearing sensitivity, exhibit dose- and time-dependent uptake and accumulation of G418-TR in hair cells. Using ORC-13661, an orally available small molecule that acts as a high-affinity permeant blocker of the mechanoelectrical transduction (MET) channel (Kitcher et al., 2019) and preserves hearing in rats treated with the aminoglycoside amikacin (Chowdhury et al., 2018), we demonstrate that hair cell uptake of G418-TR is inhibited *in vivo* in mammals. Our results show that neonatal mice injected with G418-TR can be used as a translational tool to better understand *in vivo* mammalian ototoxicity and characterize the efficacy of otoprotective therapeutics that block aminoglycoside uptake. These results also confirm a mechanism of action for ORC-13661 predicted from zebrafish and mammalian *in vitro* studies (Kitcher et al., 2019).

MATERIALS AND METHODS

Animals

C57BL/6J wild-type mice were used in all experiments. Both male and female mice were used in all experiments. All procedures involving animals were carried out in accordance with the National Institutes of Health guide for care and use of laboratory animals and approved by the Institutional Animal Care and Use Committee of the University of Washington.

Synthesis of G418-TR

A modified synthesis of geneticin (G418) conjugated Texas Red (TR) was performed based on previously published protocols (Liu et al., 2015). TR-NHS ester was dissolved in anhydrous N,N-dimethylformamide and added to a solution of 1.377 mmol G418 disulfate in a 100 mM potassium carbonate solution. The resulting solution was mixed in darkness at 4°C for 48 h. G418-TR was purified by Reverse-phase chromatography connected to a UV-Vis detector monitoring a wavelength at 214 nm. The analyte was gradient eluted from a Waters delta-pak C18 (300 angstrom) 19 mm × 30 cm column using buffers of 0.1% trifluoroacetic acid (by volume in water) for "A" and acetonitrile/0.08% trifluoroacetic acid (by volume) for "B." Fractions were collected every thirty seconds between 15 and 38 min using a gradient as follows: 0 min at 5% "B," followed by a 5-min hold at 5% "B," then ramping up to 20% "B" in 1 min, followed by a linear gradient to 50% "B" in 25 min, followed by another linear ramp to 95% "B" in 2 min and holding at 95% "B" for 5 min, and finally ramping down to 5% "B" in 2 min and column equilibration at 5% "B" over another 5–10 min. Up to 1/3 of the sample volume was loaded onto the column and purified in three successive HPLC runs. Those fractions in which the m/z value corresponding to the analyte of interest were pooled, lyophilized, and stored in the dark at −20°C with a final yield of 68%.

G418-TR Uptake

G418, an aminoglycoside structurally related to gentamicin, was used for all experiments because unlike gentamicin, which is supplied as a variable mixture of aminoglycosides, G418 is a purified single aminoglycoside without batch-to-batch variation (O'Sullivan et al., 2020). G418-TR has previously been used to study aminoglycoside trafficking in zebrafish hair cells and it has been shown to be similar to gentamicin, both in toxicity and intracellular trafficking (Hailey et al., 2017). G418-TR in saline (2 mg/kg), TR-hydrazide (2 mg/kg; Invitrogen, Waltham, MA, United States), or sterilized saline were injected s.c. into P5 neonatal mice and P25-30 adult mice. Neonatal mice were returned to cages with dams and euthanized 30 min to 72 h following injection. At time of euthanasia, whole blood was collected, and otic capsules were isolated in cold PBS. Otic capsules were fixed in 4% paraformaldehyde in PBS for 1 h at room temperature in the dark. Tissue was washed 3× with PBS, and the organ of Corti was dissected in PBS at room temperature. Basal, middle, and apical turns were isolated and transferred to a 48-well plate. The tissues were permeabilized and immunolabeled with anti-myosin VIIa antibodies (1:1000, Proteus Biosciences, Ramona, CA, United States) in 0.1% Triton X-100, 10% normal horse serum, and PBS overnight at 4°C. After washing with PBS 3×, tissues were incubated with goat anti-rabbit Alexa 488 secondary antibody (1:750, Invitrogen, Waltham, MA, United States) and DAPI (1:2500, Thermo Scientific, Waltham, MA, United States) for 90 min at room temperature. Tissues were washed with PBS 3× and mounted in Fluoromount-G (Southern Biotech, Birmingham, AL, United States).

A similar procedure was carried out in adult animals. P25-30 mice were injected subcutaneously G418-TR in saline (2 mg/kg), TR-hydrazide (2 mg/kg), or sterilized saline. Animals were euthanized 6 h after injection and whole blood was collected. Otic capsules were removed and immediately transferred to cold 4% PFA. An insulin syringe with 27 G needle was used to carefully make an apical cochleostomy, the round window was then pierced with the needle, and cold PFA was slowly infused into the cochlea. Otic capsules were then fixed at room temperature for 90 min. Tissues were washed with PBS 3× and then transferred to 500 mM EDTA for overnight decalcification at 4°C. Tissue was washed with PBS, and the organ of Corti was dissected in PBS at room temperature. Immunolabeling and staining was the performed as above for the neonates.

ORC-13661 Uptake Inhibition

ORC-13661 was obtained from Oricula therapeutics. Compound was dissolved in sterile saline immediately prior to use. Animals were injected i.p. with ORC-13661 at 10–100 mg/kg 2 h prior to receiving aminoglycoside treatment. After 2 h, animals were dosed with G418-TR s.c. at 10 mg/kg. Animals were returned to their cages, and then sacrificed at 3 and 6 h after receiving G418-TR. For booster experiments animals received a booster dose of ORC-13661 3 h following G418-TR administration. Animals and tissues were processed as described above.

Cryostat Sectioning

Cochlea, kidneys, and livers were collected for cryostat sectioning. Animals were treated as indicated above, and after sacrifice the otic capsule was dissected in cold PBS and fixed in 4% PFA for 1 h. Kidneys were also removed from animals at the time of sacrifice and immerse in 10% formalin. After washing in PBS, samples were sequentially dehydrated and equilibrated in 30% sucrose, 1:1 sucrose to OCT compound, and OCT compound overnight. Embedded tissue was frozen at −18°C and sectioned at a thickness of 12 μm. Slides were prepared with sectioned tissue. Cochlea, kidneys, and livers were labeled with phalloidin-Alexa 488 (1:200, Invitrogen, Waltham, MA, United States) for 2 h at room temperature and DAPI (1:100) for 45 min at room temperature. Cochlea sections were also immunolabeled with rabbit anti-β3 tubulin (1:1000; clone TUJ1, Biolegend, San Diego, CA, United States) overnight at 4°C followed by goat anti-rabbit Alexa-488 (1:200, Invitrogen, Waltham, MA, United States) for 2 h at room temperature and DAPI (1:100) for 45 min at room temperature. All dilutions were in 5% normal goat serum and 0.1% Triton X-100 in PBS.

Confocal Imaging

Slides were imaged with a Zeiss LSM 880 microscope (Zeiss, Oberkochen, Germany). For whole mount specimens, a 40× water objective was used to obtain 8-bit 1024 × 1024 pixel images of the mid-basal, mid-middle, and mid-apical turns. Confocal images were obtained using identical imaging parameters to compare fluorescence between images. For cryostat sectioned tissues, a 40× water objective was used to obtain 8-bit 1024 × 1024 pixel images of the organ of Corti, stria vascularis, spiral ganglia, and renal cortex. Identical imaging parameters were used for cochlea tissues, but laser intensity was decreased to avoid oversaturation when imaging renal cortex.

Fluorescence Quantification

For whole mount fluorescence quantification, ImageJ software was used for image processing and fluorescence quantification. For neonatal hair cells, a single 256 × 165 pixel region of interest (ROI) was selected from the stack in the z-plane that captured all three rows of outer hair cells (OHCs) between the nucleus and cuticular plate. A similar ROI measuring 256 × 55 pixels was selected for the inner hair cells, again at a z-plane between the nucleus and cuticular plate. Inner hair cell (IHC) and OHC ROIs were processed with a custom macro based on previously reported image analysis techniques (Makabe et al., 2020). Otsu thresholding was applied to the green channel to obtain a hair cell specific mask. This mask was then applied to the red channel image, and hair cell ROI mean fluorescence was calculated.

For cryostat sectioned tissue Phalloidin was used as a marker for hair cells, pillar cells, and stria vascularis tissue. OHC fluorescence was quantified by manually drawing an ROI for the region between the nucleus and the apical stereocilia. The ROI was then applied to the red channel, and mean fluorescence was quantified. Similarly, a manually segmented ROI for the pillar cells was used to quantify PC mean fluorescence. The stria vascularis ROI was also manually generated, and care was taken not to include acellular regions such as capillary lumens. For spiral ganglia neuron uptake quantification of tissue stained with Tuj1, a custom macro was generated that applied Otsu thresholding to the green channel to generate a mask which was then applied to the red channel to quantify mean fluorescence.

Statistics

Statistical analyses were done using GraphPad Prism 9.1.2. All statistics were performed comparing values from individual animals. When both cochlea were examined a mean value for the animal was calculated and used for analysis. Specific analyses are indicated in the figure legends. ANOVA was used to evaluate dose responses. Two-way ANOVA was used when multiple variables were analyzed for effect. When tissues from the same animal was compared, sample matching and a mixed effects model was used to account for any missing values. *P*-values less than 0.05 were considered significant.

Study Approval

All experiments were approved by the University of Washington Institution Animal Care and Use Committee.

RESULTS

Dose-Dependent Uptake of Systemically Administered G418-TR in Neonatal Mouse Hair Cells

To assess whether mammalian hair cells take up systemically injected geneticin (G418) tagged with Texas Red (TR), neonatal P5 C57/BL6 mice were subcutaneously (SC) injected with G418-TR (2.5–10 mg/kg), Texas Red-hydrazide (10 mg/kg) as a non-ototoxic control, or saline and sacrificed 6 h after injection. The selected doses of G418-TR were not toxic to neonatal mice and hair cell damage was not evident in cochlear whole mount preparations. G418-TR, like gentamicin-TR (GTTR) (Dai et al., 2006; Wang and Steyger, 2009; Makabe et al., 2020), was detectable within neonatal hair cells 6 h following SC injection with confocal microscopy of whole mount preparations (**Figure 1A**). Confocal microscopy demonstrates a dose-dependent increase in hair cell cytoplasmic accumulation of G418-TR. Control animals injected with 10 mg/kg unconjugated TR hydrazide demonstrate no significant hair cell fluorescence (**Supplementary Figure 1A**).

In order to quantify the dose-dependent uptake of G418-TR, we measured TR fluorescence present in mouse sera and cochlear hair cells. At time of euthanasia, blood was collected, serum was separated, and fluorescence was analyzed. A significant dose-dependent increase in serum fluorescence was observed in all treated animals (**Figure 1B**) after 6 h of treatment.

Quantification of IHC and OHC mean fluorescence was performed utilizing myosin VIIa immunolabeling as a hair cell-specific mask. Given the three-dimensional nature of the organ of Corti, regions of interest were calculated from different images within a stack to include the cytoplasm between the nucleus and cuticular plate for OHCs (**Figure 1A**) and IHCs (**Supplementary Figure 2**). Hair cells were analyzed from the apical, middle, and basal turns of each cochlea to assess for tonotopic differences in uptake. Following systemic administration of G418-TR in neonatal mice, both IHCs and OHCs demonstrated dose dependent increases in hair cell fluorescence (**Figures 1C,D**). When evaluating IHCs, all regions of the cochlea demonstrate a dose-dependent increase in uptake. Mixed-effect analysis with matching across tonotopic regions demonstrates a significant dose-effect ($P < 0.0001$), but no significant variation in IHC uptake across tonotopic regions ($P = 0.1090$). OHCs demonstrated dose-dependent uptake across base, middle, and apex. Mixed-effect analysis with matching across tonotopic regions demonstrates significant interaction between dose and tonotopic region ($P < 0.001$). Hair cells from animals treated with TR-hydrazide

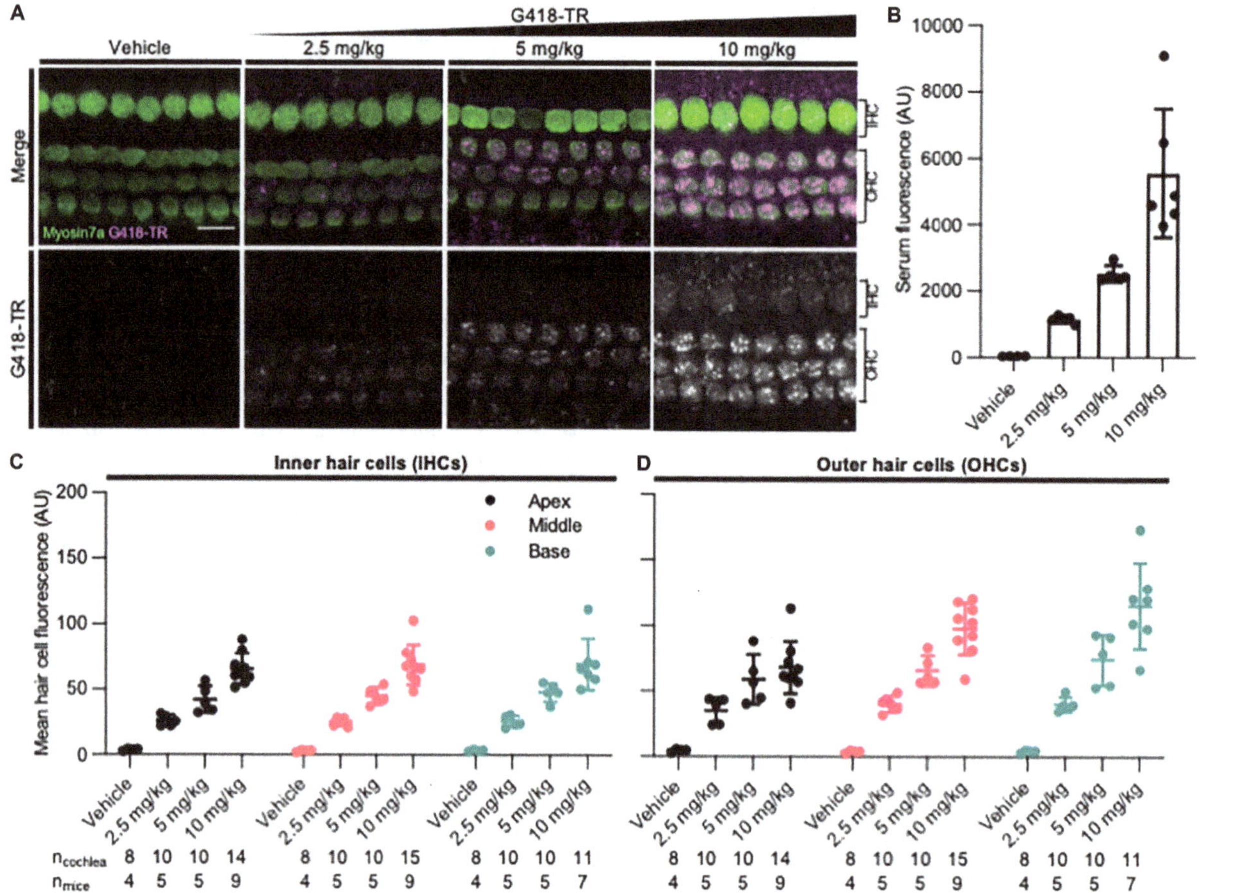

FIGURE 1 | G418-TR is taken up by neonatal mammalian hair cells following systemic administration. **(A)** At 6 h after systemic injection with G418-TR, neonatal mice (P5) were sacrificed, cochlear sensory epithelia was dissected and fixed, and tissue was immunolabeled for myosin VIIa. Representative single z-plane images captured from the middle turn of the cochlea in the region between the cuticular plate and nucleus demonstrate dose-dependent uptake of G418-TR in OHCs. Scale bar = 10 μm. **(B)** 6 h after systemic administration of G418-TR, blood was collected from neonatal mice, serum was extracted, and fluorescence was quantified with a fluorescence plate reader. Increasing doses of G418-TR results in a dose-dependent increase in serum fluorescence [One-way ANOVA; $F_{(3,16)}$ = 25.02, $P < 0.0001$]. **(C)** Mean G418-TR fluorescence intensity of IHCs by tonotopic region 6 h after systemic treatment. IHCs demonstrate similar dose-dependent uptake of G418-TR in base, middle, and apex. **(D)** Mean G418-TR fluorescence intensity of OHCs by tonotopic region 6 h after systemic treatment. OHCs demonstrate significant dose-dependent and tonotopic G418-TR uptake [Mixed effects analysis; $F_{(6,36)}$ = 5.127, P = 0.0007]. $n_{cochlea}$ and n_{mice} represent the number of cochlea and mice examined, respectively. When two cochlea from the same animal were analyzed, the animal mean was calculated and used for all statistics and graphs. Error bars are standard deviations. AU, arbitrary unit.

showed minimal background fluorescence that was not significantly different when compared to vehicle treated animals (**Supplementary Figure 1B**).

Dose-Dependent Uptake of Systemically Administered G418-TR in Mature Mouse Hair Cells Is Similar to Observed Neonatal Hair Cell Uptake

Rodent cochlear hair cells are immature at birth and only begin to acquire the morphological and biophysical specializations characterizing mature hair cells during postnatal development (He et al., 1994; Marcotti and Kros, 1999; Abe et al., 2007; Jeng et al., 2020). Hearing onset in mice is generally thought to begin at approximately P12 and roughly corresponds with maturation of specializations related to hair cell type and location as well as other biophysical properties such as the endocochlear potential. In mice, the cochlea appears fully mature between P25-30 (Rubel, 1978; Kros et al., 1998; Marcotti et al., 2003; Rubel and Fay, 2012). To evaluate whether G418-TR uptake in mature hair cells was similar to that observed in neonatal mouse hair cells, juvenile C57/BL6 mice (25–30 days old) were subcutaneously (SC) injected with G418-TR (5–20 mg/kg), Texas Red-hydrazide (20 mg/kg), or saline and sacrificed 6 h after injection.

Similar to neonatal hair cells, we observed that juvenile mouse hair cells readily take up systemically injected G418-TR (**Figure 2A**). Quantification of fluorescence from serum samples showed a significant dose-dependent increase in serum fluorescence ($P < 0.0001$) (**Figure 2B**). Both juvenile IHCs and OHCs demonstrated a dose-dependent increase in fluorescence across all tonotopic regions examined. Mixed-effect analysis with matching across tonotopic regions demonstrated

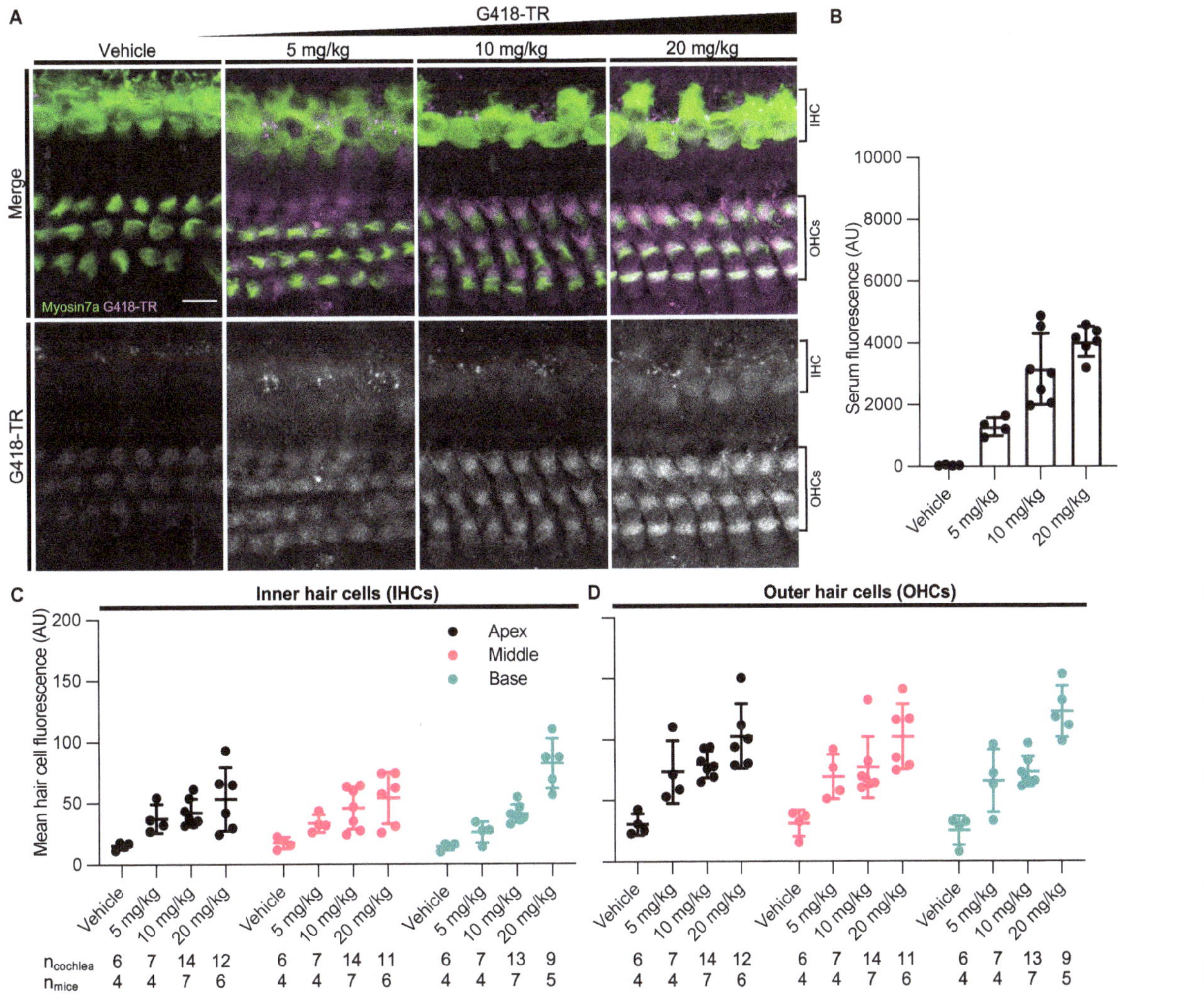

FIGURE 2 | G418-TR is taken up by mature mammalian hair cells following systemic administration. **(A)** At 6 h after systemic injection with G418-TR, juvenile mice (P25-30) were sacrificed, cochlear sensory epithelia was dissected and fixed, and tissue was immunolabeled for myosin VIIa. Representative maximum projection images captured from the middle turn of the cochlea demonstrate dose-dependent uptake of G418-TR in inner and outer hair cells. Scale bar = 10 μm. **(B)** 6 h after systemic administration of G418-TR, blood was collected from juvenile mice, serum was extracted, and fluorescence was quantified with a fluorescence plate reader. Increasing doses of G418-TR results in a dose-dependent increase in serum fluorescence [One-way ANOVA; $F_{(3,17)} = 28.28$, $P < 0.0001$]. **(C)** Mean G418-TR fluorescence intensity of IHCs by tonotopic region 6 h after systemic treatment. IHCs demonstrate low uptake at most doses of G418-TR with no significant tonotopic variation. **(D)** Mean G418-TR fluorescence intensity of OHCs by tonotopic region 6 h after systemic treatment. OHCs demonstrate dose-dependent uptake but not tonotopic variation in G418-TR uptake. $n_{cochlea}$ and n_{mice} represent the number of cochlea and mice examined, respectively. When two cochlea from the same animal were analyzed, the animal mean was calculated and used for all statistics and graphs. Error bars are standard deviations. AU, arbitrary unit.

significant dose-effects for IHCs or OHCs ($P < 0.001$ and $P < 0.0001$, respectively) but no significant variation from by tonotopic region for IHCs or OHCs ($P = 0.5924$ and $P = 9312$). Animals treated with TR-hydrazide demonstrated minimal fluorescence over background, which was similar to that observed in vehicle treated animals (**Supplementary Figures 1C,D**).

Characteristics of G418-TR Hair Cell Accumulation

Aminoglycoside-induced hair cell toxicity typically initially occurs in basal OHCs, and extends apically and to IHCs with increasing cumulative dosing (Forge and Schacht, 2000). We sought to determine whether this pattern of differential toxicity correlated with levels of G418-TR uptake. In P5 neonatal mice treated with 10 mg/kg G418-TR for 6 h, we observed dramatic tonotopic variation in uptake in OHCs, but not IHCs (**Figures 1C,D**). Basal turn OHCs demonstrated nearly twice the mean fluorescence compared to apical OHCs (115.8 and 68.2 AU, respectively). However, IHCs from the basal, middle, and apical turns from the same animals showed similar levels of fluorescence (69.7, 68.8, and 65.5 AU, respectively). In older mice with mature hearing (P25-30) treated with 20 mg/kg G418-TR for 6 h, we observed a much small but significant increase in IHC and OHC fluorescence in the basal turn only (**Figures 2C,D**).

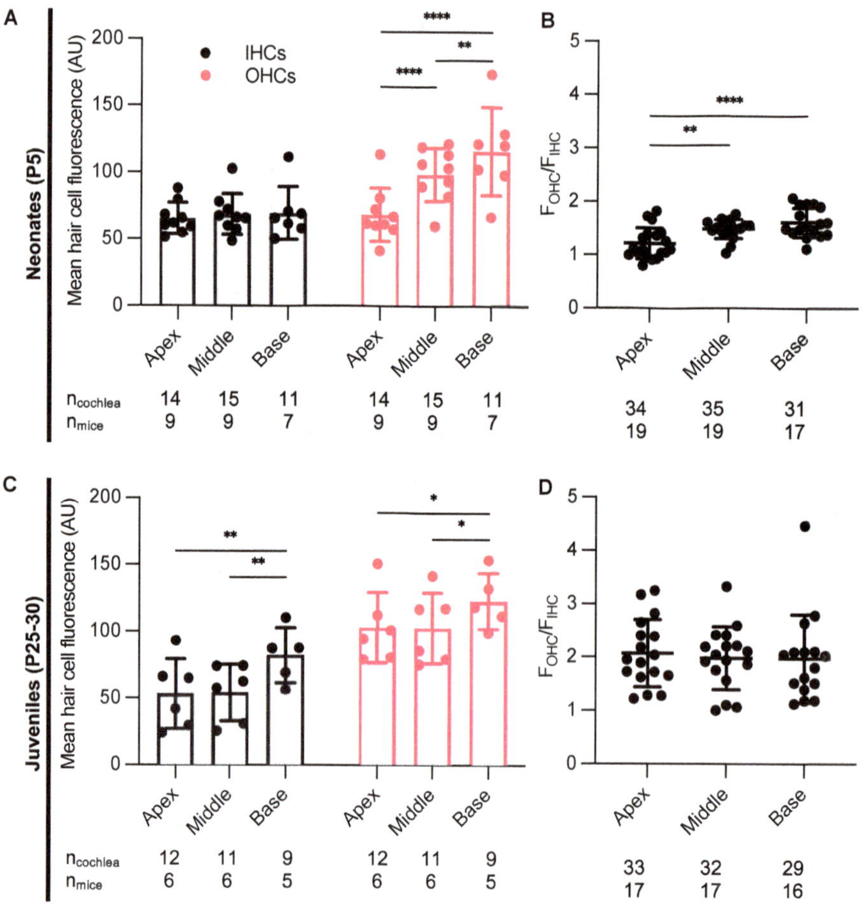

FIGURE 3 | Characteristics of G418-TR uptake in neonatal and juvenile hair cells. **(A)** Pooled analysis of the ratio of OHC to IHC uptake (F_{OHC}/F_{IHC}) was calculated for all neonatal animals treated with G418-TR (2.5, 5, and 10 mg/kg) and sorted by tonotopic region. In neonatal hair cells, there is significant variation in F_{OHC}/F_{IHC} by region [Mixed-effects Analysis; $F_{(2,52)} = 11.81$, $P < 0.0001$]. **(B)** Pooled analysis for all juvenile animals treated with G418-TR (5, 10, and 20 mg/kg) demonstrates no significant tonotopic variation in F_{OHC}/F_{IHC} [Mixed-effects Analysis; $F_{(2,31)} = 0.1442$, $P = 0.8662$]. $n_{cochlea}$ and n_{mice} represent the number of cochlea and mice examined, respectively. When two cochlea from the same animal were analyzed, the animal mean was calculated and used for all statistics and graphs. Error bars are standard deviations. $^{**}P < 0.01$, $^{****}P < 0.0001$; *P*-values generated from multiple comparisons *post hoc* test (Tukey's multiple comparison test).

In each cochlea we directly compared the ratio of OHC fluorescence to IHC fluorescence (F_{OHC}/F_{IHC}) in each tonotopic region. Apical, middle, and basal hair cells demonstrated significantly higher fluorescence in OHCs compared to IHCs (**Figures 3A,B**). When we analyzed data from all neonates treated with G418-TR (2.5–10 mg/kg) for 6 h, the ratio between OHC and IHC uptake increased from a mean of 1.21 at the apex to 1.61 at base. When the same analysis was applied to specimens collected from older animals (P25-30), mean F_{OHC}/F_{IHC} were 2.18, 2.11, and 2.02 in the apex, middle and base, respectively. Note as well that only 5 of 55 neonatal cochlea samples and 0 of the 50 juvenile cochlea samples examined in this way had F_{OHC}/F_{IHC} ratio < 1.0.

Neonatal Hair Cells Accumulate and Retain G418-TR

We also studied the relationship between G418-TR serum kinetics and hair cell uptake. We treated neonatal P5 mice with 10 mg/kg G418-TR and sacrificed cohorts of animals 30 min–72 h after injection. At the time of sacrifice, whole blood was collected from animals and serum was isolated for fluorescence quantification. Serum fluorescence was converted to concentration using a calibration curve of G418-TR diluted in fetal bovine serum. Serum kinetics for G418-TR demonstrate a peak at 3 h post-injection with a $t_{1/2}$ of 2.5 h, resembling the parameters previously reported for gentamicin-TR (Wang and Steyger, 2009; **Figure 4B**).

We also evaluated the kinetics of hair cell uptake and accumulation of G418-TR in hair cells from the same animals over 72 h. After subcutaneous injection with 10 mg/kg G418-TR, both OHCs and IHCs accumulate G418-TR over 6 h, and then retain that fluorescence for at least 72 h post-injection (**Figure 4A**). Quantification of middle turn hair cell fluorescence demonstrates that IHC and OHC fluorescence peaks at 6 h, and then plateaus with no significant decrease from 12 to 72 h post-injection (**Figure 4C**). IHC and OHC fluorescence is similar for the first 3 h, but after 6 h the difference between IHC

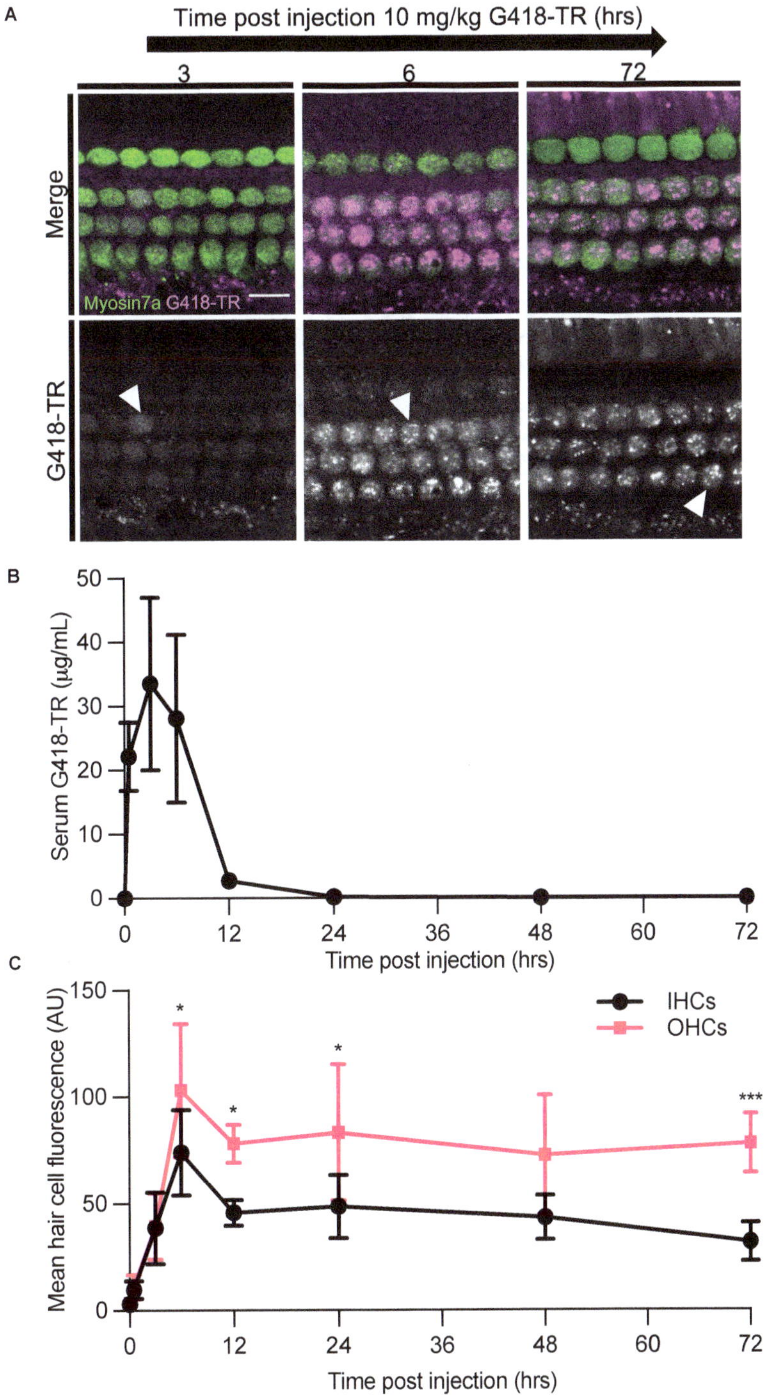

FIGURE 4 | Hair cells accumulate and retain G418-TR after systemic injection. **(A)** 30 min–72 h after systemic injection with 10 mg/kg G418-TR, neonatal mice (P5) were sacrificed, cochlear sensory epithelia was dissected and fixed, and tissue was immunolabeled for myosin VIIa. Representative images captured from the middle turn of the cochlea demonstrate uptake and retention of G418-TR. Images shown are single z-plane images capturing the region between the nucleus and cuticular plate. Arrowhead highlights transition from diffuse G418-TR distribution to accumulation in puncta with time. Scale bar = 10 μm. **(B)** Serum kinetics of G418-TR after systemic injection. After systemic injection with 10 mg/kg G418-TR, neonatal mice were sacrificed at different time points, serum was collected, and fluorescence was quantified. Fluorescence was converted to concentration in μg/mL utilizing a calibration curve of G418-TR diluted in fetal bovine serum. Quantification shows that serum levels of G418-TR peak at 3 h and are undetectable 24 h post-injection. **(C)** Mean hair cell fluorescence from the middle turn of the cochlea was calculated over 72 h. Both IHCs and OHCs show uptake and retention. Animals examined [t (hours), n] = (0,4), (0.5,4), (3,5), (6,6), (12,5), (24,5), (48,5), (72,5). Error bars are standard deviations. AU, arbitrary unit. Significant differences between IHC and OHCs denoted with: $^{*}P < 0.05$, $^{***}P < 0.001$. P-values calculated from multiple comparisons *post hoc* test (Šidák's multiple comparison test).

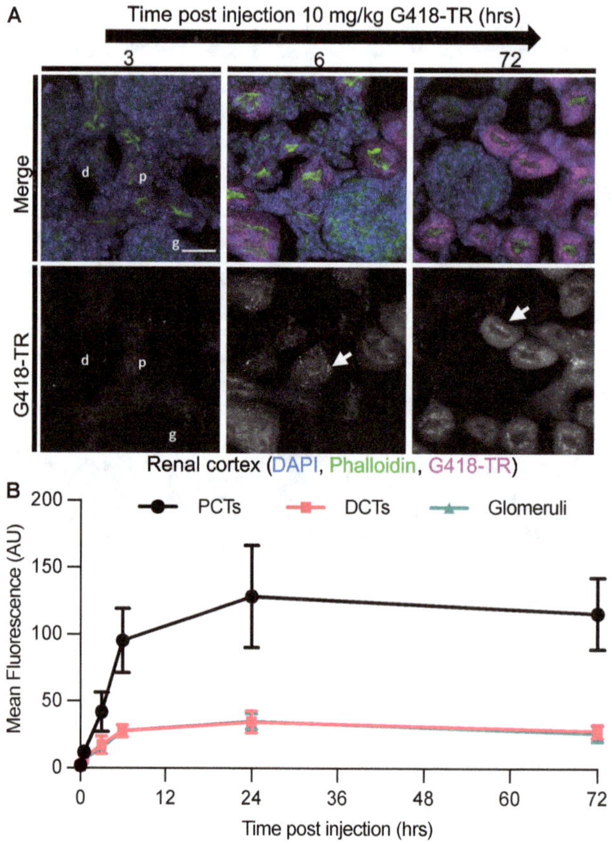

FIGURE 5 | Selective aminoglycoside retention in proximal convoluted tubule cells of the kidney. **(A)** 0 min–72 h after systemic injection with G418-TR, neonatal mice (P5) were sacrificed, and kidneys were removed. Tissues were fixed, embedded and cryostat sectioned at a thickness of 12 μm. Tissue sections were stained with phalloidin and DAPI. Representative maximum projection images from the renal cortex show proximal convoluted tubule (p) uptake and retention, but minimal uptake in the distal convoluted tubule (d) and glomeruli (g). Like hair cells, PCT cells also show apical puncta (arrow) accumulation of G418-TR. Scale bar = 20 μm. **(B)** Mean fluorescence from proximal convoluted tubules (PCTs), distal convoluted tubules (DCTs), and glomeruli was calculated over 72 h. PCTs demonstrate G418-TR uptake and retention like that observed in cochlear hair cells. Animals examined $n = 4$ for each time point. Error bars are standard deviations. AU, arbitrary unit.

and OHC mean fluorescence increases and remains significantly different. Statistical analysis demonstrates significant interaction between time since injection and hair cell population [two-way ANOVA, $F_{(7,62)} = 2.440$; $P < 0.05$]. *Post hoc* testing for multiple comparisons demonstrates significant differences between IHC and OHC values at 6, 12, 24, and 72 h post-injection ($P < 0.05$, $P < 0.05$, $P < 0.05$, and $P < 0.001$, respectively).

G418-TR Accumulation in the Kidney

Aminoglycoside nephrotoxicity is attributed to cytotoxic affects within the tubular epithelium (Lopez-Novoa et al., 2011). Within the nephron, the PCT cells, but not the glomerulus or distal convoluted tubule (DCT) cells, show unique susceptibility to aminoglycosides (Mingeot-Leclercq and Tulkens, 1999). Previous work using GTTR demonstrated that PCT cells rapidly take up aminoglycoside *in vivo* (Dunn et al., 2002; Dai et al., 2006). Kidneys were harvested from animals treated with 10 mg/kg G418-TR in order to evaluate renal aminoglycoside uptake and retention over 72 h (**Figure 5**). Similar to findings for hair cells, PCT epithelial cells rapidly accumulate G418-TR over 24 h and retain that fluorescence for up to 72 h. DCT cells and glomeruli show less accumulation of G418-TR, but it should still be noted that these cell populations demonstrate measurable G418-TR accumulation and retention. Additionally, it is worth noting that the intensity of the G418-TR signal was significantly brighter within the kidney compared to the cochlea, and the excitation laser intensity needed to be decreased in order to prevent over saturation of the detectors used. Because aminoglycosides are renally excreted, the nephrons of the kidney are exposed to significantly more aminoglycoside than the cochlea, accounting for this notable difference in overall fluorescence levels.

Aminoglycoside hepatotoxicity is rare (Aminoglycosides, 2012). Whether this is due to dose limiting toxicity in other organs (e.g., nephrotoxicity) or an intrinsic property of the liver that renders it less susceptible to aminoglycoside toxicity is unknown. When livers from animals treated with G418-TR were examined, we observed low levels of fluorescence analogous to that observed in the DCT and glomeruli of the kidney (**Supplementary Figure 3**). This complements previous analyses that noted low-level aminoglycoside uptake in the liver of animals treated with radioisotope labeled aminoglycosides (Huy et al., 1986).

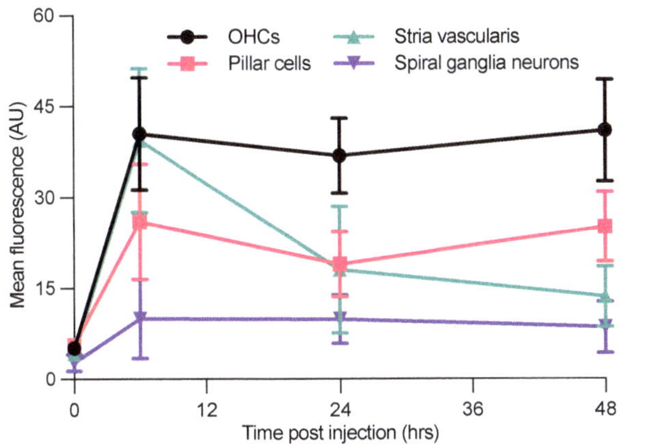

FIGURE 6 | Differential aminoglycoside uptake and retention within the cochlea. Cochlea from neonatal mice treated with G418-TR were fixed, cryostat sectioned, and signed in order to analyze the organ of Corti, stria vascularis, and spiral ganglia neurons. In order to compare relative G418-TR uptake between specific tissue types, fluorescence was quantified for outer hair cells (OHCs), pillar cells, stria vascularis, and spiral ganglia neurons. Note that while OHCs take up and retain G418-TR fluorescence, stria vascularis tissue has an early peak but then declines while SGNs show consistent low level uptake. PCs display an intermediate level of uptake with some retention. Error bars are standard deviations. Animal numbers [time (hours), *n*] = (0,3), (6,4), (24,4), and (48,4).

G418-TR Accumulation in Non-sensory Cochlear Tissues

In addition to hair cells, systemically administered aminoglycosides have been shown to accumulate in the non-sensory tissues of the inner ear (Bareggi et al., 1986; Imamura and Adams, 2003; Kitahara et al., 2005; Wang and Steyger, 2009). In neonatal mice treated with a single dose of 10 mg/kg G418-TR, we observed fluorescence in cryostat sectioned cochlear tissues in the organ of Corti, stria vascularis, and spiral ganglia neurons (**Supplementary Figure 4**).

The organ of Corti includes both the mechanosensory hair cells as well as numerous supporting cell populations and neuronal tissues. Analysis of OHCs in cross section supports the findings reported above for whole mount images; OHCs accumulate G418-TR in a diffuse pattern over 6 h, and at later time points G418-TR fluorescence is sequestered in apical regions (**Supplementary Figure 4A**). In neonatal mice, we observed a transient increase in stria vascularis fluorescence following systemic administration (**Supplementary Figure 4B**). Aminoglycosides have also been localized to spiral ganglia neurons following systemic injection (Imamura and Adams, 2003; Kitahara et al., 2005). Unlike the vascular stria vascularis, spiral ganglia neurons demonstrated consistent low-level fluorescence (**Supplementary Figure 4C**).

To compare the relative uptake of different tissues within the cochlea, we quantified mean tissue fluorescence at 0, 6, 24, and 48 h in each region (**Figure 6**). OHCs show a similar pattern as shown in whole mount imaging and quantification (**Figure 4**), with a peak at 6 h followed by retention of AG at later time points. Stria vascularis fluorescence demonstrated a peak in fluorescence at 6 h post-injection followed by a decrease to near background levels by 48 h. Pillar cells, located between IHCs and OHCs demonstrate relatively low-level uptake and retention of G418-TR, while spiral ganglion neurons demonstrated minimal uptake at all time points.

ORC-13661 Blocks the Uptake of G418-TR *in vivo* in Mammalian Hair Cells

ORC-13661 is a novel therapeutic that protects hair cells from aminoglycoside toxicity in fish and mammals (Chowdhury et al., 2018; Kitcher et al., 2019). Mechanistic studies in zebrafish and mouse cochlear cultures demonstrate that ORC-13661 reversibly blocks MET channel currents and uptake of fluorescently labeled aminoglycosides (Kitcher et al., 2019). To test whether ORC-13661 blocks uptake of aminoglycosides *in vivo* in mice, neonatal mice were pre-treated with saline or ORC-13661 (10–100 mg/kg; i.p.). Two hours after this treatment mice were injected with G418-TR (10 mg/kg; s.c.). Animals were sacrificed at either 3 or 6 h after exposure to G418-TR to test both 3 h ("short") and 6 h ("long") G418-TR exposure paradigms (**Supplementary Figures 5A,B**).

Analysis of the mid-basal turn hair cells demonstrated inhibition of uptake by ORC-13661 in both treatment schemes (**Figures 7A,B**). When animals are pre-treated with vehicle and injected with G418-TR, robust hair cell uptake is observed in both treatment schemes. When pretreated with increasing doses of ORC-13661 followed by injection with G418-TR, the short G418-TR exposure scheme demonstrates significant uptake inhibition at all doses of ORC-13661. Interestingly, the long G418-TR exposure scheme showed uptake inhibition at only the 100 mg/kg ORC-13661 dose.

To compare results between experiments, hair cell fluorescence was normalized to intra-experimental vehicle treated animals. By normalizing within experimental groups, we were able to minimize the variability between experimental groups (as observed in neonates treated with 10 mg/kg G418-TR [**Figures 1C,D**]) and discriminate smaller effects on hair cell uptake. We quantified relative fluorescence for mid-basal turn OHCs and observed a significant dose-dependent inhibition of uptake for increasing doses of ORC-13661 in the short exposure scheme with significant uptake inhibition compared to vehicle treated animals detected at all ORC-13661 dose levels (**Figure 7A**). For animals treated in the long exposure paradigm, significant uptake inhibition was only noted at the highest dose of ORC-13661 (**Figure 7B**). Kidneys from animals in the 100 mg/kg ORC-13661 dose group of the long exposure scheme demonstrated no change in PCT G418-TR uptake (**Supplementary Figure 6**). This supports the hypothesis that ORC-13661 protects hair cells through selective inhibition of MET-dependent aminoglycoside uptake, as opposed to endocytosis.

When comparing the two different treatment schemes with a two-way ANOVA, there is no significant difference in OHC uptake inhibition [$F_{(3,50)} = 1.989$, $P = 0.1276$] however

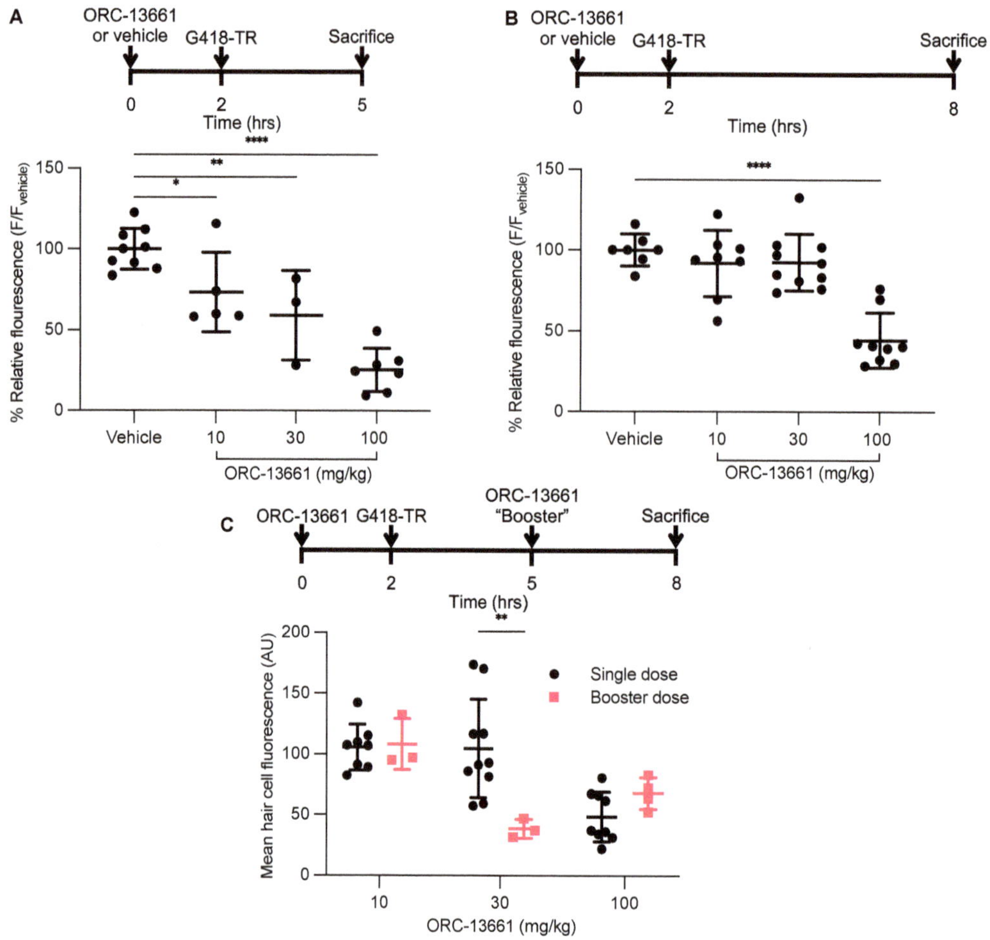

FIGURE 7 | ORC-13661 blocks G418-TR accumulation in mammalian hair cells. **(A)** Short (3 h) G418-TR exposure paradigm. Neonatal mice were pretreated with ORC-13661 or vehicle for 2 h, injected with 10 mg/kg G418-TR, and sacrificed 3 h after aminoglycoside injection. Basal turn OHC mean fluorescence for animals treated with either vehicle or ORC-13661 followed by 10 mg/kg G418-TR. OHC mean fluorescence was quantified and normalized to animals pre-treated with vehicle within each experimental replicate. [One-way ANOVA; $F_{(3,20)} = 23.55$, $P < 0.0001$]. **(B)** Long (6 h) G418-TR exposure paradigm. Neonatal mice were pretreated with ORC-13661 or vehicle for 2 h, injected with 10 mg/kg G418-TR, and sacrificed 6 h after aminoglycoside injection. [One-way ANOVA; $F_{(3,30)} = 19.62$, $P < 0.0001$]. **(C)** Booster dosing strategy with a single pretreatment injection of ORC-13661 followed by a second booster dose 3 h after G418-TR injection. Basal turn OHC mean fluorescence for animals treated with a pretreatment dose ORC-13661 (10–100 mg/kg) followed by 10 mg/kg G418-TR with an additional booster of ORC-13661 (same as pretreatment dose) 3 h after aminoglycoside administration. Note that data for single dose are non-normalized data from part **B**. Error bars are standard deviations. $^{*}P < 0.05$, $^{**}P < 0.01$, $^{***}P < 0.001$, $^{****}P < 0.0001$; P-values generated from multiple comparisons *post hoc* test (**A,B**: Dunnett's multiple comparison test; **C:** Šídák's multiple comparison test).

component analysis demonstrates a significant impact from dose [$F_{(3,50)} = 39.75$, $P < 0.0001$] and treatment scheme [$F_{(1,50)} = 13.45$, $P = 0.0006$]. These findings suggest that inhibition of aminoglycoside uptake by ORC-13661 in neonatal mice is both dose- and time-dependent.

We hypothesized that the difference between the short and long exposure paradigms was due to different pharmacokinetics for G418-TR and ORC-13661. At 6 h, we observed high levels or circulating G418-TR (**Figure 4B**). If the elimination kinetics of ORC-13661 in the neonatal mouse are rapid, this might explain the difference between the short and long G418-TR exposure paradigms. To test this hypothesis, we developed a "booster" treatment scheme. Neonatal mice were treated with a single pretreatment of ORC-13661 (10, 30, or 100 mg/kg), then injected with 10 mg/kg G418-TR, and given a booster dose of ORC-13661 (same dose as pretreatment) 3 h after G418-TR (**Figure 7C**). When compared to animals that received a single pretreatment dose of ORC-13661, animals that received 30 mg/kg ORC-13661 pretreatment and a 30 mg/kg ORC-13661 booster showed significantly more uptake inhibition. The 10 mg/kg and 100 mg/kg ORC-1366 booster schemes showed no significant difference when compared to single doses, suggesting that the 10 mg/kg dose is not enough to generate uptake inhibition while the 100 mg/kg dose may be reaching a plateau and an additional booster does not increase uptake inhibition. These findings support our hypothesis and further demonstrating the translational utility of this *in vivo* system.

DISCUSSION

Numerous drugs and therapeutic compounds are known to be toxic to the inner ear and adversely affect hearing and balance, however our understanding of the mechanisms driving ototoxicity remains incomplete. Challenges in studying ototoxicity have led to a paucity of protective therapeutics. The zebrafish lateral line and rodent explants have proven useful in screening and mechanistic studies, but translating these discoveries to adult mammals *in vivo* remains a difficult and costly endeavor. We present the development of low-cost and rapid *in vivo* mammalian model for studying ototoxic compounds and candidate protective therapeutics.

Biomarker

In mammals, diagnosis of ototoxicity is usually limited to functional evaluations such as behavioral paradigms, ABR thresholds, and otoacoustic emissions analysis or post-mortem histologic evaluation. These methods are expensive and time consuming, and they generally only detect ototoxic effects after irreversible damage has occurred. Some *in vivo* mammalian ototoxicity protocols also require cotreatment with loop diuretics, a class of therapeutics that are both independently ototoxic and show synergistic toxicity with other compounds (Rybak, 1993; Ding et al., 2016). While these protocols allow for rapid induction of *in vivo* ototoxicity, the introduction of a second therapeutic agent with independent effects on numerous organ systems confounds analysis and clinical relevance. Indeed, concomitant use of loop diuretics with aminoglycosides or cisplatin in humans is generally cautioned against in all but the most exceptional of circumstances (UpToDate, 2021; Huxel et al., 2021). We hypothesized that by injecting neonatal mice with G418-TR, we could develop a rapid and sensitive technique for evaluating *in vivo* aminoglycoside toxicity. In this study, we demonstrate that systemic injection of G418-TR into neonatal mice results in quantifiable, dose-dependent hair cell uptake of the aminoglycoside. Further evaluation of tonotopic and cell specific uptake patterns demonstrates that basal regions of the cochlea take up more aminoglycoside compared to apical regions, and OHCs take up significantly more aminoglycoside than immediately adjacent IHCs. These findings are consistent with the hypothesis that differential aminoglycoside toxicity within the inner ear is due to differential exposure of the hair cells. Whether this increased exposure is due to characteristics of aminoglycoside trafficking within the cochlea or local hair cell specific properties such as MET channel permeability remains unknown.

Because mice are born with immature cochlear hair cells and functional hearing only develops around P12, we compared neonatal hair cell uptake with that of mature hair cells from juvenile animals P25-30. Slightly higher doses of G418-TR were required in juvenile animals to achieve a similar dose-dependent increase in hair cell aminoglycoside accumulation, however the apicobasal gradient and OHC predilection were again observed. The lower doses required in neonates is consistent with the previously described "sensitive period" during rodent development when neonates are more sensitive to aminoglycosides than older animals (Chen and Saunders, 1983; Nakai et al., 1983; Prieve and Yanz, 1984).

Additionally, it is worth noting that in both neonates and juveniles we observed no animal mortality and no significant hair cell death. This is due to the fact that our studies utilized sublethal dosing of G418-TR (maximum of 10 mg/kg in neonates and 20 mg/kg in juveniles) far lower than previously described aminoglycoside ototoxicity protocols that require multiple sequential doses of 0.5–1 g/kg (Wu et al., 2001; Chowdhury et al., 2018; Horvath et al., 2019).

With similar hair cell uptake patterns observed in neonates and juveniles, albeit requiring slightly different dosing, we elected to pursue the remainder of our experiments in neonates. By using neonates we estimate we saved 80–90% on animal fees (housing only breeding animals), used 1/10th as much reagent (treating 2 g neonates vs. 20 g adults), and decreased our tissue processing time by about 50% (no decalcification required). The significant time and cost savings, coupled with faithful recapitulation of results observed in older animals, makes the neonate an attractive system for rapid and higher throughput translation of preclinical discoveries into mammalian systems designed to evaluate hearing loss and protection.

Characterization of *in vivo* Mammalian Hair Cell Uptake and Retention of G418-TR

In mammalian cochlear explant models there is clear evidence that aminoglycosides act as permeant blockers of MET channels, rapidly gaining entry into hair cells and accumulating without means of egress (Marcotti et al., 2005; Alharazneh et al., 2011; Vu et al., 2013). Aminoglycoside uptake and retention has also been documented *in vivo* (Hiel et al., 1993; Imamura and Adams, 2003; Dai et al., 2006). We sought to quantify the *in vivo* mammalian kinetics of aminoglycoside uptake in hair cells. Neonatal hair cells demonstrate rapid uptake of G418-TR from 0 to 6 h post-injection. Interestingly, we noted differences between IHC and OHC uptake and retention. Between 0 and 3 h, IHCs and OHCs demonstrate nearly identical levels of uptake. From 3 to 6 h post-injection, OHCs demonstrate a greater rate of uptake compared to IHCs which results in a significant difference in peak fluorescence between the two populations at 6 h. After reaching peak hair cell fluorescence levels at 6 h post-injections, OHCs demonstrate no significant loss by 72 h while IHCs show a moderate reduction in fluorescence. When correlated with measured serum fluorescence, we noted that hair cell uptake corresponds to the peak in serum G418-TR levels; when circulating G418-TR is maximal, the hair cells readily accumulate aminoglycoside. Once serum levels of aminoglycoside begin to drop, OHCs retain aminoglycoside while IHCs demonstrate a slow loss of signal. The mechanism of aminoglycoside egress from IHCs is undetermined as these charged molecules are unlikely to cross membranes by passive diffusion.

Our studies are consistent with previous studies using autoradiography and immunolabeling that have established that hair cells rapidly take up aminoglycosides and retain them for extended durations (Portmann et al., 1974; de Groot et al.,

1990; Imamura and Adams, 2003; Dai et al., 2006). Previous studies have noted that aminoglycoside uptake similarly shows a basal OHC predilection using qualitative and semi-quantitative methods of analysis (Hiel et al., 1993; Imamura and Adams, 2003; Dai et al., 2006). An almost universal finding is that outer hair cells are more susceptible to aminoglycoside ototoxicity than IHCs. This difference in ototoxicity remains poorly understood. It is sometimes attributed to the higher metabolic rate of outer hair cells (given their contribution to the active process of the cochlear amplifier), but there is also conflicting evidence for differential aminoglycoside uptake and accumulation in IHCs and OHCs (Lim, 1986; Hiel et al., 1993; Forge and Schacht, 2000; Imamura and Adams, 2003; Taylor et al., 2008; Wang and Steyger, 2009). Our findings support the hypothesis that differential aminoglycoside susceptibility between IHCs and OHCs is in part due to differential exposure. Explant studies have demonstrated differential rates of labeled aminoglycoside uptake in OHCs and IHCs (Alharazneh et al., 2011), but *in vivo* uptake of GTTR previously implied comparable IHC and OHC fluorescence at 3 h post-injection (Wang and Steyger, 2009; Makabe et al., 2020). In agreement with these previous studies, our results demonstrate similar IHC and OHC uptake from 0 to 3 h, but we find that a significant difference between OHCs and IHCs develops at 6 h and persists out to 72 h. We suspect that this difference is due in part to the difference in resting potentials between the hair cell populations, with a more negative OHC resting potential resulting in more favorable electrostatic uptake of positive aminoglycosides (Pickles, 1998). We also demonstrate that IHCs, unlike OHCs, show some level of aminoglycoside egress which could also be contributing to this differential susceptibility. It is worth noting that previous work has also suggested different isoforms of the MET channel could also contribute to differences between OHCs and IHCs (Beurg et al., 2006; Fettiplace, 2009), and certainly these differences could also impact aminoglycoside uptake. Quantification of aminoglycoside levels after an initial peak at 6 h also allowed for evaluation of aminoglycoside retention in hair cells. This process is an ideal application of the neonate system, because hair cell addition and turnover in aquatic vertebrates complicates prolonged analysis and in adult mammals the cost of a cross sectional study with adequate numbers is prohibitive to most research programs. We also observe not only differential accumulation, but also clearance of aminoglycoside. Despite the fact that mechanosensory hair cells and renal proximal tubule cells are known to retain aminoglycoside (Imamura and Adams, 2003; Dai et al., 2006), aminoglycoside clearance at the cellular level has not been well studied. The biologic relevance of this observation is unclear, but certainly warrants additional investigation.

Histologic evaluation of the kidneys from G418-TR treated mice corroborates previous studies which demonstrated rapid and sustained aminoglycoside uptake by the PCT cells (Dunn et al., 2002; Dai et al., 2006). While quantification of fluorescence from the PCT reveals a similar pattern of uptake and retention compared to that observed in cochlear hair cells, qualitatively there are also similarities in the cellular distribution of G418-TR. Both PCTs and hair cells show a pattern of diffuse uptake at early time points, followed by what appears to sequestration in apical puncta. Despite these similarities, hair cells and PCTs are thought to uptake aminoglycosides *via* distinct pathways. Hair cells accumulate aminoglycosides primarily through MET channel transport, with a relatively minor contribution from endocytosis (Huth et al., 2011; Hailey et al., 2017; Makabe et al., 2020). In the nephron, mutation of the PCT endocytic receptor megalin blocks aminoglycoside uptake and protects against nephrotoxicity (Schmitz et al., 2002). Given the differences in uptake mechanisms, the similarities in aminoglycoside uptake and localization in hair cells and PCTs suggest there is convergence of similar mechanisms of intracellular aminoglycoside handling and sequestration. This hypothesis is supported by the observation that aminoglycosides accumulate in lysosomal compartments within both hair cells (Hashino et al., 1997; Hailey et al., 2017) and PCT cells (Silverblatt and Kuehn, 1979). The biologic significance of aminoglycoside sequestration in puncta within hair cells and PCT cells remains to be determined and follow up studies are needed.

Evaluation of non-sensory tissues from the cochlea, including the supporting cells, spiral ganglia neurons, and the stria vascularis further demonstrates the unique pattern of uptake observed in hair cells. Cross sectional analysis of cryostat sections demonstrated once again that hair cells take up G418-TR over 6 h and then retain the aminoglycoside load. Qualitatively, we again observe aminoglycoside entering the hair cells in a diffuse pattern before localizing to puncta toward the apex and cuticular plate at later time points. This is reminiscent of the aminoglycoside loading we observed in zebrafish hair cells, where fluorescently labeled neomycin distributes within hair cells in a diffuse pattern after entry, before becoming sequestered in lysosomes (Hailey et al., 2017). Further characterization of these puncta in mammalian hair cells is needed to better understand their role in aminoglycoside toxicity. Previous *in vivo* evaluations utilizing GTTR demonstrated the intracochlear trafficking pattern of aminoglycosides, including *trans*-strial uptake into the endolymph before entering hair cells (Wang and Steyger, 2009). Indeed a recent study demonstrated *via* real-time imaging using GTTR that aminoglycoside enters the cochlea *via* the stria vascularis (Kim and Ricci, 2022). Consistent with this analysis, we observe a transient increase in stria vascularis fluorescence before fluorescence returns to near baseline levels by 48 h post-injection. Aminoglycoside uptake in spiral ganglia neurons (SGNs) has previously been observed (Bareggi et al., 1986; Imamura and Adams, 2003; Kitahara et al., 2005), however in our study we did not observe significant fluorescence in the cell bodies of the SGNs. It should, however, be noted that the cumulative dose of aminoglycoside used in these prior *in vivo* studies was 75–2000 fold higher than the 10 mg/kg administered in this analysis.

An additional extension of this work is the correlation between hair cell aminoglycoside uptake and circulating, systemic levels of aminoglycoside. Clinically, numerous trials have examined the impact of dosing schemes on aminoglycoside toxicity (Barza et al., 1996; Hatala et al., 1996; Munckhof et al., 1996; Rybak et al., 1999; Contopoulos-Ioannidis et al., 2004). Unfortunately, none of these aminoglycoside administration regimens appear to reduce incidence of ototoxicity. In this analysis, we directly correlate plasma levels of G418-TR with G418-TR fluorescence in hair cells and non-sensory tissues of the cochlea. After a single subcutaneous injection of G418-TR, hair cells rapidly accumulate the aminoglycoside at all time points that the G418-TR is detected at any significant level in the serum. While not examined closely in this analysis, the relationship between serum aminoglycoside and hair cell accumulation is likely to be of clinical relevance when considering dosing schemes such as bolus dosing, divided doses, and infusions.

ORC-13661 Blocks G418-TR Uptake *in vivo*

Therapeutic inhibition of aminoglycoside uptake is a promising strategy to combat ototoxicity. A recent analysis of gentamicin subtypes demonstrated that chemical modification of the traditional gentamicin mixtures to produce more potent MET channel-blocking analogues can diminishes ototoxicity without compromising antimicrobial activity (O'Sullivan et al., 2020). While aminoglycoside modification remains a promising strategy, multiple previous studies have utilized zebrafish-based screens to identify compounds that inhibit aminoglycoside uptake and protect hair cells (Owens et al., 2008; Kruger et al., 2016; Kirkwood et al., 2017; Chowdhury et al., 2018; Kitcher et al., 2019; Kenyon et al., 2021). Translating preliminary leads from zebrafish to a mammalian model remains challenging given the resources-intensive techniques required for *in vivo* mammalian assessment of ototoxicity. Here, we demonstrate that the drug ORC-13661 blocks aminoglycoside uptake *in vivo* in mammals, and we further highlight the utility of the neonatal mouse system to rapidly evaluate ORC-13661 dosing paradigms.

ORC-13661 is a small molecule therapeutic that protects against aminoglycoside ototoxicity in zebrafish and mammals (Chowdhury et al., 2018; Kitcher et al., 2019). Evidence from zebrafish lateral line hair cells and mammalian cochlear cultures suggests that hair cell protection occurs by blocking MET-dependent aminoglycoside uptake (Kitcher et al., 2019). Here, we extend this conclusion to the mammalian inner ear *in vivo*, demonstrating pharmacologic inhibition of aminoglycoside uptake. We examined two different dosing paradigms and observed a significant dose-dependent reduction in uptake with the short G418-TR exposure paradigm but not the long paradigm. We attribute the observed differences between the two tested schemes to the MET channel block kinetics of ORC-13661. From previous work, we know that ORC-13661 blocks MET-channel currents and MET-dependent aminoglycoside uptake, but this block is readily reversible with washout (Kitcher et al., 2019). Unlike previous *in vitro* experiments, ORC-13661 is subjected to dynamic *in vivo* pharmacokinetics in these studies. If the $t_{1/2}$ for ORC-13661 within the plasma or the endolymph of the neonatal mouse is short, the expected therapeutic window following a single injection would also be of limited duration. To test this hypothesis, we developed an ORC-13661 booster treatment scheme. We found that an additional dose of ORC-13661 rescued G418-TR uptake inhibition for animals treated with 30 mg/kg ORC-13661. Our findings suggest that ORC-13661 blocks the uptake of aminoglycosides through reversible inhibition of MET-dependent uptake, and that multiple doses of ORC-13661 may be needed to provide optimal protection from aminoglycosides.

It is worthwhile noting that the doses of ORC-13661 administered in this study (10–100 mg/kg) were larger than those used previously to protect rats (1–5 mg/kg) from aminoglycoside-induced hearing loss (Chowdhury et al., 2018; Kitcher et al., 2019). While this could be due differences between neonatal mice and adult rats, it also raises the question of how much aminoglycoside uptake inhibition is relevant from a hair cell death perspective and a measurable auditory threshold perspective. The association between aminoglycoside uptake and hair cell death is also poorly understood in mammals, in part because the molecular mechanisms of aminoglycoside-induced hair cell death are not completely understood (Forge and Schacht, 2000; Cheng et al., 2005; Rizzi and Hirose, 2007; Jiang et al., 2017). The developing blood-labyrinth barrier (BLB) is also an important consideration when comparing neonatal animals to mature adults. In particular, the role of the BLB in facilitating aminoglycoside ototoxicity, and its impact on the delivery of otoprotective therapeutics to mechanosensory hair cells are poorly understood but areas of active investigation. The characteristics of uptake inhibition, and specifically whether level of absolute inhibition, manipulation of rate of uptake, and/or altering the subcellular uptake and localization of aminoglycoside are driving protection are also unknown. Further work to begin correlating aminoglycoside uptake and accumulation with hair cell death and hearing threshold shifts, and conversely aminoglycoside uptake inhibition with hair cell survival and hearing protection is needed to better characterize the therapeutic window for uptake inhibition.

Translational Significance

The ability to rapidly evaluate the effects of ototoxins *in vivo* within the mammalian cochlea will not only enable further characterizations of ototoxins and also novel protective therapeutics. Here, we demonstrate that neonatal mice can treated with the aminoglycoside G418-TR and the kinetics of aminoglycoside uptake can be monitored within the cochlea. We find that cochlear hair cells, especially OHCs, uniquely retain G418-TR for days after a single injection without significant efflux or clearance. Further work is needed to better characterize hair cell retention of aminoglycoside in mammals and correlate aminoglycoside uptake and retention with clinical manifestations of ototoxicity. We further demonstrate that mammalian hair cell uptake of G418-TR can be modulated utilizing ORC-13661, a novel otoprotective therapeutic. These findings support the hypothesis that ORC-13661 protects against aminoglycoside ototoxicity by inhibiting MET-dependent uptake without causing any adverse effect on hearing (Kitcher et al., 2019). Finally, we demonstrate the translational utility of this system by testing a novel ORC-13661 dosing scheme which appears to provide significant and sustained aminoglycoside uptake inhibition. Important limitations of this model include the use of neonatal mice as opposed to adult animals with functional hearing and the paucity of data correlating *in vivo* mammalian aminoglycoside uptake with hearing loss, and conversely aminoglycoside uptake inhibition with hearing protection. In addition, there are likely significant differences in the distribution and metabolism of both aminoglycosides and protective compounds such as ORC-13661 across mammalian species including humans. Caution should be used in directly translating dose and timing of treatments to clinical settings. Utilizing the neonatal mouse, we will continue further characterization of additional ototoxic compounds and optimization of protective therapeutic strategies, with the goal of ultimately translating these findings to human clinical trials.

AUTHOR CONTRIBUTIONS

JB, JAS, EWR, and DWR designed the studies. JB, VR, and LT performed the all experiments. AW and JAS provided the reagents. JB and PW acquired the data. JB and DWR analyzed the data and wrote the manuscript. All authors contributed to the article and approved the submitted version.

ACKNOWLEDGMENTS

We are deeply grateful to our laboratory for insightful discussion on the manuscript and T. Linbo for his excellent technical support.

REFERENCES

Abe, T., Kakehata, S., Kitani, R., Maruya, S., Navaratnam, D., Santos-Sacchi, J., et al. (2007). Developmental expression of the outer hair cell motor prestin in the mouse. *J. Membr. Biol.* 215, 49–56. doi: 10.1007/s00232-007-9004-5

Alharazneh, A., Luk, L., Huth, M., Monfared, A., Steyger, P. S., Cheng, A. G., et al. (2011). Functional hair cell mechanotransducer channels are required for aminoglycoside ototoxicity. *PLoS One* 6:e22347. doi: 10.1371/journal.pone.0022347

Aminoglycosides (2012). *LiverTox: Clinical and Research Information on Drug-Induced Liver Injury.* Bethesda, MD: National Institute of Diabetes and Digestive and Kidney Diseases.

Bailey, T. C., Little, J. R., Littenberg, B., Reichley, R. M., and Dunagan, W. C. (1997). A meta-analysis of extended-interval dosing versus multiple daily dosing of aminoglycosides. *Clin. Infect. Dis.* 24, 786–795. doi: 10.1093/clinids/24.5.786

Bareggi, R., Narducci, P., Grill, V., Mallardi, F., Zweyer, M., and Fusaroli, P. (1986). Localization of an aminoglycoside (streptomycin) in the inner ear after its systemic administration. *Histochemistry* 84, 237–240. doi: 10.1007/BF00495788

Barza, M., Ioannidis, J. P., Cappelleri, J. C., and Lau, J. (1996). Single or multiple daily doses of aminoglycosides: a meta- analysis. *BMJ* 312, 338–344. doi: 10.1136/bmj.312.7027.338

Beurg, M., Evans, M. G., Hackney, C. M., and Fettiplace, R. (2006). A large-conductance calcium-selective mechanotransducer channel in mammalian cochlear hair cells. *J. Neurosci.* 26, 10992–11000. doi: 10.1523/JNEUROSCI.2188-06.2006

Chen, C.-S., and Saunders, J. C. (1983). The sensitive period for ototoxicity of kanamycin in mice: morphological evidence. *Arch. Otorhinolaryngol.* 238, 217–223. doi: 10.1007/BF00453932

Cheng, A. G., Cunningham, L. L., and Rubel, E. W. (2003). Hair cell death in the avian basilar papilla: characterization of the in vitro model and caspase activation. *J. Assoc. Res. Otolaryngol.* 4, 91–105. doi: 10.1007/s10162-002-3016-8

Cheng, A. G., Cunningham, L. L., and Rubel, E. W. (2005). Mechanisms of hair cell death and protection. *Curr. Opin. Otolaryngol. Head Neck Surg.* 13, 343–348. doi: 10.1097/01.moo.0000186799.45377.63

Chowdhury, S., Owens, K. N., Herr, R. J., Jiang, Q., Chen, X., Johnson, G., et al. (2018). Phenotypic optimization of urea-thiophene carboxamides to yield potent, well tolerated and orally active protective agents against aminoglycoside-induced hearing loss. *J. Med. Chem.* 61, 84–97. doi: 10.1021/acs.jmedchem.7b00932

Coffin, A. B., Williamson, K. L., Mamiya, A., Raible, D. W., and Rubel, E. W. (2013). Profiling drug-induced cell death pathways in the zebrafish lateral line. *Apoptosis* 18, 393–408. doi: 10.1007/s10495-013-0816-8

Contopoulos-Ioannidis, D. G., Giotis, N. D., Baliatsa, D. V., and Ioannidis, J. P. A. (2004). Extended-interval aminoglycoside administration for children: a meta-analysis. *Pediatrics* 114, e111–e118. doi: 10.1542/peds.114.1.e111

Dai, C. F., Mangiardi, D., Cotanche, D. A., and Steyger, P. S. (2006). Uptake of fluorescent gentamicin by vertebrate sensory cells in vivo. *Hear. Res.* 213, 64–78. doi: 10.1016/j.heares.2005.11.011

de Groot, J. C. M. J., Meeuwsen, F., Ruizendaal, W. E., and Veldman, J. E. (1990). Ultrastructural localization of gentamicin in the cochlea. *Hear. Res.* 50, 35–42. doi: 10.1016/0378-5955(90)90031-J

Ding, D., Liu, H., Qi, W., Jiang, H., Li, Y., Wu, X., et al. (2016). Ototoxic effects and mechanisms of loop diuretics. *J. Otol.* 11, 145–156. doi: 10.1016/j.joto.2016.10.001

Dunn, K. W., Sandoval, R. M., Kelly, K. J., Dagher, P. C., Tanner, G. A., Atkinson, S. J., et al. (2002). Functional studies of the kidney of living animals using multicolor two-photon microscopy. *Am. J. Physiol. Cell Physiol.* 283, C905–C916. doi: 10.1152/ajpcell.00159.2002

Durante-Mangoni, E., Grammatikos, A., Utili, R., and Falagas, M. E. (2009). Do we still need the aminoglycosides? *Int. J. Antimicrob. Agents* 33, 201–205. doi: 10.1016/j.ijantimicag.2008.09.001

Esterberg, R., Hailey, D. W., Rubel, E. W., and Raible, D. W. (2014). ER–mitochondrial calcium flow underlies vulnerability of mechanosensory hair cells to damage. *J. Neurosci.* 34, 9703–9719. doi: 10.1523/JNEUROSCI.0281-14.2014

Esterberg, R., Linbo, T., Pickett, S. B., Wu, P., Ou, H. C., Rubel, E. W., et al. (2016). Mitochondrial calcium uptake underlies ROS generation during aminoglycoside-induced hair cell death. *J. Clin. Invest.* 126, 3556–3566. doi: 10.1172/JCI84939

FDA-NIH Biomarker Working Group (2016). *BEST (Biomarkers, Endpoints, and other Tools) Resource.* Silver Spring, MD: Food and Drug Administration.

Fettiplace, R. (2009). Defining features of the hair cell mechanoelectrical transducer channel. *Pflugers Arch.* 458, 1115–1123. doi: 10.1007/s00424-009-0683-x

Forge, A., and Schacht, J. (2000). Aminoglycoside antibiotics. *Audiol. Neurootol.* 5, 3–22. doi: 10.1159/000013861

UpToDate (2021). *Furosemide: Drug Information.* Available online at: https://www.uptodate.com/contents/furosemide-drug-information [accessed November 22, 2021].

Guo, X., and Nzerue, C. (2002). How to prevent, recognize, and treat drug-induced nephrotoxicity. *Cleve. Clin. J. Med.* 69, 289–290, 293–294, 296–297 passim. doi: 10.3949/ccjm.69.4.289

Hailey, D. W., Esterberg, R., Linbo, T. H., Rubel, E. W., and Raible, D. W. (2017). Fluorescent aminoglycosides reveal intracellular trafficking routes in mechanosensory hair cells. *J. Clin. Invest.* 127, 472–486. doi: 10.1172/JCI85052

Hashino, E., Shero, M., and Salvi, R. J. (1997). Lysosomal targeting and accumulation of aminoglycoside antibiotics in sensory hair cells. *Brain Res.* 777, 75–85. doi: 10.1016/S0006-8993(97)00977-3

Hatala, R., Dinh, T., and Cook, D. J. (1996). Once-daily aminoglycoside dosing in immunocompetent adults. *Ann. Intern. Med.* 124, 717–725. doi: 10.7326/0003-4819-124-8-199604150-00003

He, D. Z., Evans, B. N., and Dallos, P. (1994). First appearance and development of electromotility in neonatal gerbil outer hair cells. *Hear. Res.* 78, 77–90. doi: 10.1016/0378-5955(94)90046-9

Hiel, H., Erre, J.-P., Aurousseau, C., Bouali, R., Dulon, D., and Aran, J.-M. (1993). Gentamicin uptake by cochlear hair cells precedes hearing impairment during chronic treatment. *Audiology* 32, 78–87. doi: 10.3109/00206099309072930

Hirose, K., Hockenbery, D. M., and Rubel, E. W. (1997). Reactive oxygen species in chick hair cells after gentamicin exposure in vitro. *Hear. Res.* 104, 1–14. doi: 10.1016/S0378-5955(96)00169-4

Horvath, L., Bächinger, D., Honegger, T., Bodmer, D., and Monge Naldi, A. (2019). Functional and morphological analysis of different aminoglycoside treatment regimens inducing hearing loss in mice. *Exp. Ther. Med.* 18, 1123–1130. doi: 10.3892/etm.2019.7687

Huth, M. E., Ricci, A. J., and Cheng, A. G. (2011). Mechanisms of aminoglycoside ototoxicity and targets of hair cell protection. *Int. J. Otolaryngol.* 2011:e937861. doi: 10.1155/2011/937861

Huxel, C., Raja, A., and Ollivierre-Lawrence, M. D. (eds). (2021). "Loop diuretics," in *StatPearls* (Treasure Island, FL: StatPearls Publishing).

Huy, P. T. B., Bernard, P., and Schacht, J. (1986). Kinetics of gentamicin uptake and release in the rat. Comparison of inner ear tissues and fluids with other organs. *J. Clin. Invest.* 77, 1492–1500. doi: 10.1172/JCI112463

Imamura, S., and Adams, J. C. (2003). Distribution of gentamicin in the guinea pig inner ear after local or systemic application. *J. Assoc. Res. Otolaryngol.* 4, 176–195. doi: 10.1007/s10162-002-2036-8

Jeng, J., Ceriani, F., Hendry, A., Johnson, S. L., Yen, P., Simmons, D. D., et al. (2020). Hair cell maturation is differentially regulated along the tonotopic axis of the mammalian cochlea. *J. Physiol.* 598, 151–170. doi: 10.1113/JP279012

Jiang, H., Sha, S.-H., Forge, A., and Schacht, J. (2006). Caspase-independent pathways of hair cell death induced by kanamycin in vivo. *Cell Death Differ.* 13, 20–30. doi: 10.1038/sj.cdd.4401706

Jiang, M., Karasawa, T., and Steyger, P. S. (2017). Aminoglycoside-induced cochleotoxicity: a review. *Front. Cell. Neurosci.* 11:308. doi: 10.3389/fncel.2017.00308

Kalinec, G. M., Webster, P., Lim, D. J., and Kalinec, F. (2003). A cochlear cell line as an in vitro system for drug ototoxicity screening. *Audiol. Neurootol.* 8, 177–189. doi: 10.1159/000071059

Kenyon, E. J., Kirkwood, N. K., Kitcher, S. R., Goodyear, R. J., Derudas, M., Cantillon, D. M., et al. (2021). Identification of a series of hair-cell MET channel blockers that protect against aminoglycoside-induced ototoxicity. *JCI Insight* 6:e145704. doi: 10.1172/jci.insight.145704

Kim, J., and Ricci, A. J. (2022). In vivo real-time imaging reveals megalin as the aminoglycoside gentamicin transporter into cochlea whose inhibition is otoprotective. *Proc. Natl. Acad. Sci. U.S.A.* 119:e2117946119. doi: 10.1073/pnas.2117946119

Kirkwood, N. K., O'Reilly, M., Derudas, M., Kenyon, E. J., Huckvale, R., van Netten, S. M., et al. (2017). d-Tubocurarine and berbamine: alkaloids that are permeant blockers of the hair cell's mechano-electrical transducer channel and protect from aminoglycoside toxicity. *Front. Cell. Neurosci.* 11:262. doi: 10.3389/fncel.2017.00262

Kitahara, T., Li, H.-S., and Balaban, C. D. (2005). Changes in transient receptor potential cation channel superfamily V (TRPV) mRNA expression in the mouse inner ear ganglia after kanamycin challenge. *Hear. Res.* 201, 132–144. doi: 10.1016/j.heares.2004.09.007

Kitcher, S. R., Kirkwood, N. K., Camci, E. D., Wu, P., Gibson, R. M., Redila, V. A., et al. (2019). ORC-13661 protects sensory hair cells from aminoglycoside and cisplatin ototoxicity. *JCI Insight* 4:e126764. doi: 10.1172/jci.insight.126764

Kros, C. J., Ruppersberg, J. P., and Rüsch, A. (1998). Expression of a potassium current in inner hair cells during development of hearing in mice. *Nature* 394, 281–284. doi: 10.1038/28401

Kruger, M., Boney, R., Ordoobadi, A. J., Sommers, T. F., Trapani, J. G., and Coffin, A. B. (2016). Natural bizbenzoquinoline derivatives protect zebrafish lateral line sensory hair cells from aminoglycoside toxicity. *Front. Cell. Neurosci.* 10:83. doi: 10.3389/fncel.2016.00083

Lee, S. H., Ju, H. M., Choi, J. S., Ahn, Y., Lee, S., and Seo, Y. J. (2018). Circulating serum miRNA-205 as a diagnostic biomarker for ototoxicity in mice treated with aminoglycoside antibiotics. *Int. J. Mol. Sci.* 19:2836. doi: 10.3390/ijms19092836

Lim, D. J. (1986). Effects of noise and ototoxic drugs at the cellular level in the cochlea: a review. *Am. J. Otolaryngol.* 7, 73–99. doi: 10.1016/S0196-0709(86)80037-0

Liu, J., Kachelmeier, A., Dai, C., Li, H., and Steyger, P. S. (2015). Uptake of fluorescent gentamicin by peripheral vestibular cells after systemic administration. *PLoS One* 10:e0120612. doi: 10.1371/journal.pone.0120612

Lopez-Novoa, J. M., Quiros, Y., Vicente, L., Morales, A. I., and Lopez-Hernandez, F. J. (2011). New insights into the mechanism of aminoglycoside nephrotoxicity: an integrative point of view. *Kidney Int.* 79, 33–45. doi: 10.1038/ki.2010.337

Makabe, A., Kawashima, Y., Sakamaki, Y., Maruyama, A., Fujikawa, T., Ito, T., et al. (2020). Systemic fluorescent gentamicin enters neonatal mouse hair cells predominantly through sensory mechanoelectrical transduction channels. *J. Assoc. Res. Otolaryngol.* 21, 137–149. doi: 10.1007/s10162-020-00746-3

Marche, P., Koutouzov, S., and Girard, A. (1983). Impairment of membrane phosphoinositide metabolism by aminoglycoside antibiotics: streptomycin, amikacin, kanamycin, dibekacin, gentamicin and neomycin. *J. Pharmacol. Exp. Ther.* 227, 415–420.

Marcotti, W., Johnson, S. L., Holley, M. C., and Kros, C. J. (2003). Developmental changes in the expression of potassium currents of embryonic, neonatal and mature mouse inner hair cells. *J. Physiol.* 548, 383–400. doi: 10.1113/jphysiol.2002.034801

Marcotti, W., and Kros, C. J. (1999). Developmental expression of the potassium current IK,n contributes to maturation of mouse outer hair cells. *J. Physiol.* 520, 653–660. doi: 10.1111/j.1469-7793.1999.00653.x

Marcotti, W., Netten, S. M. V., and Kros, C. J. (2005). The aminoglycoside antibiotic dihydrostreptomycin rapidly enters mouse outer hair cells through the mechano -electrical transducer channels. *J. Physiol.* 567, 505–521. doi: 10.1113/jphysiol.2005.085951

Mingeot-Leclercq, M.-P., and Tulkens, P. M. (1999). Aminoglycosides: nephrotoxicity. *Antimicrob. Agents Chemother.* 43, 1003–1012.

Munckhof, W. J., Grayson, M. L., and Turnidge, J. D. (1996). A meta-analysis of studies on the safety and efficacy of aminoglycosides given either once daily or as divided doses. *J. Antimicrob. Chemother.* 37, 645–663. doi: 10.1093/jac/37.4.645

Nakai, Y., Chang, K. C., Ohashi, K., and Morisaki, N. (1983). Ototoxic effect of an aminoglycoside drug on an immature inner ear. *Acta Otolaryngol. Suppl.* 393, 1–5. doi: 10.3109/00016488309129570

Naples, J., Cox, R., Bonaiuto, G., and Parham, K. (2018). Prestin as an otologic biomarker of cisplatin ototoxicity in a guinea pig model. *Otolaryngol. Head Neck Surg.* 158, 541–546. doi: 10.1177/0194599817742093

O'Sullivan, M. E., Song, Y., Greenhouse, R., Lin, R., Perez, A., Atkinson, P. J., et al. (2020). Dissociating antibacterial from ototoxic effects of gentamicin C-subtypes. *Proc. Natl. Acad. Sci. U.S.A.* 117, 32423–32432. doi: 10.1073/pnas.2013065117

Owens, K. N., Santos, F., Roberts, B., Linbo, T., Coffin, A. B., Knisely, A. J., et al. (2008). Identification of genetic and chemical modulators of zebrafish mechanosensory hair cell death. *PLoS Genet.* 4:e1000020. doi: 10.1371/journal.pgen.1000020

Pickett, S. B., and Raible, D. W. (2019). Water waves to sound waves: using zebrafish to explore hair cell biology. *J. Assoc. Res. Otolaryngol.* 20, 1–19. doi: 10.1007/s10162-018-00711-1

Pickles, J. (1998). *An Introduction to the Physiology of Hearing*, 4th Edn. Leiden: Brill.

Portmann, M., Darrouzet, J., and Coste, C. (1974). Distribution within the cochlea of dihydrostreptomycin injected into the circulation. An autoradiographic and electron microscopic study. *Arch. Otolaryngol.* 100, 473–475. doi: 10.1001/archotol.1974.00780040487014

Prieve, B. A., and Yanz, J. L. (1984). Age-dependent changes in susceptibility to ototoxic hearing loss. *Acta Otolaryngol.* 98, 428–438. doi: 10.3109/00016488409107584

Priuska, E. M., and Schacht, J. (1995). Formation of free radicals by gentamicin and iron and evidence for an iron/gentamicin complex. *Biochem. Pharmacol.* 50, 1749–1752. doi: 10.1016/0006-2952(95)02160-4

Qian, X., He, Z., Wang, Y., Chen, B., Hetrick, A., Dai, C., et al. (2021). Hair cell uptake of gentamicin in the developing mouse utricle. *J. Cell. Physiol.* 236, 5235–5252. doi: 10.1002/jcp.30228

Qian, Y., and Guan, M.-X. (2009). Interaction of aminoglycosides with human mitochondrial 12S rRNA carrying the deafness-associated mutation. *Antimicrob. Agents Chemother.* 53, 4612–4618. doi: 10.1128/AAC.00965-08

Richardson, G. P., and Russell, I. J. (1991). Cochlear cultures as a model system for studying aminoglycoside induced ototoxicity. *Hear. Res.* 53, 293–311. doi: 10.1016/0378-5955(91)90062-e

Rizzi, M. D., and Hirose, K. (2007). Aminoglycoside ototoxicity. *Curr. Opin. Otolaryngol. Head Neck Surg.* 15, 352–357. doi: 10.1097/MOO.0b013e3282ef772d

Rubel, E. W. (1978). "Ontogeny of structure and function in the vertebrate auditory system," in *Development of Sensory Systems Handbook of Sensory Physiology*, eds C. M. Bate, V. M. C. M. Carr, P. P. C. Graziadei, H. V. B. Hirsch, A. Hughes, D. Ingle, et al. (Berlin: Springer), 135–237. doi: 10.1007/978-3-642-66880-7_5

Rubel, E. W., and Fay, R. R. (2012). *Development of the Auditory System.* Berlin: Springer Science & Business Media.

Rybak, L. P. (1993). Ototoxicity of Loop Diuretics#. *Otolaryngol. Clin. North Am.* 26, 829–844. doi: 10.1016/S0030-6665(20)30770-2

Rybak, L. P., Talaska, A. E., and Schacht, J. (2008). "Drug-induced hearing loss," in *Auditory Trauma, Protection, and Repair Springer Handbook of Auditory Research*, eds J. Schacht, A. N. Popper, and R. R. Fay (Boston, MA: Springer), 219–256. doi: 10.1007/978-0-387-72561-1_8

Rybak, M. J., Abate, B. J., Kang, S. L., Ruffing, M. J., Lerner, S. A., and Drusano, G. L. (1999). Prospective evaluation of the effect of an aminoglycoside dosing regimen on rates of observed nephrotoxicity and ototoxicity. *Antimicrob. Agents Chemother.* 43, 1549–1555. doi: 10.1128/AAC.43.7.1549

Schmitz, C., Hilpert, J., Jacobsen, C., Boensch, C., Christensen, E. I., Luft, F. C., et al. (2002). Megalin deficiency offers protection from renal aminoglycoside accumulation *. *J. Biol. Chem.* 277, 618–622. doi: 10.1074/jbc.M109959200

Seyhan, A. A. (2019). Lost in translation: the valley of death across preclinical and clinical divide - identification of problems and overcoming obstacles. *Transl. Med. Commun.* 4:18. doi: 10.1186/s41231-019-0050-7

Silverblatt, F. J., and Kuehn, C. (1979). Autoradiography of gentamicin uptake by the rat proximal tubule cell. *Kidney Int.* 15, 335–345. doi: 10.1038/ki.1979.45

Taylor, R. R., Nevill, G., and Forge, A. (2008). Rapid hair cell loss: a mouse model for cochlear lesions. *J. Assoc. Res. Otolaryngol.* 9, 44–64. doi: 10.1007/s10162-007-0105-8

Van Boeckel, T. P., Gandra, S., Ashok, A., Caudron, Q., Grenfell, B. T., Levin, S. A., et al. (2014). Global antibiotic consumption 2000 to 2010: an analysis of national pharmaceutical sales data. *Lancet Infect. Dis.* 14, 742–750. doi: 10.1016/S1473-3099(14)70780-7

Vu, A. A., Nadaraja, G. S., Huth, M. E., Luk, L., Kim, J., Chai, R., et al. (2013). Integrity and regeneration of mechanotransduction machinery regulate aminoglycoside entry and sensory cell death. *PLoS One* 8:e54794. doi: 10.1371/journal.pone.0054794

Wang, Q., and Steyger, P. S. (2009). Trafficking of systemic fluorescent gentamicin into the cochlea and hair cells. *J. Assoc. Res. Otolaryngol.* 10, 205–219. doi: 10.1007/s10162-009-0160-4

Wu, W.-J., Sha, S.-H., McLaren, J. D., Kawamoto, K., Raphael, Y., and Schacht, J. (2001). Aminoglycoside ototoxicity in adult CBA, C57BL and BALB mice and the Sprague–Dawley rat. *Hear. Res.* 158, 165–178. doi: 10.1016/S0378-5955(01)00303-3

4

Phenotypic Profiling of People with Subjective Tinnitus and without a Clinical Hearing Loss

Dongmei Tang[1,2*†], Xiaoling Lu[1,2†], Ruonan Huang[1,2], Huiqian Yu[1,2] and Wenyan Li[1,2*]

[1] State Key Laboratory of Medical Neurobiology and MOE Frontiers Center for Brain Science, ENT Institute and Department of Otorhinolaryngology, Eye & ENT Hospital, Fudan University, Shanghai, China, [2] NHC Key Laboratory of Hearing Medicine, Fudan University, Shanghai, China

***Correspondence:**
Dongmei Tang
tang.dongm@163.com
Wenyan Li
_wenyan_li2000@126.com_

† These authors have contributed equally to this work and share first authorship

Our objective was to study the characteristics of patients with subjective tinnitus and normal hearing and to investigate whether the features correlated to different shapes on audiograms. In this retrospective study, 313 patients with subjective tinnitus and clinically normal hearing were enrolled from the tinnitus outpatient department of the Eye and ENT Hospital of Fudan University. The following phenotypic variables were collected: age, dominant tinnitus pitch (TP), tinnitus loudness, tinnitus duration, tinnitus severity, sex, education, hearing thresholds, tinnitus position, and tinnitus condition. The dominant TPs of patients with normal hearing were mostly high-pitched, with a mean of 4866.8 ± 2579.6 Hz; thus, we speculated that the condition is related to high-frequency hearing threshold elevations. We further divided the patients into four subgroups based on the matched TP: (i) TP $\leq$ 500 Hz (n = 34), (ii) 500 Hz $<$ TP $\leq$ 3,000 Hz (n = 15), (iii) 3,000 Hz $<$ TP $\leq$ 8,000 Hz (n = 259), and (iv) TP $>$ 8,000 Hz (n = 5). We studied the phenotypic profiling of different audiograms and found that the group with TP of $\leq$500 Hz had an average "inverted-U" shaped audiogram, and the group with TP between 500 and 3,000 Hz had a slowly ascending slope audiogram below 2,000 Hz, followed by a drastically descending slope audiogram ranging from 2,000 to 8,000 Hz; further, the high-frequency (3,000–8,000 Hz) and ultra-high-frequency ($>$8,000 Hz) groups had flat curves below 2,000 Hz and steeper slope audiograms over 2,000 Hz. Our findings confirmed a consistency ratio between the distributions of dominant TPs and the frequencies of maximum hearing thresholds in both ears. The dominant TP was positively correlated with the maximum hearing threshold elevation frequency (left ear: $r = 0.277$, $p < 0.05$; right ear: $r = 0.367$, $p < 0.001$). Hearing threshold elevations, especially in high frequency, might explain the appearance of dominant high-frequency TP in patients without clinically defined hearing loss. This is consistent with the causal role of high-frequency coding in the generation of tinnitus.

Keywords: tinnitus, normal hearing, audiogram, threshold elevation, high pitch

INTRODUCTION

Tinnitus is the auditory perception of sound in the absence of a corresponding external acoustic or electric stimulus. The commonly described sounds of tinnitus are chirping, buzzing, ringing, and hissing. More often, tinnitus is a tonal-like sensation, but in few cases, it sounds like a noise. Tinnitus affects 5–43% of people worldwide (McCormack et al., 2016). The risk of developing tinnitus increases with age, noise exposure, and hearing loss (Baguley et al., 2013; Langguth et al., 2013). It is widely accepted that the generation of tinnitus is often triggered by peripheral hearing damage and involves a central mechanism (Norena and Eggermont, 2003; Eggermont and Roberts, 2004). In people with hearing loss and tinnitus, the dominant tinnitus pitch (TP) is consistently associated with the region of hearing loss (Konig et al., 2006; Pan et al., 2009; Moore et al., 2010; Sereda et al., 2011, 2015; Schecklmann et al., 2012). However, clinical audiometric hearing loss does not occur in all cases of tinnitus. The percentage of tinnitus patients without clinical hearing loss is estimated at 20% (Jastreboff and Jastreboff, 2003).

One of the most frequently asked questions by patients suffering from tinnitus is "Why did I get tinnitus?," and the answer is more challenging in the presence of patients with normal hearing. A study assessing the reported lifetime noise exposure found some evidence for cochlear pathology associated with tinnitus and a normal audiogram (≤20 dB HL at 0.25–8 kHz). Guest et al. (2017) conducted a prospective study of 20 people with tinnitus and 20 controls closely matched for sex, age, and audiometric thresholds. Reported lifetime noise exposure was the only factor that differed between groups (Guest et al., 2017). Nevertheless, high-frequency hearing loss also provides some evidence for cochlear pathology associated with tinnitus and a normal audiogram (≤15 dB HL at 0.125 Hz–8 kHz). For example, by conducting a retrospective split of a sample of 75 people with tinnitus, Vielsmeier et al. (2015) found that those with hearing thresholds over 15 dB HL in at least one frequency from 10 to 16 kHz reported higher tinnitus symptom severity as measured by the Tinnitus Questionnaire (TQ) and Tinnitus Handicap Inventory (THI), compared with those with thresholds below 15 dB HL. In our previous study, we reported that extended high-frequency and average hearing thresholds across 4–16 kHz were significantly higher in the tinnitus group than in the matched volunteers without tinnitus (Song et al., 2021). In addition, some researchers have revealed that patients with normal hearing may have missed or hidden hearing loss. One study reported missed hearing loss in patients with normal audiograms when using fine frequency resolution in 1/24 octave step, suggesting that a more sophisticated pure-tone test should be considered to identify mild hearing impairment in patients with normal hearing (Xiong et al., 2019). Another study performed pure-tone audiometry (125 Hz–16 kHz), speech audiometry, transient evoked otoacoustic emissions (TEOAEs), distortion product otoacoustic emissions (DPOAEs), threshold equalizing noise (TEN) test (500 Hz–4 kHz), and electrocochleography (ECochG) for 9 individuals with tinnitus and normal hearing and 13 controls with normal hearing but no tinnitus, and the results showed that the SP/AP ratio in the ECochG test, together with the detection of dead regions in the TEN test, might be valuable in diagnosing hidden hearing loss, while the between-group differences in DPOAE and TEOAE were not significant (Kara et al., 2020).

According to this brief review of the literature, studies on tinnitus patients with normal hearing are mostly limited to detecting abnormalities of cochlear or auditory nerves; however, few studies have attempted to demonstrate the characteristics of pitch, loudness, and severity of tinnitus in patients with normal hearing (Savastano, 2008). Further, few studies have focused on the association between TP and audiogram features in patients with normal hearing. In this study, we focused on phenotypic profile of patients presenting with the primary complaint of subjective tinnitus and clinically normal hearing and confirmed that dominant TP was positively correlated with the maximum hearing threshold elevation frequency, which indicated that a more sophisticated pure-tone test, including extended high frequency, might be needed in evaluating the audiological features of dominant high-frequency TP in patients without clinically defined hearing loss.

MATERIALS AND METHODS

Participants

The study was conducted between January 2014 and October 2017 in tinnitus outpatients of the Eye and ENT Hospital of Fudan University, Shanghai. The recruited patients had a chief complaint of subjective tinnitus. We excluded patients who had pulsatile tinnitus and major health issues that impacted or prevented attendance. Patients with risk factors for tinnitus, such as noise exposure, sudden hearing loss, head or temporal trauma, tympanitis, and emotional disorders, were also identified and excluded. Finally, 313 patients with tinnitus and clinically normal hearing were identified from the database of all tinnitus patients, according to the World Health Organization [WHO] Programme for the Prevention of Deafness and Hearing Impairment (1997) definition of "the pure-tone threshold average across octave frequencies from 0.5 to 4 kHz ≤ 25 dB HL in each ear." In addition, 71 sex-matched volunteers with normal hearing and without tinnitus were also recruited in this study to compare the audiometric characteristics between the participants with and without tinnitus.

All tests were approved by the ethical committee of Fudan University. The sensitive information relevant to patient privacy was removed before analysis and all participants gave written informed consent to scientific research.

Audiometry Examination

A pre-exam otoscopic screening was performed to identify abnormalities in the external ear, including the ear canal and eardrum. Excessive or impacted cerumen was immediately cleared. All patients accepted the acoustic immittance measurement, and those with type "C" or type "B" diagram were ruled out. Pure-tone air conduction for both ears was measured between 0.25 and 8 kHz (0.25, 0.5, 1, 2, 4, and 8 kHz).

A standard Hughson-Westlake procedure (steps: 10 dB down, 5 dB up; 2 out of 3) was used to determine hearing thresholds.

Tinnitus Evaluation

A detailed tinnitus evaluation was performed on all participants (see below). We also recorded general information such as age, sex, educational background, self-reported laterality (unilateral, bilateral, or in the head), duration of tinnitus, and sound properties of tinnitus. Both intermittent and continuous tinnitus were included.

Symptom Severity

Tinnitus severity category was suggested according to the previous report (Biesinger et al., 1998). In brief, Grade I was defined as no impairment, Grade II as a mild complaint with passive emotional impact in certain defined conditions, Grade III as a permanent annoyance due to tinnitus (e.g., insomnia and anxiety), and Grade IV as severe impairment with severe negative impacts on work, study, or daily life.

To comprehensively evaluate the severity of tinnitus, three questionnaires were administered: the THI (Newman et al., 1996, 2008), Fear of Tinnitus Questionnaire (FTQ) (McCracken et al., 1992; Roelofs et al., 2007), and Athens Insomnia Scale (AIS) (Soldatos et al., 2000). The scoring criteria were as follows: (1) THI: slight (0–16), mild (18–36), moderate (38–56), and severe (58–100); (2) AIS: no insomnia (<4), suspicious insomnia (4–6), and insomnia (7–24); and (3) FTQ: 17 items in total, with 1 score per item; the higher the score, the more severe the tinnitus.

Pitch Matching

We established a "trinomial forced-choice method" for TP matching (China invention patent: ZL 201510165976.9). The first three frequencies were 2, 4, and 8 kHz, which were at least 5 dB above all the corresponding hearing thresholds, and each lasted 500 ms with a 1-s interval. Patients were instructed to identify the frequency closest to their TP and to judge whether it was higher, lower, or equal to their tinnitus. If 2 kHz was selected, then the upper limit frequency of tinnitus was 4 kHz − 1/3 octaves; if 4 kHz was selected, then the frequency of tinnitus was between 2 kHz + 1/3 octaves and 8 kHz − 1/3 octaves; and if 8 kHz was selected, then the lower limit frequency of tinnitus was 8 kHz − 1/3 octaves. In this way, the given sound range was gradually narrowed to the closest frequency by a final step of 1/3 octaves. A threefold repetition was performed to clearly distinguish between each of the three acoustic stimuli. When a final pitch match was selected, an octave confusion test was conducted to avoid selection bias. The octave confusion test conducted in the present study was 1/3 octaves above and 1/3 octaves below the selected pitch (±1 octave when below 1,000 Hz) whenever such frequencies were available. The final confirmed pitch was recorded as the dominant pitch of tinnitus. There were 15 frequencies in total for TP matching, namely, 0.25, 0.5, 1, 1.26, 1.58, 2, 2.52, 3.18, 4, 5.04, 6.35, 8, 10.08, 12.7, and 16 kHz.

Loudness Matching

The loudness matching was performed in a manner similar to that in the pitch-matching test, and the final gap difference was narrowed to the nearest 1 dB step size. The loudness of tinnitus was reflected in the sensation level (dB SL). Sensation level was defined as the loudness value above the hearing threshold at the TP.

The tinnitus testing devices for pitch and loudness were calibrated twice a year at the Shanghai Institute of Measurement and Testing Technology[1], which were authorized by the Administration of Quality Supervision, Inspection and Quarantine and accredited by the China National Accreditation Service for Conformity Assessment.

Data Analysis

The continuous variables are expressed as mean ± standard deviation, while the categorical variables are expressed as number (%). Group comparisons were performed using one-way analysis of variance and Fisher's exact test with RStudio software (version 4.0.3). Correlation analysis was performed between the dominant TP and corresponding frequency of maximum hearing threshold using the Spearman rank test. All the statistics and plotting were performed with RStudio software (version 4.0.3). The distribution of TP and frequency of maximum hearing threshold was mapped with Excel. The level of statistical significance was defined as a p-value of <0.05.

RESULTS

Clinical and Demographical Characteristics

According to the WHO grades of hearing impairment (version 1997), 313 subjects conformed to the criteria of clinically normal hearing with standard audiometry. The mean age was 40.2 ± 12.8 years, the male-to-female ratio was 54.3% (n = 170): 45.7% (n = 143), and nearly half of the patients (47.6%) had a college degree or higher. The mean dominant TP was 4866.8 ± 2579.6 Hz, demonstrating a common dominant high-frequency TP. The pitch-matching analysis showed that most of the matched frequencies (308/313) were no more than 8 kHz, while only five patients reported a dominant TP at 10.08 kHz. To further analyze the data, we divided the participants into four subgroups based on the dominant TP: low-pitched (≤500 Hz), middle-pitched (500–3,000 Hz), high-pitched (3,000–8,000 Hz), and ultra-high-pitched (>8,000 Hz). As shown in **Table 1**, the four groups were significantly different in terms of age (p = 0.037), tinnitus loudness (p < 0.001), and sex composition (p = 0.025). However, they were homogeneous in terms of duration (p = 0.940), severity (p = 0.965), position (p = 0.334), educational background (p = 0.166), and persistence (p = 0.089) of tinnitus. The mean duration of tinnitus was 30.7 ± 53.7 months, implying that most patients had chronic tinnitus. There was preponderance of bilateral tinnitus reported by the majority of participants (59.1% in total; 44.1, 66.7, 60.2, and 60.0% in the low, middle, high-, and ultra-high-pitched groups, respectively), with only a few reporting unilateral tinnitus (left 21.1%, right 18.2% in total; left 32.4% vs. right 23.5%, left 6.7%

[1]http://english.simt.com.cn

TABLE 1 | Demographic characteristics of patients with tinnitus and clinically normal hearing.

	Total (n = 313)	≤500 Hz (n = 34)	500–3,000 Hz (n = 15)	3,000–8,000 Hz (n = 259)	>8,000 Hz (n = 5)	p-value
Continuous variable, mean (SD)						
Age (years)	40.2 (12.8)	40.9 (13.9)	36.0 (15.4)	40.6 (12.4)	25.6 (13.1)	**0.037***
Dominant tinnitus pitch (Hz)	4866.8 (2579.6)	397.1 (124.9)	1869.3 (484.4)	5526.6 (1978.3)	1,0080 (0)	/
Tinnitus loudness (dB SL)	9.1 (5.2)	10.9 (6.1)	12.1 (9.1)	8.5 (4.6)	16.0 (6.5)	**<0.001***
Tinnitus duration (months)	30.7 (53.7)	25.8 (38.4)	32.3 (37.7)	31.4 (56.7)	24.4 (23.5)	0.940
THI score	31.0 (23.3)	30.5 (19.8)	35.1 (27.0)	31.0 (23.6)	21.2 (17.5)	0.716
AIS score	5.9 (5.3)	5.8 (5.7)	7.3 (4.7)	5.8 (5.3)	3 (3.7)	0.454
FTQ score	8.1 (4.0)	7.9 (3.5)	9.7 (4.1)	8.0 (4.0)	6.4 (4.3)	0.306
Categorical variable, n (%)						
Sex						
Male	170 (54.3%)	11 (32.4%)	7 (46.7%)	150 (57.9%)	3 (60.0%)	**0.025***
Female	143 (45.7%)	23 (67.6%)	8 (53.3%)	109 (42.1%)	2 (40.0%)	
Education						
Below high school	95 (30.4%)	15 (44.1%)	2 (13.3%)	78 (30.1%)	0 (0)	
High school or technical school	69 (22.0%)	8 (23.5%)	4 (26.7%)	55 (21.2%)	2 (40.0%)	0.166
College degree or above	149 (47.6%)	11 (32.4%)	9 (60.0%)	126 (48.7%)	3 (60.0%)	
Tinnitus position						
Left ear	66 (21.1%)	11 (32.4%)	1 (6.7%)	53 (20.5%)	1 (20.0%)	
Right ear	57 (18.2%)	8 (23.5%)	3 (20.0%)	46 (17.8%)	1 (20.0%)	0.334
Bilateral ears	185 (59.1%)	15 (44.1%)	10 (66.7%)	156 (60.2%)	3 (60.0%)	
In head	5 (1.6%)	0 (0)	1 (6.6%)	4 (1.5%)	0 (0)	
Tinnitus severity						
Grade I	5 (1.6%)	1 (2.9%)	0 (0)	4 (1.5%)	0 (0)	
Grade II	124 (39.6%)	12 (35.3%)	6 (40.0%)	103 (39.8%)	3 (60.0%)	0.965
Grade III	140 (44.7%)	17 (50.0%)	7 (46.7%)	114 (44.0%)	2 (40.0%)	
Grade IV	44 (14.1%)	4 (11.7%)	2 (13.3%)	38 (14.7%)	0 (0)	
Tinnitus condition						
Intermittent	45 (14.4%)	8 (23.5%)	4 (26.7%)	32 (12.4%)	1 (20.0%)	0.089
Continuous	268 (85.6%)	26 (76.5%)	11 (73.3%)	227 (87.6%)	4 (80.0%)	

The bold values represent the variable items compared between the four subgroups. n means number and SD means standard deviation.
**P < 0.05.*

vs. right 20.0%, left 20.5% vs. right 17.8%, and left 20.0% vs. right 20.0% in the low, middle, high-, and ultra-high-pitched groups, respectively). The overall education level of the patients varied; 47.6% had a college degree or higher, 22.0% finished high school or technical school, and 30.4% received primary education or were illiterate. Most patients (85.6%) reported continuous tinnitus, with the remaining patients reporting intermittent tinnitus (**Table 1**).

Tinnitus Loudness and Severity

The mean tinnitus loudness was 9.1 ± 5.2 dB SL above the threshold for all patients with tinnitus and normal hearing. To be visualized, the level of loudness was mid-range; hence, the tinnitus was hardly masked by the surrounding ambient sounds, causing disruption to patients' daily lives, sleep, and work. The mean loudness measured by sensation level was 10.9 ± 6.1, 12.1 ± 9.1, 8.5 ± 4.6, and 16.0 ± 6.5 in the low, middle, high-, and ultra-high-pitched groups, respectively ($p < 0.001$). According to the Biesinger classification, 1.6% of patients had no impairment (Grade I), 39.6% had slight impairment (Grade II), 44.7% had permanent annoyance (Grade III), and 14.1% had severe impairment (Grade IV), with no differences between the four subgroups. This implied that most patients with tinnitus and normal hearing were slightly or severely disturbed in private and professional areas. These findings were reconfirmed by the three questionnaire assessments: the THI global score was 31.0 ± 23.3, AIS score was 5.9 ± 5.3, and FTQ score was 8.1 ± 4.0 (**Table 1**).

Dominant Tinnitus Pitch of Clinically Normal Hearing Might Be Associated With Hearing Threshold Elevations

In previous studies, TP has been found to be consistent with the region of hearing loss (Sereda et al., 2011, 2015; Schecklmann et al., 2012). However, the cause of tinnitus without a clinical hearing loss remains unclear, especially for those who do not have any hearing deficits at all test frequencies ranging from 250 to 8,000 Hz. Among all the features of tinnitus with normal hearing, the average high-pitched-matching result was the most salient and intriguing. We speculated that the generation of tinnitus and the dominant TP in patients with normal hearing might be related to different audiogram types. We drew the average pure-tone audiograms for each ear in the low, middle, high-, and ultra-high-pitched subgroups. As a contrast, 71 volunteers with normal hearing and without tinnitus also received the standard pure-tone audiometry in the same audiometric environment with the patients with tinnitus.

As shown in **Figure 1** and **Table 2**, the control group totally had flat audiograms both in right ears and left ears, and the average pure-tone thresholds were all less than those in patients with tinnitus from 250 to 8,000 Hz. To clearly compare the audiogram curves between tinnitus patients and the controls, the average pure-tone audiogram of volunteers without tinnitus was presented repeatedly in the four subgroups. The average pure-tone audiograms in the low-pitched (≤500 Hz) group presented an inverted-U shape in both left and right ears, indicating that dominant low-pitched tinnitus may be associated with hearing threshold elevations ranging from 250 to 500 Hz (**Figure 1A**). The inclination and intensity of threshold elevations in low frequencies were attenuated in the middle-pitched (500–3,000 Hz) subgroup when compared to the low-pitched subgroup, demonstrating a slowly ascending slope audiogram below 2,000 Hz, followed by a drastically descending slope audiogram ranging from 2,000 to 8,000 Hz (**Figure 1B**). In the high- (3,000–8,000 Hz) and ultra-high- (above 8,000 Hz) pitched subgroups, both the audiogram curves below 2,000 Hz were flat without any severe threshold elevations, while the audiograms over 2,000 Hz revealed steeper slopes in both ears (**Figures 1C,D**). Therefore, widespread threshold elevations in high frequencies (over 2,000 Hz) were found in all the four subgroups, which might contribute to reasonable explanation for our observation that the majority of patients with normal hearing had a dominant high-frequency TP. However, the threshold elevations in low frequencies (250–500 Hz) and the elevated degrees would control the final distribution of TP. The inverted-U-shaped audiogram in patients with normal hearing might indicate a low-pitched tinnitus.

We further examined the association between TP and the frequencies of hearing threshold elevation and found that TP was correlated to the frequency of maximum hearing threshold in both ears, with a coefficient of association of 0.277 in the left ears (p = 0.015) (**Figure 2A**) and 0.367 in the right ears ($p < 0.001$) in the high-pitched subgroup (**Figure 2B**). This finding confirmed that the dominant TP might be speculated by the different audiograms of patients, indicating that minor pure-tone threshold elevation ranging from 250 to 8,000 Hz might be responsible for the generation of tinnitus in individuals with normal hearing.

Moreover, we analyzed the distribution of dominant TP vs. the distribution of maximum threshold-elevating frequencies in both ears and found that the distributions of threshold-elevating frequencies in both ears were consistent with the distribution of dominant TP. Furthermore, of the 313 participants, 259 had high-pitched tinnitus, 251 had maximum hearing threshold in the high frequency range (3,000–8,000 Hz) in their left ears, and 249 had maximum hearing threshold in the high frequency range (3000–8000 Hz) in their right ears. These results confirmed our explanation that the matched dominant TP was mostly high-pitched in patients without clinical hearing loss (**Figure 3**). Our findings provide noteworthy links between tinnitus pitch and subclinical threshold elevations in the audiometric profile within the testing range of conventional audiometer at the first time, indicating a causal role of mild threshold elevation in the generation of tinnitus. Additionally, the pitch of tinnitus might be predicted from different types of audiograms.

DISCUSSION

It is well-known that the presence of tinnitus is strongly associated with hearing loss, and that the dominant TP is often within the region of hearing loss. However, tinnitus is not limited to individuals with a clinically measurable hearing loss. To date, only a few studies have examined the association between tinnitus and "subclinical" threshold elevations in the audiometric profile. Previous research mainly focused on discovering the existence of ultra- or extended high-frequency (above 8 kHz) hearing loss in patients with tinnitus and normal hearing, as well as the age-, sex-, and audiometry-matched controls without tinnitus; however, they failed to find a close relationship between TP and the frequency of maximum hearing loss or edge frequency. The possible reason might be partially attributed to the absence of TP-matching procedure in extended high-frequency regions. In the present study, we performed the "trinomial forced-choice method" for tinnitus matching, with 16 frequency measurement points ranging from 250 Hz to 16 kHz. Nevertheless, 308 of the 313 participants reported matched TPs no higher than 8 kHz, indicating that ultra-high frequency hearing loss might be insufficient evidence for the generation of tinnitus in patients with normal hearing and that the profiling of conventional audiometry (125 Hz–8 kHz) data should be investigated further. Hence, this study sought to verify whether minor audiometric deficits up to 8 kHz play a defining role in the phenotypic profiling of tinnitus in patients with normal hearing.

Our results found that the dominant TP of patients with clinically normal hearing was almost within the high-frequency range (especially at 4 and 8 kHz), with a mean of 4866.8 ± 2579.6 Hz. In several studies, Paglialonga et al. (2010, 2011) have established that normal hearing (with mean thresholds ≤ 20 dB HL at 0.5–4 kHz and ≤ 40 dB at 8 kHz) in patients with tinnitus does not preclude a completely normal hearing level for someone with cochlear dead regions or outer hair cell damage, particularly at high frequencies. This pattern is frequently observed when compared to controls (Paglialonga et al., 2010, 2011). In the present study, we demonstrated a more direct correspondence between TPs and the frequencies of hearing deficits according to the audiometric profiles. The participants were divided into four groups based on the pitch-matching results: low-frequency (≤500 Hz), middle-frequency (500–3,000 Hz), high-frequency (3,000–8,000 Hz), and ultra-high-frequency (>8,000 Hz). Interestingly, 82.7% of the participants had high-pitched tinnitus in the 3–8 kHz range, with audiograms characterized by dramatical threshold elevations above 2 kHz in a sharp descending slope and flat curve below 2 kHz with no obvious threshold elevations. A similar phenotypic profiling of audiograms

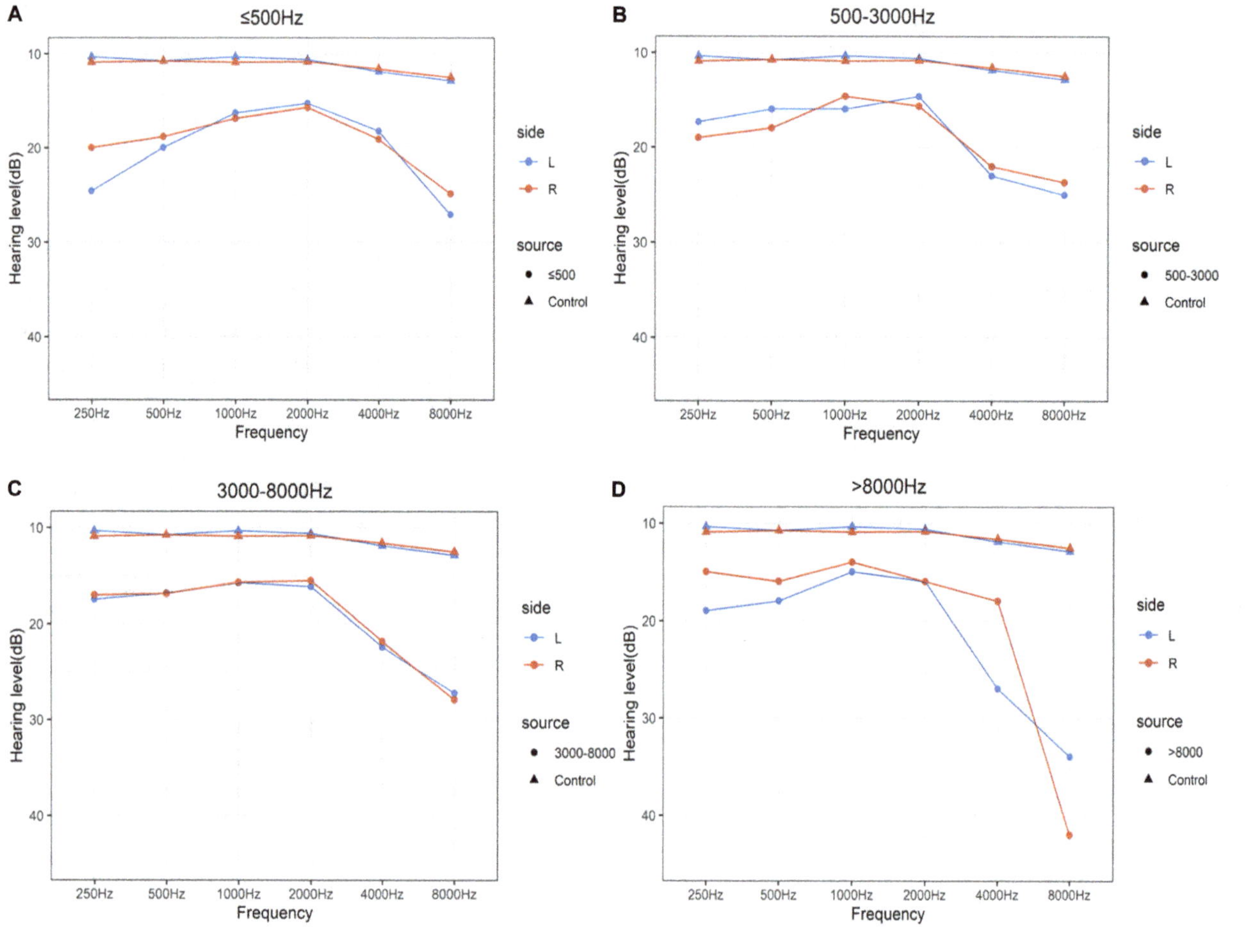

FIGURE 1 | Average pure-tone audiograms of patients with clinically normal hearing and volunteers without tinnitus using a 250–8,000 Hz conventional audiometer. **(A–D)** Mean values of average hearing thresholds for the controls with normal hearing and without tinnitus and patients with clinically normal hearing in dominant tinnitus pitch ≤500 Hz **(A)**, 500 Hz–3 kHz **(B)**, 3–8 kHz **(C)**, and >8,000 Hz **(D)**. Blue solid lines and dots represent left ears and red solid lines and dots represent right ears in patients with tinnitus. Blue solid lines and triangles represent left ears and red solid lines and triangles represent right ears in volunteers with normal hearing and without tinnitus.

TABLE 2 | The average pure tone thresholds (mean) and the corresponding standard deviations (SD) in different subgroups with tinnitus and the control group without tinnitus.

Frequency		Hearing thresholds [mean (SD), dB HL]				
		Control (*n* = 71)	≤500 Hz (*n* = 34)	500–3,000 Hz (*n* = 15)	3,000–8,000 Hz (*n* = 259)	>8,000 Hz (*n* = 5)
250 Hz	L	10.4 (4.7)	24.6 (18.4)	17.3 (3.7)	17.5 (5.1)	19.0 (7.4)
	R	10.9 (4.3)	20.0 (5.9)	19.0 (3.4)	17.0 (4.9)	15.0 (5.0)
500 Hz	L	10.8 (5.0)	20.0 (7.4)	16.0 (3.4)	16.9 (4.4)	18.0 (5.7)
	R	10.8 (3.9)	18.8 (4.8)	18.0 (3.7)	16.9 (4.3)	16.0 (4.2)
1,000 Hz	L	10.4 (3.9)	16.3 (4.3)	16.0 (7.1)	15.8 (4.1)	15.0 (3.5)
	R	10.9 (3.9)	16.9 (4.4)	14.7 (3.0)	15.7 (3.8)	14.0 (4.2)
2,000 Hz	L	10.6 (3.3)	15.3 (4.8)	14.7 (4.4)	16.2 (5.1)	16.0 (5.5)
	R	10.8 (3.4)	15.7 (5.5)	15.7 (3.7)	15.5 (4.5)	16.0 (6.5)
4,000 Hz	L	11.9 (5.4)	18.2 (6.4)	23.0 (11.9)	22.5 (10.0)	27.0 (12.5)
	R	11.6 (4.1)	19.1 (8.4)	22.0 (12.6)	21.9 (9.9)	18.0 (5.7)
8,000 Hz	L	12.9 (4.6)	27.1 (16.7)	25.0 (13.0)	27.2 (14.1)	34.0 (16.4)
	R	12.5 (4.6)	24.9 (14.0)	23.7 (11.1)	27.9 (14.9)	42.0 (29.7)

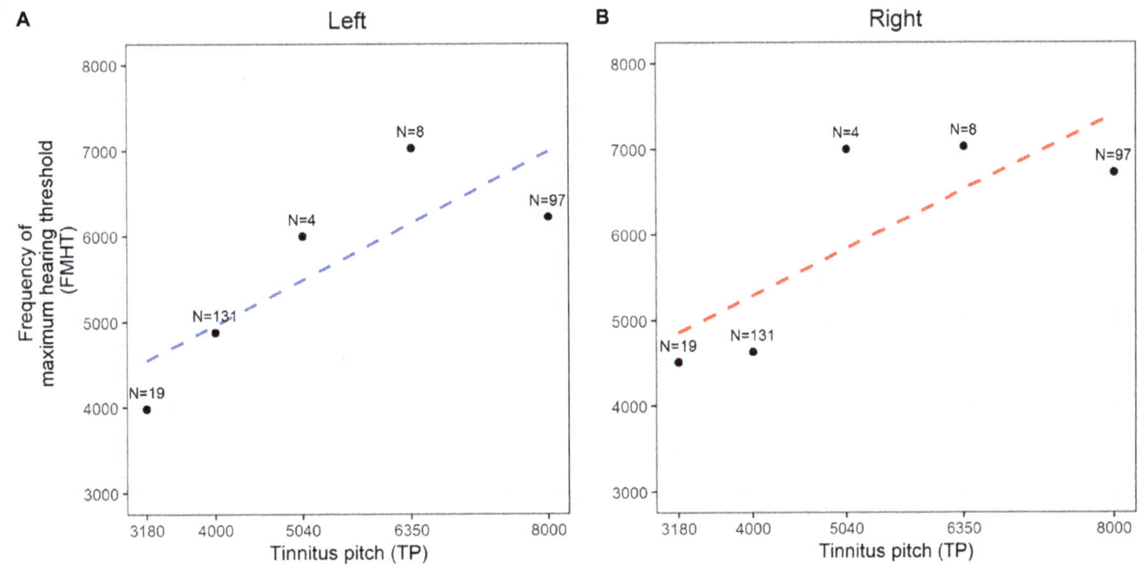

FIGURE 2 | Spearman rank correlation between dominant tinnitus pitch (TP) and frequency of maximum hearing threshold (FMHT). **(A,B)** The correlation coefficient and generalized linear regression between the matched tinnitus pitch and the frequency of maximum hearing threshold were demonstrated in the left ears (**A**, blue dotted line) and right ears (**B**, red dotted line). N means the counts of each data.

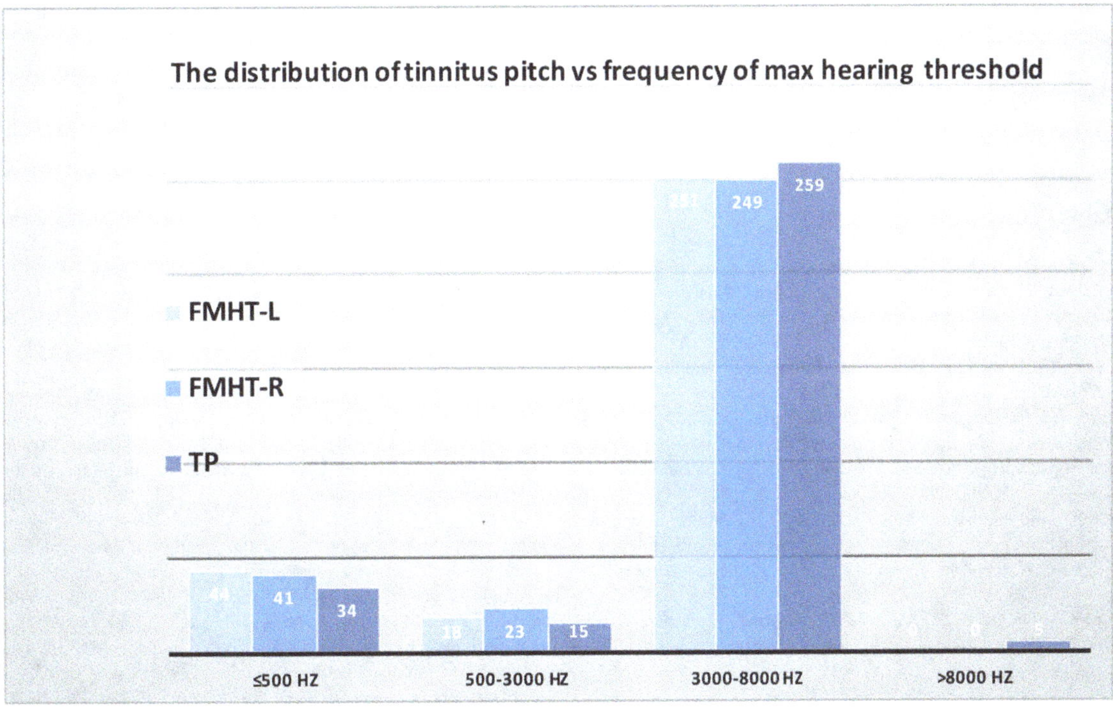

FIGURE 3 | Association between the distribution of tinnitus pitch and the distribution of maximum threshold corresponding frequency in patients with tinnitus and normal hearing. The distribution of threshold-elevated frequencies in both the left ears and right ears was consistent with the distribution of dominant tinnitus pitch.

was examined in patients with ultra-high-pitched tinnitus. Approximately 10.9% of the individuals presented low-pitched tinnitus with distinctive inverted-U-shaped audiograms in both ears, suggesting comparable threshold elevations in the low-frequency region (≤500 Hz) vs. the high-frequency region (4–8 kHz). Furthermore, we confirmed a positive correlation between TP and frequency of maximum hearing threshold in both right and left ears. Additionally, the distribution of TP was proven to be consistent with the distribution of maximum hearing threshold corresponding frequency. Therefore, our results indicated that minor hearing deficits might be the cause of tinnitus in patients with normal hearing and that the TP might be predicted by different audiograms.

Tinnitus severity and subjective tinnitus-related discomfort are often more severe in subjects with hearing loss than in those with normal hearing. However, Yenigun et al. (2014) found that the tinnitus severity index and THI results are significantly similar between the groups with normal hearing and hearing loss. Our data did not show a significant between-group difference in THI score when the patients were divided into subgroups based on the TP ($p = 0.716$). The mean score for THI was 31.0 ± 23.3, and according to the scoring criterion for THI, the majority of patients with tinnitus and normal hearing experienced mild to moderate disturbance. The assessment of tinnitus also requires multi-dimensional psychoacoustic evaluation. Furthermore, we used AIS and FTQ to evaluate sleep disorders and fear of tinnitus in patients with normal hearing, and the results were similar to those obtained with THI, with no significant between-group difference ($p = 0.454$ for AIS and $p = 0.306$ for FTQ).

In summary, we expound the characteristics of tinnitus in patients with clinically normal hearing in terms of age, sex, education, hearing threshold, tinnitus duration, tinnitus severity, dominant TP, laterality, tinnitus loudness, multi-dimensional evaluation scales, and intermittent vs. continuous tinnitus. We discovered that the dominant TP was mostly in the high-frequency range, and that the dominant TP in patients with tinnitus and normal hearing might be related to threshold elevations up to 8 kHz. On dividing the patients into four subgroups based on the TP, we identified different types and distinctive audiograms in the low-pitched ($\leq$500 Hz), middle-pitched (500 Hz–3 kHz), high-pitched (3–8 kHz), and ultra-high-pitched subgroups. Therefore, our results suggest that the details of conventional audiogram should be well-studied in patients with tinnitus and normal hearing. We believe that our results at least partially explicit the common question "Why did I get tinnitus?" in patients with normal hearing from the aspect of audiogram. The efficacy of tinnitus management involving different subgroups in patients with normal hearing is worthy to study in the future.

AUTHOR CONTRIBUTIONS

DT and XL performed the experiments and drafted the manuscript. DT, RH, and HY analyzed the data and approved the final manuscript. DT and WL conceived and designed the study, interpreted and analyzed the data, and approved the final manuscript. All authors contributed to the article and approved the submitted version.

ACKNOWLEDGMENTS

We thank Deborah Hall, University of Nottingham, for providing scientific guidance on the manuscript preparation.

REFERENCES

Baguley, D., Mcferran, D., and Hall, D. (2013). Tinnitus. *Lancet* 382, 1600–1607.

Biesinger, E., Heiden, C., Greimel, V., Lendle, T., Hoing, R., and Albegger, K. (1998). [Strategies in ambulatory treatment of tinnitus]. *HNO* 46, 157–169. doi: 10.1007/s001060050215

Eggermont, J. J., and Roberts, L. E. (2004). The neuroscience of tinnitus. *Trends Neurosci.* 27, 676–682.

Guest, H., Munro, K. J., Prendergast, G., Howe, S., and Plack, C. J. (2017). Tinnitus with a normal audiogram: relation to noise exposure but no evidence for cochlear synaptopathy. *Hear. Res.* 344, 265–274. doi: 10.1016/j.heares.2016.12.002

Jastreboff, P. J., and Jastreboff, M. M. (2003). Tinnitus retraining therapy for patients with tinnitus and decreased sound tolerance. *Otolaryngol. Clin. North Am.* 36, 321–336. doi: 10.1016/s0030-6665(02)00172-x

Kara, E., Aydın, K., Akbulut, A. A., Karakol, S. N., Durmaz, S., Yener, H. M., et al. (2020). Assessment of hidden hearing loss in normal hearing individuals with and without tinnitus. *J. Int. Adv. Otol.* 16, 87–92. doi: 10.5152/iao.2020.7062

Konig, O., Schaette, R., Kempter, R., and Gross, M. (2006). Course of hearing loss and occurrence of tinnitus. *Hear. Res.* 221, 59–64. doi: 10.1016/j.heares.2006.07.007

Langguth, B., Kreuzer, P. M., Kleinjung, T., and De Ridder, D. (2013). Tinnitus: causes and clinical management. *Lancet Neurol.* 12, 920–930. doi: 10.1016/S1474-4422(13)70160-1

McCormack, A., Edmondson-Jones, M., Somerset, S., and Hall, D. (2016). A systematic review of the reporting of tinnitus prevalence and severity. *Hear. Res.* 337, 70–79. doi: 10.1016/j.heares.2016.05.009

McCracken, L. M., Zayfert, C., and Gross, R. T. (1992). The pain anxiety symptoms scale: development and validation of a scale to measure fear of pain. *Pain* 50, 67–73. doi: 10.1016/0304-3959(92)90113-p

Moore, B. C. J., Vinay, C., and Sandhya, B. (2010). The relationship between tinnitus pitch and the edge frequency of the audiogram in individuals with hearing impairment and tonal tinnitus. *Hear. Res.* 261, 51–56. doi: 10.1016/j.heares.2010.01.003

Newman, C. W., Jacobson, G. P., and Spitzer, J. B. (1996). Development of the tinnitus handicap inventory. *Arch. Otolaryngol. Head Neck Surg.* 122, 143–148.

Newman, C. W., Sandridge, S. A., and Bolek, L. (2008). Development and psychometric adequacy of the screening version of the tinnitus handicap inventory. *Otol. Neurotol.* 29, 276–281. doi: 10.1097/MAO.0b013e31816569c4

Norena, A. J., and Eggermont, J. J. (2003). Changes in spontaneous neural activity immediately after an acoustic trauma: implications for neural correlates of tinnitus. *Hear. Res.* 183, 137–153. doi: 10.1016/s0378-5955(03)00225-9

Paglialonga, A., Del Bo, L., Ravazzani, P., and Tognola, G. (2010). Quantitative analysis of cochlear active mechanisms in tinnitus subjects with normal hearing sensitivity: multiparametric recording of evoked otoacoustic emissions and contralateral suppression. *Auris Nasus Larynx* 37, 291–298. doi: 10.1016/j.anl.2009.09.009

Paglialonga, A., Fiocchi, S., Del Bo, L., Ravazzani, P., and Tognola, G. (2011). Quantitative analysis of cochlear active mechanisms in tinnitus subjects with normal hearing sensitivity: time-frequency analysis of transient evoked otoacoustic emissions and contralateral suppression. *Auris Nasus Larynx* 38, 33–40. doi: 10.1016/j.anl.2010.04.006

Pan, T., Tyler, R. S., Ji, H., Coelho, C., Gehringer, A. K., and Gogel, S. A. (2009). The relationship between tinnitus pitch and the audiogram. *Int. J. Audiol.* 48, 277–294. doi: 10.1080/14992020802581974

Roelofs, J., Sluiter, J. K., Frings-Dresen, M. H., Goossens, M., Thibault, P., Boersma, K., et al. (2007). Fear of movement and (re)injury in chronic musculoskeletal pain: evidence for an invariant two-factor model of the Tampa Scale for Kinesiophobia across pain diagnoses and Dutch, Swedish, and Canadian samples. *Pain* 131, 181–190. doi: 10.1016/j.pain.2007.01.008

Savastano, M. (2008). Tinnitus with or without hearing loss: are its characteristics different? *Eur. Arch. Otorhinolaryngol.* 265, 1295–1300. doi: 10.1007/s00405-008-0630-z

Schecklmann, M., Vielsmeier, V., Steffens, T., Landgrebe, M., Langguth, B., and Kleinjung, T. (2012). Relationship between Audiometric slope and tinnitus pitch in tinnitus patients: insights into the mechanisms of tinnitus generation. *PLoS One* 7:e34878. doi: 10.1371/journal.pone.0034878

Sereda, M., Edmondson-Jones, M., and Hall, D. A. (2015). Relationship between tinnitus pitch and edge of hearing loss in individuals with a narrow tinnitus bandwidth. *Int. J. Audiol.* 54, 249–256. doi: 10.3109/14992027.2014.979373

Sereda, M., Hall, D. A., Bosnyak, D. J., Edmondson-Jones, M., Roberts, L. E., Adjamian, P., et al. (2011). Re-examining the relationship between audiometric profile and tinnitus pitch. *Int. J. Audiol.* 50, 303–312. doi: 10.3109/14992027.2010.551221

Soldatos, C. R., Dikeos, D. G., and Paparrigopoulos, T. J. (2000). Athens insomnia scale: validation of an instrument based on ICD-10 criteria. *J. Psychosom. Res.* 48, 555–560. doi: 10.1016/s0022-3999(00)00095-7

Song, Z., Wu, Y., Tang, D., Lu, X., Qiao, L., Wang, J., et al. (2021). Tinnitus is associated with extended high-frequency hearing loss and hidden high-frequency damage in young patients. *Otol. Neurotol.* 42, 377–383. doi: 10.1097/MAO.0000000000002983

Vielsmeier, V., Lehner, A., Strutz, J., Steffens, T., Kreuzer, P. M., Schecklmann, M., et al. (2015). The relevance of the high frequency audiometry in tinnitus patients with normal hearing in conventional pure-tone audiometry. *Biomed. Res. Int.* 2015, 302515. doi: 10.1155/2015/302515

World Health Organization [WHO] Programme for the Prevention of Deafness and Hearing Impairment (1997). *Future Programme Developments for Prevention of Deafness and Hearing Impairments: Report of the First Informal Consultation, Geneva, 23-24 January 1997.* Geneva: World Health Organization.

Xiong, B., Liu, Z., Liu, Q., Peng, Y., Wu, H., Lin, Y., et al. (2019). Missed hearing loss in tinnitus patients with normal audiograms. *Hear. Res.* 384, 107826. doi: 10.1016/j.heares.2019.107826

Yenigun, A., Dogan, R., Aksoy, F., Akyuz, S., and Dabak, H. (2014). Assessment of tinnitus with tinnitus severity index, tinnitus handicap inventory and distortion product otoacoustic emissions in patients with normal hearing and hearing loss. *Kulak Burun Bogaz Ihtis Derg.* 24, 11–16. doi: 10.5606/kbbihtisas.2014.60783

5

Effects of Inter-Stimulus Interval on Speech-Evoked Frequency-Following Response in Elderly Adults

Dongxin Liu[1], *Jiong Hu*[2], *Ruijuan Dong*[1], *Jing Chen*[1], *Gabriella Musacchia*[2] *and Shuo Wang*[1]*

[1]*Otolaryngology—Head & Neck Surgery, Beijing Tongren Hospital, Beijing Institute of Otolaryngology, Capital Medical University, Beijing, China,* [2]*Department of Audiology, University of the Pacific, San Francisco, CA, United States*

Correspondence:
Shuo Wang
shannonwsh@aliyun.com

Background: The speech-evoked frequency following response (FFR) has shown to be useful in assessing complex auditory processing abilities and in different age groups. While many aspects of FFR have been studied extensively, the effect of timing, as measured by inter-stimulus-interval (ISI), especially in the older adult population, has yet to be thoroughly investigated.

Objective: The purpose of this study was to examine the effects of different ISIs on speech evoked FFR in older and younger adults who speak a tonal language, and to investigate whether the older adults' FFR were more susceptible to the change in ISI.

Materials and Methods: Twenty-two normal hearing participants were recruited in our study, including 11 young adult participants and 11 elderly participants. An Intelligent Hearing Systems Smart EP evoke potential system was used to record the FFR in four ISI conditions (40, 80, 120 and 160 ms). A recorded natural speech token with a falling tone /yi/ was used as the stimulus. Two indices, stimulus-to-response correlation coefficient and pitch strength, were used to quantify the FFR responses. Two-way analysis of variance (ANOVA) was used to analyze the differences in different age groups and different ISI conditions.

Results: There was no significant difference in stimulus-to-response correlation coefficient and pitch strength among the different ISI conditions, in either age groups. Older adults appeared to have weaker FFR for all ISI conditions when compared to their younger adult counterparts.

Conclusion: Shorter ISIs did not result in worse FFRs from older adults or younger adults. For speech-evoked FFR using a recorded natural speech token that is 250 ms in length, an ISI of as short as 40 ms appeared to be sufficient and effective to record FFR for elderly adults.

Keywords: evoked potential, frequency-following response, lexical tone, aging, inter-stimulus intervals

INTRODUCTION

The frequency-following response (FFR) recorded from the human scalp is an electrophysiological potential which follows the periodicity of the stimuli (Moushegian et al., 1973). It is a far-field potential recorded from surface electrodes, reflecting the synchronous activity of axonal and dendritic potentials generated primarily by populations of neurons in the lateral lemniscus and inferior colliculus of the brainstem (Smith et al., 1975; Møeller, 1998). In recent years, the FFR has seen a renewed interested in the research realm due to its unique ability to assess various auditory functions using complex stimuli (Skoe and Kraus, 2010). One reason that the FFR has been successful in this regard is that the frequency information that is extracted from the FFR waveform corresponds to the spectrum of the stimulus. By examining the spectral property of FFR, one can have a means to assess the processing of complex sounds in the auditory system (Cunningham et al., 2001; Aiken and Picton, 2008; Skoe and Kraus, 2010; White-Schwoch et al., 2013). For example, Krishnan et al. (2004, 2005) used four different Mandarin Chinese tones to evoke FFR in young adult native speakers of Mandarin to examine the effect of language background on pitch processing. Another application of FFR is to use a consonant-vowel (CV) complex, typically /da/, to evaluate various aspects of the auditory processing function, such as the effect of maturation (Anderson et al., 2010), auditory training (Song et al., 2008), music training (Musacchia et al., 2008), language and/or reading issues (Banai et al., 2009) and speech perception in noise (Banai et al., 2009). Germane to the current study, the FFR has been utilized to assess how aging affects the physiological process of auditory function. For example, Clinard et al. (2010) demonstrated that older adults, even with normal hearing sensitivity, have auditory perceptual deficits relative to their young counterparts. Similarly, Wang et al. (2016) demonstrated that pitch processing ability at the brainstem level of the elderly were not as strong as younger adults in tonal language speakers.

Results from previous FFR studies in older adults showed that aging may lead to the degradation of the FFR. However, poor FFR stimulus representation in the elderly might stem from age-related neural degeneration, or simply because of the overlapping response caused by the inter-stimulus interval (ISI) used in those studies. As the cumulative neural fatigue, adaption time and incomplete recovery involving hair-cell-cochlear nerve junctions and synaptic transmission in the elderly may be more inferior than that of the young, longer ISIs may be required.

The purpose of this study is to expand on our previous work on the speech-evoked FFR in older adults who speak a tonal language, and to examine the effect of different ISIs on the older adults' FFR. Results from this study should help answer the important question of whether ISI has a different impact on older adults' FFR compared to its impact on younger adults. It can also help bridge the gap between the laboratory research and clinical utility of FFR by recommending an appropriate length of ISI for future FFR usage in the clinical application, especially for the older population.

MATERIALS AND METHODS

This research has received approval from the Ethics Committee of Beijing Tongren Hospital Affiliated to Capital Medical University and Beijing Institute of Otolaryngology. All subjects participated in this research on their own accord. They had signed the informed consent and were compensated for their participation. All operations throughout the research did no harm on the subjects.

Participants

Eleven young adults (five males) and eleven elderly (four male) participants were recruited from Beijing Tongren Hospital. The younger adults were 20–26 years old (mean ± SD = 22.90 ± 2.79) and the elderly adults were 60–65 years old (mean ± SD = 62.83 ± 2.82). All participants were native speakers of Mandarin Chinese, reported no neurological or otological symptoms or illnesses. They all presented normal tympanometric measurements (Type A tympanograms and present acoustic reflexes). The older adult group had slightly elevated thresholds at higher audiometric frequencies. Still, all participants were considered to have clinically normal hearing, defined as thresholds ≤25 dB HL at octave frequencies from 250 Hz to 4000 Hz (**Figure 1**). All participants had normal click ABR latencies and thresholds, measured with a 100 μs click stimulus at a rate of 20.1 Hz.

Experiment Equipment, Stimulation and Recording

All experiments were conducted in a sound-treated chamber with anechoic walls with an ambient noise ≤20 dB(A). The Smart EP instrument (Intelligent Hearing Systems, Miami, FL, USA) was used to record FFR. An electromagnetically shielded insert earphone (ER-3) was used for monoaural stimulation to the right ear. A recorded natural speech stimulus /yi/ with a falling fundamental frequency contour whose f0 ranged from 185 Hz to 135 Hz was presented at the level of 70 dB SPL. The stimulus had a duration of 250 ms, including a 5 ms rise time at the onset and a 5 ms fall time at the end. Four different ISIs (40, 80, 120 and 160 ms) were used in this study. For each ISI condition, one of

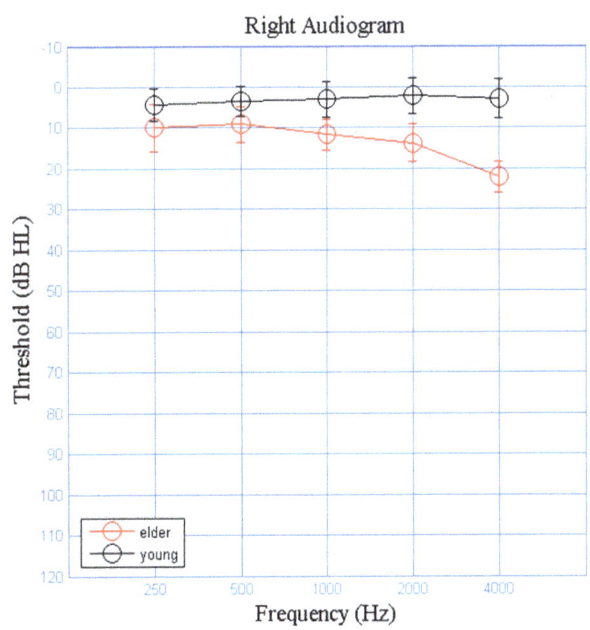

FIGURE 1 | Averaged audiograms for the young (black) and older (red) participants on the right ears. Air conduction audiometric hearing threshold were denoted by circles, where error bars represent the standard deviations.

the four ISIs was inserted between presentations of the speech stimulus, which resulted in an effective stimulation rate of 3.45, 3.03, 2.70 and 2.44 samples/s, respectively.

Throughout recording sessions, participants laid in bed with their eyes closed and in a calm and steady state. Three gold-plated recording electrodes were placed accordingly: high forehead as non-inverting, right mastoid as inverting and low forehead as ground (all impedances kept $\leq 3k\Omega$). The four ISI conditions were presented in random order for each participant. In each ISI condition, there were two repetitions of 2,000 accepted sweeps of the speech stimulus. The artifact rejection criteria were set at ± 30 μV and the band-pass filter was set between 70 Hz and 1,500 Hz.

At the end of each experiment session, a control condition (earphone tube occluded and removed from the participant's ear while stimulation was still present) was conducted. The recordings from the control conditions were analyzed to detect and eliminate any potential stimulus artifact.

Data Analysis

All data were analyzed using MatLab (Mathworks, Natick, MA, USA). EEGs were filtered through a 100–1500 Hz bandpass filter with a linear phase of 500 poles. After averaging the EEG, a cross-correlation between the stimulus and recorded waveforms was carried out to identify the time shift point, that corresponds to the maximum cross-correlation value. Starting from this time point, a segment of 250 ms was extracted from the averaged data as the FFR response.

Two indices were used in this study, namely, stimulus-to-response correlation coefficient and pitch strength. The stimulus-to-response correlation coefficient, ranging from 0 to 1, is the result of cross-correlation function of stimulus waveform and FFR waveform, representing the faithfulness of pitch tracking. For discrete signals, the cross-correlation function is defined as $R(n) = (1/N)^* \sum([x(m)^*y(m+n)])$, where n is time, N is the number of sampling points and m ranges from 0 to $N - 1$. The maximum of R(n) is defined as the stimulus-to-response correlation coefficient. The other index is the pitch strength of FFR, ranging from 0 to 1 too. It is the result of the autocorrelation function to the FFR waveform itself, representing the robustness of neural phase-locking. Pitch strength is defined as the distance between of the maximum of and the minimum of the autocorrelation function. For detailed discussion on these two indices, please refer to our previous work in Jeng and Warrington (2011) and Wang et al. (2016).

Statistical analysis was carried out with a two-way analysis of variance (ANOVA), where aging (young and older adults) and the duration of inter-stimuli intervals on FFR (40, 80, 120 and 160 ms) were evaluated as independent variables, and stimulus-to-response cross correlation coefficient and pitch strength as dependent variables.

RESULTS

In the older adult group, grand averaged results of stimulus-to-response correlation coefficient under the four different ISIs (40, 80, 120, 160 ms) were 0.7 ± 0.24, 0.68 ± 0.20, 0.65 ± 0.23, 0.69 ± 0.23, respectively. Similarly, grand averaged results of pitch strength under the four different ISIs were 0.38 ± 0.09, 0.45 ± 0.07, 0.39 ± 0.09, 0.39 ± 0.09, respectively. In the younger group, grand averaged results of stimulus-to-response correlation coefficient under the four different ISIs were 0.95 ± 0.03, 0.94 ± 0.04, 0.95 ± 0.07, 0.96 ± 0.03, respectively. In the same age group, grand averaged results of pitch strength under the four ISIs were 0.57 ± 0.13, 0.61 ± 0.11, 0.59 ± 0.13, 0.60 ± 0.14, respectively.

Comparisons among the ISI levels and age groups, as well as their interactions, were calculated using two-way ANOVA. For the index stimulus-to-response correlation coefficient, two-way ANOVA showed that the four levels of ISI were not significantly different ($F_{(3,80)} = 0.13$, $p > 0.05$) from each other (**Figure 2**), while there was a significant different tween the two age groups (**Figure 3**, $F_{(1,80)} = 61.59$, $p < 0.01$), and there was no significant interaction between factors age and ISI ($F_{(3,80)} = 0.08$, $p > 0.05$). Similarly, for pitch strength, there was no significant difference among the four ISI levels (**Figure 4**, $F_{(3,80)} = 0.95$, $p > 0.05$), while a significant difference was found between the two age groups (**Figure 5**, $F_{(1,80)} = 68.8$, $p < 0.05$), and there was no significant interaction between factors age and ISI ($F_{(3,80)} = 0.15$, $p > 0.05$).

DISCUSSION

Effect of ISI in Older Adults

Results from this study suggest that different ISIs, at least for those used in the study, did not seem to impact the speech-evoked FFR. Our data revealed that although the responses were weaker than the younger adults, older adults' FFR did not appear to be more susceptible to differing ISI lengths, some as short

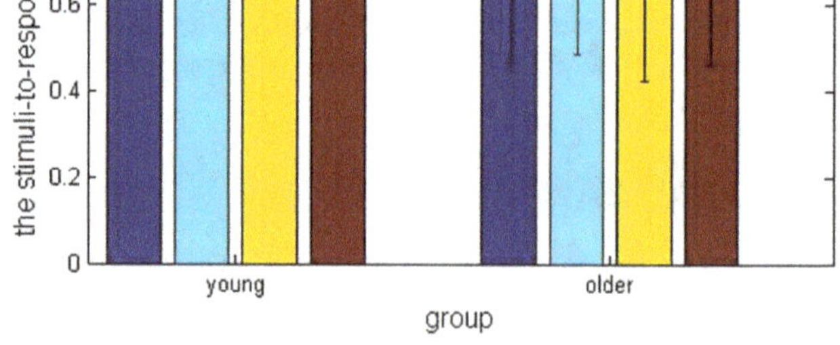

FIGURE 2 | The stimulus-to-response correlation coefficients obtained under the four different inter-stimulus intervals (ISIs) of 40 ms (blue), 80 ms (cyan), 120 ms (amber) and 160 ms (crimson), respectively, and divided into the young (left) and older (right) adult groups.

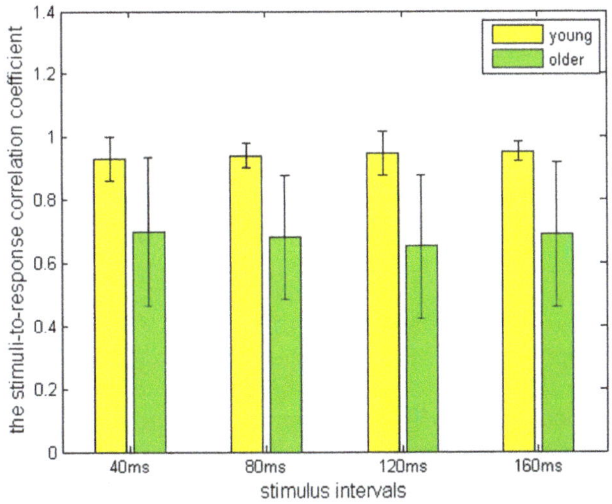

FIGURE 3 | The stimulus-to-response correlation coefficients obtained from the young (yellow) and the elderly (green) groups, grouped by different ISIs.

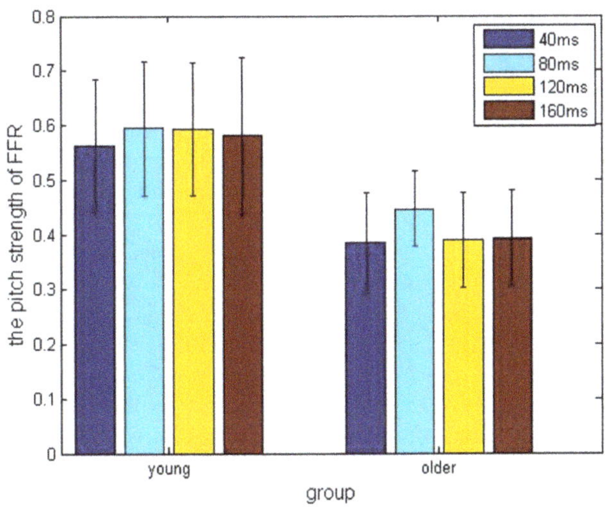

FIGURE 4 | Pitch strength results obtained under different ISIs of 40 ms (blue), 80 ms (cyan), 120 ms (amber) and 160 ms (crimson), respectively, and divided into the young (left) and older (right) adult groups.

as 40 ms. The 40 ms ISI has been widely used in the FFR literature for Mandarin Chinese speech stimuli in younger adults (Krishnan et al., 2004, 2005; Jeng et al., 2011; Wang et al., 2016). In the current study, it did not seem to be too short for the older adults' FFR, reflected by the two indices, stimulus-to-response correlation coefficient and the pitch strength.

This is an interesting finding in that one might think due the aging effect, the auditory pathways in older adults might need a longer ISI than their younger counterparts. Since FFR are evoked by longer and more spectro-temporally complex stimuli, which are strongly influenced by rostral brainstem and midbrain generators (Swaminathan et al., 2008), a different ISI may have been needed for older adults, as

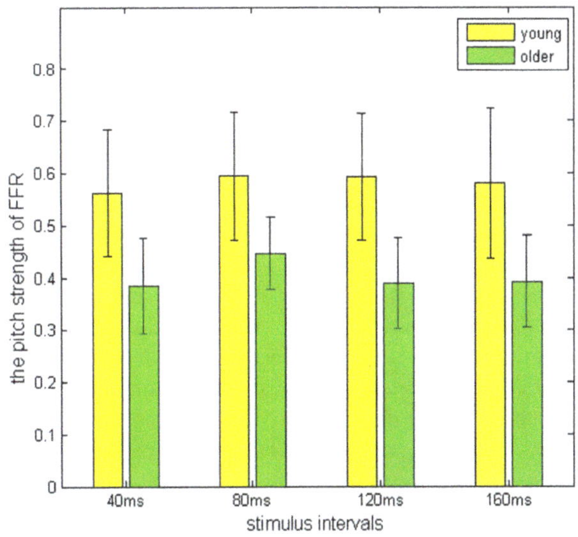

FIGURE 5 | The pitch strength result obtained from the young (yellow) and the elderly (green) groups, under different ISIs.

they may have decreased neural timing during transmission and processing auditory information. However, our data does not seem to support that thought. One possibility might have been that 40 ms is still long enough for the older adults to have adequate neural adaptation during the FFR recordings. Perhaps, with an ISI that is even shorter than 40 ms, one might be able to observe degraded FFR in the older groups, which can only be answered in future studies.

The result from this study is also somewhat in contrast with previous works on cortical response (Tremblay et al., 2004), where older adults showed prolonged N1 and P2 latencies when speech stimuli were presented at a higher rate. One possible explanation may be that cortical responses such as N1/P2 are compound far-field potentials that may origin from multiple neuro generators (Lightfoot, 2016). Increased stimulus rate may negatively impact the activation and transmission in some or all of those neural generators, especially in an aged auditory system. The collective result of such negative impact may manifest as a reduced evoked potential, like the N1/P2 in older adults. On the other hand, brainstem responses like the FFR have comparably simpler sources of neural activities, and that may be part of the reason why the older adults in our study did not appear to be more susceptible to the change in ISI. Our results are also a little different from Clinard and Cotter (2015), where they found that using tonal-sweep to elicit FFR, older adults seemed to have weaker responses when the stimulus rate is higher. This may be explained by the fact that the older adults in our study were all native speakers of Mandarin Chinese, and this population has been shown to have enhanced pitch processing ability and stronger FFR, which may in turn help them become less sensitive to a fast stimulus rate or a shorter ISI. Regardless, more research is needed to find out the effect on ISI or stimulus rate for different electrophysiological tests in the older adult populations, with different language backgrounds.

In short, the fact that with longer (80 ms, 120 ms and 160 ms) ISI, older adults still had poorer speech-evoked FFR compared to the younger adults, suggest that the effect of ISI, at least as short as 40 ms for speech-evoked FFR, may have played little, if any, role in the reduced response reported in this study and previous studies. Although the current study did not find significant differences in the ISIs in older adults, it does not mean that isn't one that is too short for them. Further, there may also be one ISI where the older adults would start to have degraded response, while the younger adults still present relatively robust FFR. Future studies are need to answer these questions, as well as to compare the ISI used in FFR to those used in other auditory evoked potential tests.

Effect of Aging on the FFR

The significant difference in older adults' and younger adults' FFR reaffirmed our previous work (Wang et al., 2016) and those of others (Anderson et al., 2012). These studies have demonstrated the effect of aging on the auditory system, even with "normal" audiogram, and many theories have been proposed to explain such effects. For example, elderly population have shown to have degraded temporal processing ability (Gordon-Salant and Fitzgibbons, 1999), which had been proposed to contribute to why they often complain of hearing the sounds without desired clarity, especially in the presence of background noise (Anderson et al., 2012). One explanation for poor speech discrimination and impaired speech understanding is that aging adversely affects synchronized nerve fiber firing, temporal processing and phase-locking ability (Frisina and Frisina, 1997; Burkard and Sims, 2001; Clinard et al., 2010). Other studies (Schatteman et al., 2008; Bidelman et al., 2014) showed that both brainstem and cortical speech-evoked brain responses were impacted by the aging process too, resulting in the atypical neural information processing and speech information transformation between functional levels of the auditory neural system.

Our results revealed that after controlling for the ISI, older adults still showed significantly weaker pitch processing ability at the brainstem level compared to the younger adults. Future research on FFR in older adults is needed to further investigate the underlining reason of such deficit.

Choosing an Appropriate Inter-Stimulus-Interval for Recording Speech-Evoked FFR in Older Adults

As previously mentioned, the choice of ISI for voice-evoked FFR is an important consideration to ensure the separation of adjacent responses and completing a testing within a reasonable time frame. For recorded speech tokens such as the Mandarin Chinese syllable /yi/, which is typically 250 ms, a recording session with 2,000 repetitions can last as short as nearly 10 min with an ISI of 40 ms, and as long as 14 min with an ISI of 160 ms. In a real clinical setting, 14 min per recording session for an electrophysiological test would be too long. Fortunately, as the results of this study suggested, a 40 ms ISI yield similar responses to those longer ISIs, which means that within 10 min, a speech FFR can be obtained from typical clinical population such as older adults.

The only other study to date on the effect of ISI on speech-evoked FFR was conducted by Jeng et al. (2011), where they suggested a 35–45 ms ISI to be used in younger adults when FFR is evoked using Mandarin Chinese syllable /yi/. Our data suggest a similar recommendation: that an ISI around 40 ms is appropriate for the same FFR technique, and it can be extended to be used in both younger and older adults. With future studies, this finding fills the gap in current understanding of speech-evoked FFR, and may help paving the way for speech-evoked FFR into wilder clinical utility.

LIMITATIONS

Although both groups had clinically normal hearing thresholds (defined as $\leq$25 dB HL at octave frequencies from 250 Hz to 4000 Hz), there was a difference at higher frequencies, which may have affected our result. However, had the older adults in our study actually had "better" thresholds, it would only have helped them process speech sounds better and become even less sensitive to the shorter ISIs. Regardless, since such limitations have also been reported in similar studies where auditory brainstem and cortical responses were utilized to examine the effect of aging (Tremblay et al., 2004; Anderson et al., 2012; Clinard and Cotter, 2015; Wang et al., 2016), the difference in peripheral hearing should definitely be carefully examined, considered and/or controlled for future studies in the field.

Last but least, the recommended 40 ms ISI should only be considered for speech tokens, e.g., Mandarin Chinese syllables, that are around 250 ms long. Considering that there are many types of stimuli that can licit FFR, such as CVs, tonal sweeps or even simple tones, this recommendation has its limitation in its ability to be generalized into other FFR tokens.

CONCLUSION

As previously demonstrated, under different ISI conditions, older adults have weaker neurophysiological responses compared to their younger counterparts. Thus, an ISI around 40 ms could serve as a reasonable choice for future studies in the field of speech-evoked FFR in the elderly population.

AUTHOR CONTRIBUTIONS

DL was in charge of collecting data, analyzing statistics and writing the article. JH was in charge of designing the research and correcting the article. RD and JC were in charge of contacting the subjects and collecting data. GM were in charge of proofreading the manuscript for several times. The corresponding author SW was in charge of designing the research and correcting the article.

REFERENCES

Aiken, S. J., and Picton, T. W. (2008). Envelope and spectral frequency-following responses to vowel sounds. *Hear. Res.* 245, 35–47. doi: 10.1016/j.heares.2008.08.004

Anderson, S., Parbery-Clark, A., White-Schwoch, T., and Kraus, N. (2012). Aging affects neural precision of speech encoding. *J. Neurosci.* 32, 14156–14164. doi: 10.1523/JNEUROSCI.2176-12.2012

Anderson, S., Skoe, E., Chandrasekaran, B., Zecker, S., and Kraus, N. (2010). Brainstem correlates of speech-in-noise perception in children. *Hear. Res.* 270, 151–157. doi: 10.1016/j.heares.2010.08.001

Banai, K., Hornickel, J., Skoe, E., Nicol, T., Zecker, S., and Kraus, N. (2009). Reading and subcortical auditory function. *Cereb. Cortex* 19, 2699–2707. doi: 10.1093/cercor/bhp024

Bidelman, G. M., Villafuerte, J. W., Moreno, S., and Alain, C. (2014). Age-related changes in the subcortical-cortical encoding and categorical perception of speech. *Neurobiol. Aging* 35, 2526–2540. doi: 10.1016/j.neurobiolaging.2014.05.006

Burkard, R. F., and Sims, D. (2001). The human auditory brain-stem response to high click rates: aging effects. *Am. J. Audiol.* 10, 53–61. doi: 10.1044/1059-0889(2001/008)

Clinard, C. G., and Cotter, C. M. (2015). Neural representation of dynamic frequency is degraded in older adults. *Hear. Res.* 323, 91–98. doi: 10.1016/j.heares.2015.02.002

Clinard, C. G., Tremblay, K. L., and Krishnan, A. R. (2010). Aging alters the perception and physiological representation of frequency: evidence from human frequency-following response recordings. *Hear. Res.* 264, 48–55. doi: 10.1016/j.heares.2009.11.010

Cunningham, J., Nicol, T., Zecker, S., Bradlow, A. R., and Kraus, N. (2001). Neurobiologic responses to speech in noise in children with learning problems: deficits and strategies for improvement. *Clin. Neurophysiol.* 112, 758–767. doi: 10.1016/s1388-2457(01)00465-5

Frisina, D. R., and Frisina, R. D. (1997). Speech recognition in noise and presbycusis: relations to possible neural mechanisms. *Hear. Res.* 106, 95–104. doi: 10.1016/s0378-5955(97)00006-3

Gordon-Salant, S., and Fitzgibbons, P. J. (1999). Profile of auditory temporal processing in older listeners. *J. Speech Lang. Hear. Res.* 42, 300–311. doi: 10.1044/jslhr.4202.300

Jeng, F.-C., Hu, J., Dickman, B., Montgomery-Reagan, K., Tong, M., Wu, G., et al. (2011). Cross-linguistic comparison of frequency-following responses to voice pitch in american and chinese neonates and adults. *Ear Hear.* 32, 699–707. doi: 10.1097/aud.0b013e31821cc0df

Jeng, F.-C., and Warrington, R. P. (2011). Effects of silent interval on human frequency-following responses to voice pitch. *J. Acoust. Soc. Am.* 130:2545. doi: 10.1121/1.3655173

Krishnan, A., Xu, Y., Gandour, J. T., and Cariani, P. A. (2004). Human frequency-following response: representation of pitch contours in chinese tones. *Hear. Res.* 189, 1–12. doi: 10.1016/s0378-5955(03)00402-7

Krishnan, A., Xu, Y., Gandour, J. T., and Cariani, P. A. (2005). Encoding of pitch in the human brainstem is sensitive to language experience. *Cogn. Brain Res.* 25, 161–168. doi: 10.1016/j.cogbrainres.2005.05.004

Lightfoot, G. (2016). Summary of the N1–P2 cortical auditory evoked potential to estimate the auditory threshold in adults. *Semin. Hear.* 37, 1–8. doi: 10.1055/s-0035-1570334

Møeller, A. R. (1998). Neural generators of the brainstem auditory evoked potentials. *Semin. Hear.* 19, 11–27. doi: 10.1055/s-0028-1082955

Moushegian, G., Rupert, A. L., and Stillman, R. D. (1973). Laboratory note. Scalp-recorded early responses in man to frequencies in the speech range. *Electroencephalogr. Clin. Neurophysiol.* 35, 665–667. doi: 10.1016/0013-4694(73)90223-x

Musacchia, G., Strait, D., and Kraus, N. (2008). Relationships between behavior, brainstem and cortical encoding of seen and heard speech in musicians and non-musicians. *Hear. Res.* 241, 34–42. doi: 10.1016/j.heares.2008.04.013

Schatteman, T. A., Hughes, L. F., and Caspary, D. M. (2008). Aged-related loss of temporal processing: altered responses to amplitude modulated tones in rat dorsal cochlear nucleus. *Neuroscience* 154, 329–337. doi: 10.1016/j.neuroscience.2008.02.025

Skoe, E., and Kraus, N. (2010). Auditory brain stem response to complex sounds: a tutorial. *Ear Hear.* 31, 302–324. doi: 10.1097/aud.0b013e3181cdb272

Smith, J. C., Marsh, J. T., and Brown, W. S. (1975). Far-field recorded frequency-following responses: evidence for the locus of brainstem sources. *Electroencephalogr. Clin. Neurophysiol.* 39, 465–472. doi: 10.1016/0013-4694(75)90047-4

Song, J. H., Skoe, E., Wong, P. C. M., and Kraus, N. (2008). Plasticity in the adult human auditory brainstem following short-term linguistic training. *J. Cogn. Neurosci.* 20, 1892–1902. doi: 10.1162/jocn.2008.20131.

Swaminathan, J., Krishnan, A., Gandour, J. T., and Xu, Y. (2008). Applications of static and dynamic iterated rippled noise to evaluate pitch encoding in the human auditory brainstem. *IEEE Trans. Biomed. Eng.* 55, 281–287. doi: 10.1109/tbme.2007.896592

Tremblay, K. L., Billings, C., and Rohila, N. (2004). Speech evoked cortical potentials: effects of age and stimulus presentation rate. *J. Am. Acad. Audiol.* 15, 226–237. doi: 10.3766/jaaa.15.3.5

Wang, S., Hu, J., Dong, R., Liu, D., Chen, J., Musacchia, G., et al. (2016). Voice pitch elicited frequency following response in Chinese older adults. *Front. Aging Neurosci.* 8:286. doi: 10.3389/fnagi.2016.00286

White-Schwoch, T., Woodruff Carr, K., Anderson, S., Strait, D. L., and Kraus, N. (2013). Older adults benefit from music training early in life: biological evidence for long-term training-driven plasticity. *J. Neurosci.* 33, 17667–17674. doi: 10.1523/JNEUROSCI.2560-13.2013

6

Glutathione Peroxidase 1 Protects Against Peroxynitrite-Induced Spiral Ganglion Neuron Damage through Attenuating NF-κB Pathway Activation

Xue Wang[1,2†], Yuechen Han[1,2†], Fang Chen[1,2†], Man Wang[1,2], Yun Xiao[1,2], Haibo Wang[1,2], Lei Xu[1,2] and Wenwen Liu[1,2*]*

[1] Department of Otolaryngology-Head and Neck Surgery, Shandong Provincial ENT Hospital, Cheeloo College of Medicine, Shandong University, Jinan, China, [2] Shandong Institute of Otorhinolaryngology, Jinan, China

***Correspondence:**
Lei Xu
sdphxl@126.com
Wenwen Liu
wenwenliu_1@yahoo.com

† These authors have contributed equally to this work

Glutathione peroxidase 1 (GPX1) is a crucial antioxidant enzyme that prevented the harmful accumulation of intra-cellular hydrogen peroxide. GPX1 might contribute in limiting cochlear damages associated with aging or acoustic overexposure, but the function of GPX1 in the inner ear remains unclear. The present study was designed to investigate the effect of GPX1 on cochlear spiral ganglion neurons (SGNs) against oxidative stress induced by peroxynitrite, a versatile oxidant generated by the reaction of superoxide anion and nitric oxide. Here, we first found that the expression of GPX1 in cultured SGNs was downregulated after peroxynitrite exposure. Then, the GPX1 mimic ebselen and the *gpx1* knockout ($gpx1^{-/-}$) mice were used to investigate the role of GPX1 in SGNs treated with peroxynitrite. The pretreatment with ebselen significantly increased the survived SGN numbers, inhibited the apoptosis, and enhanced the expression of 4-HNE in the cultured SGNs of peroxynitrite + ebselen group compared with the peroxynitrite-only group. On the contrary, remarkably less survived SGNs, more apoptotic SGNs, and the higher expression level of 4-HNE were detected in the peroxynitrite + $gpx1^{-/-}$ group compared with the peroxynitrite-only group. Furthermore, rescue experiments with antioxidant N-acetylcysteine (NAC) showed that the expression of 4-HNE and the apoptosis in SGNs were significantly decreased, while the number of surviving SGNs was increased in peroxynitrite + NAC group compared the peroxynitrite-only group and in peroxynitrite + $gpx1^{-/-}$ + NAC group vs. peroxynitrite + $gpx1^{-/-}$ group. Finally, mechanistic studies showed that the activation of nuclear factor-kappa B (NF-κB) was involved in the SGNs damage caused by peroxynitrite and that GPX1 protected SGNs against peroxynitrite-induced damage, at least in part, *via* blocking the NF-κB pathway activation. Collectively, our findings suggest that GPX1 might serve as a new target for the prevention of nitrogen radical-induced SGNs damage and hearing loss.

Keywords: glutathione peroxidase 1, spiral ganglion neuron, peroxynitrite, oxidative stress, nuclear factor-kappa B, hearing loss

INTRODUCTION

In mammals, cochlea spiral ganglion neurons (SGNs) are the primary sensory neurons on the auditory conduction pathway. SGNs transmit complex acoustic information from sensory hair cells (HCs) to the second-order sensory neurons in the cochlear nucleus for sound processing. The survival of SGNs is essential for hearing preservation and, conversely, as SGN cannot regenerate spontaneously, the impairment and irreversible loss of SGNs result in permanent sensorineural hearing loss (SNHL) (Liu et al., 2019a; Leake et al., 2020; Pavlinkova, 2020), which seriously affects the human social and cognitive development. Multiple stimuli, such as excessive noise, ototoxic drugs, hereditary defects, and aging process, can cause SGNs damage. Although the pathogenic mechanisms by which these factors lead to SGN damage are various, researches have documented that the oxidative stress is a basic mechanism involved in SGNs death (Liu et al., 2011, 2012, 2019b, 2021; Xiong et al., 2011; Yamasoba et al., 2013; Wang et al., 2019, 2021). Oxidative stress is the disturbance in the balance between the generation of free radicals, such as reactive oxygen species (ROS) and reactive nitrogen species (RNS), and antioxidant defenses, and can cause oxidative damage to diverse cellular components, such as membranes, proteins, and DNA. Among RNS molecules, peroxynitrite, a product of superoxide anion and nitric oxide, is one of the most prominent one (Liu et al., 2011, 2012; Labbe et al., 2016; Cao et al., 2017; Ramdial et al., 2017). Peroxynitrite can oxidize a wide variety of biomolecules, which, in turn, modulates cell signal transduction pathways, interferes with mitochondrial function, impairs DNA, and finally mediates necrosis and apoptosis in different cell types (Korkmaz et al., 2009). Peroxynitrite participates in the occurrence and development of the varieties of pathological conditions, but data about the effects of peroxynitrite on auditory cells in the cochlea are still very limited. In our previous studies, we found that peroxynitrite induced cytotoxicity in rat SGNs (Liu et al., 2011, 2012) and mouse cochlear HCs (Cao et al., 2017). However, the effect of peroxynitrite on SGNs has not yet been fully elucidated, and it is important to eliminate the excessive peroxynitrite so as to counteract its toxic effect to protect cells from oxidative injuries.

Studies have shown that organisms can activate a series of defense responses, such as improving the activity of antioxidant enzymes in the body and initiating lysosomal degradation pathways, to prevent oxidative damage. Glutathione peroxidase 1 (GPX1) is one of the most abundant members of the GPXs family that protects cell from oxidative damage and maintains the balance of intracellular redox systems (Brigelius-Flohé, 1999). Glutathione peroxidase 1 has been reported for its effect in modulating many pathophysiologic processes in which oxidative stress play a vital role (Lubos et al., 2011). For example, GPX1 might play a protective role in alleviating oxidative stress as a neuromodulator in neurodegenerative disorders (Sharma et al., 2021a), GPX1 is a gatekeeper restraining the oncogenic power of mitochondrial ROS generated by superoxide dismutase 2 (SOD2) (Ekoue et al., 2017), and the upregulation of the GPX1 activity allows the mitochondrial-defective cells to survive oxidative stress and cisplatin treatment (Lu et al., 2012). In the auditory system, a previous study reported that a single nucleotide polymorphism in GPX1 might be associated with the vulnerability to noise-induced hearing loss (NIHL) among the Chinese Han population (Wen et al., 2014). Kil et al. (2007) have declared that GPX1 is the dominant isoform of GPXs family and is highly expressed in HCs, supporting cells, SGNs, stria vascularis, and spiral ligament in the rat cochlea. Additionally, the mice by knockout of GPX1 are more susceptible to NIHL compared with wild type mice (Ohlemiller et al., 2000; McFadden et al., 2001). Nevertheless, the effect of GPX1 on SGNs damage induced by oxidative stress remains unclear.

Ebselen [2-phenyl-1,2-benzoisoselenazol-3(2H)-one] is a synthetic organoselenium radical scavenger compound that has GPX-like activity, and it can directly increase GPX1 activity to mimic the effect of GPX1 overproduction. Generally, ebselen is capable of reducing oxidative stress levels in various cell types potentially through a variety of mechanisms. It has been demonstrated that ebselen possesses otoprotective activity and alleviated NIHL in rat *via* preventing the loss of outer HCs and reduces the acute swelling of the stria vascularis (Kil et al., 2007), it can also attenuate cisplatin-induced ROS generation through Nrf2 activation in auditory cells (Kim et al., 2009). Besides, a phase 2 clinical trial declared the safety and efficacy of ebselen for the prevention of NIHL in human (Kil et al., 2017). Here, we used ebselen, as a GPX1 mimic, and the *gpx1* knockout ($gpx1^{-/-}$) mice to investigate the role of GPX1 in SGNs treated with peroxynitrite.

In this study, we first identified the expression change of GPX1 in mouse cochlea SGNs through the *in vitro* peroxynitrite-damaged SGNs model, then we investigated the neuroprotective effect of GPX1 against peroxynitrite-induced SGN damage. Finally, we explored the possible underlying mechanism by which GPX1 was involved in protecting SGNs against peroxynitrite damage. Our findings demonstrated that GPX1 protected against peroxynitrite-induced SGNs damage by inhibiting oxidative stress and apoptosis, at least partially, through inhibiting the activation of nuclear factor-kappa B (NF-κ B) pathway.

MATERIALS AND METHODS

Experimental Animals and Genotyping

The C57BL/6 wide type (WT) mice were purchased from the Animal Center of Shandong University (Jinan, China). The *gpx1* knockout mice ($gpx1^{-/-}$) in the C57BL/6 background (KOCMP-14775-Gpx1-B6N-VA) were constructed by Cyagen Biosciences Inc. (Suzhou, China). The genotyping for $gpx1^{-/-}$ mice with PCR was performed according to the Cyagen Biosciences recommendations. The genotyping primers are listed in **Table 1**. All animal experiments were performed according to protocols approved by the Animal Care Committee of Shandong University (No. ECAESDUSM 20123011) and were consistent with the National Institute of Health's Guide for the Care and Use of Laboratory Animals.

TABLE 1 | PCR primer sequences used in the experiments.

Gene	Forward sequence	Reverse sequence
Gpx1-WT	TTACACAATATAAGGGAGCTGTGC	ATACCTGGTGTCCGAACTGATTG
Gpx1-Mut	TTACACAATATAAGGGAGCTGTGC	TTAAGGCACTGAGTAGCAGTGTG
Bax	CGTGGTTGCCCTCTTCTACT	TTGGATCCAGACAAGCAGCC
Bcl-2	TGACTTCTCTCGTCGCTACCG	GTGAAGGGCGTCAGGTGCAG
p53	GGTGCTGACGAAGAAGAGGA	AGCCCAACTGTGATGAAGCA
Bcl-xL	GGAGCTGGTGGTTGACTTTCT	CCGGAAGAGTTCATTCACTAc
Gapdh	AGGTCGGTGTGAACGGATTTG	TGTAGACCATGTAGTTGAGGTCA

Organotypic Culture of Neonatal Mouse Cochleae Spiral Ganglion Neurons and Drug Treatments

The C57BL/6 WT mice or $gpx1^{-/-}$ mice were decapitated at postnatal day (P) 3, and only the middle turn segments of mouse cochleae were collected and cultured for all experiments to keep sampling consistence between groups. The tissue dissection procedure was carried out as described in our previous report (Wang et al., 2019; Liu et al., 2021). Briefly, after cutting off the temporal bones of two sides and removing the cochlear capsule and stria vascularis, the middle turn cochlear explants containing SGNs were then adhered onto 10 mm glass coverslips (Fisher Scientific, PA) pre-coated with CellTak (Corning, 354241). Isolated SGNs explants were cultured in Dulbecco's Modified Eagle Medium/F12 (DMEM/F12, Gibco, 11330032) supplemented with 10% fetal bovine serum (FBS, Gibco, 10099133C) and ampicillin (50 mg/ml, Sigma, A5354) overnight at 37°C in a 5% CO_2 atmosphere.

On the following day, samples were changed into fresh culture media containing peroxynitrite (Cayman, 81565) alone for 24 or 48 h, or with the following drugs for 48 h as indicated in the text: ebselen (30 μM, Sigma-Aldrich, E3520); NAC (2 mM, Sigma-Aldrich, A7250); BAY 11-7082 (10 μM, Med Chem Express, HY-13453). After incubation, samples were used in the immunostaining or other assays.

Cryosection

Cochleae from P3, P14, and P30 C57BL/6 WT mice were dissected out and fixed with 4% paraformaldehyde (PFA) in PBS at 4°C overnight. Tissues were then incubated in 10, 20, and 30% sucrose in 1 × PBS, embedded in OCT compound (Tissue-Tek, Sakura Finetek, 4583), snap frozen on dry ice, and then stored frozen at −80°C. Frozen sections were cut into 7 μm using a cryostat (Leica CM 1850; Leica, Germany).

Immunostaining

After organotypic culture or cryosection, the cochlear explants or tissue sections were fixed with 4% PFA, permeabilized with 1% TritonX-100 in PBS, and blocked by incubation in PBT-1 solution (0.1% Triton X-100, 8% donkey serum, 1% bovine serum albumin, and 0.02% sodium azide in PBS) at room temperature for 1 h. The samples were then incubated with the following primary antibodies: anti-Tuj 1 (1:1,000 dilution; Neuromics, MO15013), anti-GPX1 (1:500 dilution, GeneTex, GTX116040), anti-C-caspase 3 (1:400 dilution, Cell Signaling Technology, 9664), anti-NeuN (1:500, Cell Signaling Technology,12943), anti-4-HNE (1:500 dilution, Abcam, ab48506, United States), or anti-NF-κB p65 (1:500 dilution, Cell Signaling Technology, 6956) diluted in the blocking solution at 4°C overnight. The next day, samples were incubated with FITC-conjugated, TRITC-conjugated, or Cy5-conjugated (1:1000, Invitrogen, United States) secondary antibody along with 4′,6-diamidino-2-phenylindole (DAPI) (1:1000, Sigma-Aldrich, United States) at room temperature for 1 h. Then, coverslips were mounted and the samples were observed under a laser scanning confocal microscope (Leica SP8; Leica, Germany).

Western Blot

After the drug treatment, the proteins from the cultured SGNs were extracted with radioimmunoprecipitation assay buffer (RIPA) buffer (Protein Biotechnology, China). The mixture was centrifuged at 4°C and 12,000 × *g* in a refrigerated centrifuge and the supernatant was collected. A total of 30 μg of each protein sample was denatured and separated by 12% sodium dodecyl sulfate–polyacrylamide gel electrophoresis (SDS-PAGE) gels. The primary antibodies were anti-GPX1 (1:1,000 dilution, GeneTex, GTX116040), anti-C-caspase 3 (1:500 dilution, Cell Signaling Technology, 9664), anti-4-HNE (1:1000, Abcam, ab46545), anti-phosphorylated (p)-NFκB p65 (1:1,000 dilution, Cell Signaling Technology, 3033), and anti-β-actin (1:2,000 dilution, ZSGB-BIO, TA-09). The protein signals were detected using an ECL kit (Millipore, United States) and analyzed by Image J software. The relative optical density ratio was calculated by comparison to β -actin.

Real Time-Polymerase Chain Reaction

After drug treatment for 48 h, total RNA of different groups was isolated from middle turn cochlear explants using TRIzol reagent (Life Technologies, 15596026) following manufacturer's instructions. The cDNA was synthesized from each RNA sample by reverse transcription using the Revert Aid First Strand cDNA Synthesis Kit (Thermo Fisher Scientific, K1622). A SYBR Premix Ex Taq (TaKaRa Bio, RR420A) was used to quantify the mRNA levels of related genes. *Gapdh* was amplified as the housekeeping gene. All data were analyzed using an Eppendorf Realplex 2 and the relative expression levels were calculated using the $2^{-\Delta\Delta CT}$ method. PCR primers for the genes were listed in **Table 1**.

Spiral Ganglion Neuron Counting

The counting of SGNs was performed according to our previous researches (Wang et al., 2019; Liu et al., 2021). Briefly, SGNs were immunolabeled with the Tuj 1 antibody that specifically labels both SGN bodies and neurites. The images of cultured middle turn cochlear explants were taken using a Leica confocal fluorescence microscope. Spiral ganglion neurons in which the nucleus comprised 40% of the soma area were counted using the Image J software and the total number of SGNs in each spiral ganglion explant was obtained by adding the SGN counts in all consecutive sections. The density of SGNs was then calculated per unit area (0.01 mm^2).

Statistical Analysis

All experiments were repeated at least three times and the data were presented as mean ± SEM. Two-tailed, unpaired Student's *t*-tests were used to determine statistical significance in comparisons between two groups. When comparing more than two groups, data were statistically analyzed by one-way ANOVA followed by a Dunnett multiple comparisons test. A value of $p < 0.05$ was considered to indicate a statistically significant result. Scale bars and *n* values are defined in the respective figures and legends and *n* represents the number of independent cochlear samples from each sub-group.

RESULTS

Glutathione Peroxidase 1 Expression Is Decreased in Spiral Ganglion Neurons After Peroxynitrite Injury

First, we characterized the expression of GPX1 in postnatal cochlear SGNs with mice at different ages. Immunofluorescence staining was performed on the frozen cochlear cryosections of P3, P14, and P30 C57BL/6 mouse cochleae (**Figure 1A**), and Tuj 1, a neuron-specific marker which specifically labels both the cytoplasm and neurite of SGN, was used to mark SGN. As the expression pattern of GPX1 was the same in all three turns of cochlea SGNs, the middle turn was presented as the representative sample in **Figure 1B**. The results showed that robust GPX1 labeling was observed in cochlear SGNs of P3, P14, and P30 mice, and it appeared that the expression of GPX1 was mainly in the cytoplasm but not in the nuclei of SGNs (**Figure 1B**).

Next, to determine the neurotoxic effect of peroxynitrite on cultured SGNs, the cultured SGNs were treated with different concentrations (100 or 200 μM) of peroxynitrite for 24 or 48 h, respectively (**Figure 2A**). As shown in **Figure 2B**, after the administration of peroxynitrite, the SGN morphology was disrupted and pyknotic, cells arrangement was disordered, nerve fibers were disordered, broken, or lost. Quantitative analysis showed that the numbers of survived SGNs were reduced significantly in peroxynitrite-treated groups in a dose- and time-dependent manner compared with the control group (**Figure 2B**), that is, the higher concentration of peroxynitrite and the longer processing time induced more SGNs loss. In detail, treatment with 100 μM peroxynitrite for 24 h induced minor SGN loss (75.4 ± 2.49% SGNs survived after treatment) and the higher concentration of 200 μM peroxynitrite treatment for 48 h caused approximately only 32.7 ± 1.84% SGNs survival compared with controls. The treatment of 100 μM peroxynitrite exposure for 48 h resulted in an obvious but moderate SGN loss, as there were 59.3 ± 3.71% SGNs left compared with the control group (**Figure 2B**), and it was selected as the peroxynitrite treatment condition for all subsequent experiments.

Then, the expression change of GPX1 in SGNs was analyzed after peroxynitrite damage. The cultured SGNs were exposed to 100 μM peroxynitrite for 48 h (**Figure 2C**) and immunostaining illustrated that the fluorescence intensity of GPX1 in the peroxynitrite group was significantly reduced compared with that of the control group (**Figure 2D**). Western blot showed that the protein level of GPX1 was significantly decreased in peroxynitrite group compared with the control group (**Figure 2E**). Together, these results indicated that the administration of peroxynitrite caused a reduced expression of GPX1 in cochlear SGNs, thus suggesting that GPX1 might play a role in peroxynitrite-induced SGN damage.

Glutathione Peroxidase 1 Promotes the Survival of Spiral Ganglion Neurons After Peroxynitrite Damage

To clarify the role of GPX1 in the process of SGN injury caused by peroxynitrite, we performed experiments by increasing or inhibiting the expression of GPX1 in SGNs with the GPX1 mimic ebselen or using the $gpx1^{-/-}$ mouse model. Immunofluorescence staining and western blot results verified that GPX1 expression was absent in the cochlear SGNs of $gpx1^{-/-}$ mice (**Supplementary Figures 1A,C**), and there was no significant difference in SGNs number between the $gpx1^{-/-}$ mice and WT mice (**Supplementary Figure 1B**), which indicated that the absence of GPX1 in normal SGNs would not affect the survival of SGNs. Next, we examined the effect of regulating GPX1 expression by ebselen or GPX1 deficiency on peroxynitrite-induced SGNs loss. The cultured SGNs from P3 WT mice were incubated with 100 μM peroxynitrite for 48 h with or without the pretreatment of 30 μM ebselen for 1 h, or the SGNs from $gpx1^{-/-}$ mice were cultured and exposed to 100 μM peroxynitrite for 48 h. The dose of ebselen was chosen according to our published study (Liu et al., 2021), which shows that 30 μM ebselen treatment protects against cisplatin-induced oxidative stress in SGNs. As illustrated in **Figure 3**, the protein expressions of GPX1 were significantly increased in peroxynitrite + ebselen group compared with the peroxynitrite-only group, while it was absent in the peroxynitrite + $gpx1^{-/-}$ group (**Figures 3A–C**). Immunostaining and cell counting results showed that the number of surviving SGNs was significantly increased after the pretreatment with ebselen compared with the peroxynitrite-only group, while remarkably less survived SGNs were detected in $gpx1^{-/-}$ mice group compared with WT mice after peroxynitrite treatment (**Figures 3D,E**). These results suggested that the upregulation of GPX1 promotes, while the deficiency of GPX1 suppresses, the survival of SGNs after peroxynitrite injury.

Glutathione Peroxidase 1 Inhibits Apoptosis of Spiral Ganglion Neurons After Peroxynitrite Injury

The role of GPX1 in regulating the peroxynitrite-induced apoptosis of cochlear SGNs was investigated by immunostaining and western blot. After the drug treatment (**Figure 4A**), cleaved-Caspase3 (C-CASP3) immunostaining results showed that

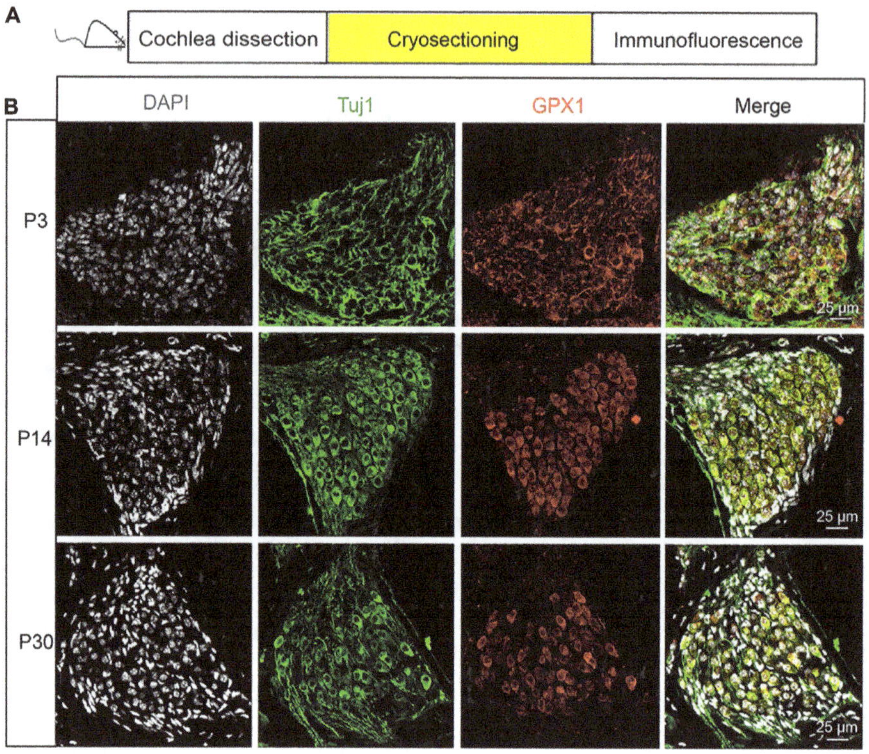

FIGURE 1 | The expression of GPX1 in postnatal cochlear spiral ganglion neurons (SGNs) with mice at different ages. **(A)** Immunofluorescence staining was performed on the frozen cochlear cryosection of P3, P14, and P30 C57BL/6 mouse cochlea. **(B)** Immunostaining images of the middle turn cochlea showed that robust GPX1 labeling was observed in cochlear SGNs of P3, P14, and P30 mice, and it appeared that the expression of GPX1 was mainly in the cytoplasm but not in the nuclei of SGNs. Scale bar = 25 μm.

distinct C-CASP3-positive SGNs were observed in peroxynitrite group, but not in the control group. The number of C-CASP3-positive SGNs was downregulated in the presence of ebselen, while it was further increased in *gpx1*$^{-/-}$ mice compared with the peroxynitrite-only group (**Figure 4B**). Western blot analysis of C-CASP3 protein was consistent with the above results, i.e., the expression level of C-CASP3 was significantly reduced in the peroxynitrite + ebselen group, while it was significantly increased in the peroxynitrite + *gpx1*$^{-/-}$ group compared with the peroxynitrite-only group (**Figure 4C**). Therefore, these results revealed that the Caspase 3-mediated apoptosis was inhibited by ebselen and was aggravated by the lack of GPX1 in SGNs after peroxynitrite injury.

Glutathione Peroxidase 1 Attenuates Peroxynitrite-Induced Oxidative Stress in Spiral Ganglion Neurons

Glutathione peroxidase 1 is known as a major intracellular peroxide-scavenging enzyme to eliminate the damage of ROS to cells, proteins, and liposomes through the reduction of glutathione. In this study, we also investigated the relationship between GPX1 and ROS generation in peroxynitrite damaged SGNs. The cultured SGN explants from WT or *gpx1*$^{-/-}$ mice were exposed to peroxynitrite with or without ebselen pretreatment, and the expression changes of 4-HNE were examined to evaluate the oxidative stress level in SGNs (**Figure 5A**). The results of immunostaining and western blot showed that an obvious increased protein expression of 4-HNE was found in peroxynitrite treated SGNs, while it was significantly decreased in peroxynitrite + ebselen group but further increased in peroxynitrite + *gpx1*$^{-/-}$mice compared with the peroxynitrite-only group (**Figures 5B,C**).

Antioxidant Treatment Rescues the Aggravated Spiral Ganglion Neurons Loss and Apoptosis Induced by Glutathione Peroxidase 1 Deficiency After Peroxynitrite Injury

To explore whether GPX1 plays a protective role in peroxynitrite-induced SGNs damage by reducing intracellular ROS, we conducted a rescue experiment by using the antioxidant N-acetylcysteine (NAC). The cultured SGN explants from WT or *gpx1*$^{-/-}$ mice were treated with peroxynitrite and 2 mM NAC for 48 h (**Figures 6A, 7A**). The dose of NAC was chosen according to our published studies (Liu et al., 2019b, 2021), which show that 2 mM NAC treatment successfully rescues the SGN loss from cisplatin damage. Immunostaining results illustrated that the immunofluorescence of 4-HNE was weaker in the peroxynitrite + NAC group compared

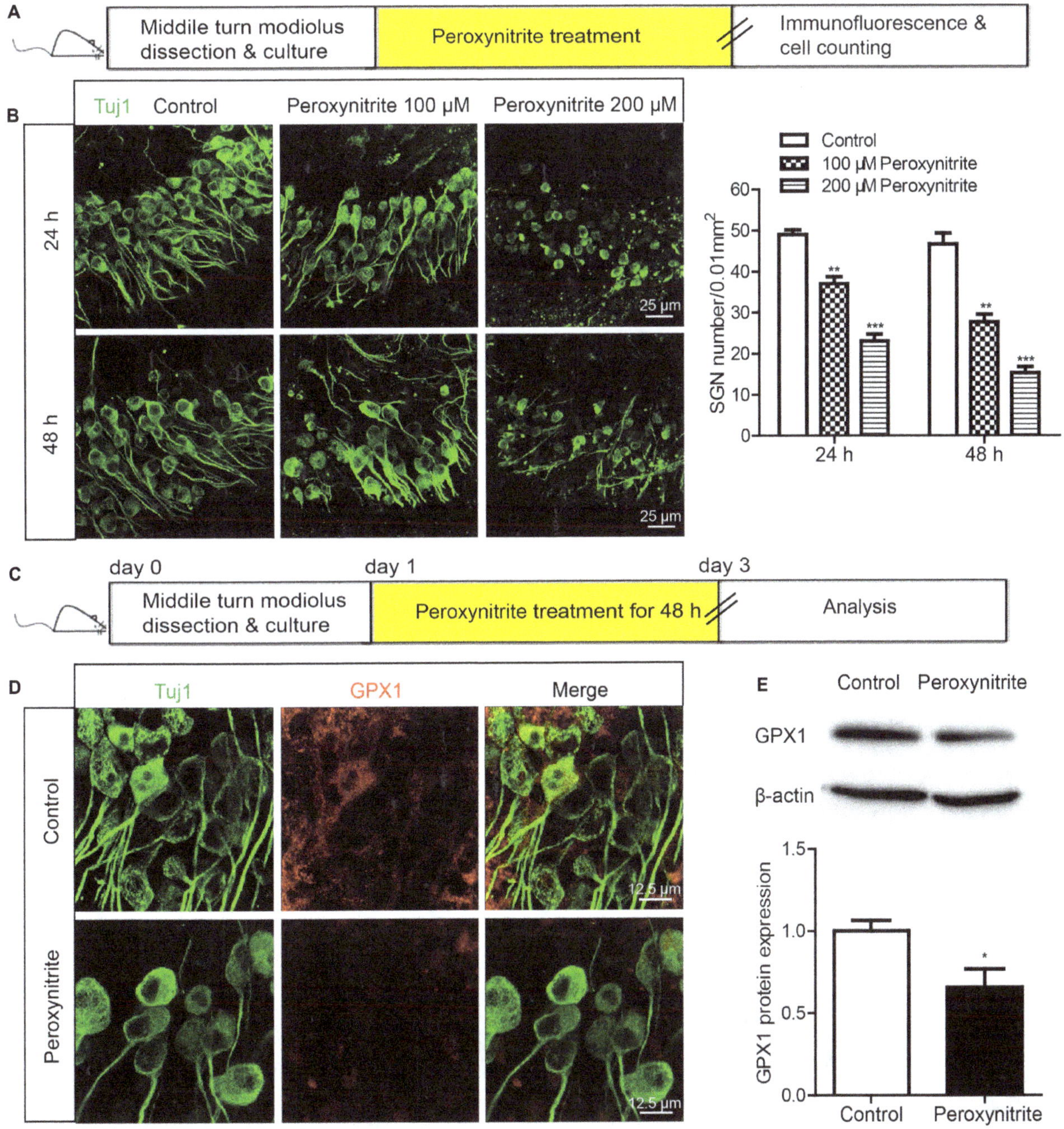

FIGURE 2 | The expression of GPX1 is decreased in cochlear SGNs after peroxynitrite injury. **(A)** The cultured SGNs from WT C57BL/6 mice were treated with different concentrations (100 or 200 μM) of peroxynitrite for 24 or 48 h, respectively. **(B)** Immunostaining images showed that the SGN morphology was disrupted, cells arrangement was disordered, and nerve fibers were disordered or lost after peroxynitrite administration. Quantitative analysis verified that the numbers of survived SGNs were reduced significantly in peroxynitrite-treated groups in a dose- and time-dependent manner compared with the control group. Scale bar = 25 μm. **(C)** The cultured SGNs were exposed to 100 μM peroxynitrite for 48 h. **(D)** Immunostaining illustrated that the fluorescence intensity of GPX1 in peroxynitrite group was significantly reduced compared with control group. Scale bar = 12.5 μm. **(E)** Western blot showed that the protein level of GPX1 was significantly decreased in peroxynitrite group compared with the control group. $^{*}p < 0.05$, $^{**}p < 0.01$, and $^{***}p < 0.001$, $n = 3$ for each group.

with the peroxynitrite-only group, and it was also lower in the peroxynitrite + $gpx1^{-/-}$ + NAC group compared with the peroxynitrite + $gpx1^{-/-}$ group (**Figure 6B**). Western blot and statistical analysis of the protein expression level of 4-HNE were consistent with the immunostaining results (**Figure 6C**). Correspondingly, we found that the NAC treatment largely increased the number of surviving SGNs in the peroxynitrite + NAC group compared with the peroxynitrite-only group, as well as in the peroxynitrite + $gpx1^{-/-}$ + NAC group compared with the peroxynitrite + $gpx1^{-/-}$ group (**Figure 6D**).

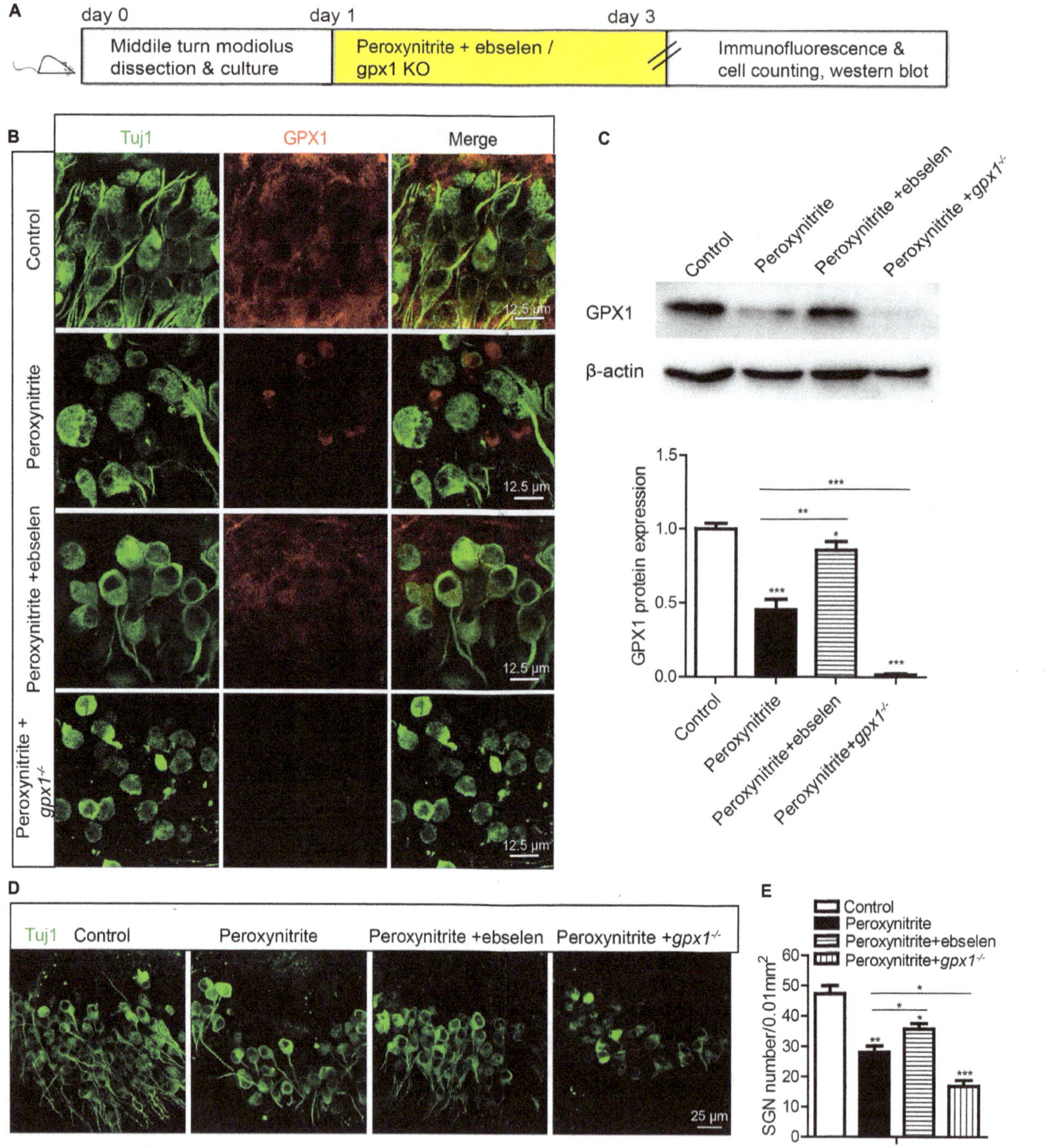

FIGURE 3 | Glutathione peroxidase promotes the survival of SGNs after peroxynitrite damage. The cultured SGNs from P3 WT mice were incubated with 100 μM peroxynitrite for 48 h with or without pretreatment of 30 μM ebselen for 1 h, or the SGNs from $gpx1^{-/-}$ mice were cultured and exposed to 100 μM peroxynitrite for 48 h. **(A–C)** Immunofluorescence staining and western blot results showed that the protein expressions of GPX1 were significantly increased in peroxynitrite + ebselen group compared with the peroxynitrite-only group, while it was absent in the peroxynitrite + $gpx1^{-/-}$ group. Scale bar = 12.5 μm. **(D,E)** Immunostaining and cell counting showed that the number of surviving SGNs was significantly increased after pretreatment with ebselen compared with the peroxynitrite-only group, while remarkably less survived SGNs were detected in $gpx1^{-/-}$ mice group compared with WT mice after peroxynitrite treatment. Scale bar = 25 μm. $^*p < 0.05$, $^{**}p < 0.01$, $^{***}p < 0.001$, and $n = 3$ for each group.

Furthermore, the apoptosis of SGNs detected by C-CASP3 immunostaining and western blot showed that there was much less C-CASP3-positive SGNs and remarkable reduction of the C-CASP3 protein levels in the NAC co-treated groups compared with the peroxynitrite-only groups, and it was also lower in the peroxynitrite + $gpx1^{-/-}$ + NAC group compared

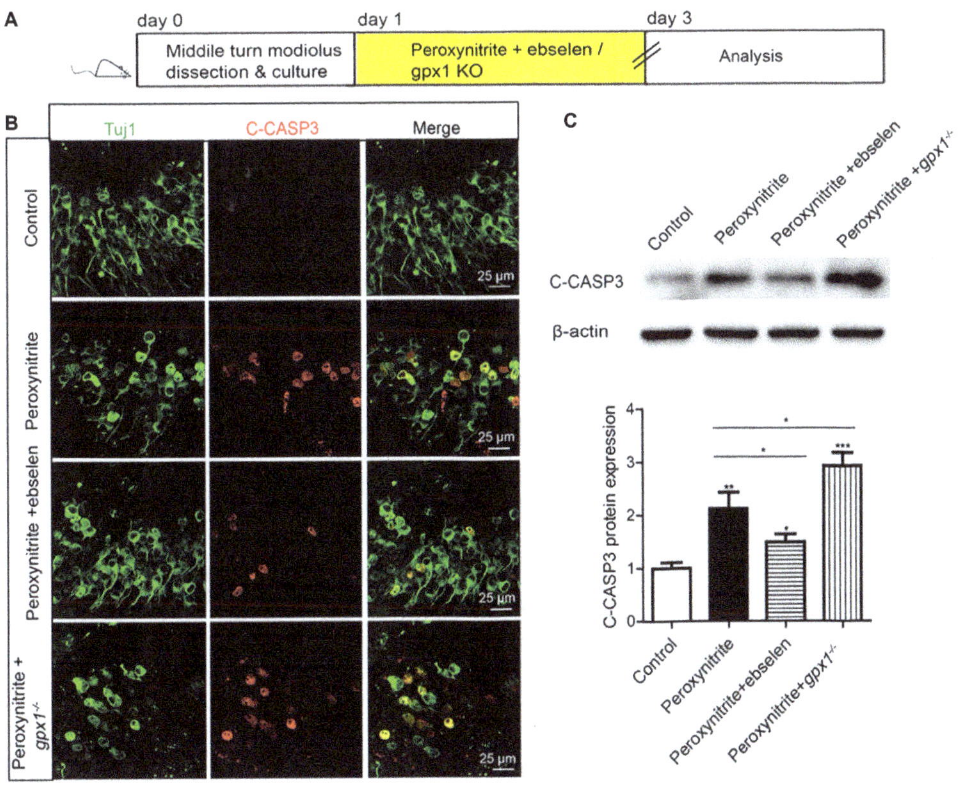

FIGURE 4 | Glutathione peroxidase inhibits the apoptosis of SGNs after peroxynitrite injury. **(A)** The cultured SGNs from P3 WT mice were incubated with 100 μM peroxynitrite for 48 h with or without the pretreatment of 30 μM ebselen for 1 h, or the SGNs from *gpx1*$^{-/-}$ mice were cultured and exposed to 100 μM peroxynitrite for 48 h. **(B)** Immunostaining results showed that distinct C-CASP3-positive SGNs were observed in the peroxynitrite group, but not in the control group. The number of C-CASP3-positive SGNs was downregulated in the presence of ebselen, while it was further increased in *gpx1*$^{-/-}$ mice compared with the peroxynitrite-only group. Scale bar = 25 μm. **(C)** The western blot analysis of C-CASP3 protein verified that the expression level of C-CASP3 was significantly reduced in the peroxynitrite + ebselen group, while it was significantly increased in the peroxynitrite + *gpx1*$^{-/-}$ group compared with the peroxynitrite-only group. $^{*}p < 0.05$, $^{**}p < 0.01$, and $^{***}p < 0.001$, $n = 3$ for each group.

with the peroxynitrite + *gpx1*$^{-/-}$ group (**Figures 7B,C**). Collectively, these findings suggest that the antioxidant NAC treatment successfully rescued the exacerbated ROS generation, SGNs loss, and apoptosis caused by GPX1-deficiency after peroxynitrite damage.

Glutathione Peroxidase 1 Inhibits the NF-κB Pathway to Protect Against Peroxynitrite-Induced Spiral Ganglion Neurons Damage

The transcription factor NF-κB plays a vital role in cellular death and survival under oxidative stress conditions (Li and Karin, 1999), and the activation of NF-κB can promote cell death (Schneider et al., 1999; Zhang et al., 2005). Recently, the correlation between GPX1 and NF-κB pathway has been declared (Koeberle et al., 2020; Sharma et al., 2021b). Therefore, to identify the role of NF-κB and the regulative mechanism between GPX1 and NF-κB in SGNs damage induced by peroxynitrite, we measured the NF-κB pathway in SGNs after peroxynitrite administration with GPX1 upregulation or deficiency (**Figure 8A**). As illustrated in **Figure 8B**, the anti-NeuN antibody was used to label the nucleus of SGN and the fluorescence of NF-κB p65 was mainly detected in the cytoplasm of SGNs in control group (**Figure 8B**). Peroxynitrite induced obvious nuclear distribution of NF-κB p65 in SGNs and pretreatment with ebselen significantly reduced it, whereas the lack of GPX1 intensified the nuclear fluorescence of NF-κB p65 in SGNs of peroxynitrite + *gpx1*$^{-/-}$ group (**Figure 8B**). Furthermore, we found that the expression of the p-NF-κB p65 protein was upregulated in peroxynitrite-exposed SGNs compared with the untreated controls, and the pretreatment with ebselen significantly reduced it while the lack of GPX1 increased it (**Figure 8C**). Besides, to further confirm peroxynitrite-mediated activation of the NF-κB pathway, we also measured the mRNA expression levels of known NF-κB p65 target genes *Bax*, *P53*, *Bcl2*, and *Bcl-xL*. Real time-PCR (RT-PCR) results revealed that peroxynitrite treatment caused significant increases in the mRNA expression of proapoptotic genes *Bax* and *P53*, and decreases in the mRNA expression of antiapoptotic genes *Bcl2* and *Bcl-xL* compared with controls (**Figure 8D**). In addition, the lower mRNA expression levels of *Bax* and *P53* and the higher expression levels of *Bcl2* and *Bcl-xL* were detected in the

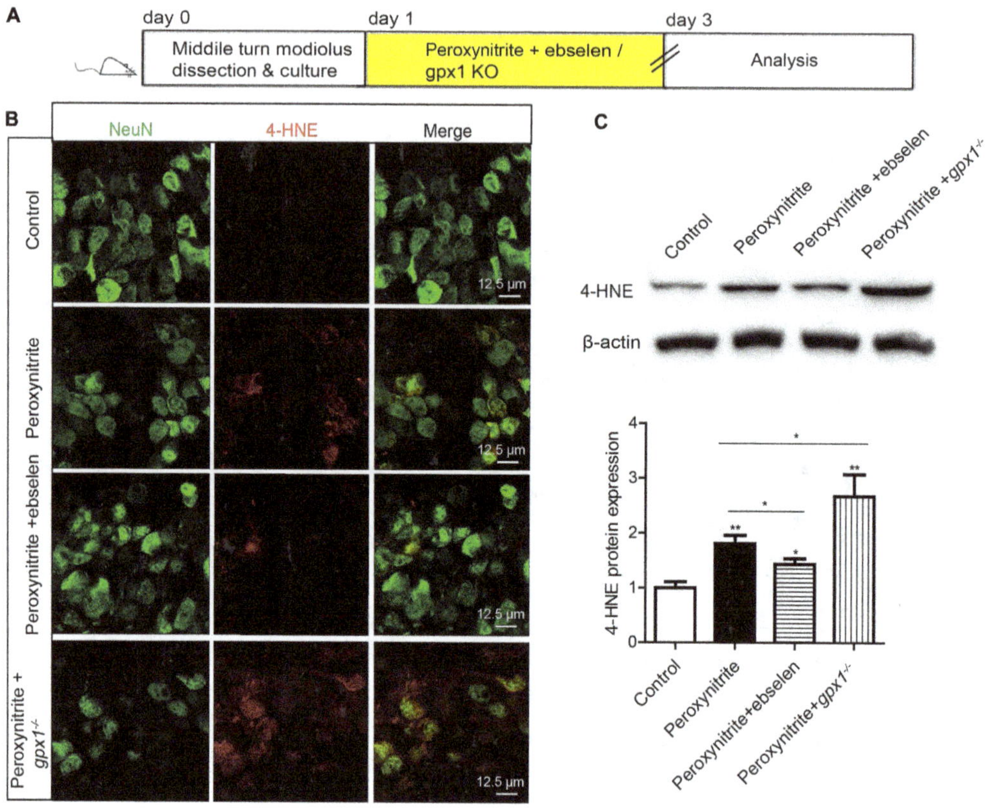

FIGURE 5 | Glutathione peroxidase attenuates peroxynitrite-induced oxidative stress in SGNs. **(A)** The cultured SGNs from P3 WT mice were incubated with 100 μM peroxynitrite for 48 h with or without the pretreatment of 30 μM ebselen for 1 h, or the SGNs from *gpx1*$^{-/-}$ mice were exposed to 100 μM peroxynitrite for 48 h. **(B,C)** Immunostaining and western blot results showed that obvious increased protein expression of 4-HNE was found in peroxynitrite treated SGNs, while it was significantly decreased in the peroxynitrite + ebselen group but further increased in the peroxynitrite + *gpx1*$^{-/-}$ mice compared with the peroxynitrite-only group. Scale bar = 12.5 μm. $^{*}p < 0.05$, and $^{**}p < 0.01$, $n = 3$ for each group.

peroxynitrite + ebselen group compared with the peroxynitrite-only group, while the lack of GPX1 in SGNs from *gpx1*$^{-/-}$ mice led to an opposite pattern (**Figure 8D**). These data, taken together, suggest that the NF-κB pathway is activated in SGNs after peroxynitrite treatment and GPX1 can partially block the nuclear translocation of NF-κB/p65 and inhibit the activation of the NF-κ B signaling.

Next, we used a highly potent NF-κB inhibitor, BAY 11-7082, to further verify the role of NF-κB pathway in SGNs damage induced by peroxynitrite (**Figure 9**). The cultured SGN explants from WT or *gpx1*$^{-/-}$ mice were treated with peroxynitrite and 10 μM BAY 11-7082 for 48 h. The dose of BAY11-7082 was chosen based on our preliminary results of dose response, which showed that 10 μM BAY11-7082 significantly increased the number of surviving SGNs after cisplatin damage *in vitro* (**Supplementary Figure 2**). Our results showed that 10 μM BAY 11-7082 effectively inhibited the nuclear translocation of NF-κB p65 and the mRNA expression of *Bax* and *P53*, but increased the mRNA expression of *Bcl2* and *Bcl-xL* in the peroxynitrite + BAY 11-7082 group compared with the peroxynitrite-only group, as well as in the peroxynitrite + *gpx1*$^{-/-}$ + BAY 11-7082 group compared with the peroxynitrite + *gpx1*$^{-/-}$ group (**Figures 9A–C**). Correspondingly, the inhibition of NF-κB by BAY 11-7082 significantly increased the survived SGN numbers, while decreased the C-CASP3 positive SGN numbers and the C-CASP3 expression in peroxynitrite + BAY 11-7082 group compared with the peroxynitrite group (**Figures 9D–F**). More importantly, BAY 11-7082 treatment also rescued the aggravated SGN loss and apoptosis induced by the deficiency of GPX1 after peroxynitrite injury, as the number of SGNs was added, whereas the C-CASP3 expression was reduced in the peroxynitrite + *gpx1*$^{-/-}$ + BAY 11-7082 group vs. the peroxynitrite + *gpx1*$^{-/-}$ group (**Figures 9D–F**). Therefore, these results indicate that the inhibition of NF-κB pathway contributes to promote SGNs survived from peroxynitrite injury, and that GPX1 protects SGNs against peroxynitrite-induced damage, at least in part, *via* blocking the NF-κB pathway activation.

DISCUSSION

Glutathione peroxidase is a crucial antioxidant enzyme that participate in restraining the harmful accumulation of intracellular hydrogen peroxide and is more effective than catalase at eliminating intracellular peroxides under various physiological conditions (Antunes et al., 2002; Lubos et al., 2011).

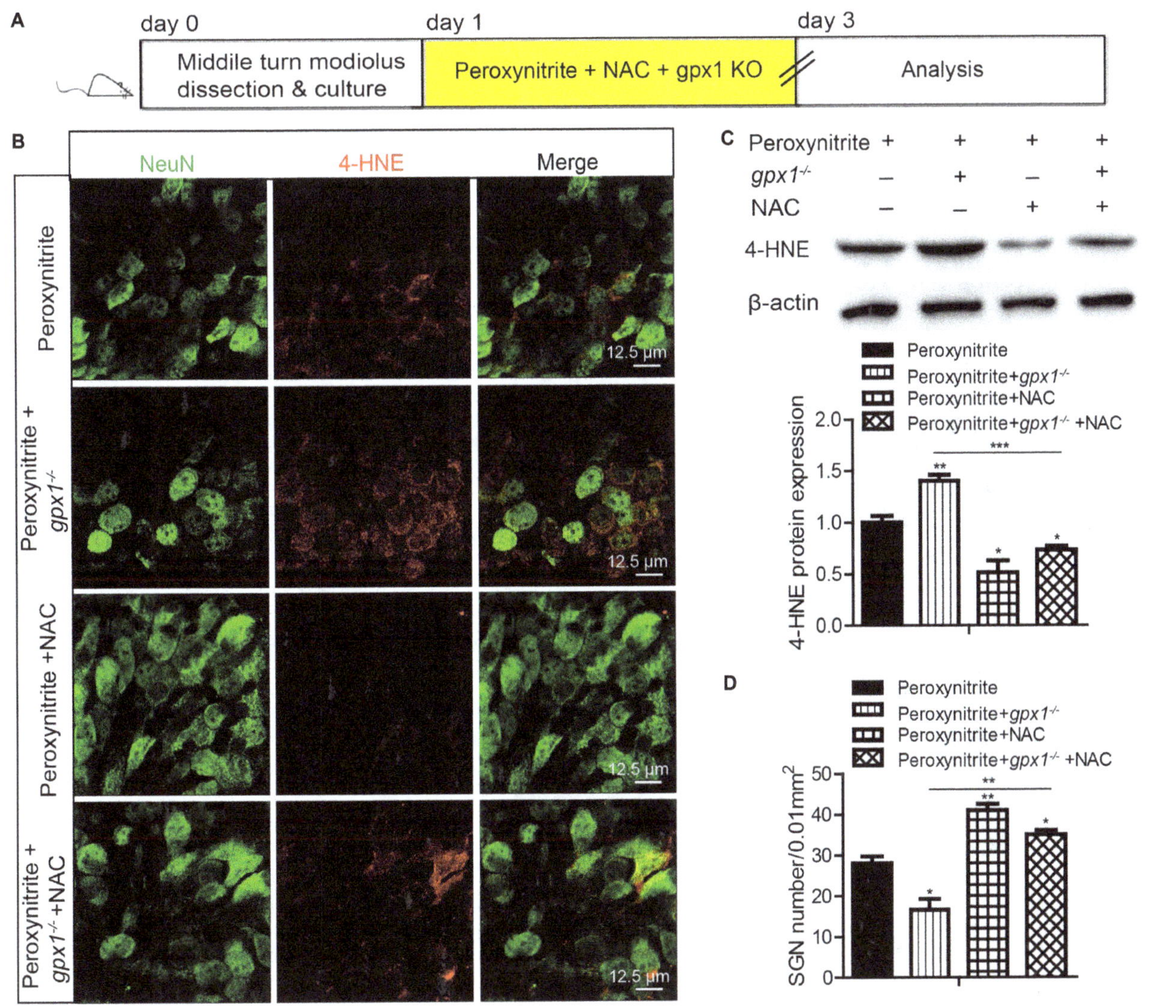

FIGURE 6 | Antioxidant treatment rescues the aggravated SGNs loss and ROS accumulation induced by GPX1 deficiency after peroxynitrite injury. **(A)** The cultured SGNs from WT or *gpx1*$^{-/-}$ mice were treated with peroxynitrite and 2 mM NAC for 48 h. **(B,C)** Immunostaining results illustrated that the immunofluorescence of 4-HNE was weaker in the peroxynitrite + NAC group compared with the peroxynitrite-only group, and it was also lower in the peroxynitrite + *gpx1*$^{-/-}$ + NAC group compared with the peroxynitrite + *gpx1*$^{-/-}$ group. Western blot results verified that the protein expression level of 4-HNE was consistent with the immunostaining results. Scale bar = 12.5 μm. **(D)** Cell counting and statistical analysis showed that the NAC treatment largely increased the number of surviving SGNs in the peroxynitrite + N-acetylcysteine (NAC) group compared with the peroxynitrite-only group, as well as in the peroxynitrite + *gpx1*$^{-/-}$ + NAC group compared with the peroxynitrite + *gpx1*$^{-/-}$ group. $^{*}p < 0.05$, $^{**}p < 0.01$, and $^{***}p < 0.001$, $n = 3$ for each group.

Here, for the first time, we reported that the expression of GPX1, which was observed robustly distributed in SGNs cytoplasm, was significantly reduced after peroxynitrite damage. Our finding is consistent with previous studies indicated that a decrease of GPX1 activity was found in mouse cochlea HCs and stria vascular after noise induced hearing loss (McFadden et al., 2001; Kil et al., 2007), and suggested that the antioxidant enzyme GPX1 might play a role in the oxidative injury of SGNs induced by peroxynitrite.

In the present study, the role of GPX1 in SGNs treated with peroxynitrite was explored *via* using ebselen and GPX1 deficient mice. Ebselen was found to increase the expression of GPX1 in SGNs after peroxynitrite damage, which is consistent with the reports that ebselen can increase the expression of GPX1 in cochlea after electrical stimulation (Liang et al., 2019) and in stria vascularis after noise exposure (Kil et al., 2007). Ebselen effectively promotes SGN survival and prevents SGN apoptosis after peroxynitrite injury by reducing SGNs oxidative stress, while the absence of GPX1 in *gpx1*$^{-/-}$ mice leads to the aggravated SGN injury (cell loss and apoptosis) induced by peroxynitrite, although it might cause no effect on SGN development as SGNs presented normal morphology and cell number in *gpx1*-deficient mice. These results suggest a neuroprotective effect of GPX1 against the peroxynitrite-induced SGN damage. It is

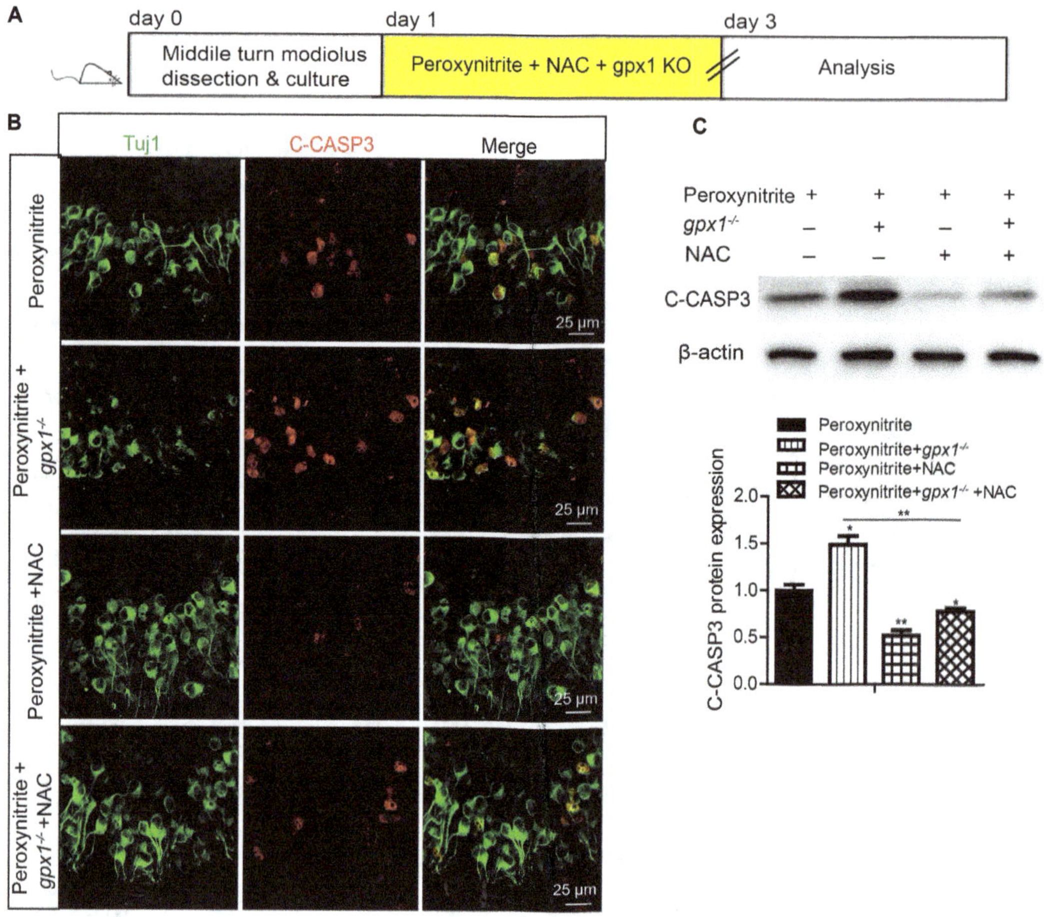

FIGURE 7 | N-acetylcysteine treatment reduced the apoptosis of SGNs in the lacking of GPX1 expression after peroxynitrite injury. **(A)** The cultured SGNs from WT or *gpx1*$^{-/-}$ mice were treated with peroxynitrite and 2 mM NAC for 48 h. **(B)** Immunostaining results illustrated that there was much less C-CASP3-positive SGNs in the peroxynitrite + NAC group compared with the peroxynitrite-only group, as well as in the peroxynitrite + *gpx1*$^{-/-}$ + NAC group compared with the peroxynitrite + *gpx1*$^{-/-}$ group. Scale bar = 12.5 μm. **(C)** Western blot results verified that the protein expression level of C-CASP3 was weaker in the peroxynitrite + NAC group compared with the peroxynitrite-only group, and it was also lower in the peroxynitrite + *gpx1*$^{-/-}$ + NAC group compared with the peroxynitrite + *gpx1*$^{-/-}$ group. $^{*}p < 0.05$, and $^{**}p < 0.01$, $n = 3$ for each group.

important to note that ebselen mimics the activities of all the selenium-dependent mammalian GPXs, not only to GPX1, and has other effects on redox status. Thus, its protective effects overlap those of GPX1. Other types of GPXs have been shown to be expressed in the cochlea, for instance, GPX2 protein is greatly increased in chicken utricle HC expression during HC differentiation (Zhu et al., 2019) and cisplatin injury leads to the decreased GPX2 expression in HEI-OC1 cells (Youn et al., 2017; Jo et al., 2019). It has been reported that GPX3 and GPX4 labeling are absent in the spiral ganglia, while GPX1 is the major isoform of GPXs family that highly expressed in cochlear SGNs in adult rat (Kil et al., 2007). In this study, we also examined the expression of GPX2 and GPX4 in mouse SGNs, and relative low expressions of GPX2 and GPX4 were found in mouse SGNs (**Supplementary Figure 3**). Moreover, ebselen increased the expression of GPX2 and GPX4 in SGNs after peroxynitrite injury (**Supplementary Figure 3**), which is consistent with previous studies that ebselen can increase the expression of GPX2 or GPX4 in rat stomach (Kumar et al., 2010), gastric cancer cells (Xu et al., 2018), or cochlea (Liang et al., 2019). GPX2 and GPX4 serve a distinct function in antioxidant and cellular protection in some tissues that complements that of GPX1 and experimental evidence hints that the expression of GPX2 and GPX4 is less sensitive to variations in selenium levels compared with GPX1 (Lubos et al., 2011). However, to date, studies about the specific function of GPX2 or GPX4 in SGN are still lacking. Our preliminary data suggest that they might also play a part in SGNs against oxidative stress, which is worthy to be investigated in future studies.

With regard to how GPX1 influences the apoptotic outcome, the pieces of evidence indicate that GPX1 may influence several steps in apoptotic cascades *via* regulating oxidant accumulation. For example, one study revealed that an overexpression of GPX1 inhibited the nucleus-translocation of apoptosis-inducing factor (AIF) from mitochondria in

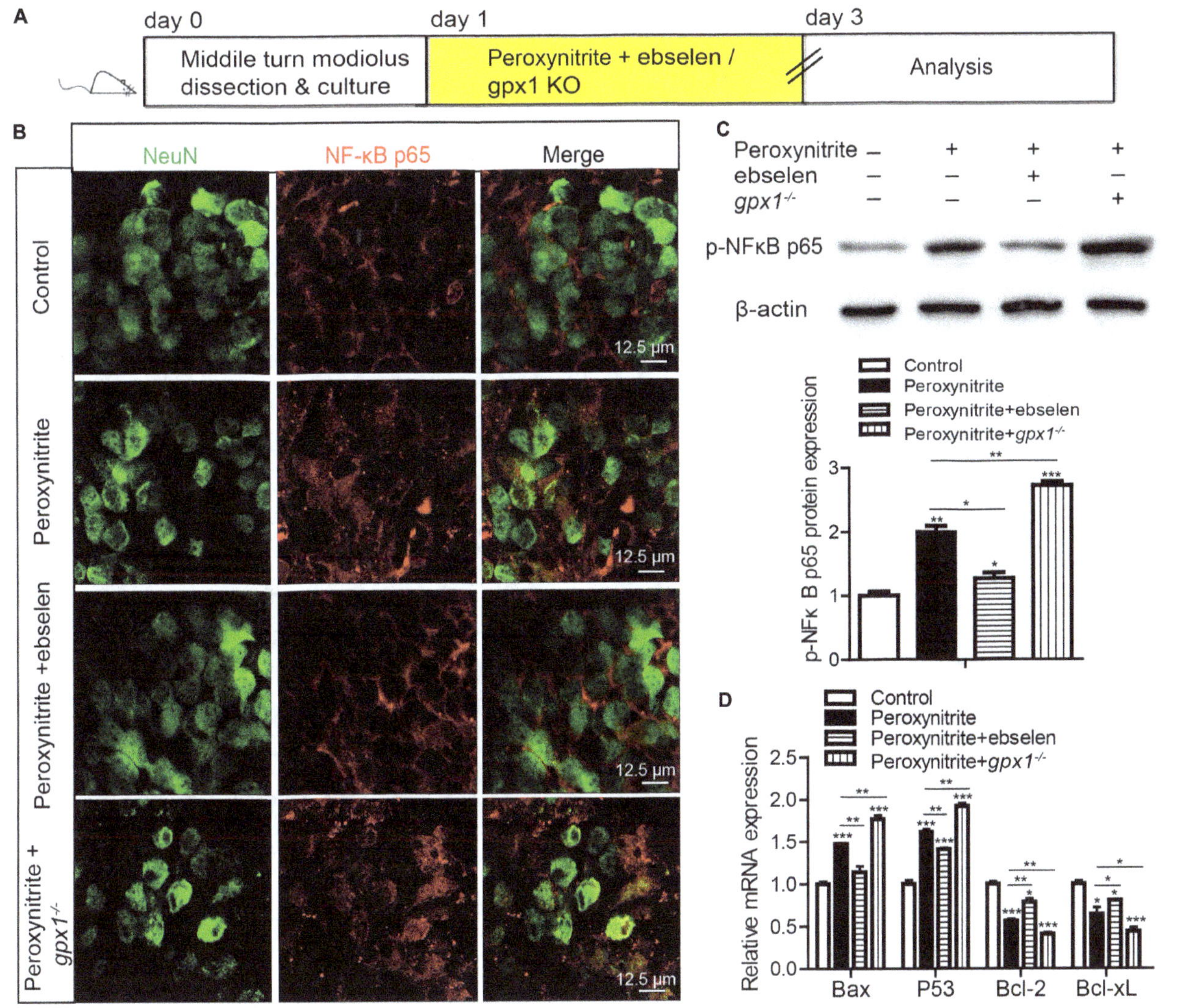

FIGURE 8 | The activated nuclear factor-kappa B (NF-κB) pathway is inhibited by GPX1 in SGNs after peroxynitrite damage. **(A)** The cultured SGNs from P3 WT mice were incubated with 100 μM peroxynitrite for 48 h with or without the pretreatment of 30 μM ebselen for 1 h, or the SGNs from *gpx1*$^{-/-}$ mice were exposed to 100 μM peroxynitrite for 48 h. **(B)** The anti-NeuN antibody was used to label the nucleus of SGN, and the immunostaining results showed that the fluorescence of NF-κB p65 was mainly detected in the cytoplasm of SGNs in the control group. Peroxynitrite induced obvious nuclear distribution of NF-κB p65 in SGNs and pretreatment with ebselen significantly reduced it, whereas the lack of GPX1 intensified the nuclear fluorescence of NF-κB p65 in SGNs of the peroxynitrite + *gpx1*$^{-/-}$ group. Scale bar = 12.5 μm. **(C)** Western blot results verified that the expression of the p-NF-kB p65 protein was upregulated in peroxynitrite-exposed SGNs compared with the untreated controls, and the pretreatment with ebselen significantly reduced it while the lack of GPX1 increased it. **(D)** Real-time PCR (RT-PCR) results revealed that peroxynitrite treatment caused significant increases in the microRNA (mRNA) expression of proapoptotic genes *Bax* and *P53*, and decreased the expression of antiapoptotic genes *Bcl2*, *Bcl-xL* compared with controls. The lower mRNA expression levels of *Bax* and *P53* and the higher expression levels of *Bcl2* and *Bcl-xL* were found in the peroxynitrite + ebselen group compared with the peroxynitrite-only group, while the lack of GPX1 in SGNs from *gpx1*$^{-/-}$ mice led to an opposite pattern. $^{*}p < 0.05$, $^{**}p < 0.01$, and $^{***}p < 0.001$, $n = 3$ for each group.

neuronal cells after ischemia-induced apoptosis (Zemlyak et al., 2009), another analysis showed that GPX1 decreased the ratio of Bax:Bcl-2 to create a more antiapoptotic environment in human endothelial cells (Faucher et al., 2005). It is known that the intrinsic pathway of apoptosis involves the mitochondria release of pro-apoptotic factors, such as AIF or cytochrome c, and these processes can be activated by ROS. Therefore, it is possible that GPX1, as an essential antioxidant enzyme, attenuates AIF release and enhances the expression of Bcl-2 to inhibit cell apoptosis, by reducing ROS level. In the current study, our results suggest that GPX1 protects against peroxynitrite-induced SGNs damage by suppressing ROS accumulation in SGNs. Interestingly, we have reported that intranuclear localization of AIF involves in the peroxynitrite-induced apoptosis of SGNs (Liu et al., 2012), whether GPX1 regulates the intranuclear localization of mitochondrial AIF to alleviate apoptosis in SGNs after peroxynitrite injury deserved further exploration.

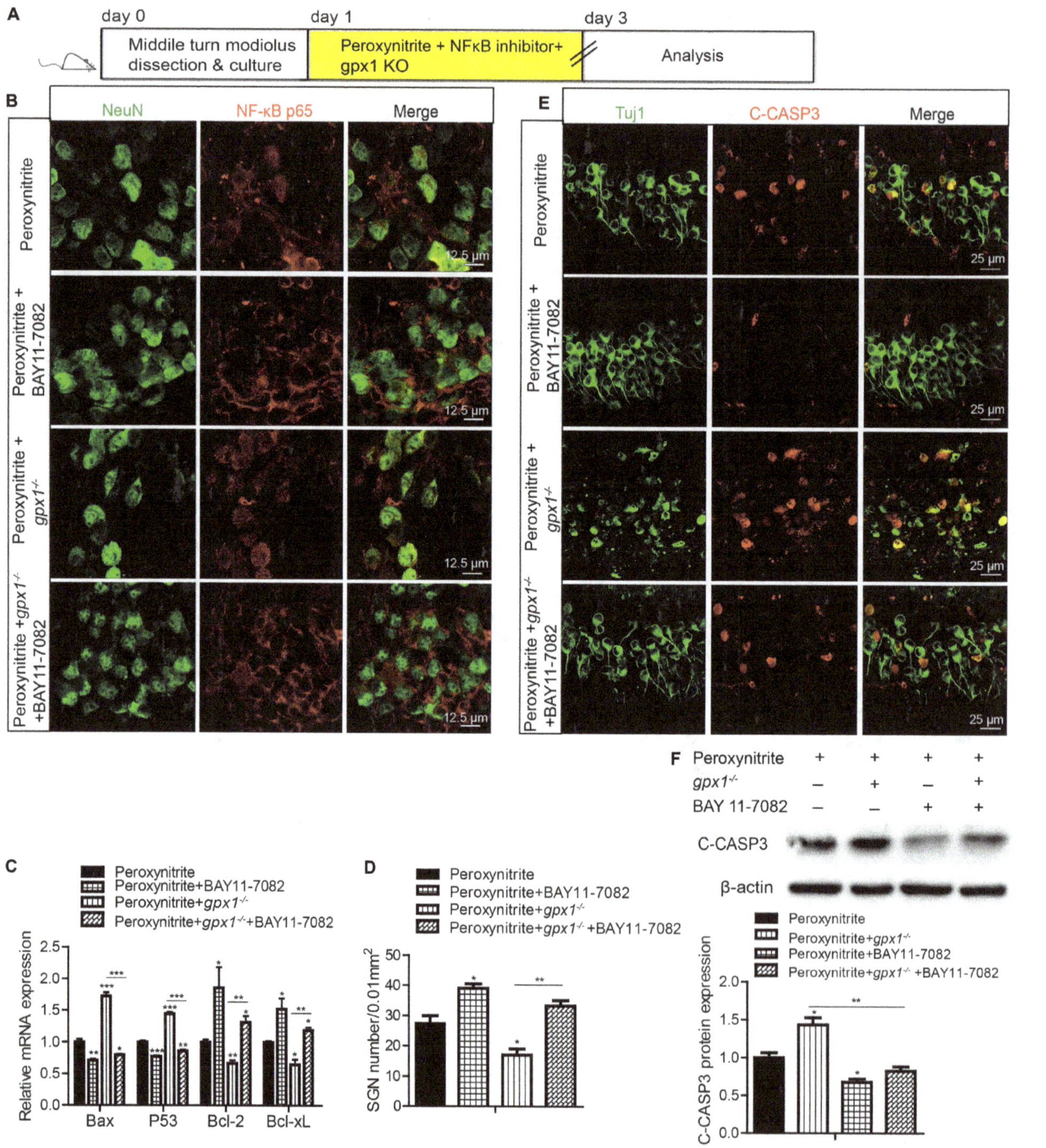

FIGURE 9 | Glutathione peroxidase inhibits the NF-κB pathway to protect against peroxynitrite-induced SGNs damage. **(A)** The cultured SGN explants from WT or *gpx1*$^{-/-}$ mice were treated with peroxynitrite and 10 μM BAY 11-7082 for 48 h. **(B,C)** Immunostaining and RT-PCR results showed that BAY 11-7082 effectively inhibited the nuclear translocation of NF-κB p65 and the mRNA expression of *Bax* and *P53*, but increased the mRNA expression of *Bcl2* and *Bcl-xL*, in the peroxynitrite + BAY 11-7082 group compared with the peroxynitrite-only group, as well as in the peroxynitrite + *gpx1*$^{-/-}$ + BAY 11-7082 group compared with the peroxynitrite + *gpx1*$^{-/-}$ group. Scale bar = 12.5 μm. **(D–F)** Immunostaining, cell counting, and western blot results showed that the inhibition of NF-κB by BAY 11-7082 significantly increased the survived SGN numbers, while decreased the C-CASP3 positive SGNs numbers and the C-CASP3 expression in the peroxynitrite + BAY 11-7082 group compared with the peroxynitrite group. Moreover, BAY 11-7082 treatment also increased the number of SGNs, whereas reduced the C-CASP3 expression in the peroxynitrite + *gpx1*$^{-/-}$ + BAY 11-7082 group vs. the peroxynitrite + *gpx1*$^{-/-}$ group. Scale bar = 25 μm. $^{*}p < 0.05$, $^{**}p < 0.01$, and $^{***}p < 0.001$, $n = 3$ for each group.

Finally, we explored the possible signaling pathways by which GPX1 was involved in protecting SGNs against peroxynitrite-induced injury. It has been shown that GPX1 can alter the activation of NF-κB (Li et al., 2001), modulate Akt pathways (Handy et al., 2009) to affect cellular proliferation and survival, and modify the ratio of Bax:Bcl-2 to create a more antiapoptotic environment (Faucher et al., 2005). NF-κB is known to be a redox-sensitive transcription factor in several cell types and involved in cellular death and survival under oxidative stress conditions (Li and Karin, 1999; Song et al., 2021). In this study, we found that the NF-κB pathway is activated in SGNs after peroxynitrite treatment and that the inhibition of NF-κB pathway contributes to promote SGNs survived from peroxynitrite injury. More importantly, we discovered that GPX1 can partially block the nuclear translocation of NF-κB p65 and inhibit the activation of the NF-κB signaling to protect SGNs against peroxynitrite damage. This observation is interesting that NF-κB activation is considered anti-apoptotic and pro-survival, partially due to augment the expression of IAPs and thus attenuating the activation of caspase. For instance, a study reported that the NF-κB signaling pathway is activated in noise-exposed cochleae to protect against inducible nitric oxide synthase-triggered oxidative stress and apoptosis (Tamura et al., 2016). We speculate the controversial effect of NF-κB pathway activation on inner ear cells, i.e., protecting or damaging cells, might rely on the cell and stimuli types. Furthermore, one possible explanation for the pro-apoptotic effect of NF-κB activation is that in the context of GPX1 deficiency, excess accumulation of cellular ROS might alter NF-κB responses. Evidence showed that excess intracellular hydrogen peroxide regulates the expression of various NF-κB component proteins, and the alterations in the composition or quantity of the NF-κB dimer can change down-stream target gene expression, and conduce to the upregulation of pro-inflammatory genes and a pro-apoptotic environment (Li et al., 2001; Oliveira-Marques et al., 2009; Lubos et al., 2011).

In summary, we investigated the role of GPX1 in protecting SGNs against oxidative stress by upregulating or inhibiting the expression of GPX1 in SGNs *via* the GPX1 mimic ebselen or the *gpx1* knockout mouse model, and further determined the mechanistic details behind the neuroprotective effect of GPX1 in SGNs against peroxynitrite injury. We found that the ebselen could significantly promote SGN survival, decrease SGN apoptosis, and reduce intracellular ROS levels after peroxynitrite exposure *in vitro*, while the deficiency of GPX1 led to opposite patterns of the above effects. Moreover, we showed that the protective mechanism of GPX1 involves inhibiting the activation of NF-κB pathway in SGNs exposed to peroxynitrite. These findings suggest that GPX1 might serve as a novel target for the prevention of oxidative stress-induced SGNs damage and hearing loss.

AUTHOR CONTRIBUTIONS

WL and LX designed and supervised the project. XW, YH, FC, MW, and YX performed the experiments and acquired the data. WL, LX, XW, FC, YX, and HW analyzed the results and performed the statistical analysis. WL, LX, and HW wrote the manuscript. All authors contributed to the article and approved the submitted version.

SUPPLEMENTARY MATERIAL

Supplementary Figure 1 | GPX1 expression was absent in the cochlear SGNs of *gpx1*$^{-/-}$ mice. Immunofluorescence staining and western blot results verified that GPX1 expression was absent in the cochlear SGNs of *gpx1*$^{-/-}$ mice. Cell counting and statistical analysis showed that there was no significant difference in SGNs number between the *gpx1*$^{-/-}$ mice and WT mice. $^{**}p < 0.01$. Scale bar = 12.5 μm.

Supplementary Figure 2 | Dose responses of BAY11-7082 co-treated with peroxynitrite in cultured SGNs. The cultured cochlear SGNs were treated with different doses of BAY11-7082 (5 μM, 10 μM and 20 μM) and co-treated with 100 μM peroxynitrite for 48 h. **(A,B)** Immunostaining and cell counting results showed that co-treatment with 10 μM BAY11-7082 effectively increased the number of surviving SGNs after peroxynitrite damage, while the co-treatment with 5 μM or 20 μM BAY11-7082 showed no significant differences in SGN number compared to the peroxynitrite-only group. All data are presented as the mean ± SEM, $^{*}p < 0.05$, $^{**}p < 0.01$. Scale bars: 25 μm.

Supplementary Figure 3 | Effects of ebselen on expressions of GPX2 and GPX4 in SGNs after peroxynitrite injury. **(A,C)** Immunofluorescence staining was performed on cochlear frozen cryosection to determine the expression of GPX2 and GPX4 in P3 C57BL/6 mouse cochlea. The Immunofluorescence labeling of GPX2 **(A)** and GPX4 **(C)** was observed in cochlear SGNs of P3 mice. Scale bars: 25 μm. **(B,D)**The cultured middle turn cochleae were treated with peroxynitrite (100 μM) alone, or cotreated with ebselen (30 μM) for 48 h. The immunostaining result showed that the fluorescence intensity of GPX2 **(B)** and GPX4 **(D)** in the peroxynitrite group was reduced compared to that of the control group, while it was increased in the peroxynitrite + ebselen group compared with the peroxynitrite-only group. Scale bars: 12.5 μm.

REFERENCES

Antunes, F., Han, D., and Cadenas, E. (2002). Relative contributions of heart mitochondria glutathione peroxidase and catalase to H(2)O(2) detoxification in *in vivo* conditions. *Free Radic. Biol. Med.* 33, 1260–1267. doi: 10.1016/s0891-5849(02)01016-x

Brigelius-Flohé, R. (1999). Tissue-specific functions of individual glutathione peroxidases. *Free Radic. Biol. Med.* 27, 951–965. doi: 10.1016/s0891-5849(99)00173-2

Cao, Z., Yang, Q., Yin, H., Qi, Q., Li, H., Sun, G., et al. (2017). Peroxynitrite induces apoptosis of mouse cochlear hair cells *via* a Caspase-independent pathway in vitro. *Apoptosis* 22, 1419–1430. doi: 10.1007/s10495-017-1417-8

Ekoue, D. N., He, C., Diamond, A. M., and Bonini, M. G. (2017). Manganese superoxide dismutase and glutathione peroxidase-1 contribute to the rise and fall of mitochondrial reactive oxygen species which drive oncogenesis. *Biochim. Biophys. Acta Bioenerg.* 1858, 628–632. doi: 10.1016/j.bbabio.2017.01.006

Faucher, K., Rabinovitch-Chable, H., Cook-Moreau, J., Barrière, G., Sturtz, F., and Rigaud, M. (2005). Overexpression of human GPX1 modifies Bax to Bcl-2 apoptotic ratio in human endothelial cells. *Mol. Cell Biochem.* 277, 81–87. doi: 10.1007/s11010-005-5075-8

Handy, D. E., Lubos, E., Yang, Y., Galbraith, J. D., Kelly, N., Zhang, Y. Y., et al. (2009). Glutathione peroxidase-1 regulates mitochondrial function to modulate redox-dependent cellular responses. *J. Biol. Chem.* 284, 11913–11921. doi: 10.1074/jbc.M900392200

Jo, E. R., Youn, C. K., Jun, Y., and Cho, S. I. (2019). The protective role of ferulic acid against cisplatin-induced ototoxicity. *Int. J. Pediatr. Otorhinolaryngol.* 120, 30–35. doi: 10.1016/j.ijporl.2019.02.001

Kil, J., Lobarinas, E., Spankovich, C., Griffiths, S. K., Antonelli, P. J., Lynch, E. D., et al. (2017). Safety and efficacy of ebselen for the prevention of noise-induced hearing loss: a randomised, double-blind, placebo-controlled, phase 2 trial. *Lancet* 390, 969–979. doi: 10.1016/s0140-6736(17)31791-9

Kil, J., Pierce, C., Tran, H., Gu, R., and Lynch, E. D. (2007). Ebselen treatment reduces noise induced hearing loss *via* the mimicry and induction of glutathione peroxidase. *Hear Res.* 226, 44–51. doi: 10.1016/j.heares.2006.08.006

Kim, S. J., Park, C., Han, A. L., Youn, M. J., Lee, J. H., Kim, Y., et al. (2009). Ebselen attenuates cisplatin-induced ROS generation through Nrf2 activation in auditory cells. *Hear Res.* 251, 70–82. doi: 10.1016/j.heares.2009.03.003

Koeberle, S. C., Gollowitzer, A., Laoukili, J., Kranenburg, O., Werz, O., Koeberle, A., et al. (2020). Distinct and overlapping functions of glutathione peroxidases 1 and 2 in limiting NF-kappaB-driven inflammation through redox-active mechanisms. *Redox. Biol.* 28:101388. doi: 10.1016/j.redox.2019.101388

Korkmaz, A., Oter, S., Seyrek, M., and Topal, T. (2009). Molecular, genetic and epigenetic pathways of peroxynitrite-induced cellular toxicity. *Interdiscip. Toxicol.* 2, 219–228. doi: 10.2478/v10102-009-0020-4

Kumar, B. S., Tiwari, S. K., Saikant, R., Manoj, G., Kunwar, A., Sivaram, G., et al. (2010). Antibacterial and ulcer healing effects of organoselenium compounds in naproxen induced and *Helicobacter* pylori infected Wistar rat model. *J. Trace Elem. Med. Biol.* 24, 263–270. doi: 10.1016/j.jtemb.2010.04.003

Labbe, D., Bloch, W., Schick, B., and Michel, O. (2016). Hearing impairment, cochlear morphology, and peroxynitrite (ONOO(-)) formation in adult and aging NOS II knockout mice. *Acta Otolaryngol.* 136, 991–998. doi: 10.1080/00016489.2016.1183167

Leake, P. A., Akil, O., and Lang, H. (2020). Neurotrophin gene therapy to promote survival of spiral ganglion neurons after deafness. *Hear Res.* 394:107955. doi: 10.1016/j.heares.2020.107955

Li, N., and Karin, M. (1999). Is NF-kappaB the sensor of oxidative stress? *FASEB J.* 13, 1137–1143.

Li, Q., Sanlioglu, S., Li, S., Ritchie, T., Oberley, L., and Engelhardt, J. F. (2001). GPx-1 gene delivery modulates NFkappaB activation following diverse environmental injuries through a specific subunit of the IKK complex. *Antioxid. Redox. Signal.* 3, 415–432. doi: 10.1089/15230860152409068

Liang, Q., Shen, N., Lai, B., Xu, C., Sun, Z., Wang, Z., et al. (2019). Electrical Stimulation Degenerated Cochlear Synapses Through Oxidative Stress in Neonatal Cochlear Explants. *Front. Neurosci.* 13:1073. doi: 10.3389/fnins.2019.01073

Liu, W., Fan, Z., Han, Y., Lu, S., Zhang, D., Bai, X., et al. (2011). Curcumin attenuates peroxynitrite-induced neurotoxicity in spiral ganglion neurons. *Neurotoxicology* 32, 150–157. doi: 10.1016/j.neuro.2010.09.003

Liu, W., Fan, Z., Han, Y., Zhang, D., Li, J., and Wang, H. (2012). Intranuclear localization of apoptosis-inducing factor and endonuclease G involves in peroxynitrite-induced apoptosis of spiral ganglion neurons. *Neurol. Res.* 34, 915–922. doi: 10.1179/1743132812y.0000000098

Liu, W., Wang, X., Wang, M., and Wang, H. (2019a). Protection of Spiral Ganglion Neurons and Prevention of Auditory Neuropathy. *Adv. Exp. Med. Biol.* 1130, 93–107. doi: 10.1007/978-981-13-6123-4_6

Liu, W., Xu, X., Fan, Z., Sun, G., Han, Y., Zhang, D., et al. (2019b). Wnt Signaling Activates TP53-Induced Glycolysis and Apoptosis Regulator and Protects Against Cisplatin-Induced Spiral Ganglion Neuron Damage in the Mouse Cochlea. *Antioxid. Redox. Signal.* 30, 1389–1410. doi: 10.1089/ars.2017.7288

Liu, W., Xu, L., Wang, X., Zhang, D., Sun, G., Wang, M., et al. (2021). PRDX1 activates autophagy *via* the PTEN-AKT signaling pathway to protect against cisplatin-induced spiral ganglion neuron damage. *Autophagy* 17, 4159–4181. doi: 10.1080/15548627.2021.1905466

Lu, W., Chen, Z., Zhang, H., Wang, Y., Luo, Y., and Huang, P. (2012). ZNF143 transcription factor mediates cell survival through upregulation of the GPX1 activity in the mitochondrial respiratory dysfunction. *Cell Death Dis.* 3:e422. doi: 10.1038/cddis.2012.156

Lubos, E., Loscalzo, J., and Handy, D. E. (2011). Glutathione peroxidase-1 in health and disease: from molecular mechanisms to therapeutic opportunities. *Antioxid Redox. Signal.* 15, 1957–1997. doi: 10.1089/ars.2010.3586

McFadden, S. L., Ohlemiller, K. K., Ding, D., Shero, M., and Salvi, R. J. (2001). The Influence of Superoxide Dismutase and Glutathione Peroxidase Deficiencies on Noise-Induced Hearing Loss in Mice. *Noise Health* 3, 49–64.

Ohlemiller, K. K., McFadden, S. L., Ding, D. L., Lear, P. M., and Ho, Y. S. (2000). Targeted mutation of the gene for cellular glutathione peroxidase (Gpx1) increases noise-induced hearing loss in mice. *J. Assoc. Res. Otolaryngol.* 1, 243–254. doi: 10.1007/s101620010043

Oliveira-Marques, V., Marinho, H. S., Cyrne, L., and Antunes, F. (2009). Role of hydrogen peroxide in NF-kappaB activation: from inducer to modulator. *Antioxid Redox. Signal* 11, 2223–2243. doi: 10.1089/ars.2009.2601

Pavlinkova, G. (2020). Molecular Aspects of the Development and Function of Auditory Neurons. *Int. J. Mol. Sci.* 22:131. doi: 10.3390/ijms22010131

Ramdial, K., Franco, M. C., and Estevez, A. G. (2017). Cellular mechanisms of peroxynitrite-induced neuronal death. *Brain Res. Bull.* 133, 4–11. doi: 10.1016/j.brainresbull.2017.05.008

Schneider, A., Martin-Villalba, A., Weih, F., Vogel, J., Wirth, T., and Schwaninger, M. (1999). NF-kappaB is activated and promotes cell death in focal cerebral ischemia. *Nat. Med.* 5, 554–559. doi: 10.1038/8432

Sharma, G., Shin, E. J., Sharma, N., Nah, S. Y., Mai, H. N., Nguyen, B. T., et al. (2021a). Glutathione peroxidase-1 and neuromodulation: Novel potentials of an old enzyme. *Food Chem. Toxicol.* 148:111945. doi: 10.1016/j.fct.2020.111945

Sharma, N., Shin, E. J., Pham, D. T., Sharma, G., Dang, D. K., Duong, C. X., et al. (2021b). GPx-1-encoded adenoviral vector attenuates dopaminergic impairments induced by methamphetamine in GPx-1 knockout mice through modulation of NF-kappaB transcription factor. *Food Chem. Toxicol.* 154:112313. doi: 10.1016/j.fct.2021.112313

Song, Y., Wu, Z., and Zhao, P. (2021). The protective effects of activating Sirt1/NF-κB pathway for neurological disorders. *Rev. Neurosci.* [Epub Online ahead of print] doi: 10.1515/revneuro-2021-0118

Tamura, A., Matsunobu, T., Tamura, R., Kawauchi, S., Sato, S., and Shiotani, A. (2016). Photobiomodulation rescues the cochlea from noise-induced hearing loss *via* upregulating nuclear factor kappaB expression in rats. *Brain Res.* 1646, 467–474. doi: 10.1016/j.brainres.2016.06.031

Wang, M., Han, Y., Wang, X., Liang, S., Bo, C., Zhang, Z., et al. (2021). Characterization of EGR-1 Expression in the Auditory Cortex Following Kanamycin-Induced Hearing Loss in Mice. *J. Mol. Neurosci.* 71, 2260–2274. doi: 10.1007/s12031-021-01791-0

Wang, X., Han, Y., Wang, M., Bo, C., Zhang, Z., Xu, L., et al. (2019). Wnt Signaling Protects against Paclitaxel-Induced Spiral Ganglion Neuron Damage in the Mouse Cochlea In Vitro. *Biomed. Res. Int.* 2019:7878906. doi: 10.1155/2019/7878906

Wen, X., Qiu, C., Li, X., Lin, H., and Huang, Y. (2014). [Association between GPX-1 single nucleotide polymorphisms and susceptibility to noise-induced hearing loss among Chinese Han population]. *Zhonghua Lao Dong Wei Sheng Zhi Ye Bing Za Zhi.* 32, 568–572.

Xiong, M., He, Q., Lai, H., and Wang, J. (2011). Oxidative stress in spiral ganglion cells of pigmented and albino guinea pigs exposed to impulse noise. *Acta Otolaryngol.* 131, 914–920. doi: 10.3109/00016489.2011.577448

Xu, L., Gong, C., Li, G., Wei, J., Wang, T., Meng, W., et al. (2018). Ebselen suppresses inflammation induced by *Helicobacter* pylori lipopolysaccharide *via* the p38 mitogen-activated protein kinase signaling pathway. *Mol. Med. Rep.* 17, 6847–6851. doi: 10.3892/mmr.2018.8641

Yamasoba, T., Lin, F. R., Someya, S., Kashio, A., Sakamoto, T., and Kondo, K. (2013). Current concepts in age-related hearing loss: epidemiology and mechanistic pathways. *Hear Res.* 303, 30–38. doi: 10.1016/j.heares.2013.01.021

Youn, C. K., Jo, E. R., Sim, J. H., and Cho, S. I. (2017). Peanut sprout extract attenuates cisplatin-induced ototoxicity by induction of the Akt/Nrf2-mediated redox pathway. *Int. J. Pediatr. Otorhinolaryngol.* 92, 61–66. doi: 10.1016/j.ijporl.2016.11.004

Zemlyak, I., Brooke, S. M., Singh, M. H., and Sapolsky, R. M. (2009). Effects of overexpression of antioxidants on the release of cytochrome c and apoptosis-inducing factor in the model of ischemia. *Neurosci. Lett.* 453, 182–185. doi: 10.1016/j.neulet.2009.02.020

Zhang, W., Potrovita, I., Tarabin, V., Herrmann, O., Beer, V., Weih, F., et al. (2005). Neuronal activation of NF-kappaB contributes to cell death in cerebral ischemia. *J. Cereb. Blood Flow Metab.* 25, 30–40. doi: 10.1038/sj.jcbfm.9600004

Zhu, Y., Scheibinger, M., Ellwanger, D. C., Krey, J. F., Choi, D., Kelly, R. T., et al. (2019). Single-cell proteomics reveals changes in expression during hair-cell development. *Elife* 8:e50777 doi: 10.7554/eLife.50777

7

The Mechanotransduction Channel and Organic Cation Transporter are Critical for Cisplatin Ototoxicity in Murine Hair Cells

*Jinan Li, Chang Liu, Samuel Kaefer, Mariam Youssef and Bo Zhao**

Department of Otolaryngology-Head and Neck Surgery, Indiana University School of Medicine, Indianapolis, IN, United States

Correspondence:
Bo Zhao
zhaozb@iu.edu

Cisplatin is one of the most widely used chemotherapeutic drugs across the world. However, the serious ototoxic effects, leading to permanent hair cell death and hearing loss, significantly limit the utility of cisplatin. In zebrafish, the functional mechanotransduction channel is required for cisplatin ototoxicity. However, it is still unclear the extent to which the mechanotransduction channel is involved in cisplatin uptake and ototoxicity in mammalian hair cells. Herein, we show that genetically disrupting mechanotransduction in mouse partially protects hair cells from cisplatin-induced hair cell death. Using a fluorescent-dye conjugated cisplatin, we monitored cisplatin uptake in cochlear explants and found that functional mechanotransduction is required for the uptake of cisplatin in murine hair cells. In addition, cimetidine, an inhibitor of the organic cation transporter, also partially protects hair cells from cisplatin ototoxicity. Notably, the otoprotective effects of cimetidine do not require mechanotransduction. These findings suggest that both the mechanotransduction channel and the organic cation transporter are critical for cisplatin ototoxicity in murine hair cells.

Keywords: cisplatin, ototoxicity, mechanotransduction, TMIE, organic cation transporter

INTRODUCTION

Hair cells, the sensory receptors of auditory system, are susceptible to numerous insults such as noise, ototoxic drugs, trauma and aging. Cisplatin is a chemotherapeutic drug widely used to treat various types of cancers, including testicular, ovarian, bladder, head and neck, lung, and cervical cancers. However, patients treated with cisplatin frequently suffer from nausea, vomiting, fatigue, serious kidney problems, tinnitus and hearing loss. The strong ototoxicity of cisplatin, which leads to the permanent hair cell death and irreversible hearing loss in 22–77% of patients, significantly limits its usage in clinics (Knight et al., 2005; Kushner et al., 2006; Coradini et al., 2007; Sheth et al., 2017; Kros and Steyger, 2019; Meijer et al., 2021).

Over the years, the understanding of the ototoxic mechanisms of cisplatin has increased (Sheth et al., 2017; Hazlitt et al., 2018; Kros and Steyger, 2019; Rybak et al., 2019; Prayuenyong et al., 2021). Systemically administrated cisplatin traffics across the blood–labyrinth barrier, enters hair cells predominantly from their apical surface, and remains in the cochlea for months to years (Chu et al., 2016; Breglio et al., 2017). After entry into hair cells, cisplatin induces an accumulation of platinated DNA and reactive oxygen species (ROS), activation of BRAF/MEK/ERK cellular pathway, and ultimately leads to hair cell damage and permanent hearing loss (Sheth et al., 2017; Kros and Steyger, 2019; Ingersoll et al., 2020; Ramkumar et al., 2021). However, the entry routes of cisplatin into hair cells are still not very clear. In cancer cells, copper transport 1 (CTR1) and organic cation transporter 2 (OCT2) have been revealed to mediate cisplatin uptake (Harrach and Ciarimboli, 2015). In HEI-OC1 cells, an auditory cell line derived from the mouse organ of Corti, as well as in neonatal rat cochlear explants, CTR1 and OCT2 mediate cisplatin-induced ototoxicity, suggesting that the influx of cisplatin into hair cells occurs *via* the above two proteins (Ciarimboli et al., 2010; More et al., 2010; Ding et al., 2011). Notably, mice lacking organic cation transporters are insusceptible to cisplatin ototoxicity (Ciarimboli et al., 2010). However, inhibiting CTR1 or OCT2 does not completely protect hair cells from cisplatin-induced hair cell death (Ding et al., 2011), indicating that there are some other proteins involved in cisplatin uptake and ototoxicity. Interestingly, in the lateral line hair cells of zebrafish, functional mechanotransduction but not CTR1 or OCT2 is required for cisplatin-induced hair cell death (Thomas et al., 2013). Several other studies have also indicated a potential role of the mechanotransduction channel in cisplatin ototoxicity (Waissbluth and Daniel, 2013). ORC-13661, a high-affinity permeant blocker of the mechanotransduction channel, protects murine hair cells from cisplatin ototoxicity (Kitcher et al., 2019). In addition, in chicken hair cells, high doses of cisplatin are able to block mechanotransduction currents (Kimitsuki et al., 1993). However, direct evidence of an essential role of mechanotransduction in cisplatin uptake and ototoxicity in murine hair cells is still missing.

The mechanotransduction machinery of hair cells is localized within the stereocilia that protrude from the apical surface of hair cells. The mechanotransduction machinery in hair cells is formed by several distinctive proteins, including transmembrane channel-like 1 and 2 (TMC1/2), LHFPL tetraspan subfamily member 5 protein (LHFPL5; previously named TMHS), transmembrane inner ear protein (TMIE), calcium and integrin-binding family member 2 (CIB2), and tip link proteins (Protocadherin-15 and Cadherin-23) (Siemens et al., 2004; Sollner et al., 2004; Kazmierczak et al., 2007; Kawashima et al., 2011; Xiong et al., 2012; Zhao et al., 2014; Giese et al., 2017; Pan et al., 2018; Pacentine and Nicolson, 2019; Cunningham et al., 2020). Previous studies have found that TMIE is an essential subunit of the mechanotransduction channel defining its pore and gating properties (Zhao et al., 2014; Cunningham et al., 2020). Notably, murine hair cells that lack TMIE have no mechanotransduction currents (Zhao et al., 2014; Cunningham et al., 2020).

In this study, we compared the murine hair cell death caused by cisplatin in wild-type and TMIE-deficient cochlear explants. Furthermore, using commercially available Texas Red-conjugated cisplatin (TR–cisplatin), we investigated the cisplatin uptake in wild-type and TMIE-deficient hair cells. Since OCT2 has been reported to mediate the toxicity of cisplatin in cancer cells and murine hair cells (Harrach and Ciarimboli, 2015), we studied the otoprotective effects of cimetidine on wild-type and TMIE-deficient hair cells. Our results suggest that both the mechanotransduction channel and OCT2 are critical for cisplatin ototoxicity in murine hair cells.

MATERIALS AND METHODS

Animal Models and Animal Care

Tmie$^{-/-}$ mice (MGI: 5784557) have been described previously (Zhao et al., 2014). More than three mice per group, including both male and female mice, were used. All of the animal experiments were carried out in accordance with the National Institutes of Health Guide and were approved by the Institutional Animal Care and Use Committee of Indiana University School of Medicine (IACUC; Protocol #19075).

Cochlear Explants Culture and TR-Cisplatin Uptake Assay

Cochlear explants were dissected from P3 mice and cultured in DMEM/F12 medium (Cat.# 21041025, Life Technologies Corporation) overnight at 37°C in a 5% CO2 humidified atmosphere. Then, the samples were incubated in DMEM/F12 medium containing various concentrations of cisplatin (Cat.# 232120, Millipore Sigma, dissolved in DMEM/F12) for 2 days at 37°C. Cimetidine (Cat.# AAJ6282506, Fisher Scientific) was also dissolved in DMEM/F12 and added to the cochlear explants prior to adding of cisplatin. To monitor the cisplatin uptake in hair cells, the cochlear explants were incubated in DMEM/F12 medium containing 2 μg/mL of TR–cisplatin (Ursa BioScience) for various amounts of time. Stacked images were then captured using a deconvolution microscope (Leica) with a 63 × objective (HCX APO L63X/0.90 Water). The images were then deconvoluted using the blind deconvolution method.

Immunostaining

Immunostaining was performed as described previously (Liu et al., 2018). In brief, the cochlear explants were fixed in 4% PFA for 20 min at room temperature and then washed three times for 5 min each in HBSS. The tectorial membrane was then removed and the samples were blocked in blocking buffer (5% bovine serum albumin and 0.5% Triton X-100 in HBSS solution) for 20 min at room temperature. Then, the samples were incubated with primary antibodies diluted in antibody dilution buffer (1% BSA and 0.1% Triton X-100 in HBSS solution) overnight at 4°C. After being washed with HBSS, the samples were incubated with secondary antibodies for 2 h at room temperature. Then, the samples were mounted in ProLong® Antifade Reagents (Cat.# P36971, Life technologies Corporation). Stacked images were then captured using a deconvolution microscope (Leica) with a 20 × objective (HC PL FLUOTAR 20x/0.55) or a 100 × objective (HCX PL APO 100x/1.40-0.70 OIL). Antibodies used in this study were anti-β2 spectrin (1:200, Cat.# sc-136074, Santa Cruz) and Alexa Fluor 488 goat anti-mouse (1:2,000, Cat.# A11017, Life technologies Corporation).

Data Analysis

At least three different animals, including both genders, were used for each experiment. The precise numbers, sample size, repetitions, and statistical tests are indicated in the figures and figure legends. The Kolmogorov–Smirnov test was used to determine the normality of data distribution. Then two-way ANOVA followed by Bonferroni *post hoc* test or two-tailed unpaired Student's *t*-test was used to determine statistical significance ($^{*}p < 0.05$, $^{**}p < 0.01$, and $^{***}p < 0.001$).

RESULTS

Cisplatin Dose-Dependently Kills Wild-Type Murine Hair Cells

To investigate the extent to which functional mechanotransduction affects cisplatin ototoxicity, we first determined the concentration at which cisplatin effectively kills wild-type hair cells. Mouse cochlear explants dissected from postnatal day 3 (P3) wild-type C57/BL6J mice were cultured overnight and then exposed to cisplatin at a range of concentrations from 0 to 50 μM for 2 days. Then, the samples were fixed and labeled with an antibody against β2-spectrin, a protein highly expressed in cochlear hair cells (Holley and Ashmore, 1990; Scheffer et al., 2015; Liu et al., 2019). Without cisplatin exposure, we observed a highly organized cochlear epithelium with three rows of outer hair cells (OHCs) on the external side of the tunnel of Corti and one row of inner hair cells (IHCs) on the internal side (**Figure 1A**). Cisplatin caused a reliable dose-dependent loss of hair cells (**Figures 1A,B**). The loss of hair cells, mainly OHCs, was observed in the cochlear explants exposed to cisplatin at a concentration as low as 5 μM. Furthermore, we found that 20 μM of cisplatin led to an ~80% reduction of hair cells in the middle region of the cochlea. Cisplatin at a 30 μM or higher concentration killed almost all of the hair cells from the apical to basal regions of the cochlea (**Figures 1A,B**). Consistent with previous findings (Anniko and Sobin, 1986; Cardinaal et al., 2000; Rainey et al., 2016), the OHCs were more sensitive to cisplatin ototoxicity compared to the IHCs (**Figure 1A**). In addition, the hair cells in the basal region were also more susceptible to cisplatin ototoxicity compared to the hair cells in the apical region (**Figures 1A,B**). Due to the tonotopic susceptibility of the hair cells to cisplatin toxicity, in the following studies, we imaged and analyzed the hair cells in the middle region of the cochlear explants.

Abolishing Mechanotransduction Partially Protects Hair Cells From Cisplatin Ototoxicity

We next sought to determine whether murine hair cells lacking mechanotransduction are more resistant to cisplatin ototoxicity. The cochlear explants were dissected from P3 *Tmie* homozygous (*Tmie*$^{-/-}$) mice, which have no mechanotransduction current in their hair cells (Zhao et al., 2014). The samples were then exposed to various concentrations of cisplatin for 2 days. Similar to that in the wild-type hair cells, 20 μM of cisplatin killed ~80% of the hair cells in the *Tmie* heterozygous (*Tmie*$^{\pm}$) cochlear explants. Interestingly, we did not observe any significant hair cell loss in the *Tmie*$^{-/-}$ mice after exposure to 20 μM of cisplatin (**Figures 2A,B**). Notably, there was significant *Tmie*$^{-/-}$ hair cell death after exposure to 30 μM of cisplatin, but much less compared to that of the *Tmie*$^{\pm}$ mice (**Figures 2A,B**). At concentrations of 50 μM or higher, cisplatin killed almost all of the hair cells in both the *Tmie*$^{\pm}$ and *Tmie*$^{-/-}$ (**Figures 2A,B**), suggesting that abolishing mechanotransduction partially protects hair cells from cisplatin ototoxicity.

Abolishing Mechanotransduction Blocks Cisplatin Uptake

Impaired mechanotransduction partially protects hair cells from cisplatin ototoxicity, suggesting that functional mechanotransduction might be critical for cisplatin uptake into murine hair cells. Fluorophore–cisplatin conjugates have been widely used to study the cellular uptake of cisplatin (Thomas et al., 2013; Chu et al., 2016). Thus, wild-type and *Tmie*$^{-/-}$ hair cells were incubated with Texas Red-conjugated cisplatin (TR–cisplatin). Fifteen minutes after the exposure to TR–cisplatin, a robust fluorescent signal was detected in the cell body of the wild-type hair cells, but not in the *Tmie*$^{-/-}$ hair cells (**Figure 3A**). Two hours after the exposure to TR–cisplatin, we still did not detect a fluorescent signal in the cell body of the *Tmie*$^{-/-}$ hair cells (**Figure 3B**), suggesting an essential role of mechanotransduction in cisplatin uptake. A very weak fluorescent signal at the stereociliary region was observed in the *Tmie*$^{-/-}$ hair cells, as well as in the wild-type hair cells (**Figures 3A,B**).

Otoprotective Effects of Cimetidine Do Not Require Mechanotransduction

Although OCT2 is not involved in cisplatin uptake and ototoxicity in zebrafish hair cells (Thomas et al., 2013), it might play a significant role in murine hair cells, as suggested by several studies (Ding et al., 2011). To investigate the extent to which OCT2 is involved in protecting hair cells from cisplatin ototoxicity, wild-type and *Tmie*$^{-/-}$ hair cells were exposed to different concentrations of cisplatin with/without 1 mM cimetidine for 2 days. Cimetidine prevented hair cell death in the wild-type cochlear explants exposed to low concentrations of cisplatin (**Figures 4A,B**). Notably, higher concentrations of cisplatin still efficiently killed wild-type hair cells even in the presence of cimetidine (**Figures 4A,B**). Then, we asked whether the protection effects of cimetidine rely on mechanotransduction. Thus, *Tmie*$^{-/-}$ hair cells were exposed to 50, 70, 100, and 120 μM of cisplatin with/without 1 mM cimetidine for 2 days. Remarkably, cimetidine also protected the *Tmie*$^{-/-}$ hair cells from cisplatin ototoxicity (**Figures 5A,B**), suggesting that the otoprotective effects of cimetidine occur *via* other mechanisms instead of affecting mechanotransduction.

DISCUSSION

Sensorineural hearing loss occurs in 22–77% of patients treated with cisplatin (Knight et al., 2005; Kushner et al., 2006; Coradini et al., 2007; Sheth et al., 2017; Kros and Steyger, 2019). Patients suffering hearing loss nowadays benefit from

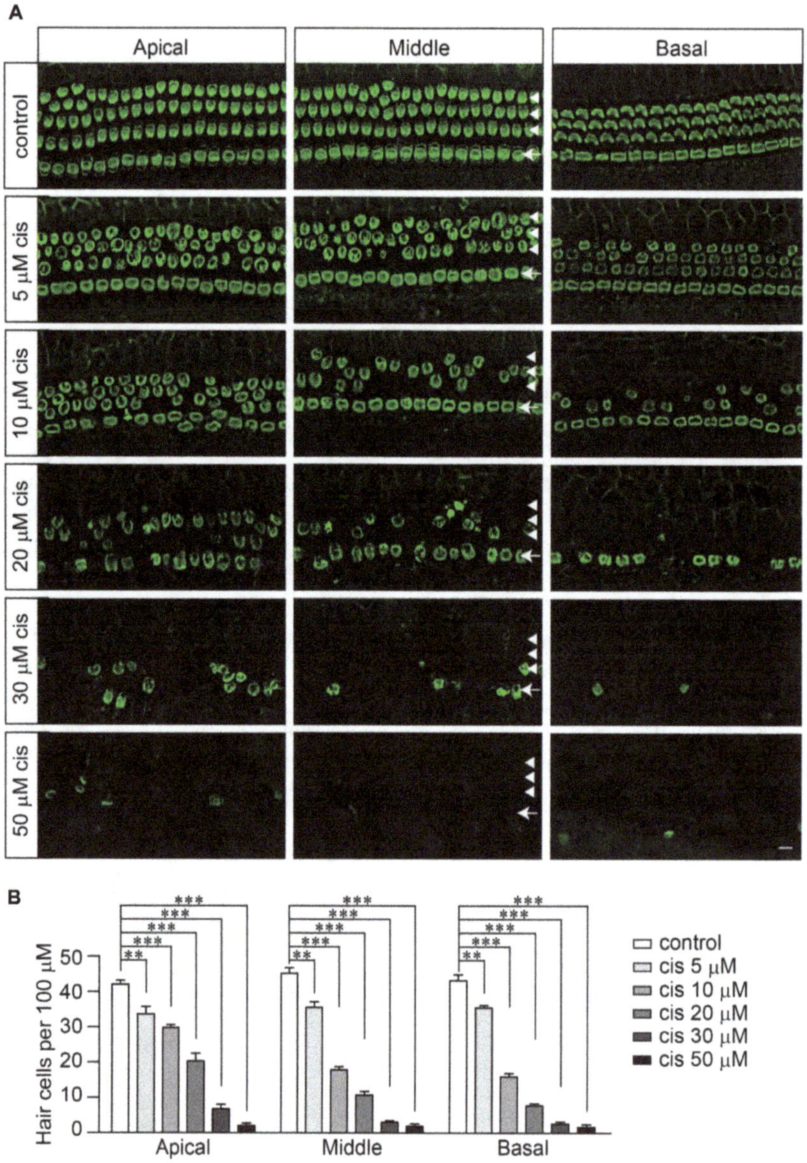

FIGURE 1 | Cisplatin dose-dependently kills wild-type murine hair cells. **(A)** Cochlear explants were dissected from P3 wild-type C57/BL6J mice and cultured overnight in DMEM/F12 culture medium. Then, the cochlear explants were exposed to cisplatin at different concentrations for 2 days. The samples were fixed and labeled with an antibody against β2-spectrin, a hair cell marker. Note, OHCs (arrowheads) were more susceptible to cisplatin than IHCs (arrows). Scale bar: 10 μm. **(B)** Numbers of hair cells per 100 μm (3 mice per group). Data are represented as the mean ± standard error (SE). Two-way ANOVA followed by Bonferroni *post hoc* test was performed ($^{**}p < 0.01$ and $^{***}p < 0.001$).

the use of hearing aids and cochlear implants (Brant et al., 2021). With the upgrade in hearing aids and the improvement in cochlear implant surgery to reduce the discomfort of patients (Freni et al., 2020), outcomes will continue to improve in the future. To restore natural hearing, it will be of interest to study the molecular mechanisms underlying cisplatin ototoxicity. The uptake of cisplatin in murine hair cells is not clear. Taking advantage of *Tmie* mutant mouse, we found that genetic abolishing mechanotransduction in hair cells prevents cisplatin uptake and partially prevents cisplatin-induced hair cell death, suggesting an essential role of the functional mechanotransduction channel in cisplatin uptake and toxicity in murine hair cells. In addition, we also found that cimetidine, an OCT2 inhibitor, protects murine hair cells from cisplatin ototoxicity *via* a mechanism that does not require mechanotransduction in hair cells.

Our results show that functional mechanotransduction is critical for cisplatin uptake in murine hair cells, similar to that in the zebrafish hair cells (Thomas et al., 2013). Cisplatin at high concentrations blocks mechanotransduction current (Kimitsuki et al., 1993). The uptake kinetics of TR–cisplatin and cisplatin in hair cells might be slightly different due

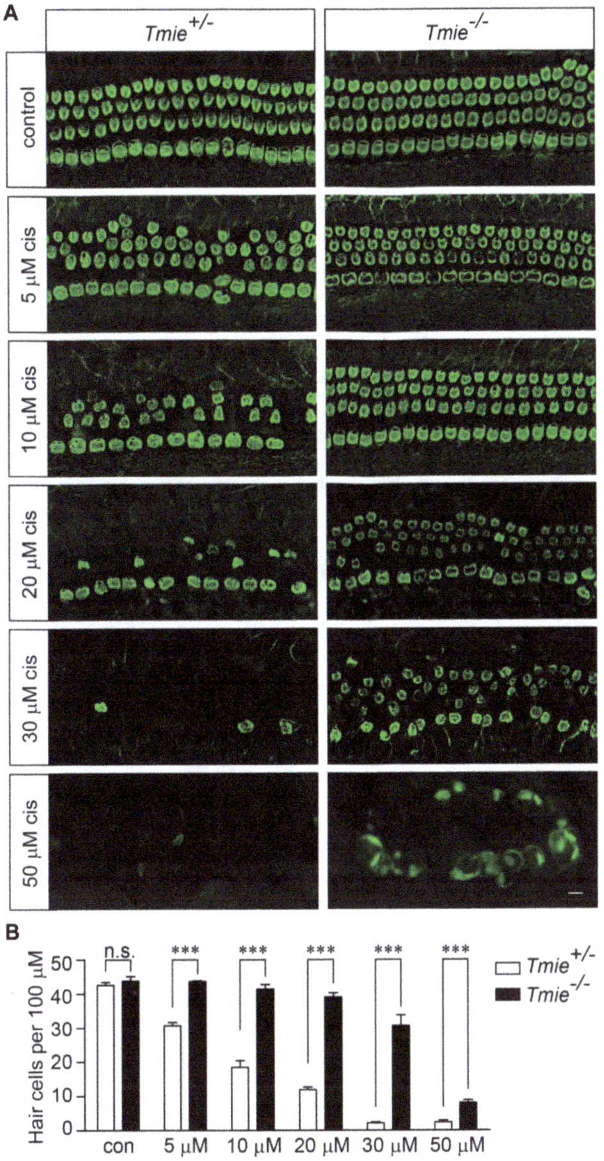

FIGURE 2 | *Tmie* mutant hair cells are more resistant to cisplatin ototoxicity. **(A)** Cochlear explants were dissected from P3 *Tmie*$^{\pm}$ and *Tmie*$^{-/-}$ mice and then exposed to cisplatin at different concentrations for 2 days. The samples were fixed and labeled with an antibody against β2-spectrin. The majority of the *Tmie*$^{-/-}$ hair cells were dead with a few swollen hair cells in the explants, after the exposure to 50 μM of cisplatin for 2 days. Note, the *Tmie*$^{-/-}$ hair cells are more resistant to cisplatin ototoxicity. Scale bar: 10 μm. **(B)** Numbers of hair cells per 100 μm in the middle region of the cochlea (5 mice per group, control; 3 mice per group, 5 μM cisplatin; 7 mice per group, 10 μM cisplatin; 4 mice per group, 20 μM cisplatin; 4 mice per group, 30 μM cisplatin; 3 mice per group, 50 μM cisplatin). Data are represented as the mean ± SE. n.s., not significant; ***$p < 0.001$ by Student's *t*-test.

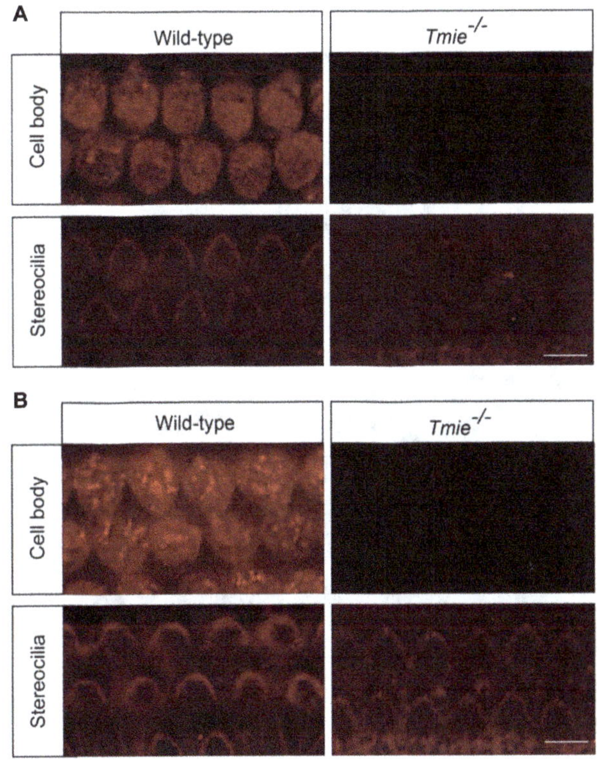

FIGURE 3 | Cisplatin uptake relies on functional mechanotransduction. Cochlear explants dissected from P3 wild-type and *Tmie*$^{-/-}$ mice were incubated with Texas Red-conjugated cisplatin (TR–cisplatin) for 15 min **(A)** or 2 h **(B)**. Note, a robust TR–cisplatin signal was detected in the cell body of the wild-type OHCs. A weak cisplatin signal was detected in the stereocilia in the wild-type and *Tmie*$^{-/-}$ hair cells. Scale bars: 10 μm.

to their different sizes. In our studies, we did not observe a significant TR-cisplatin signal in the cell body of hair cells lacking mechanotransduction, even after a long-term incubation with TR-cisplatin (**Figure 3**). Consistently, abolishing mechanotransduction protects hair cells from cisplatin ototoxicity (**Figure 2**). These results strongly implicate the mechanotransduction channel as being a major entry route of cisplatin into murine hair cells. However, we could not exclude the possibility that cisplatin enters hair cells *via* another channel that is regulated by mechanotransduction (Thomas et al., 2013). It will be important to reconstitute the mechanotransduction machinery in a heterologous system (Zhao and Muller, 2015) and then investigate whether the mechanotransduction channel is responsible for cisplatin uptake. A very weak fluorescent signal at the stereociliary region was observed in the *Tmie*$^{-/-}$ hair cells, as well as in wild-type hair cells (**Figures 3A,B**). Consistently, in zebrafish hair cells with impaired mechanotransduction, a weak cisplatin signal was also detected in the stereociliary region (Thomas et al., 2013). It is possible that some cisplatin entered hair cells *via* another route and was then retained in the stereociliary region. Another possibility is that cisplatin did not cross the cell membrane, but instead bound to the extracellular region of some stereociliary proteins. Unfortunately, the stereocilia are very tiny structures, which makes it extremely difficult to determine the detailed subcellular localization of cisplatin in stereocilia using fluorescent microscopy.

In our studies, we found that cimetidine, an inhibitor of the organic cation transporter, protected *Tmie*$^{-/-}$ hair cells

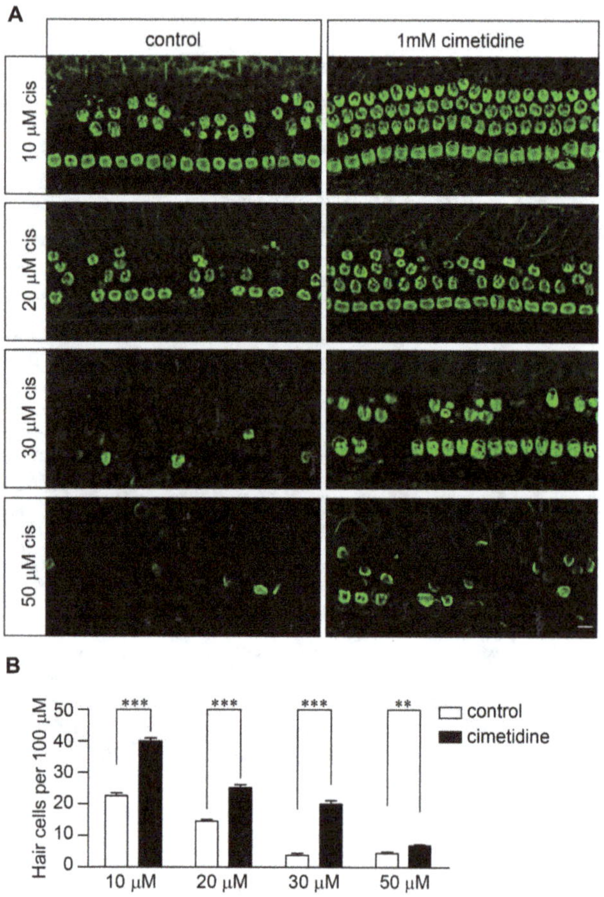

FIGURE 4 | Cimetidine protects wild-type hair cells from cisplatin ototoxicity. **(A)** Cochlear explants were dissected from P3 wild-type mice and then exposed to different concentrations of cisplatin with/without 1 mM cimetidine for 2 days. The samples were then fixed and labeled with an antibody against β2-spectrin. Note, 1 mM cimetidine partially protected hair cells from cisplatin ototoxicity. Scale bar: 10 μm. **(B)** Numbers of hair cells per 100 μm in the middle region of the cochlea (5 mice per group, 10 μM cisplatin; 6 mice per group, 20 μM cisplatin; 3 mice per group, 30 μM cisplatin; 3 mice per group, 50 μM cisplatin). Data are represented as the mean ± SE. $^{**}p < 0.01$ and $^{***}p < 0.001$ by Student's *t*-test.

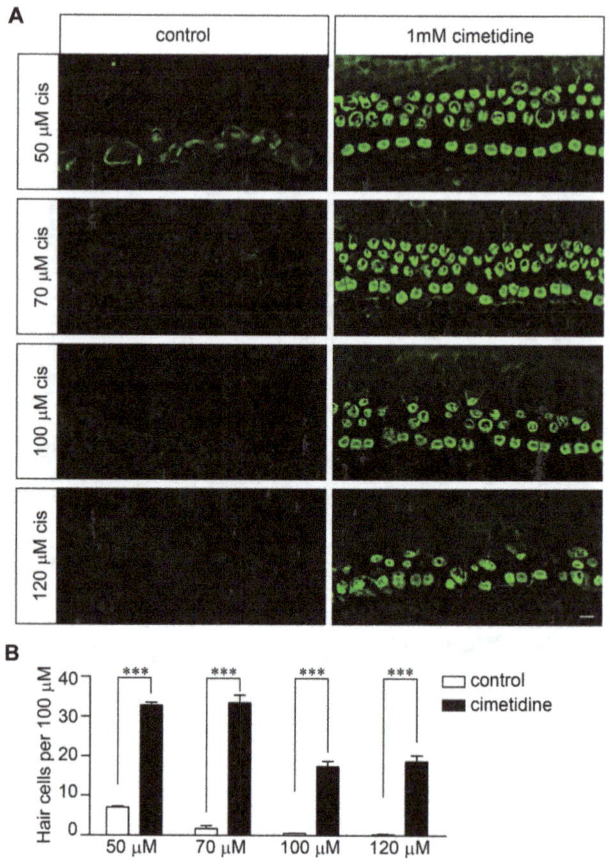

FIGURE 5 | Cimetidine protects $Tmie^{-/-}$ hair cells from cisplatin ototoxicity. **(A)** Cochlear explants were dissected from P3 $Tmie^{-/-}$ mice and then exposed to cisplatin at the indicated doses with/without 1 mM cimetidine for 2 days. The samples were fixed and labeled with an antibody against β2-spectrin. Note, cimetidine protected the *Tmie* mutant hair cells from cisplatin ototoxicity. Scale bar: 10 μm. **(B)** Numbers of hair cells per 100 μm in the middle region of cochlea (5 mice per group, 50 μM cisplatin; 4 mice per group, 70 μM cisplatin; 3 mice per group, 100 μM cisplatin; 3 mice per group, 120 μM cisplatin). Data are represented as the mean ± SE. $^{***}p < 0.001$ by Student's *t*-test.

from cisplatin ototoxicity, suggesting that the otoprotective effects of cimetidine occur *via* other mechanisms instead of affecting mechanotransduction. Interestingly, previous studies found that OCT2 is highly expressed in both IHCs and OHCs in murine inner ear and mice lacking OCT1/2 are insusceptible to cisplatin ototoxicity (Ciarimboli et al., 2010). These results suggest an essential role of OCT2 in cisplatin ototoxicity. Other studies found that cimetidine could also inhibit histamine H2 receptor, which is expressed in the inner ear (Takumida et al., 2016). Thus, it is possible that histamine receptors might also be involved in cisplatin ototoxicity and characterization of mice lacking histamine receptor(s) would be informative. In our studies, we found that blocking both mechanotransduction and OCT2 did not provide complete protection against cisplatin (**Figure 5**), implicating the possibility of additional entry routes of cisplatin into murine hair cells. Thus, it will be of interest to investigate the extent to which other candidates such as TRP channels (Sheth et al., 2017; Jiang et al., 2019) are involved in cisplatin uptake and ototoxicity in murine hair cells.

Mechanotransduction channel is essential for auditory perception. Mutations of TMIE lead to permanent hearing loss in humans and mice (Mitchem et al., 2002; Naz et al., 2002; Zhao et al., 2014). Disrupting mechanotransduction protects hair cells from cisplatin-induced hair cell death (**Figure 2**). Notably, some compounds, such as d-Tubocurarine and Berbamine, could reversibly block the mechanotransduction channel, suggesting that transiently blocking the mechanotransduction channel in hair cells is a potential therapeutic method to prevent cisplatin ototoxicity (Kirkwood et al., 2017).

Besides hair cells, spiral ganglion neurons that innervate hair cells and stria vascularis cells that generate the endocochlear potential are another two major targets of cisplatin in the inner ear (Van Ruijven et al., 2004, 2005; Taukulis et al., 2021). Before entering hair cells, systemically administered cisplatin enters the stria vascularis through the blood-labyrinth barrier (Chu et al., 2016; Breglio et al., 2017; Prayuenyong et al., 2021). Revealed by LacZ staining, the expression level of *Tmie* is low in mouse stria vascularis or spiral ganglion neurons (Zhao et al., 2014). Interestingly, specific OCT2 expression was detected in the stria vascularis cells and spiral ganglion neurons (Ciarimboli et al., 2010; Hellberg et al., 2015), suggesting that OCT2 is a potential target for protecting stria vascularis cells and spiral ganglion neurons against cisplatin ototoxicity.

In summary, we found that both mechanotransduction and the organic cation transporter are critical for cisplatin ototoxicity in murine hair cells. Extensively illustrating the entry routes and ototoxic mechanisms of cisplatin in murine hair cells may lead to the development of novel therapeutic approaches to prevent cisplatin-induced hearing loss.

AUTHOR CONTRIBUTIONS

JL, CL, SK, and BZ: methodology and investigation. MY and JL: counting survived cells. JL, CL, and BZ: writing manuscript. BZ: conceptualization and supervision. All authors contributed to the article and approved the submitted version.

ACKNOWLEDGMENTS

Tmie mutant mice were generated in Ulrich Müller's lab, and we would like to thank Müller for his support.

REFERENCES

Anniko, M., and Sobin, A. (1986). Cisplatin: evaluation of its ototoxic potential. *Am. J. Otolaryngol.* 7, 276–293. doi: 10.1016/s0196-0709(86)80050-3

Brant, J. A., Adewole, D. O., Vitale, F., and Cullen, D. K. (2021). Bioengineering applications for hearing restoration: emerging biologically inspired and biointegrated designs. *Curr. Opin. Biotechnol.* 72, 131–138. doi: 10.1016/j.copbio.2021.11.002

Breglio, A. M., Rusheen, A. E., Shide, E. D., Fernandez, K. A., Spielbauer, K. K., Mclachlin, K. M., et al. (2017). Cisplatin is retained in the cochlea indefinitely following chemotherapy. *Nat. Commun.* 8:1654. doi: 10.1038/s41467-017-01837-1

Cardinaal, R. M., De Groot, J. C., Huizing, E. H., Veldman, J. E,, and Smoorenburg, G. F. (2000). Cisplatin-induced ototoxicity: morphological evidence of spontaneous outer hair cell recovery in albino guinea pigs? *Hear Res.* 144, 147–156. doi: 10.1016/s0378-5955(00)00060-5

Chu, Y. H., Sibrian-Vazquez, M., Escobedo, J. O., Phillips, A. R., Dickey, D. T., Wang, Q., et al. (2016). Systemic Delivery and Biodistribution of Cisplatin in Vivo. *Mol. Pharm.* 13, 2677–2682. doi: 10.1021/acs.molpharmaceut.6b00240

Ciarimboli, G., Deuster, D., Knief, A., Sperling, M., Holtkamp, M., Edemir, B., et al. (2010). Organic cation transporter 2 mediates cisplatin-induced oto- and nephrotoxicity and is a target for protective interventions. *Am. J. Pathol.* 176, 1169–1180. doi: 10.2353/ajpath.2010.090610

Coradini, P. P., Cigana, L., Selistre, S. G., Rosito, L. S., and Brunetto, A. L. (2007). Ototoxicity from cisplatin therapy in childhood cancer. *J. Pediatr. Hematol. Oncol.* 29, 355–360. doi: 10.1097/MPH.0b013e318059c220

Cunningham, C. L., Qiu, X., Wu, Z., Zhao, B., Peng, G., Kim, Y. H., et al. (2020). TMIE Defines Pore and Gating Properties of the Mechanotransduction Channel of Mammalian Cochlear Hair Cells. *Neuron* 107:e128. doi: 10.1016/j.neuron.2020.03.033

Ding, D., He, J., Allman, B. L., Yu, D., Jiang, H., Seigel, G. M., et al. (2011). Cisplatin ototoxicity in rat cochlear organotypic cultures. *Hear Res.* 282, 196–203. doi: 10.1016/j.heares.2011.08.002

Freni, F., Gazia, F., Slavutsky, V., Scherdel, E. P., Nicenboim, L., Posada, R., et al. (2020). Cochlear Implant Surgery: endomeatal Approach versus Posterior Tympanotomy. *Int. J. Environ. Res. Public. Health* 17:4187. doi: 10.3390/ijerph17124187

Giese, A. P. J., Tang, Y. Q., Sinha, G. P., Bowl, M. R., Goldring, A. C., Parker, A., et al. (2017). CIB2 interacts with TMC1 and TMC2 and is essential for mechanotransduction in auditory hair cells. *Nat. Commun.* 8:43. doi: 10.1038/s41467-017-00061-1

Harrach, S., and Ciarimboli, G. (2015). Role of transporters in the distribution of platinum-based drugs. *Front. Pharmacol.* 6:85. doi: 10.3389/fphar.2015.00085

Hazlitt, R. A., Min, J., and Zuo, J. (2018). Progress in the Development of Preventative Drugs for Cisplatin-Induced Hearing Loss. *J. Med. Chem.* 61, 5512–5524. doi: 10.1021/acs.jmedchem.7b01653

Hellberg, V., Gahm, C., Liu, W., Ehrsson, H., Rask-Andersen, H., and Laurell, G. (2015). Immunohistochemical localization of OCT2 in the cochlea of various species. *Laryngoscope* 125, E320–E325.

Holley, M. C., and Ashmore, J. F. (1990). Spectrin, actin and the structure of the cortical lattice in mammalian cochlear outer hair cells. *J. Cell. Sci.* 96, 283–291. doi: 10.1242/jcs.96.2.283

Ingersoll, M. A., Malloy, E. A., Caster, L. E., Holland, E. M., Xu, Z., Zallocchi, M., et al. (2020). BRAF inhibition protects against hearing loss in mice. *Sci. Adv.* 6:eabd0561. doi: 10.1126/sciadv.abd0561

Jiang, M., Li, H., Johnson, A., Karasawa, T., Zhang, Y., Meier, W. B., et al. (2019). Inflammation up-regulates cochlear expression of TRPV1 to potentiate drug-induced hearing loss. *Sci. Adv.* 5:eaaw1836. doi: 10.1126/sciadv.aaw1836

Kawashima, Y., Geleoc, G. S., Kurima, K., Labay, V., Lelli, A., Asai, Y., et al. (2011). Mechanotransduction in mouse inner ear hair cells requires transmembrane channel-like genes. *J. Clin. Invest.* 121, 4796–4809. doi: 10.1172/JCI60405

Kazmierczak, P., Sakaguchi, H., Tokita, J., Wilson-Kubalek, E. M., Milligan, R. A., Muller, U., et al. (2007). Cadherin 23 and protocadherin 15 interact to form tip-link filaments in sensory hair cells. *Nature* 449, 87–91. doi: 10.1038/nature06091

Kimitsuki, T., Nakagawa, T., Hisashi, K., Komune, S., and Komiyama, S. (1993). Cisplatin blocks mechano-electric transducer current in chick cochlear hair cells. *Hear Res.* 71, 64–68. doi: 10.1016/0378-5955(93)90021-r

Kirkwood, N. K., O'reilly, M., Derudas, M., Kenyon, E. J., Huckvale, R., Van Netten, S. M., et al. (2017). d-Tubocurarine and Berbamine: alkaloids That Are Permeant Blockers of the Hair Cell's Mechano-Electrical Transducer Channel and Protect from Aminoglycoside Toxicity. *Front. Cell. Neurosci.* 11:262. doi: 10.3389/fncel.2017.00262

Kitcher, S. R., Kirkwood, N. K., Camci, E. D., Wu, P., Gibson, R. M., Redila, V. A., et al. (2019). ORC-13661 protects sensory hair cells from aminoglycoside and cisplatin ototoxicity. *JCI Insight* 4:e126764. doi: 10.1172/jci.insight.126764

Knight, K. R., Kraemer, D. F., and Neuwelt, E. A. (2005). Ototoxicity in children receiving platinum chemotherapy: underestimating a commonly occurring toxicity that may influence academic and social development. *J. Clin. Oncol.* 23, 8588–8596. doi: 10.1200/JCO.2004.00.5355

Kros, C. J., and Steyger, P. S. (2019). Aminoglycoside- and Cisplatin-Induced Ototoxicity: mechanisms and Otoprotective Strategies. *Cold Spring Harb. Perspect Med.* 9:a033548. doi: 10.1101/cshperspect.a033548

Kushner, B. H., Budnick, A., Kramer, K., Modak, S., and Cheung, N. K. (2006). Ototoxicity from high-dose use of platinum compounds in patients with neuroblastoma. *Cancer* 107, 417–422. doi: 10.1002/cncr.22004

Liu, C., Luo, N., Tung, C. Y., Perrin, B. J., and Zhao, B. (2018). GRXCR2 Regulates Taperin Localization Critical for Stereocilia Morphology and Hearing. *Cell. Rep.* 25, 1268.e–1280.e. doi: 10.1016/j.celrep.2018.09.063

Liu, Y., Qi, J., Chen, X., Tang, M., Chu, C., Zhu, W., et al. (2019). Critical role of spectrin in hearing development and deafness. *Sci. Adv.* 5:eaav7803. doi: 10.1126/sciadv.aav7803

Meijer, A. J. M., Li, K. H., Brooks, B., Clemens, E., Ross, C. J., Rassekh, S. R., et al. (2021). The cumulative incidence of cisplatin-induced hearing loss in young children is higher and develops at an early stage during therapy compared with older children based on 2052 audiological assessments. *Cancer* 128, 169–179. doi: 10.1002/cncr.33848

Mitchem, K. L., Hibbard, E., Beyer, L. A., Bosom, K., Dootz, G. A., Dolan, D. F., et al. (2002). Mutation of the novel gene Tmie results in sensory cell defects in the inner ear of spinner, a mouse model of human hearing loss DFNB6. *Hum. Mol. Genet.* 11, 1887–1898. doi: 10.1093/hmg/11.16.1887

More, S. S., Akil, O., Ianculescu, A. G., Geier, E. G., Lustig, L. R., and Giacomini, K. M. (2010). Role of the copper transporter, CTR1, in platinum-induced ototoxicity. *J. Neurosci.* 30, 9500–9509. doi: 10.1523/JNEUROSCI.1544-10.2010

Naz, S., Giguere, C. M., Kohrman, D. C., Mitchem, K. L., Riazuddin, S., Morell, R. J., et al. (2002). Mutations in a novel gene, TMIE, are associated with hearing loss linked to the DFNB6 locus. *Am. J. Hum. Genet.* 71, 632–636. doi: 10.1086/342193

Pacentine, I. V., and Nicolson, T. (2019). Subunits of the mechano-electrical transduction channel, Tmc1/2b, require Tmie to localize in zebrafish sensory hair cells. *PLoS Genet* 15:e1007635. doi: 10.1371/journal.pgen.1007635

Pan, B., Akyuz, N., Liu, X. P., Asai, Y., Nist-Lund, C., Kurima, K., et al. (2018). TMC1 Forms the Pore of Mechanosensory Transduction Channels in Vertebrate Inner Ear Hair Cells. *Neuron* 99, 736–753.e6. doi: 10.1016/j.neuron.2018.07.033

Prayuenyong, P., Baguley, D. M., Kros, C. J., and Steyger, P. S. (2021). Preferential Cochleotoxicity of Cisplatin. *Front. Neurosci.* 15:695268. doi: 10.3389/fnins.2021.695268

Rainey, R. N., Ng, S. Y., Llamas, J., Van Der Horst, G. T., and Segil, N. (2016). Mutations in Cockayne Syndrome-Associated Genes (Csa and Csb) Predispose to Cisplatin-Induced Hearing Loss in Mice. *J. Neurosci.* 36, 4758–4770. doi: 10.1523/JNEUROSCI.3890-15.2016

Ramkumar, V., Mukherjea, D., Dhukhwa, A., and Rybak, L. P. (2021). Oxidative Stress and Inflammation Caused by Cisplatin Ototoxicity. *Antioxidants* 10:1919. doi: 10.3390/antiox10121919

Rybak, L. P., Mukherjea, D., and Ramkumar, V. (2019). Mechanisms of Cisplatin-Induced Ototoxicity and Prevention. *Semin. Hear* 40, 197–204. doi: 10.1055/s-0039-1684048

Scheffer, D. I., Shen, J., Corey, D. P., and Chen, Z. Y. (2015). Gene Expression by Mouse Inner Ear Hair Cells during Development. *J. Neurosci.* 35, 6366–6380. doi: 10.1523/JNEUROSCI.5126-14.2015

Sheth, S., Mukherjea, D., Rybak, L. P., and Ramkumar, V. (2017). Mechanisms of Cisplatin-Induced Ototoxicity and Otoprotection. *Front. Cell. Neurosci.* 11:338. doi: 10.3389/fncel.2017.00338

Siemens, J., Lillo, C., Dumont, R. A., Reynolds, A., Williams, D. S., Gillespie, P. G., et al. (2004). Cadherin 23 is a component of the tip link in hair-cell stereocilia. *Nature* 428, 950–955. doi: 10.1038/nature02483

Sollner, C., Rauch, G. J., Siemens, J., Geisler, R., Schuster, S. C., Muller, U., et al. (2004). Mutations in cadherin 23 affect tip links in zebrafish sensory hair cells. *Nature* 428, 955–959. doi: 10.1038/nature02484

Takumida, M., Takumida, H., and Anniko, M. (2016). Localization of histamine (H1, H2, H3 and H4) receptors in mouse inner ear. *Acta Otolaryngol.* 136, 537–544. doi: 10.3109/00016489.2015.1136433

Taukulis, I. A., Olszewski, R. T., Korrapati, S., Fernandez, K. A., Boger, E. T., Fitzgerald, T. S., et al. (2021). Single-Cell RNA-Seq of Cisplatin-Treated Adult Stria Vascularis Identifies Cell Type-Specific Regulatory Networks and Novel Therapeutic Gene Targets. *Front. Mol. Neurosci.* 14:718241. doi: 10.3389/fnmol.2021.718241

Thomas, A. J., Hailey, D. W., Stawicki, T. M., Wu, P., Coffin, A. B., Rubel, E. W., et al. (2013). Functional mechanotransduction is required for cisplatin-induced hair cell death in the zebrafish lateral line. *J. Neurosci.* 33, 4405–4414. doi: 10.1523/JNEUROSCI.3940-12.2013

Van Ruijven, M. W., De Groot, J. C., Klis, S. F., and Smoorenburg, G. F. (2005). The cochlear targets of cisplatin: an electrophysiological and morphological time-sequence study. *Hear Res.* 205, 241–248. doi: 10.1016/j.heares.2005.03.023

Van Ruijven, M. W., De Groot, J. C., and Smoorenburg, G. F. (2004). Time sequence of degeneration pattern in the guinea pig cochlea during cisplatin administration. *Hear Res.* 197, 44–54. doi: 10.1016/j.heares.2004.07.014

Waissbluth, S., and Daniel, S. J. (2013). Cisplatin-induced ototoxicity: transporters playing a role in cisplatin toxicity. *Hear Res.* 299, 37–45. doi: 10.1016/j.heares.2013.02.002

Xiong, W., Grillet, N., Elledge, H. M., Wagner, T. F., Zhao, B., Johnson, K. R., et al. (2012). TMHS is an integral component of the mechanotransduction machinery of cochlear hair cells. *Cell* 151, 1283–1295. doi: 10.1016/j.cell.2012.10.041

Zhao, B., and Muller, U. (2015). The elusive mechanotransduction machinery of hair cells. *Curr. Opin. Neurobiol.* 34, 172–179. doi: 10.1016/j.conb.2015.08.006

Zhao, B., Wu, Z., Grillet, N., Yan, L., Xiong, W., Harkins-Perry, S., et al. (2014). TMIE is an essential component of the mechanotransduction machinery of cochlear hair cells. *Neuron* 84, 954–967. doi: 10.1016/j.neuron.2014.10.041

8

Connexin30-Deficiency Causes Mild Hearing Loss with the Reduction of Endocochlear Potential and ATP Release

Junmin Chen [1,2,3†], Penghui Chen [1,2,3†], Baihui He [1,2,3†], Tianyu Gong [1,2,3], Yue Li [1,2,3], Jifang Zhang [1,2,3], Jingrong Lv [1,2,3], Fabio Mammano [4,5], Shule Hou [1,2,3] and Jun Yang [1,2,3*]*

[1]*Department of Otorhinolaryngology—Head & Neck Surgery, Xinhua Hospital, Shanghai Jiaotong University School of Medicine, Shanghai, China,* [2]*Ear Institute, Shanghai Jiaotong University School of Medicine, Shanghai, China,* [3]*Shanghai Key Laboratory of Translational Medicine on Ear and Nose Diseases, Shanghai, China,* [4]*Department of Physics and Astronomy "G. Galilei", University of Padua, Padua, Italy,* [5]*Department of Biomedical Sciences, Institute of Cell Biology and Neurobiology, Italian National Research Council, Monterotondo, Italy*

***Correspondence:**
Shule Hou
houshule8562@xinhuamed.com.cn
Jun Yang
yangjun@xinhuamed.com.cn

†These authors have contributed equally to this work

GJB2 and *GJB6* are adjacent genes encoding connexin 26 (Cx26) and connexin 30 (Cx30), respectively, with overlapping expressions in the inner ear. Both genes are associated with the commonest monogenic hearing disorder, recessive isolated deafness DFNB1. Cx26 plays an important role in auditory development, while the role of Cx30 in hearing remains controversial. Previous studies found that Cx30 knockout mice had severe hearing loss along with a 90% reduction in Cx26, while another Cx30 knockout mouse model showed normal hearing with nearly half of Cx26 preserved. In this study, we used CRISPR/Cas9 technology to establish a new Cx30 knockout mouse model ($Cx30^{-/-}$), which preserves approximately 70% of Cx26. We found that the 1, 3, and 6-month-old $Cx30^{-/-}$ mice showed mild hearing loss at full frequency. Immunofluorescence and HE staining suggested no significant differences in microstructure of the cochlea between $Cx30^{-/-}$ mice and wild-type mice. However, transmission electron microscopy showed slight cavity-like damage in the stria vascularis of $Cx30^{-/-}$ mice. And Cx30 deficiency reduced the production of endocochlear potential (EP) and the release of ATP, which may have induced hearing loss. Taken together, this study showed that lack of Cx30 can lead to hearing loss with an approximately 30% reduction of Cx26 in the present Cx30 knockout model. Hence, Cx30 may play an important rather than redundant role in hearing development.

Keywords: connexin30, hearing loss, connexin26, stria vascularis, endocochlear potential

INTRODUCTION

Hearing loss is a major global health problem, which can be caused by continued excessive noise (Guo et al., 2021), ototoxic drugs (Breglio et al., 2020), aging (Guo et al., 2021), genetic factors (Fu et al., 2021), and infections (Zhang et al., 2021), among which genetic factors caused 50% of the hearing loss. *GJB2* and *GJB6* are two adjacent genes encoding connexin 26 (Cx26) and connexin 30 (Cx30) respectively which form gap junctions (GJs) between supporting cells (SCs) or exist as the hemichannels at the surface of the SCs in the cochlea (Mammano, 2019).

There are two independent GJ networks identified in the inner ear: the epithelial gap junctional network in the organ of Corti and the connective tissue gap junctional network in the cochlear lateral wall (Kikuchi et al., 1995).

Auditory development depends not only on the functional maturation of cochlear hair cells (HCs) but also on the normal differentiation and organization of nonsensory SCs. SCs are coupled through Cx26 and/or Cx30 GJ channels or hemichannels to form a supporting cell network, transmit ATP, ions, signals, and nutrient molecules (Bruzzone et al., 1996; Jagger and Forge, 2015; Verselis, 2019), and the microenvironment of surrounding HCs (Chen et al., 2018). ATP triggers cytosolic Ca^{2+} concentration oscillations and propagation of intercellular Ca^{2+} waves, which appear to play a crucial role in the normal development of the cochlear sensory epithelium, hearing acquisition and the functional maturation of HCs (Johnson et al., 2017; Mammano and Bortolozzi, 2018; Mazzarda et al., 2020). Chai et al. (He et al., 2017; Zhang et al., 2020a,b; Zhang Y. et al., 2020) further confirmed that regenerating HCs cannot achieve functional maturity in the absence of a normal and stable microenvironment by SCs.

GJB2 and *GJB6* mutations account for up to 50% of all nonsyndromic hearing loss cases (Denoyelle et al., 1997; Estivill et al., 1998; Mishra et al., 2018). Homozygous Cx26 and Cx30 deletions lead to severe hearing loss in animal models (Kelsell et al., 1997; del Castillo et al., 2002). It has been reported that Cx26 and Cx30 are both important for hearing development (Adadey et al., 2020). Notably, Cx30 knockout mice displayed severe hearing loss in the absence of endocochlear potential, accompanied by a 90% reduction in Cx26 (Teubner et al., 2003; Boulay et al., 2013). Over-expression of Cx26 in Cx30 knockout mice rescued hearing (Ahmad et al., 2007), but not *vice versa* (Qu et al., 2012). These results indicated that Cx26 is critical for hearing development since it could not be substituted by Cx30 in early cochlear development. Cx30-deficient mice with nearly 50% Cx26 expression showed normal hearing (Boulay et al., 2013). Therefore, the role of Cx30 in the cochlea remains controversial.

In this study, we used CRISPR/Cas9 technology to establish a novel Cx30 knockout mouse model ($Cx30^{-/-}$), which preserved approximately 70% of Cx26 expression in the cochlea and displayed mild hearing loss under full frequency. This new genotype model showed different morphological and functional phenotypes from the past. We believe that this model is of significant importance to explore the mechanism of hearing loss caused by Cx30 deletion.

MATERIALS AND METHODS

Creation and Genotyping of Cx30 Knockout Mice

Cx30 knockout mice ($Cx30^{-/-}$) maintained on a pure C57BL/6 background were purchased from the Shanghai Model Organisms. CRISPR/Cas9 technology was used to repair the mutation introduced by non-homologous recombination, resulting in the shift of the protein reading frame of the *Gjb6* Exon3 gene and loss of function. The mouse genotyping was identified by PCR amplification with the following primers: *Gjb6* primer 1 (P1) 5′-CTAGTGCAACAGCACCCGTA-3′, *Gjb6* P2 5′-CTAGTGCTGAAGGTGTGGGG-3′,*Gjb6* P3 5′-TGGCATTGTTTCACCGTAGT-3′, *Gjb6* P4 5′-AGGTCATGTGAATCTGTCTC-3′, Wild type (WT): *Gjb6* P1 and P2 PCR to obtain a single 2369 bp band; *Gjb6* P3 and P4 can obtain a 512 bp band; Heterozygous (HE): *Gjb6* P1 and P2 PCR to obtain both 527 bp and 2,369 bp bands; *Gjb6* P3 and P4 to obtain 512 bp band; Homozygous (HO): *Gjb6* P1 and P2 PCR obtained a single 527 bp band; *Gjb6* P3 and P4 could not obtain a band. The WT littermates served as controls in the experiment. The experimental procedures were approved by the Shanghai Xinhua Hospital's Animal Center and conducted according to the standards of the NIH Guidelines for the Care and Use of Laboratory Animals.

Assessment of Hearing Loss

Auditory brainstem response (ABR) reflects the electrical response of the cochlear ganglion neurons and the nuclei of the central auditory pathway to sound stimulation. Their threshold assesses the cochlear sensitivity and it is visually measured according to the occurrence of Wave II in a series of repeatable ABR responses obtained at various sound intensities. After 1, 3, and 6-month-old littermates were anesthetized with ketamine (80 mg/kg) and xylazine (10 mg/kg), they were subjected to sudden tones of various frequencies from 4 to 32 kHz (duration of 10 ms, rising -The fall time is 0.5 ms). The sound is generated by Tucker-Davis System II hardware and software (Tucker-Davis Technologies, Alachua, FL).

Quantitative PCR Analyses

Total RNA was extracted from the whole dissected cochlea, the basemental membrane (BM), or the stria vascularis (SV) of postnatal day 5 (P5, where P0 is the date of birth) and 1-month-old mice using the Takara MiniBEST Universal RNA Extraction Kit (Takara, 9767, Japan). Reverse transcription was performed using 1 μg of RNA. Quantitative PCR (qPCR) was conducted on cDNAs using. The primers used are as follows:

Cx30 primers: Forward 5′-AAGACCTGGAGGACATCAAA CG-3′ and

Reverse 5′-CGAAATGAAGCAGTCCACGAG-3′

Cx26 primers: Foward 5′-TCACAGAGCTGTGCTATTTG-3′ and

Reverse 5′-ACTGGTCTTTTGGACTTTCC-3′

Actin primers: Foward 5′-GAGAGGGAAATCGTGCGT GA-3′ and

Reverse 5′-ACATCTGCTGGAAGGTGGAC-3′),

using TB Green® Premix Ex Taq™ (Takara, RR420B, Japan). Samples were analyzed in triplicate on Applied Biosystems 7500 (ThermoFisher). The expression levels of mRNAs were calculated by the $2^{-\Delta\Delta CT}$ method.

Western Blot Analysis

Proteins were extracted from the whole dissected cochlea, the BM, or the SV of P5 and 1-month-old mice. The proteins were separated by SDS-PAGE and transferred to PVDF membranes (Millipore, Billerica, MA, USA). The membranes were blocked with 5% skim milk (Beyotime, Shanghai, China) at room temperature for 1 h and then incubated with primary antibodies against Tublin (Zen Bioscience, 330628, 1:1,000, China), Cx30 antibody (Invitrogen, 71-2800, 1:200, USA), and Cx26 antibody (Invitrogen, 33-5800, 1:200, USA) at 4°C overnight. After three times of washing with PBS-0.01% Tween 20 (PBS-T), the membranes were incubated with a secondary antibody, anti-rabbit IgG, or antimouse IgG (Beyotime; 1:1,000, China), for 2 h at 37°C. After washing the membranes, and adding freshly prepared chemiluminescence solution (Millipore; A:B = 1:1), the immunoreactive bands were imaged under the Bio-Rad ChemiDoc XRS+ (Bio-Rad Co., Hercules, CA, USA). Semiquantitative densitometric analysis was performed with ImageJ software.

Immunohistochemistry and Confocal Imaging

Cochleas of P5 and 1-month-old mice were fixed with 4% paraformaldehyde, decalcified, frozen, and cut by a cryostat. The tissue sections were directly mounted onto glass slides for staining and storage. The cochlear section was incubated in a blocking solution (10% goat serum and 1% BSA in the PBS) with 0.1% Triton X-100 for 1 h at room temperature. Then, the section was incubated with rabbit anti-Cx30 antibody (Invitrogen, 71-2800, 1:200, USA), the rabbit anti-Cx26 antibody (Invitrogen, 51-2800, 1:200, USA), or the mouse anti-Cx26 antibody (Invitrogen, 33-5800, 1:200, USA) in the blocking solution at 4°C overnight, following reaction with corresponding Alexa Fluor 488-, 458- or 647- secondary antibodies (Invitrogen, 1:500, USA) for 2 h at room temperature (23°C). The sections were further stained by 1% 40, 6-diamidino-2-phenylindole (DAPI, Invitrogen, 1:200, USA) for ~10 min or AlexaFluor 568 phalloidin (Servicebio, G1041, 1:500) for ~15 min following the 2nd antibody incubation to visualize cell nuclei or F-Actin. After washout, the sections were mounted and observed under a microscope.

ATP Release Measurement

The P5 mouse temporal bone was micro-dissected in ice-cold HBSS (Thermo Fisher Scientific). The inner ear was opened from its apex to base. After removal of the bone, the exposed BM and SV were dissected separately and put into an incubation chamber. For testing ATP release, the isolated BM and SV was incubated in a zero Ca^{2+} solution (ZCS) containing (in mM): 137 NaCl, 5.36 KCl, 0.44 KH2PO4, 0.18 Na2HPO4, 0.1 EGTA, 25 HEPES, and 5.55 Dextrose (pH 7.3). To quantify ATP release, the BM and SV were incubated in ZCS for 20 min at 37°C, 5% CO2. The collected incubation solutions were kept on ice. The amount of ATP was measured by a bioluminescence method with a luciferin-luciferase assay kit (FL-ASC, Sigma, USA) using a black 96-well plate to avoid optical cross-talk. The bioluminescence was read by a Biotek Synergy 4 Hybrid Microplate Reader (Biotek Instruments Inc, Winooski, VT, USA). All bioluminescence measurements reported in this article fell within the linearity range of the ATP standard curve generated according to the manufacturer's instructions.

Measurement of Endocochlear Potential

The endocochlear potential was recorded under general anesthesia on $Cx30^{-/-}$ (n = 6) mice and Wt (n = 6) mice at 1-month-old. Mice were anesthetized with ketamine (150 mg/kg, IP) and xylazine (6 mg/kg, IP). Body temperature was maintained at 37°C on a heating operating table (Harvard Apparatus, 73-3771). A mouse head holding adaptor (MA-6N, Narishige, Tokyo, Japan) was used to maintain a supine position. A tracheotomy was performed, followed by opening the auditory bulla through a ventral approach to expose the basal turn of the cochlea. A silver chloride reference electrode was placed under the skin. Access to the scala media of the basal turn was obtained by thinning the bone over the spiral ligament and making a small opening with a pick. A micropipette electrode (~2 μm) filled with 150 mM KCl was advanced through the bony aperture into the spiral ligament. Entry of the electrode tip into the endolymph is characterized by transients in recorded potentials. The electrode was advanced until a stable potential was observed. The signal was amplified through a patch-Clamp Amplifier (HEKA EPC 10 USB double, Germany). The DC potentials were recorded *via* an A-D converter (HEKA EPC 10 USB PROBE 1, Germany).

Transmission Electron Microscope Observation

After the cochlea of P5 mice was dissected, it was fixed in 2.5% glutaraldehyde for 24 h and decalcified with 10% EDTA for several days. The samples were fixed in 1% osmic acid for 2 h, dehydrated with acetone, and embedded in 812 resin. After staining the ultrathin sections with alkaline lead citrate and uranyl acetate, the structure of each cochlea under a Hitachi HF5000 transmission electron microscope (Hitachi, Tokyo, Japan) was observed.

Statistics

Several statistical methods were used to analyze the data. The Kolmogorov-Smirnov test was used to analyze the normality of the distribution. The Student t-test compared statistical means. The Mann-Whitney U test was used for non-normal distributions or distributions with different variances. All statistical analyses were performed using SPSS v19.0 (SPSS Inc. Chicago, IL). Mean values are quoted ± standard error of the mean (s.e.m.) where $p < 0.05$ was assumed as statistically significant.

RESULTS

Deletion of Cx30 in the Cochlea

In our model, CRISPR/Cas9 technology was used to repair the mutation introduced by non-homologous recombination, resulting in a shift of the protein reading frame of the *Gjb6* exon 3 gene and loss of function (**Figures 1A,B**). To test for Cx30 inactivation, we measured Cx30 expression in the inner ear by qPCR (**Figure 1C**). As expected, no Cx30 transcript was detected in $Cx30^{-/-}$ mice, whereas $Cx30^{+/-}$ mice displayed a 57.6% reduction in expression of Cx30 mRNA compared to $Cx30^{+/+}$ (WT) control mice. Consistent with the mRNA results, Western

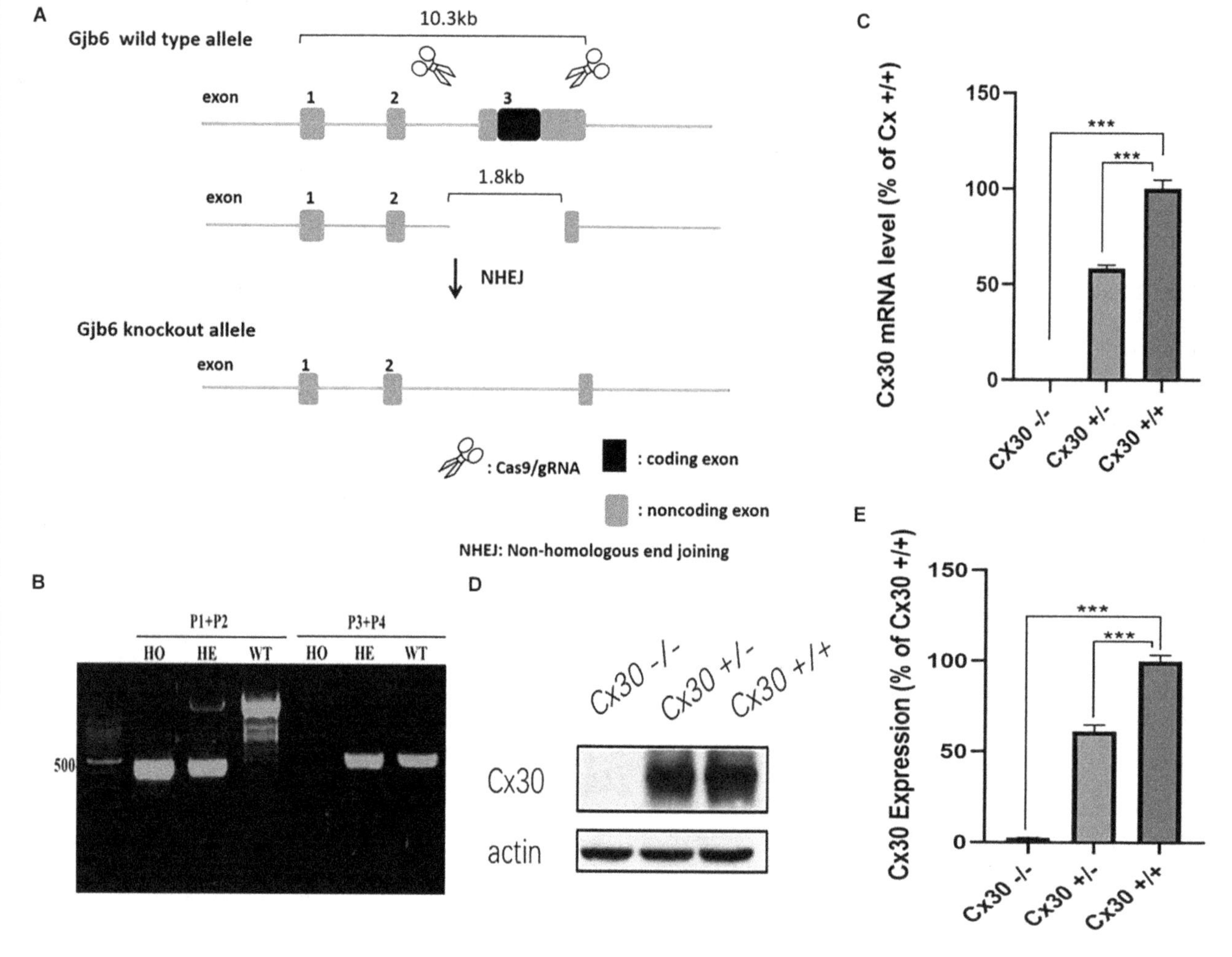

FIGURE 1 | Cx30$^{-/-}$ mice model. **(A)** CRISPR/Cas9 technology was used to repair the mutation introduced by non-homologous recombination, resulting in the shift of the protein reading frame of the *Gjb6* Exon3 gene. **(B)** PCR genotyping: Wild type (WT): *Gjb6* primer 1 (P1) and P2 PCR to obtain a single 2,369 bp band; *Gjb6* P3 and P4 can obtain a 512 bp band; Heterozygous (HE): *Gjb6* P1 and P2 PCR to obtain both 527 bp and 2,369 bp bands; *Gjb6* P3 and P4 to obtain 512 bp band; Homozygous (HO): *Gjb6* P1 and P2 PCR obtained a single 527 bp band; *Gjb6* P3 and P4 could not obtain a band. **(C–E)** Cx30 expression was quantified by qPCR **(C)** and western blot **(D,E)** in the whole cochlea. Data presented as Mean ± SEM; three independent experiments; three mice of each genotype per experiment; *t*-test. $^{***}p < 0.001$.

blot analysis of protein levels in the inner ear of Cx30 +/- mice showed a 61.1% reduction compared to WT mice, while it was undetectable in Cx30 $^{-/-}$ mice (**Figures 1D,E**).

Hearing Loss in Cx30$^{-/-}$ Mice

One-month-old, 3-month-old and 6-month-old Cx30$^{-/-}$ mice displayed mild hearing loss at the full frequency (**Figure 2**). Compared with WT mice, the ABR thresholds in 1-month-old Cx30$^{-/-}$ mice at 4, 8, 11, 16, 22, 32, and 40 kHz were elevated by 22.7 ± 2.1 ($p < 0.001$), 20 ± 4.2 ($p < 0.01$), 15 ± 5.9, 11.3 ± 3.8 ($p < 0.01$), 15.3 ± 4.2 ($p < 0.05$), and 6.8 ± 4.4 dB SPL, respectively. Compared with WT mice, the ABR thresholds in 3-month-old Cx30$^{-/-}$ mice at 4, 8, 11, 16, 22, 32, and 40 kHz were elevated by 21.8 ± 2.62 ($p < 0.001$), 17 ± 2.9 ($p < 0.001$), 18.6 ± 3.4 ($p < 0.001$), 14.3 ± 2.9 ($p < 0.001$), 15 ± 4.5 ($p < 0.01$), and 25.5 ± 3.9 ($p < 0.001$) dB SPL, respectively. Compared with WT mice, the ABR thresholds in 6-month-old Cx30$^{-/-}$ mice at 4, 8, 11, 16, 22, 32, and 40 kHz were elevated by 17.5 ± 2.9 ($p < 0.01$), 35 ± 2.9 ($p < 0.001$), 32.1 ± 1.7 ($p < 0.001$), 33.3 ± 1.7 ($p < 0.001$), 18.3 ± 4.4, and −2.5 ± 2.9 dB SPL, respectively. At 6-months of age, the high-frequency hearing thresholds in Cx30$^{-/-}$ mice and WT mice were nearly identical.

Normal Cochlea Microstructure in Cx30$^{-/-}$ Mice

Cx30$^{-/-}$ mice had no cochlear developmental disorders (**Figure 3**). Whole-mounting of the apical, middle, and basal turns of the cochlear sensory epithelium of 1-month-old Cx30$^{-/-}$ mice and WT mice showed no apparent hair cell loss (**Figures 3A,E**). HE staining of cochlear frozen sections in Cx30$^{-/-}$ mice and WT mice showed no difference in the number of SGNs and the thickness of SV (**Figures 3B–D**).

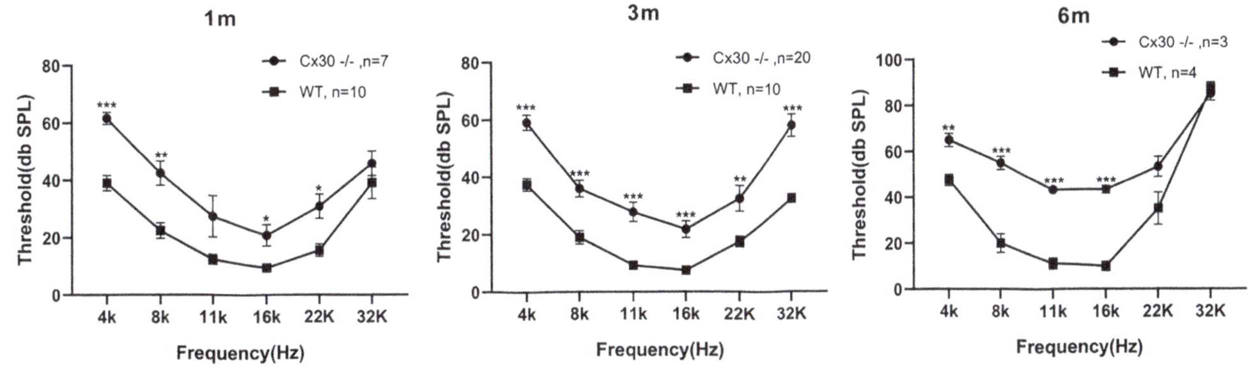

FIGURE 2 | Mild hearing loss in $Cx30^{-/-}$ mice. ABR waveforms were recorded from $Cx30^{-/-}$ and WT littermate mice at 1 m, 3 m, 6 m. 1 m: 1-month-old; 3 m: 3-month-old; 6 m: 6-month-old. Data presented as Mean ± SEM; $n > 3$ in each group. *t*-test. $^{*}p < 0.05$, $^{**}p < 0.01$, $^{***}p < 0.001$. ABR, Auditory brainstem response.

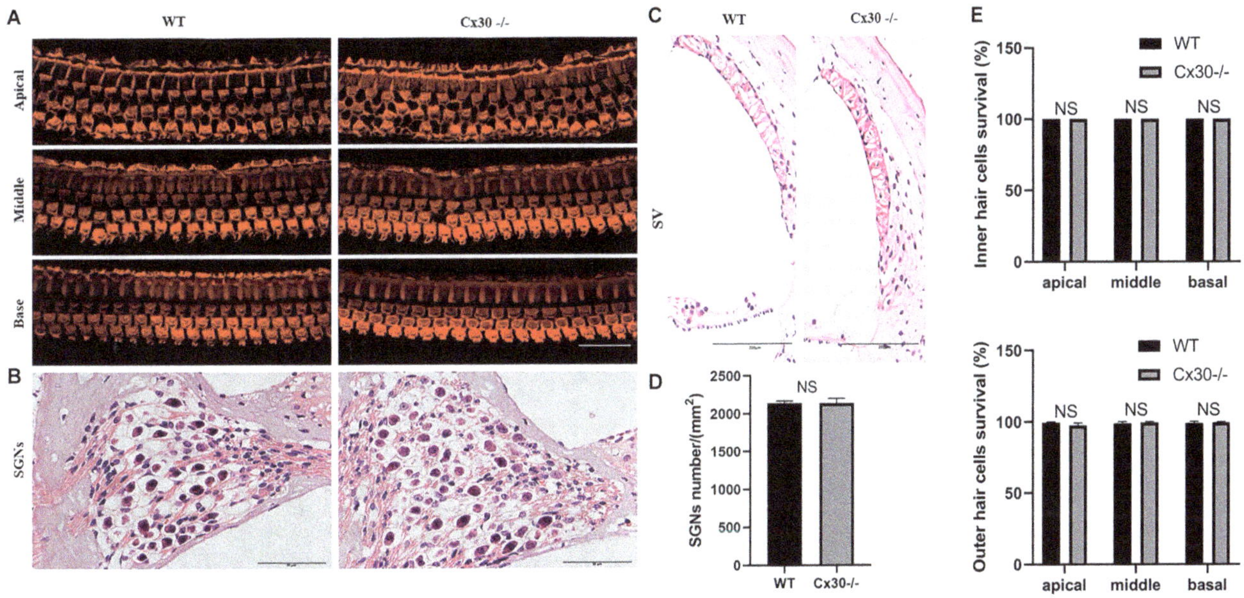

FIGURE 3 | The microscopic structure of cochlea in $Cx30^{-/-}$ mice. **(A,E)** Whole-mountings of the apical, middle and basal turns of cochlear sensory epithelium in 1-month-old $Cx30^{-/-}$ mice and WT mice were obtained by maximal intensity back-projection of 15 confocal optical sections from a 0.8 μm step through—focus sequence (z-stack); actin filaments were stained with phalloidin (red); scale bar: 50 μm. **(B,D)** HE staining of frozen sections of the cochlea in $Cx30^{-/-}$ mice and WT mice showed no difference in the number of spiral ganglions (SGNs). Scale bar: 50 μm. **(C)** HE staining of frozen sections of the cochlea in $Cx30^{-/-}$ mice and WT mice showed no difference in the thickness of SV. SV, stria vascularis. Scale bar: 50 μm. NS, not statistically significant. Data presented as Mean ± SEM. *t*-test.

Cx26 Expression in $Cx30^{-/-}$ Mice

Immunofluorescence showed that Cx26 expression in the BM of $Cx30^{-/-}$ mice was stronger than that of WT mice, and Cx26 expression in the vascular stripe of $Cx30^{-/-}$ mice was significantly lower than that of WT mice both in 1-mouth-old and P5 (**Figures 4A,B**).The mRNA and protein levels of Cx26 in the cochlea of $Cx30^{-/-}$ mice relative to that of WT mice were quantified (**Figures 4C,D**). qPCR analysis showed that the whole cochlear Cx26 mRNA levels of 1-month-old $Cx30^{-/-}$ mice decreased by 41.8% compared with WT mice; whole cochlear mRNA levels in $Cx30^{-/-}$ mice decreased by 28% compared with WT mice at P5; cochlear BM Cx26 mRNA levels in $Cx30^{-/-}$ mice increased by 36.7% compared with WT mice at P5; cochlear SV Cx26 mRNA levels in $Cx30^{-/-}$ mice decreased by 56.6% compared with WT mice in P5 (**Figure 4D**). Western blot showed that the whole cochlear Cx26 protein levels in 1-month-old $Cx30^{-/-}$ mice decreased by 25.9% compared with WT mice; whole cochlear Cx26 protein levels of $Cx30^{-/-}$ mice reduced by 9.84% compared with WT mice at P5; cochlear BM Cx26 protein levels of $Cx30^{-/-}$ mice increased by 19.8% compared with WT mice at P5; cochlear SV Cx26 protein level of $Cx30^{-/-}$ mice decreased by 25.6% compared with WT mice in P5 (**Figure 4C**).

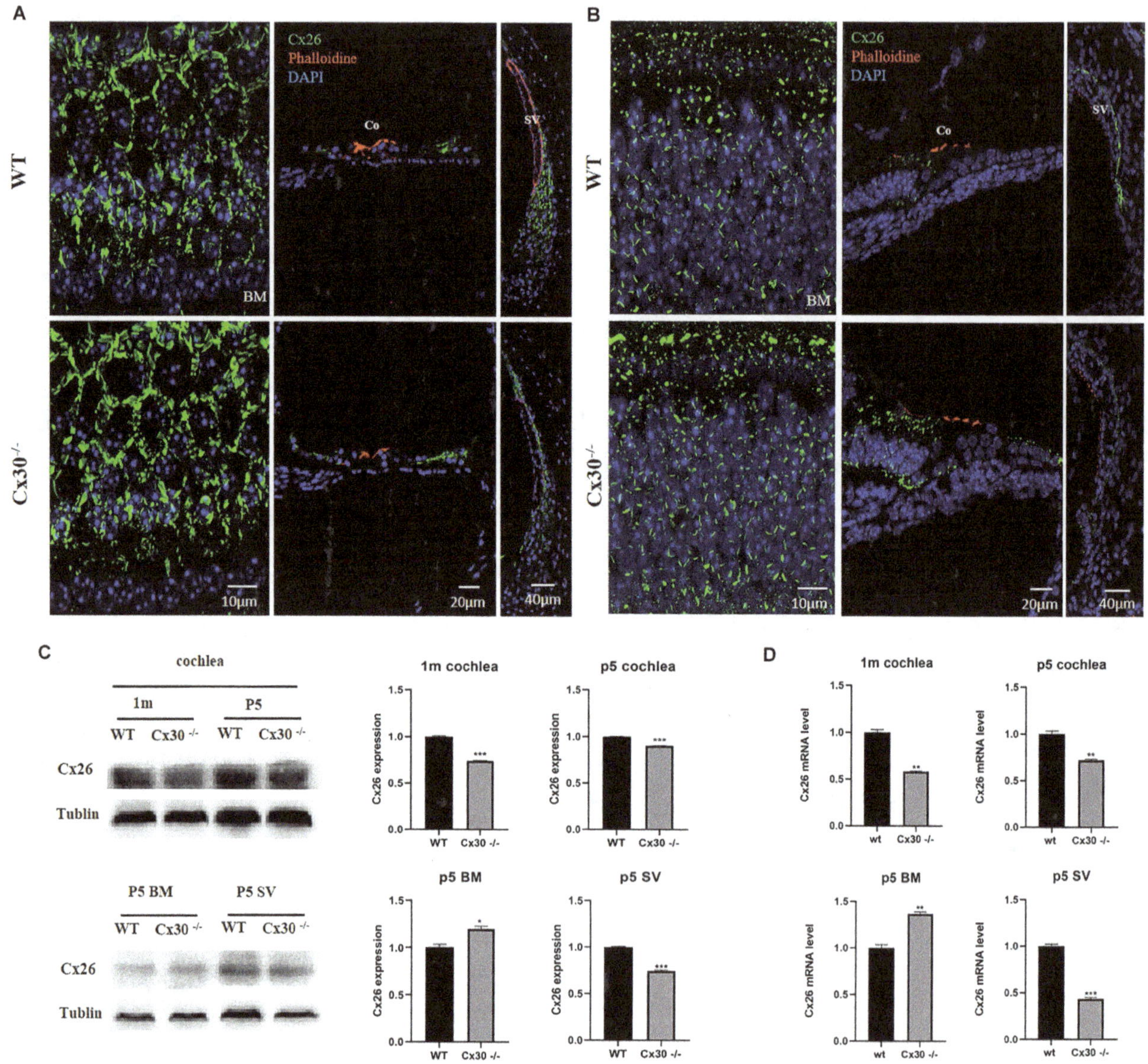

FIGURE 4 | Cx26 expression in Cx30$^{-/-}$ mice. **(A)** Immunofluorescence analysis of frozen sections and BM in the cochlea of 1-month-old mouse. **(B)** Immunofluorescence analysis of frozen sections and BM in the cochlea at P5. Both in 1-month-old and P5, Cx26 expression in the BM of Cx30$^{-/-}$ mice was stronger than that of WT mice, and Cx26 expression in the vascular stripe of Cx30$^{-/-}$ mice was significantly lower than that of WT mice. Cx26: Green, Phalloidin: Red, DAPI: Blue (for cell nuclei); scale bar: 10 μm, 20 μm, 40 μm. **(C)** Western blot analysis of the cochlea, BM, and SV in 1-month-old and P5 mice. Whole cochlear Cx26 protein levels in 1-month-old Cx30$^{-/-}$ mice showed a 25.9% decrease compared with WT mice; whole cochlear Cx26 protein levels of Cx30$^{-/-}$ mice showed 9.84% reduction compared with WT mice at P5; cochlear BM Cx26 protein levels of Cx30$^{-/-}$ mice increased by 19.8% compared with WT mice at P5; Cx26 protein level in SV of the cochlea in Cx30$^{-/-}$ mice decreased by 25.6% compared with WT mice in P5. **(D)** qPCR analysis of the cochlea, BM, and SV in 1-month-old and P5 mice. Whole cochlear Cx26 mRNA levels of 1-month-old Cx30$^{-/-}$ mice declined by 41.8% compared with WT mice; whole cochlear mRNA levels of Cx30$^{-/-}$ mice decreased by 28% compared with WT mice at P5; cochlear BM Cx26 mRNA levels in Cx30$^{-/-}$ mice increased by 36.7% compared with WT mice at P5; cochlear SV Cx26 mRNA levels in Cx30$^{-/-}$ mice reduced by 56.6% compared with WT mice at P5. Data presented as Mean ± SEM. *t*-test. $^{*}p < 0.05$, $^{**}p < 0.01$, $^{***}p < 0.001$. BM, basemental membrane; SV, stria vascularis; Co, Corti's organ.

Mild Damaged Stria Vascularis Submicroscopic Structure in Cx30$^{-/-}$ Mice

Figure 5 shows the transmission electron microscopy images of the submicroscopic structure of the SV in Cx30$^{-/-}$ mice. There was some visible vacuolar injury in the SV of Cx30$^{-/-}$ mice compared with WT mice, which suggested that Cx30 deletion might cause mild damage to the SV.

Reduction of Endocochlear Potential in Cx30$^{-/-}$ Mice

Figure 6 shows a reduction of EP in 1-month-old Cx30$^{-/-}$ mice compared with the WT mice. EPs in Cx30$^{-/-}$ mice and WT mice were 80.1 ± 2.6 mV and 104.6 ± 1.9 mV, respectively (**Figure 6B**). EP in Cx30$^{-/-}$ mice was significantly reduced by 23.4% ($p < 0.001$) relative to WT mice.

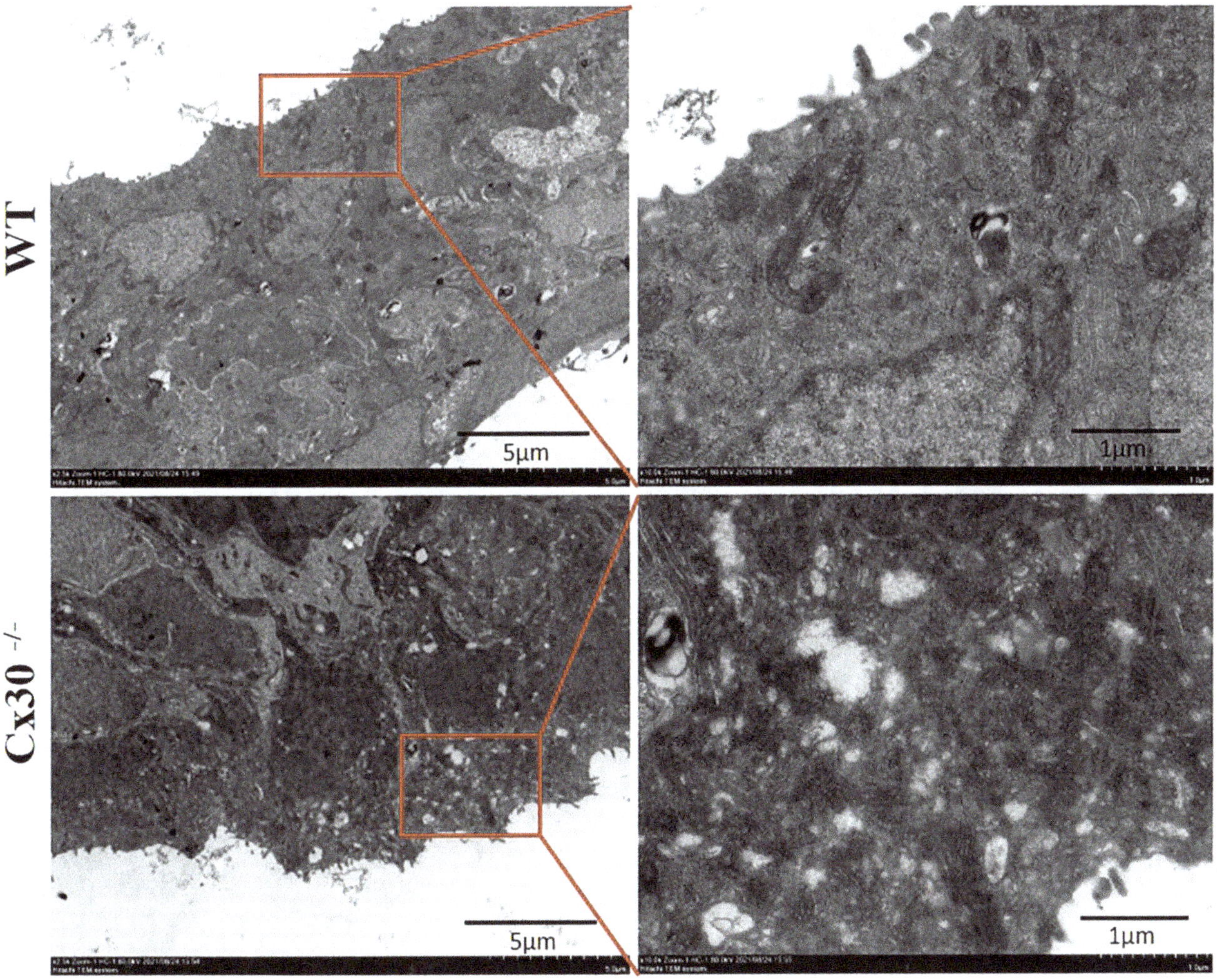

FIGURE 5 | Transmission electron microscopy of the submicroscopic structure of the stria vascularis in Cx30$^{-/-}$ mice. Visible cavity-like damage in the SV of Cx30$^{-/-}$ mice compared with WT mice. Scale bar: 5 μm, 1 μm.

Reduction of ATP Release in Cx30$^{-/-}$ Mice

Figure 7 shows reductions in ATP release of Cx30$^{-/-}$ mice relative to WT mice, both in BM and SV at P5. Compared with WT mice, ATP release in Cx30$^{-/-}$ mice was significantly reduced by 14.2% ($p < 0.05$) in BM and 37.9% ($p < 0.01$) in SV, respectively. ATP release of SV decreased more significantly than that of BM.

DISCUSSION

Seven large genomic deletions of *GJB6* have been previously reported, including >920 kb deletion (Feldmann et al., 2009), 179 kb deletion (Tayoun et al., 2016), 131 kb deletion (Wilch et al., 2010), del(*GJB6*-D13S175), del(*GJB6*-D13S1830), del(*GJB6*-D13S1854; Bliznetz et al., 2017) and del(*GJB6*-D13S1834; Pandya et al., 2020). Homozygous deletion of *GJB6* results in severe to profound hearing loss in humans, similar to the mouse model (Teubner et al., 2003; Mei et al., 2017; Pandya et al., 2020). In many cases, the large deletions of *GJB6* disrupt a 50 cis-acting element upstream of both genes, which abolishes the expression of *GJB2*, and hence is responsible for the phenotype (Rodriguez-Paris and Schrijver, 2009). A recent study reported the del (*GJB6*-D13S1830) deletion in 16.35% of all *GJB2* heterozygotes, which causes more profound hearing loss than those with bi-allelic change in *GJB2* (Pandya et al., 2003, 2020; Snoeckx et al., 2005). The more severe audiological findings in digenic probands cannot be explained by the sole theory of a putative cis-regulatory element in the deleted region (Pandya et al., 2020), suggesting that both *GJB6* and *GJB2* products may contribute to the hearing loss.

The Corti's organ is the core in the auditory system, which is composed of HCs and SCs. SCs release ATP via connexin which triggers intercellular Ca^{2+} wave propagation and might be critical for the functional maturation of HCs (Johnson et al., 2017). The function of HCs is to transduce the sound mechanical stimulation into the primary acoustic signals (Abeytunge et al., 2021), while the spiral ganglion neurons (SGNs) transmit primary acoustic information from HCs in the organ of Corti to the higher auditory centers

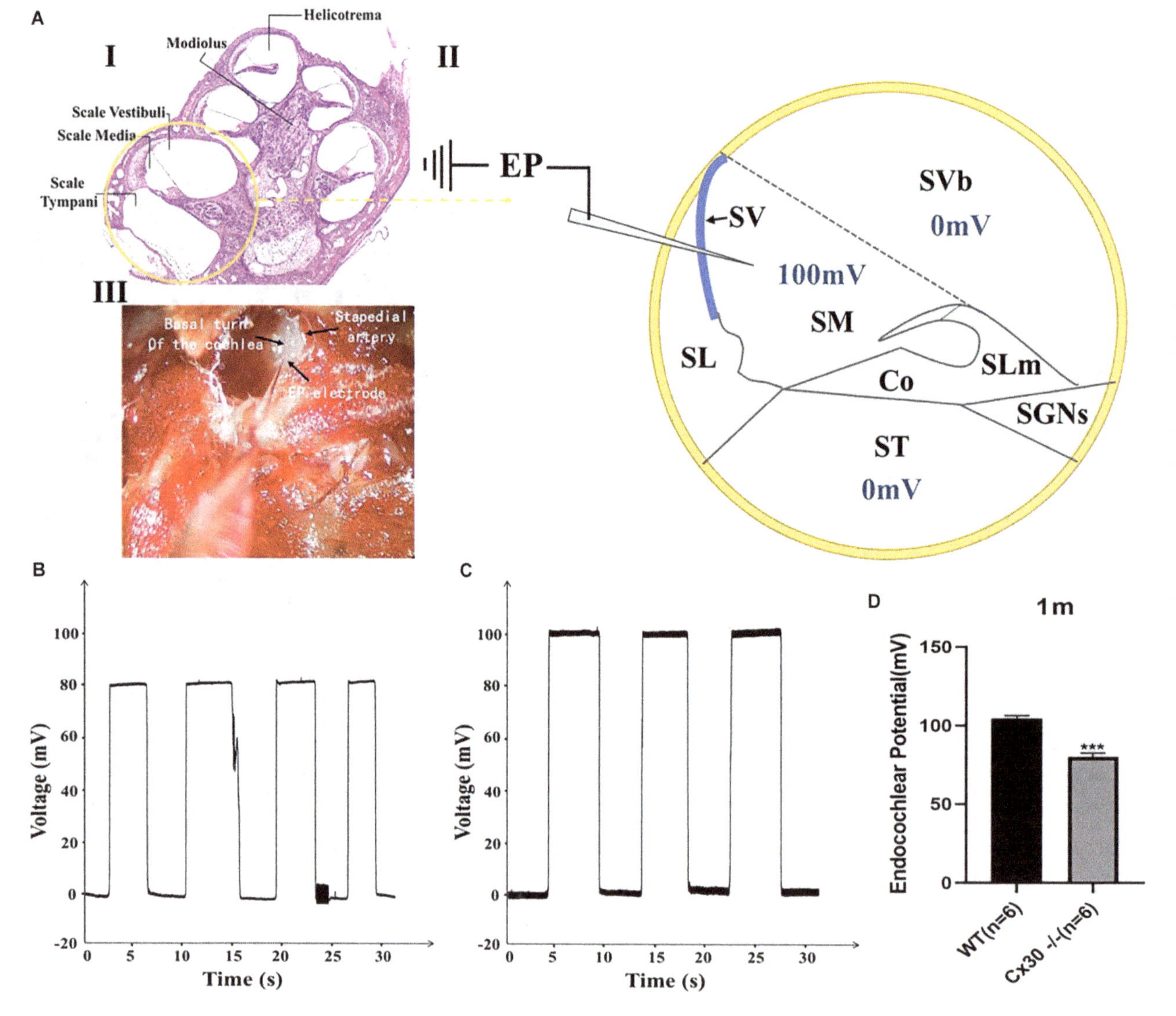

FIGURE 6 | Endocochlear potential (EP) measurements in WT and Cx30 KO mice. **(A)** (I) Cross-section of a cochlea. (II) Schematic diagram of the cross-section of the basal cochlear turn illustrating the method of EP measurement. A microelectrode filled with 3 M KCl was inserted into the endolymph-filled scala media (100 mV in a WT mouse) to record EP. (III) Photograph of a surgically exposed cochlea before EP measurement showing the location of the stapedial artery and the insertion site of the microelectrode. **(B,C)** Representative EP recordings from 1-month-old WT and Cx30 KO mice. The traces showed the voltage (mV) of the scala media as a function of time (s). **(D)** The graph illustrates a significant 23.4% reduction in the EP in 1-month-old Cx30 KO mice (80.1 ± 2.6 mV) compared with age-matched WT mice (104.6 ± 1.9 mV). Data presented as Mean ± SEM (n = 6). t-test. $^{***}p < 0.001$. Co, Corti's organ; SGNs, spinal ganglion neurons; SL, spiral ligament; SLm, spiral limbus; SM, scala media; ST, scala tympani; SV, stria vascularis; SVb, scala vestibuli.

of the central nervous system (Wei et al., 2021). *GJB6* and *GJB2* are located on the same chromosome (13q12.11) in the human genome. Due to the relative proximity of these two genes, their expressions might be controlled by the same set of regulatory elements (Wilch et al., 2006). Homozygous deletion mutations of either Cx26 or Cx30 could cause deafness in humans (Kelsell et al., 1997; del Castillo et al., 2002). Cx26 plays a critical role in auditory function and its deficiency leads to significant hearing loss in the animal model (Cohen-Salmon et al., 2002; Chen et al., 2014). Cx26 deficiency in the cochlea could cause pathological changes, including cochlear developmental disorders (Wang et al., 2009; Liang et al., 2012), HCs and SGNs degeneration (Cohen-Salmon et al., 2002; Sun et al., 2009; Wang et al., 2009), EP reduction (Chen et al., 2014), and impairment of active cochlear amplification (Zhu et al., 2013, 2015). HCs and SGNs degeneration was detected around P14 in Cx26-deficient mice (Sun et al., 2009; Wang et al., 2009). However, severe hearing loss precedes substantial hair cell loss after the deletion of Cx26 (Liang et al., 2012). Nevertheless, EP remained normal after targeted deletion of Cx26 expression in Deiters SCs and outer pillar SCs, which are located around OHCs in the cochlear sensory epithelium (Zhu et al., 2013). This indicates that impairment of the cochlear sensory GJ network may not affect EP generation in the inner

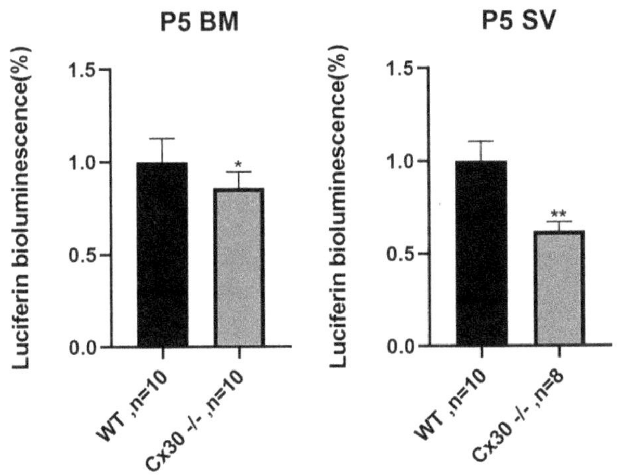

FIGURE 7 | Reduction of ATP release in the cochlea in $Cx30^{-/-}$ mice. ATP release is reduced in $Cx30^{-/-}$ mice in BM and SV at P5. Data presented as Mean ± SEM. *t*-test. $^{*}p < 0.05$, $^{**}p < 0.01$. BM, basemental membrane; SV, stria vascularis.

ear (Zhu et al., 2013; Chen and Zhao, 2014; Chen et al., 2015). However, Cx26 deficiency in the cochlear SCs can affect OHC electromotility and active cochlear amplification, since distortion product otoacoustic emission (DPOAE) was reduced (Yu and Zhao, 2009; Zhu et al., 2013, 2015). On the other hand, the cochlear tunnel opens from P5 (Kraus and Aulbach-Kraus, 1981). Cx26 deficiency before P5 can lead to occlusion of the cochlear tunnel and induce cochlear developmental disorders with congenital deafness (Chen et al., 2014). Nevertheless, cochlear development proceeded normally, the cochlear tunnel opened normally, and hearing remained normal at a young age after deletion of Cx26 after P5 (Chen et al., 2014). These findings suggest that Cx26 expression in the cochlea at the early postnatal development stage is critical for cochlear postnatal development and maturation.

Teubner et al. (2003) found that Cx30 knockout mice display severe hearing loss with the absence of EP. Whether the Cx30 deficiency itself or the accompanying significant decrease of Cx26 (approximately 90%) leads to hearing loss in this model remains unknown. Restoration of Cx26 protein level in the cochlea completely rescues hearing in Cx30 knockout mice, whereas hearing loss in the conditional Cx26 (cCx26) null mice could not be rescued by genetically over-expressing Cx30 (Ahmad et al., 2007; Qu et al., 2012). Cx26 protein expression preceded that of Cx30, and Cx26 is the only and essential GJ protein detected by immunolabeling in the organ of Corti during the early postnatal period (Qu et al., 2012). During the postnatal development, the lack of GJs in the Corti's organ leads to obstacles in intercellular material transport and communication, and failure of Corti's organ to mature, leading to hearing loss. However, the Cx26 expression of BM increased in $Cx30^{-/-}$ mice at the early postnatal period (P5) in the present study.

Boulay et al. (2013) established $Cx30^{fl/fl}$ mice, and found no significant difference in hearing between $Cx30^{fl/fl}$ mice and WT mice, however, Cx26 was decreased to 35% and Cx30 was reduced to 64%. Normal EP and DPOAE were observed in this kind of mice (Boulay et al., 2013). Crossing $Cx30^{fl/fl}$ mice with Pgk-Cre mice generated $Cx30^{\Delta/\Delta}$ mice to delete Cx30, which exhibited no hearing loss, while Cx26 was decreased to 52% (Boulay et al., 2013). The threshold level of Cx26 decline in Cx30-deficient mice that causes hearing loss remains unclear. The $Cx30^{-/-}$ mice established in this study exhibited only mild hearing loss, while cochlear Cx26 decreased to 74%. Since Cx26 did not show any major decrease through Cx30 knockout, the mechanism of hearing loss needs to be further explored.

The high positive potential of EP is critical for animal hearing and develops rapidly in the days before the onset of hearing (P4–P11; Chen et al., 2015). EP (+100–110 mV) is the driving force for the generation of auditory receptor currents and potentials by K^+ ions through transduction channels in the HCs, which are formed by a complex process in the SV of the cochlea. The widely accepted "two-cell" model suggests that EP production begins in the fibroblasts of the spiral ligament. Type II fibroblasts depolarize the cells to ~5 mV *via* Na^+/K^+ - ATPase and Na^+, K^+, $2Cl^-$ cotransport proteins. The intermediate cells of the SV are subsequently coupled by Cx26 and Cx30 *via* GJs. Thereafter, the ATP-dependent Kir4.1 K^+ channel on the apical membrane of intermediate cells (Ando and Takeuchi, 1999; Liu and Zhao, 2008; Nin et al., 2008) generates a 105–110 mV transmembrane potential (Nernst's K^+ balance potential) between the intracellular space and the intrastriatal space. This positive intrastriatal potential eventually leads to EP positivity in the middle-grade endolymph. The network of two GJs composed of Cx26 and Cx30 forms a pathway through which K^+ ions that pass through sensory cells during mechanosensory transmission can be recirculated into the endolymphatic space such that they re-enter sensory cells (Wangemann, 2002). GJs deficiency may lead to the obstruction of K^+ circulation, thus affecting the formation of EP and hearing. ATP is necessary for EP generation and K^+ recycling (Zhu and Zhao, 2010; Chen et al., 2015). The perfusion of ATP into the cochlea can significantly increase EP (Sueta et al., 2003). As described above, depolarization of fibroblasts by co-activation of Na^+/K^+ - ATPase and Na^+, K^+, $2Cl^-$-cotransporters is the first step in EP production. Although Na^+/K^+ - ATPase is primarily driven by intracellular ATP, extracellular ATP can stimulate Na^+/K^+ - ATPase activity by activating purinergic receptor and Src family kinase (SFK) as well (Shahidullah et al., 2012). In addition, the function of the primary active Na^+/K^+ - ATPase requires K-channel coupling to recycle K^+ (Muto et al., 2003). This "pump coupling" was proposed in 1958, and was subsequently confirmed by experimental data (Koefoed-Johnsen and Ussing, 1958; Dawson and Richards, 1990; Tsuchiya et al., 1992). Recently, it was found that extracellular ATP can also activate ATP-sensitive (KIR) K channels in hippocampal CA3 pyramidal neurons and lung epithelial cells, which cooperate with Na^+/K^+ - ATPase activity. ATP may initially activate the P2X receptor and subsequently activate the KIR potassium channel and Na^+/K^+ - ATPase (Telang et al., 2010; Jiang et al., 2013; Schmid and Evans, 2019).

In this study, we established a novel Cx30 complete knockout mouse model, with a mild full-frequency hearing loss as indicated by ABR. The protein level of Cx26 was decreased by less than 30% in the cochlea of these mice, which was significantly different from the previous Cx30-deficient mouse model. Moreover, both EP and ATP release showed a decreasing trend in the present mouse model. These results suggest that Cx30 may play an important role in hearing development, however, further investigation on the underlying mechanism is needed in the future.

AUTHOR CONTRIBUTIONS

JC: experimental implementation, data quality control, and wrote the manuscript. PC: immunohistochemical staining and statistical data analysis. BH: western blot and qPCR. TG: qPCR experiments. YL: collection of cochlear samples for TEM experiments. JZ: collection of cochlear samples for H&E experiments. JL: collection of cochlear samples for TEM experiments. FM: EP experiments. SH: research conception and experimental supervision. JY: research conception, manuscript review and revision. All authors contributed to the article and approved the submitted version.

REFERENCES

Abeytunge, S., Gianoli, F., Hudspeth, A. J., and Kozlov, A. S. (2021). Rapid mechanical stimulation of inner-ear hair cells by photonic pressure. *eLife* 10:e65930. doi: 10.7554/eLife.65930

Adadey, S. M., Wonkam-Tingang, E., Twumasi Aboagye, E., Nayo-Gyan, D. W., Boatemaa Ansong, M., Quaye, O., et al. (2020). Connexin genes variants associated with non-syndromic hearing impairment: a systematic review of the global burden. *Life (Basel)* 10:258. doi: 10.3390/life10110258

Ahmad, S., Tang, W., Chang, Q., Qu, Y., Hibshman, J., Li, Y., et al. (2007). Restoration of connexin26 protein level in the cochlea completely rescues hearing in a mouse model of human connexin30-linked deafness. *Proc. Natl. Acad. Sci. U S A* 104, 1337–1341. doi: 10.1073/pnas.0606855104

Ando, M., and Takeuchi, S. (1999). Immunological identification of an inward rectifier K+ channel (Kir4. 1) in the intermediate cell (melanocyte) of the cochlear stria vascularis of gerbils and rats. *Cell Tissue Res.* 298, 179–183. doi: 10.1007/s004419900066

Bliznetz, E. A., Lalayants, M. R., Markova, T. G., Balanovsky, O. P., Balanovska, E. V., Skhalyakho, R. A., et al. (2017). Update of the GJB2/DFNB1 mutation spectrum in Russia: a founder Ingush mutation del(GJB2-D13S175) is the most frequent among other large deletions. *J. Hum. Genet.* 62, 789–795. doi: 10.1038/jhg.2017.42

Boulay, A. C., del Castillo, F. J., Giraudet, F., Hamard, G., Giaume, C., Petit, C., et al. (2013). Hearing is normal without connexin30. *J. Neurosci.* 33, 430–434. doi: 10.1523/JNEUROSCI.4240-12.2013

Breglio, A. M., May, L. A., Barzik, M., Welsh, N. C., Francis, S. P., Costain, T. Q., et al. (2020). Exosomes mediate sensory hair cell protection in the inner ear. *J. Clin. Invest.* 130, 2657–2672. doi: 10.1172/JCI128867

Bruzzone, R., White, T. W., and Paul, D. L. (1996). Connections with connexins: the molecular basis of direct intercellular signaling. *Eur. J. Biochem.* 238, 1–27. doi: 10.1111/j.1432-1033.1996.0001q.x

Chen, J., Chen, J., Zhu, Y., Liang, C., and Zhao, H. B. (2014). Deafness induced by Connexin 26 (GJB2) deficiency is not determined by endocochlear potential (EP) reduction but is associated with cochlear developmental disorders. *Biochem. Biophys. Res. Commun.* 448, 28–32. doi: 10.1016/j.bbrc.2014.04.016

Chen, S., Xu, K., Xie, L., Cao, H.-Y., Wu, X., Du, A.-N., et al. (2018). The spatial distribution pattern of Connexin26 expression in supporting cells and its role in outer hair cell survival. *Cell Death Dis.* 9:1180. doi: 10.1038/s41419-018-1238-x

Chen, J., and Zhao, H. B. (2014). The role of an inwardly rectifying K(+) channel (Kir4.1) in the inner ear and hearing loss. *Neuroscience* 265, 137–146. doi: 10.1016/j.neuroscience.2014.01.036

Chen, J., Zhu, Y., Liang, C., Chen, J., and Zhao, H.-B. (2015). Pannexin1 channels dominate ATP release in the cochlea ensuring endocochlear potential and auditory receptor potential generation and hearing. *Sci. Rep.* 5:10762. doi: 10.1038/srep10762S

Cohen-Salmon, M., Ott, T., Michel, V., Hardelin, J. P., Perfettini, I., Eybalin, M., et al. (2002). Targeted ablation of connexin26 in the inner ear epithelial gap junction network causes hearing impairment and cell death. *Curr. Biol.* 12, 1106–1111. doi: 10.1016/s0960-9822(02)00904-1

Dawson, D. C., and Richards, N. W. (1990). Basolateral K conductance: role in regulation of NaCl absorption and secretion. *Am. J. Physiol.* 259, C181–C195. doi: 10.1152/ajpcell.1990.259.2.C181

del Castillo, I., Villamar, M., Moreno-Pelayo, M. A., del Castillo, F. J., Alvarez, A., Telleria, D., et al. (2002). A deletion involving the connexin 30 gene in nonsyndromic hearing impairment. *N. Engl. J. Med.* 346, 243–249. doi: 10.1056/NEJMoa012052

Denoyelle, F., Weil, D., Maw, M. A., Wilcox, S. A., Lench, N. J., Allen-Powell, D. R., et al. (1997). Prelingual deafness: high prevalence of a 30delG mutation in the connexin 26 gene. *Hum. Mol. Genet.* 6, 2173–2177. doi: 10.1093/hmg/6.12.2173

Estivill, X., Fortina, P., Surrey, S., Rabionet, R., Melchionda, S., D'Agruma, L., et al. (1998). Connexin-26 mutations in sporadic and inherited sensorineural deafness. *Lancet* 351, 394–398. doi: 10.1016/S0140-6736(97)11124-2

Feldmann, D., Le Marechal, C., Jonard, L., Thierry, P., Czajka, C., Couderc, R., et al. (2009). A new large deletion in the DFNB1 locus causes nonsyndromic hearing loss. *Eur. J. Med. Genet.* 52, 195–200. doi: 10.1016/j.ejmg.2008.11.006

Fu, X., An, Y., Wang, H., Li, P., Lin, J., Yuan, J., et al. (2021). Deficiency of Klc2 induces low-frequency sensorineural hearing loss in C57BL/6 J mice and human. *Mol. Neurobiol.* 58, 4376–4391. doi: 10.1007/s12035-021-02422-w

Guo, L., Cao, W., Niu, Y., He, S., Chai, R., and Yang, J. (2021). Autophagy regulates the survival of hair cells and spiral ganglion neurons in cases of noise, ototoxic drug and age-induced sensorineural hearing loss. *Front. Cell. Neurosci.* 15:760422. doi: 10.3389/fncel.2021.760422

He, Z., Guo, L., Shu, Y., Fang, Q., Zhou, H., Liu, Y., et al. (2017). Autophagy protects auditory hair cells against neomycin-induced damage. *Autophagy* 13, 1884–1904. doi: 10.1080/15548627.2017.1359449

Jagger, D. J., and Forge, A. (2015). Connexins and gap junctions in the inner ear-it's not just about K+ recycling. *Cell Tissue Res.* 360, 633–644. doi: 10.1007/s00441-014-2029-z

Jiang, R., Taly, A., and Grutter, T. (2013). Moving through the gate in ATP-activated P2X receptors. *Trends Biochem. Sci.* 38, 20–29. doi: 10.1016/j.tibs.2012.10.006

Johnson, S.L., Ceriani, F., Houston, O., Polishchuk, R., Polishchuk, E., Crispino, G., et al. (2017). Connexin-mediated signaling in nonsensory cells is crucial for the development of sensory inner hair cells in the mouse cochlea. *J. Neurosci.* 37, 258–268. doi: 10.1523/jneurosci.2251-16.2016

Kelsell, D. P., Dunlop, J., Stevens, H. P., Lench, N. J., Liang, J., Parry, G., et al. (1997). Connexin 26 mutations in hereditary non-syndromic sensorineural deafness. *Nature* 387, 80–83. doi: 10.1038/387080a0

Kikuchi, T., Kimura, R.S., Paul, D.L., and Adams, J.C. (1995). Gap junctions in the rat cochlea: immunsohistochemical and ultrastructural analysis. *Anat. Embryol. (Berl)* 191, 101–118. doi: 10.1007/BF00186783

Koefoed-Johnsen, V., and Ussing, H. H. (1958). The nature of the frog skin potential. *Acta Physiol. Scand.* 42, 298–308. doi: 10.1111/j.1748-1716.1958.tb01563.x

Kraus, H. J., and Aulbach-Kraus, K. (1981). Morphological changes in the cochlea of the mouse after the onset of hearing. *Hear. Res.* 4, 89–102. doi: 10.1016/0378-5955(81)90038-1

Liang, C., Zhu, Y., Zong, L., Lu, G. J., and Zhao, H. B. (2012). Cell degeneration is not a primary causer for Connexin26 (GJB2) deficiency associated hearing loss. *Neurosci. Lett.* 528, 36–41. doi: 10.1016/j.neulet.2012.08.085

Liu, Y.-P., and Zhao, H.-B. (2008). Cellular characterization of Connexin26 and Connnexin30 expression in the cochlear lateral wall. *Cell Tissue Res.* 333, 395–403. doi: 10.1007/s00441-008-0641-5

Mammano, F. (2019). Inner ear connexin channels: roles in development and maintenance of cochlear function. *Cold Spring Harb. Perspect. Med.* 9:a033233. doi: 10.1101/cshperspect.a033233

Mammano, F., and Bortolozzi, M. (2018). $Ca^{(2+)}$ signaling, apoptosis and autophagy in the developing cochlea: milestones to hearing acquisition. *Cell Calcium* 70, 117–126. doi: 10.1016/j.ceca.2017.05.006

Mazzarda, F., D'Elia, A., Massari, R., De Ninno, A., Bertani, F.R., and Businaro, L. (2020). Organ-on-chip model shows that ATP release through connexin hemichannels drives spontaneous $Ca^{(2+)}$ signaling in non-sensory cells of the greater epithelial ridge in the developing cochlea. *Lab Chip.* 20, 3011–3023. doi: 10.10.1039/d0lc00427h

Mei, L., Chen, J., Zong, L., Zhu, Y., Liang, C., Jones, R. O., et al. (2017). A deafness mechanism of digenic Cx26 (GJB2) and Cx30 (GJB6) mutations: reduction of endocochlear potential by impairment of heterogeneous gap junctional function in the cochlear lateral wall. *Neurobiol. Dis.* 108, 195–203. doi: 10.1016/j.nbd.2017.08.002

Mishra, S., Pandey, H., Srivastava, P., Mandal, K., and Phadke, S. R. (2018). Connexin 26 (GJB2) mutations associated with non-syndromic hearing loss (NSHL). *Indian J. Pediatr.* 85, 1061–1066. doi: 10.1007/s12098-018-2654-8

Muto, S., Asano, Y., Wang, W., Seldin, D., and Giebisch, G. (2003). Activity of the basolateral K+ channels is coupled to the Na+-K+-ATPase in the cortical collecting duct. *Am. J. Physiol. Renal. Physiol.* 285, F945–F954. doi: 10.1152/ajprenal.00081.2003

Nin, F., Hibino, H., Doi, K., Suzuki, T., Hisa, Y., and Kurachi, Y. (2008). The endocochlear potential depends on two K+ diffusion potentials and an electrical barrier in the stria vascularis of the inner ear. *Proc. Natl. Acad. Sci. U S A* 105, 1751–1756. doi: 10.1073/pnas.0711463105

Pandya, A., Arnos, K. S., Xia, X. J., Welch, K. O., Blanton, S. H., Friedman, T. B., et al. (2003). Frequency and distribution of GJB2 (connexin 26) and GJB6 (connexin 30) mutations in a large North American repository of deaf probands. *Genet. Med.* 5, 295–303. doi: 10.1097/01.GIM.0000078026.01140.68

Pandya, A., O'Brien, A., Kovasala, M., Bademci, G., Tekin, M., and Arnos, K. S. (2020). Analyses of del(GJB6–D13S1830) and del(GJB6–D13S1834) deletions in a large cohort with hearing loss: caveats to interpretation of molecular test results in multiplex families. *Mol. Genet. Genomic. Med.* 8:e1171. doi: 10.1002/mgg3.1171

Qu, Y., Tang, W., Zhou, B., Ahmad, S., Chang, Q., Li, X., et al. (2012). Early developmental expression of connexin26 in the cochlea contributes to its dominate functional role in the cochlear gap junctions. *Biochem. Biophys. Res. Commun.* 417, 245–250. doi: 10.1016/j.bbrc.2011.11.093

Rodriguez-Paris, J., and Schrijver, I. (2009). The digenic hypothesis unraveled: the GJB6 del(GJB6–D13S1830) mutation causes allele-specific loss of GJB2 expression in cis. *Biochem. Biophys. Res. Commun.* 389, 354–359. doi: 10.1016/j.bbrc.2009.08.152

Schmid, R., and Evans, R. J. (2019). ATP-gated P2X receptor channels: molecular insights into functional roles. *Annu. Rev. Physiol.* 81, 43–62. doi: 10.1146/annurev-physiol-020518-114259

Shahidullah, M., Mandal, A., Beimgraben, C., and Delamere, N. (2012). Hyposmotic stress causes ATP release and stimulates Na, K-ATPase activity in porcine lens. *J. Cell. Physiol.* 227, 1428–1437. doi: 10.1002/jcp.22858

Snoeckx, R. L., Huygen, P. L., Feldmann, D., Marlin, S., Denoyelle, F., Waligora, J., et al. (2005). GJB2 mutations and degree of hearing loss: a multicenter study. *Am. J. Hum. Genet.* 77, 945–957. doi: 10.1086/497996

Sueta, T., Paki, B., Everett, A., and Robertson, D. (2003). Purinergic receptors in auditory neurotransmission. *Hear. Res.* 183, 97–108. doi: 10.1016/s0378-5955(03)00221-1

Sun, Y., Tang, W., Chang, Q., Wang, Y., Kong, W., and Lin, X. (2009). Connexin30 null and conditional connexin26 null mice display distinct pattern and time course of cellular degeneration in the cochlea. *J. Comp. Neurol.* 516, 569–579. doi: 10.1002/cne.22117

Tayoun, A. N., Mason-Suares, H., Frisella, A. L., Bowser, M., Duffy, E., Mahanta, L., et al. (2016). Targeted droplet-digital PCR as a tool for novel deletion discovery at the DFNB1 locus. *Hum. Mutat.* 37, 119–126. doi: 10.1002/humu.22912

Telang, R. S., Paramananthasivam, V., Vlajkovic, S. M., Munoz, D. J., Housley, G. D., and Thorne, P. R. (2010). Reduced P2x 2 receptor-mediated regulation of endocochlear potential in the ageing mouse cochlea. *Purinergic Signal.* 6, 263–272. doi: 10.1007/s11302-010-9195-6

Teubner, B., Michel, V., Pesch, J., Lautermann, J., Cohen-Salmon, M., Sohl, G., et al. (2003). Connexin30 (Gjb6)-deficiency causes severe hearing impairment and lack of endocochlear potential. *Hum. Mol. Genet.* 12, 13–21. doi: 10.1093/hmg/ddg001

Tsuchiya, K., Wang, W., Giebisch, G., and Welling, P. (1992). ATP is a coupling modulator of parallel Na, K-ATPase-K-channel activity in the renal proximal tubule. *Proc. Natl. Acad. Sci. U S A* 89, 6418–6422. doi: 10.1073/pnas.89.14.6418

Verselis, V. K. (2019). Connexin hemichannels and cochlear function. *Neurosci. Lett.* 695, 40–45. doi: 10.1016/j.neulet.2017.09.020

Wang, Y., Chang, Q., Tang, W., Sun, Y., Zhou, B., Li, H., et al. (2009). Targeted connexin26 ablation arrests postnatal development of the organ of corti. *Biochem. Biophys. Res. Commun.* 385, 33–37. doi: 10.1016/j.bbrc.2009.05.023

Wangemann, P. (2002). K+ cycling and its regulation in the cochlea and the vestibular labyrinth. *Audiol. Neurotol.* 7, 199–205. doi: 10.1159/000063736

Wei, H., Chen, Z., Hu, Y., Cao, W., Ma, X., Zhang, C., et al. (2021). Topographically conductive butterfly wing substrates for directed spiral ganglion neuron growth. *Small* 17:e2102062. doi: 10.1002/smll.202102062

Wilch, E., Azaiez, H., Fisher, R. A., Elfenbein, J., Murgia, A., Birkenhager, R., et al. (2010). A novel DFNB1 deletion allele supports the existence of a distant cis-regulatory region that controls GJB2 and GJB6 expression. *Clin. Genet.* 78, 267–274. doi: 10.1111/j.1399-0004.2010.01387.x

Wilch, E., Zhu, M., Burkhart, K. B., Regier, M., Elfenbein, J. L., Fisher, R. A., et al. (2006). Expression of GJB2 and GJB6 is reduced in a novel DFNB1 allele. *Am. J. Hum. Gen.* 79, 174–179. doi: 10.1086/505333

Yu, N., and Zhao, H. B. (2009). Modulation of outer hair cell electromotility by cochlear supporting cells and gap junctions. *PLoS One* 4:e7923. doi: 10.1371/journal.pone.0007923

Zhang, Y., Li, Y., Fu, X., Wang, P., Wang, Q., Meng, W., et al. (2021). The detrimental and beneficial functions of macrophages after cochlear injury. *Front. Cell Dev. Biol.* 9:631904. doi: 10.3389/fcell.2021.631904

Zhang, S., Qiang, R., Dong, Y., Zhang, Y., Chen, Y., Zhou, H., et al. (2020a). Hair cell regeneration from inner ear progenitors in the mammalian cochlea. *Am. J. Stem Cells* 9, 25–35.

Zhang, S., Zhang, Y., Dong, Y., Guo, L., Zhang, Z., Shao, B., et al. (2020b). Knockdown of foxg1 in supporting cells increases the trans-differentiation of supporting cells into hair cells in the neonatal mouse cochlea. *Cell. Mol. Life Sci.* 77, 1401–1419. doi: 10.1007/s00018-019-03291-2

Zhang, Y., Zhang, S., Zhang, Z., Dong, Y., Ma, X., Qiang, R., et al. (2020). Knockdown of Foxg1 in Sox9+ supporting cells increases the trans-differentiation of supporting cells into hair cells in the neonatal mouse utricle. *Aging (Albany NY)* 12, 19834–19851. doi: 10.18632/aging.104009

Zhu, Y., Chen, J., Liang, C., Zong, L., Chen, J., Jones, R. O., et al. (2015). Connexin26 (GJB2) deficiency reduces active cochlear amplification leading to late-onset hearing loss. *Neuroscience* 284, 719–729. doi: 10.1016/j.neuroscience.2014.10.061

Zhu, Y., Liang, C., Chen, J., Zong, L., Chen, G. D., and Zhao, H. B. (2013). Active cochlear amplification is dependent on supporting cell gap junctions. *Nat. Commun.* 4:1786. doi: 10.1038/ncomms2806

Zhu, Y., and Zhao, H.-B. (2010). ATP-mediated potassium recycling in the cochlear supporting cells. *Purinergic Signal.* 6, 221–229. doi: 10.1007/s11302-010-9184-9

9

Development of Tinnitus and Hyperacusis in a Mouse Model of Tobramycin Cochleotoxicity

Ryan J. Longenecker, Rende Gu, Jennifer Homan and Jonathan Kil*

Sound Pharmaceuticals Inc., Seattle, WA, United States

Correspondence:
Ryan J. Longenecker
rlongenecker@soundpharma.com

Aminoglycosides (AG) antibiotics are a common treatment for recurrent infections in cystic fibrosis (CF) patients. AGs are highly ototoxic, resulting in a range of auditory dysfunctions. It was recently shown that the acoustic startle reflex (ASR) can assess behavioral evidence of hyperacusis and tinnitus in an amikacin cochleotoxicity mouse model. The goal of this study was to establish if tobramycin treatment led to similar changes in ASR behavior and to establish whether ebselen can prevent the development of these maladaptive neuroplastic symptoms. CBA/Ca mice were divided into three groups: Group 1 served as a control and did not receive tobramycin or ebselen, Group 2 received tobramycin (200 mg/kg/s.c.) and the vehicle (DMSO/saline/i.p.) daily for 14 continuous days, and Group 3 received the same dose/schedule of tobramycin as Group 2 and ebselen at (20 mg/kg/i.p.). Auditory brainstem response (ABR) and ASR hearing assessments were collected at baseline and 2, 6, 10, 14, and 18 weeks from the start of treatment. ASR tests included input/output (I/O) functions which assess general hearing and hyperacusis, and Gap-induced prepulse inhibition of the acoustic startle (GPIAS) to assess tinnitus. At 18 weeks, histologic analysis showed predominantly normal appearing hair cells and spiral ganglion neuron (SGN) synapses. Following 14 days of tobramycin injections, 16 kHz thresholds increased from baseline and fluctuated over the 18-week recovery period. I/O functions revealed exaggerated startle response magnitudes in 50% of mice over the same period. Gap detection deficits, representing behavioral evidence of tinnitus, were observed in a smaller subset (36%) of animals. Interestingly, increases in ABR wave III/wave I amplitude ratios were observed. These tobramycin data corroborate previous findings that AGs can result in hearing dysfunctions. We show that a 14-day course of tobramycin treatment can cause similar levels of hearing loss and tinnitus, when compared to a 14-day course of amikacin, but less hyperacusis. Evidence suggests that tinnitus and hyperacusis might be common side effects of AG antibiotics.

Keywords: hearing loss, tobramycin, hyperacusis, tinnitus, ebselen, aminoglycoside – ototoxicity

---

Abbreviations: AG, aminoglycosides; CF, cystic fibrosis; SGN, spiral ganglion neurons; ABR, auditory brainstem response; ASR, acoustic startle reflex; kHz, kilohertz; DMSO, dimethyl sulfoxide; GPIAS, gap-induced prepulse inhibition of the acoustic startle reflex; GAP, trial with gap preceding startle SO, trial with startle only; ANOVA, analysis of variance; IO, input/output; CMD, center of mass displacement.

INTRODUCTION

Aminoglycosides (AG) such as tobramycin are commonly used to treat cystic fibrosis (CF) patients with recurrent pulmonary infections and those infected with multi-drug resistant tuberculosis (Flume et al., 2009). Unfortunately, AGs are ototoxic and can often result in permanent hearing loss (Staecker, 2021). Recent prospective clinical studies demonstrated that a single course of tobramycin can lead to hearing threshold shifts, word-in-noise deficits, and tinnitus, or sound perception in the absence of a sound source (Garinis et al., 2020; Harruff et al., 2020). For those being treated with AGs for chronic conditions, the cumulative ototoxic effects present an enhanced risk of cochleotoxicity (American Speech-Language-Hearing Association, 1994; Garinis et al., 2017; Elson et al., 2020; Hong et al., 2020). While AG-induced hearing loss is now beginning to be well-documented, little is known about the auditory dysfunctions that often accompany hearing loss. However, more research into the prevalence of tinnitus and hyperacusis should be examined in animal models and clinically (Baguley and Andersson, 2007; Hammill and Campbell, 2018).

In vivo assessments of hearing functionality via auditory brainstem response (ABR) and postmortem cochlear histology are common in AG animal models, albeit with methodological inconsistency and variable reports of hearing dysfunction (Huth et al., 2011; Ogier et al., 2020). Longenecker et al. (2020) recently expanded on these traditional hearing assessments by showing that the acoustic startle reflex (ASR), a reflexed-based behavioral assay (Davis, 1984; Gómez-Nieto et al., 2020), can identify potential AG-induced changes to the central auditory system. Amikacin was also shown to induce behavioral evidence of hyperacusis, a sensitivity to loud sounds, and tinnitus, a ringing or buzzing in the ears (Longenecker et al., 2020), which has been observed in noise-induced (Auerbach et al., 2014; Shore and Wu, 2019) and salicylate-induced tinnitus animal models (Salvi et al., 2021). It is unknown if these auditory dysfunctions are specific to amikacin treatment or if they are a general side effect of AG antibiotics. Tinnitus is a prevalent side effect of many classes of drugs which include non-steroidal anti-inflammatory drugs, antibiotics, cancer drugs, diuretics, antimalarial drugs, and antidepressants. Indeed, a recent meta-analysis of clinical reports from the Cochrane library shows that tinnitus is one of the more common side effects for CF patients with recurrent AG treatments (Smith et al., 2018). Hyperacusis is under-reported clinically but is known to be debilitating and comorbid with tinnitus (Pienkowski et al., 2014), increasing with the number of years a patient has experienced tinnitus (Raj-Koziak et al., 2021; Refat et al., 2021). Thus, it is important for AG-induced auditory dysfunctions to be further investigated in animal models to develop potential therapeutics for these diseases of maladaptive plastic change.

Ebselen, a novel anti-inflammatory and anti-oxidant drug, has shown clinical efficacy for ameliorating hearing loss caused by acute noise exposure, and chronic Meniere's disease, and is now investigating therapeutic interventions for tobramycin-induced ototoxicity (Kil et al., 2021). Less is known as to whether the anti-inflammatory properties of ebselen can prevent or treat diseases of the brain (Martini et al., 2019; Sharpley et al., 2020), but it is likely that inflammation plays an important role in AG-induced auditory dysfunctions (Jiang et al., 2017b; Wood and Zuo, 2017). Encouragingly, recent work in mice has demonstrated that ebselen can reduce suprathreshold ABR wave fluctuations and hyperacusis caused by amikacin treatment (Longenecker et al., 2020). Therefore, ebselen, with its variety of proposed anti-oxidant/anti-inflammatory mechanisms of action (Wang et al., 2020), is a good candidate to investigate as a potential therapy for both peripheral and central sensory diseases.

Here we show the effects of a 14-day course of tobramycin in CBA/Ca mice. Small magnitude temporary threshold shifts were observed in many mice. The prevalence of tobramycin-induced hyperacusis and tinnitus as assessed by ASR was highest 2 weeks after treatment and observed to decrease over time. This corresponded to an increase in brain activity as measured by ABR amplitudes. In an amikacin model, ebselen provided statistically significant protection against tobramycin-induced threshold shifts and demonstrated some efficacy for protecting against tobramycin-induced tinnitus (Longenecker et al., 2020). Finally, we suggest potential mechanisms that could explain the AG-induced auditory dysfunctions we have observed in tobramycin and amikacin treated mice.

MATERIALS AND METHODS

Subjects

A total of 36 male and female CBA/Ca mice 3-6 months of age (at the start of experiments) were used in this study. Mice were born in house from parents obtained from Jackson Laboratories. Mice were housed 3 - 5 to a cage within a colony room with a 12-h light-dark cycle at 23°C. Hearing sensitivity and behavior was tracked longitudinally for each animal in a repeated measures design and animals were sacrificed for cochlear histology 18 weeks after the start of dosing following the final behavioral tests (see **Figure 1**).

Drug Formulation, Dosing, and Schedule

Stock ebselen powder was dissolved in pure dimethylsulfoxide (DMSO) at 20 mg/ml and stock tobramycin was dissolved in distilled water at 50 mg/ml and both were stored at minus 20°C. Mice were divided into three groups: Group 1 (n = 8) served as a control and did not receive tobramycin or ebselen. Group 2 (n = 14) received the vehicle i.p. and tobramycin (200 mg/kg body weight diluted in 0.2 ml saline) s.c. thirty minutes later. Group 3 (n = 14) received ebselen i.p. (20 mg/ml in DMSO at 20 mg/kg body weight was diluted in fresh 0.5 ml sterile saline) and tobramycin at s.c. thirty minutes later. The daily dosing schedules for Groups 2 and 3 was identical and was continued for 14 days. During the dosing period, the health and condition of animals were monitored by body weight, which is known to decrease during AG treatments.

Auditory Brainstem Response

Mice were anesthetized with isoflurane. Basal body temperature was maintained using a Gaymar T-pump warming pad set to 37°C and the animals' health was monitored by observation of respiration and circulation. Each ear was otoscopically inspected prior to insertion of ear tips (Nicolet Biomedical, Inc.) for

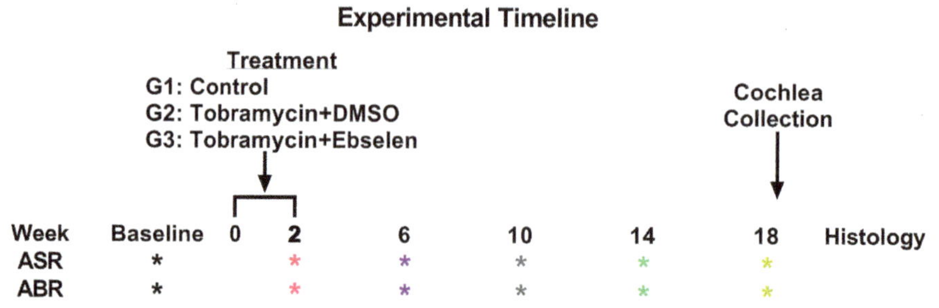

FIGURE 1 | Experimental timeline. ASR and ABR tests (* symbol) are color coded to specific weeks the tests occurred after the start of treatment. This color code is maintained throughout the manuscript. Tobramycin treatment was carried out from week 0 to 2 for two separate dosing groups. Animals were sacrificed after week 18 tests for cochlear histology.

sound delivery. Monaural closed field ABRs (Intelligent Hearing Systems) were collected before (baseline), as well as at weeks 2, 6, 10, 14, and 18 from the start of AG treatment. Subdermal platinum needle electrodes (Grass Telefactor, Inc.) were placed with the active electrode at the vertex and the reference electrode to the test ear, and the ground to the contralateral ear. Each ear was tested independently. Stimuli consisted of pure tone pips (5 ms duration, rectangular envelope) at 4, 8, 16, and 20 kHz presented for 800 repetitions (19.3 r/s) at sound levels from 80 dB SPL to 0 dB SPL (initially 20 dB steps until near threshold, then 5 dB steps) calibrated with a 0.25-inch microphone (Brüel and Kjaer, 4939). Thresholds were measured in 5 dB increments and defined visually by the presence of the most robust peak (I or III) that was reliable within 0.1 ms. Thresholds were analyzed by a scientist blind to treatment and isolated from data collection.

Behavioral Assessments of Hyperacusis, Tinnitus

Acoustic Startle Hardware/Software

Startle Reflex Hardware was purchased from Proxima Centauri Technologies (Julian, California). Each startle cabinet was lined with Sonex anechoic foam to minimize sound reflection and wave canceling sound echoes (Longenecker and Galazyuk, 2012). Sound levels from each cabinet's speakers was calibrated with a 0.5-inch microphone (Brüel and Kjaer 4939). Startle Waveforms were recorded using load-cell platforms and calibrated with 100 g weights. Offline data processing with code written in visual basic was used to evaluate whether each trial was a startle or non-startle via template matching and startle magnitude data was converted from force to center of mass displacement (CMD) (Grimsley et al., 2015). Only legitimate startles were included and used in the final data analyses (Longenecker et al., 2018).

Input/Output Functions for Hyperacusis Assessments

Startle stimuli were pseudorandomly presented between 60- and 100-dB SPL in 5 dB steps. Intertrial intervals were randomized between 4 and 6 s. Each input/output (I/O) session lasted roughly 12 min and consisted of 135 total trials in which each startle intensity was presented 15 times. I/O assessments were collected before (baseline), as well as at weeks 2, 6, 10, 14, and 18 from the start of AG treatment. For each individual animal, hyperacusis was defined by a significant increase in startle magnitude (two-way ANOVA) between baseline and any time point after dosing.

GPIAS for Tinnitus Assessment

Gap prepulse inhibition of the acoustic startle reflex was used to assess behavioral evidence of tinnitus (Longenecker and Galazyuk, 2011; Longenecker and Galazyuk, 2016). The ability of mice to detect a gap of silence preceding a startle stimulus was determined by comparing the startle magnitude in response to a startle stimulus (white noise; 100 dB SPL) presented alone (SO) and a startle stimulus paired with a preceding (100 ms before) gap (20 ms long) of silence (GAP). Both trials were presented in a continuous narrowband noise carrier presented at 5 different frequencies (4, 8, 12.5, 16, 20 kHz) at a constant intensity of 65 dB SPL. Additionally, 15 startles presented in silence were used to monitor startle habituation. Intertrial intervals were randomized between 4 and 6 s. Eight mice were excluded from GPIAS analysis because their baseline gap detection ratios did not meet criterion.

A testing session was comprised of 15 blocks comprising 150 trials, lasting roughly 15 min. A block was defined by 10 trials containing 5 pseudorandom SO and GAP trials presented in a uniform carrier frequency. Throughout the session, each carrier frequency block was represented 3 times for a total of 45 trials. On each testing day, 3 GPIAS sessions were run on each mouse lasting roughly 45 min. The best performance ratio was used to determine an individual animal's daily gap detection performance (Longenecker et al., 2018). GPIAS assessments were collected before (baseline), as well as at weeks 2, 6, 10, 14, and 18 from the start of AG treatment. For each individual animal, tinnitus was defined by a significant increase in the gap ratio (less inhibition) between baseline and any time point after dosing.

Cochlear Histology

Following the final ABR and behavioral assessments, mice (~6-12 months old) in three different groups (untreated control n = 8; tobramycin/DMSO n = 14; tobramycin/ebselen n = 14) were sacrificed with CO_2. Cochlea were collected, fixed in 4% PFA overnight, then processed for whole mount immunostaining. After the bony wall was removed carefully, the intact membranous cochlea was isolated from the modiolus. After decalcification in 0.5 M EDTA for 1 h, the membranous cochlea was permeabilized and blocked in 0.2% Triton X-100, 1% BSA and 5% donkey serum in PBS. To assess damage to inner and outer hair cells, tissue of one cochlea from each group were incubated with primary antibody: Rabbit anti-Myosin VIIa (1:200 dilution) overnight at 4°C, rinsed in PBS, and incubated with secondary antibody: Alexa Fluor 594 Donkey anti-Rabbit IgG (1:500 dilution) for 2 h at room temperature. Then the tissue was stained with FITC-Phalloidin (1:1000 dilution) for 10 min. For ribbon synapse observation, tissue of the cochlea (untreated control n = 14; tobramycin/DMSO *n* = 25; tobramycin/ebselen n = 25) were incubated with two primary antibodies: Rabbit anti-GluR2 (1:500 dilution) and Mouse anti-CtBP2 (1:500 dilution) overnight at 4°C, rinsed in PBS, and incubated with two secondary antibodies: Alexa Fluor 594 Donkey anti-Rabbit IgG (1:500 dilution), Alexa Fluor 488 Donkey anti-mouse IgG (1:500 dilution) for 2 h at room temperature. After the immunostaining was finished, the membranous cochlea was cut at the apical turn and the basal turn, then further dissected, embedded in mounting media with DAPI. Samples were examined via an epi-fluorescent microscope (Nikon Eclipse Ti), images were captured via a charge-coupled device camera (Hamamatsu C11440). Hair cells were observed as row images of the cochlea and were captured under 20X plain lens, then single images were assembled to form the whole cochlea image by using Adobe Photoshop CC 2018. For ribbon synapse observation, raw images at 16 kHz region were captured under 60X oil optical lens with a Z-stack range at 6 – 10 μm (based on the distribution of ribbon synapse / inner hair cell), in 0.2 μm steps; raw images then deconvoluted and processed with maximum intensity project.

Data Analysis

GraphPad Prism 9 was used for statistical analysis. One-way and two-way ANOVAs were used in data sets with normally distributed and equal sample sizes. Mixed models analyzed data that did not meet these assumptions. Sidak's multiple comparison or Fisher's LSD tests were used to discover individual differences at specific timepoints in the in vivo dosing study. Greyscale statistical symbols represent significance differences between dosing groups, while colored symbols represent specific significant differences between baseline and specific after dosing epochs. For each figure, the level of statistical significance is represented as: one symbol, $p \leq 0.05$; two symbols, $p \leq 0.01$; three symbols, $p \leq 0.001$; four symbols, $p \leq 0.0001$. Fisher's exact test were used to analyze clinically relevant ABR threshold, hyperacusis, and tinnitus changes. To develop clinically relevant ABR threshold shift criterion, we modified ASHA guidelines for ototoxic change using pure tone audiometry (American Speech-Language-Hearing Association, 1994; Gu et al., 2020; Longenecker et al., 2020). Here, we identified ototoxic change using the following three criteria: (1) A ≥ 10 dB shift at three adjacent tested frequencies (4, 8, 16, 20 kHz). (2) A ≥ 15 dB shift at two adjacent tested frequencies. (3) A ≥ 20 dB shift at any one tested frequency. Each ear was tested and analyzed independently. The percentage of ears which met the threshold shift criteria was calculated for each time point (weeks 2, 6, 10, 14, and 18).

RESULTS

Tobramycin Causes Temporary Threshold Shifts Without Permanent Cochlear Damage

To examine the effects of tobramycin on hearing sensitivity, we documented ABR thresholds up to 18 weeks from the start of AG treatment. Following a standard 14-day tobramycin regimen, mean ABR thresholds were elevated 10-15 dB at 16 kHz from baseline levels (**Figure 2**). ABR traces from baseline and 2 weeks following the start of dosing are shown from an untreated control (**Figure 2A**), a tobramycin/DMSO treated (**Figure 2B**, and a tobramycin/ebselen treated mouse (**Figure 2C**). A two-way ANOVA found a significant effect of dosing between subjects at 2 weeks [$F_{(2,265)} = 9.724$, $p < 0.001$] and 6 weeks [$F_{(2,264)} = 11.40$, $p < 0.001$] after the start of dosing (**Figures 2D,E**). Significant effects for frequency were also found at 2 weeks [$F_{(3,265)} = 5.363$, $p = 0.001$], 6 weeks [$F_{(3,264)} = 3.172$, $p = 0.025$], 10 weeks [$F_{(3,262)} = 3.499$, $p = 0.016$] and 14 weeks [$F_{(3,257)} = 2.820$, $p = 0.040$] after dosing. Interactions between dosing and frequency were seen at 2 weeks [$F_{(6,265)} = 3.118$, $p = 0.006$] and 6 weeks [$F_{(6,264)} = 2.660$, $p = 0.016$]. Šidák's multiple comparison tests showed highly significant differences between control and tobramycin/DMSO groups at 16 kHz during the 2-week (**Figure 2D**, $p = 0.001$) and 6-week (**Figure 2E**, $p = 0.001$) epochs. Specific differences at 16 kHz were also seen between tobramycin/DMSO and tobramycin/ebselen groups at week 2 ($p < 0.001$), week 6 ($p < 0.001$), week 10 ($p = 0.014$), and week 14 ($p = 0.021$), as well as at 20 kHz at the 6-week epoch ($p = 0.036$) (**Figures 2D-G**). Tobramycin-induced threshold shifts were resolved by week 18 after the start of dosing (**Figure 2H**). To evaluate if these ABR deficits were significant on a per ear level, we applied the recently developed clinically relevant change criteria (**Figure 2I**; Gu et al., 2020; Longenecker et al., 2020). When evaluated with the Fisher's exact test, these responder criteria revealed a significant difference between tobramycin/DMSO and tobramycin/ebselen treated ears at week 2 (39.3% vs 7.7%, $p = 0.010$) and week 6 (35.7% vs. 0%, $p < 0.001$), but not at later timepoints after dosing. These data suggest that although the mean threshold shifts were relatively mild after tobramycin treatment, a sizeable minority of mice experienced noticeable hearing impairment via a clinically relevant hearing assessment.

To investigate if the central auditory system became more reactive following tobramycin treatment, we assessed ABR wave III/wave I amplitude ratios (**Supplementary Figure 1**). We found that for most frequencies and amplitudes that there was a general increase in the wave III/wave I amplitude ratio (**Supplementary Figures 1A-F**) in tobramycin treated animals. While a significant effect of time was not found, a trend towards increased ratios over time was observed at some frequencies (reference to 100% dashed line). A between subjects mixed-effects analysis found an effect of dose for 16 kHz 40 dB ratios [$F_{(2,69)} = 3.295$, $p = 0.043$], in which subjects of the tobramycin/DMSO group ratio was higher at most epochs than the subjects of the control or tobramycin/ebselen groups

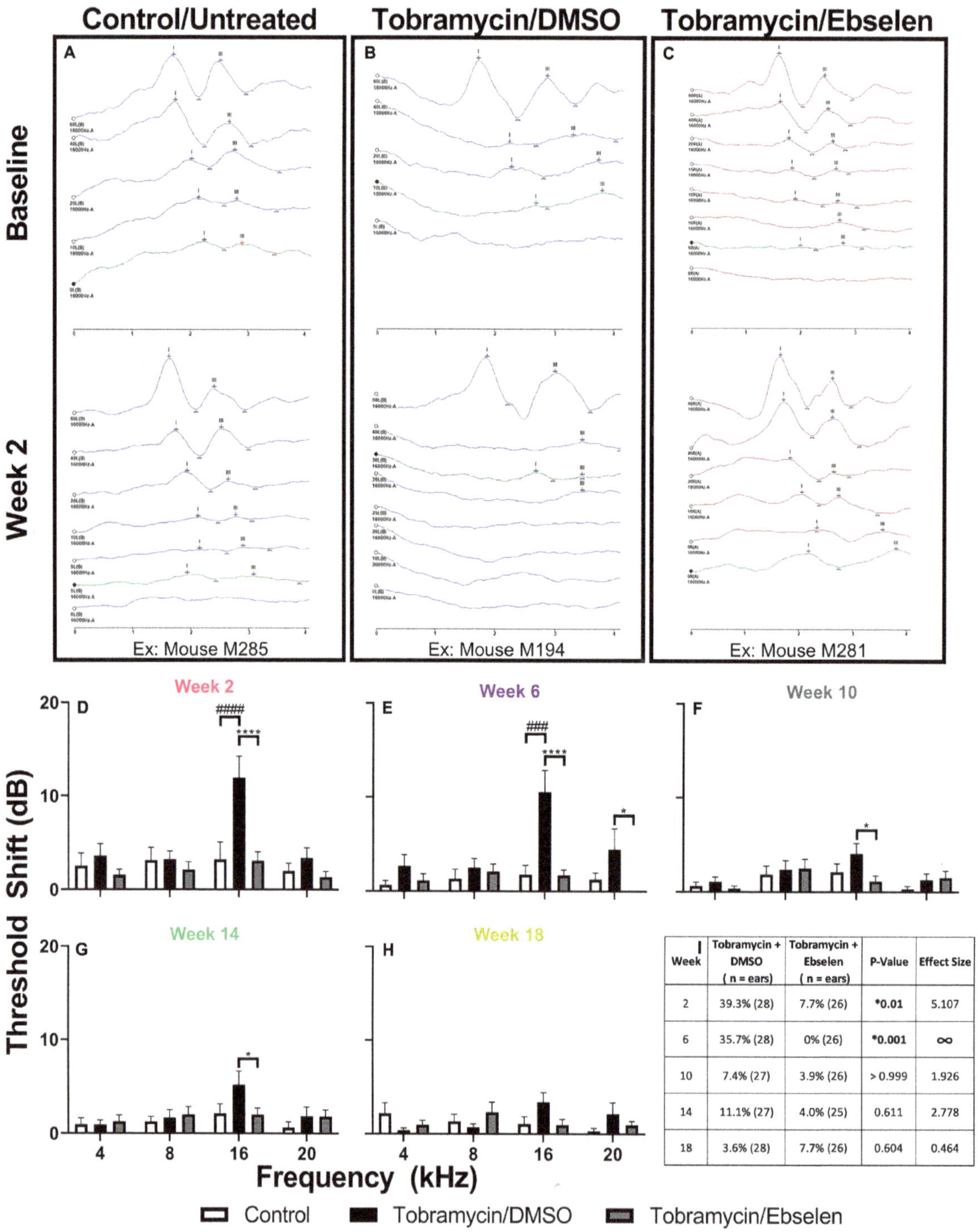

Week	Tobramycin + DMSO (n = ears)	Tobramycin + Ebselen (n = ears)	P-Value	Effect Size
2	39.3% (28)	7.7% (26)	*0.01	5.107
6	35.7% (28)	0% (26)	*0.001	∞
10	7.4% (27)	3.9% (26)	> 0.999	1.926
14	11.1% (27)	4.0% (25)	0.611	2.778
18	3.6% (28)	7.7% (26)	0.604	0.464

FIGURE 2 | Evaluation of hearing loss caused by tobramycin. ABR traces from 16 kHz stimuli collected at baseline and 2 weeks after the start of treatment showing impact of tobramycin on hearing thresholds (**(A)**: untreated control, **(B)**: tobramycin/DMSO, **(C)**: tobramycin/ebselen). Blue and red traces show ABRs from left and right ears, respectively. Green trace in each panel represents threshold. Averaged tobramycin-induced ABR threshold shifts comparing testing groups at different epochs (**(D):** week 2, **(E):** week 6, **(F):** week 10, **(G):** week 14, **(H):** week 18) after the start of treatment. ABRs were collected for 4, 8, 16, and 20 kHz. Shifts represent the specific epoch minus the baseline ABR value for each group. Data is represented by threshold shift means and standard errors. Post hoc tests determined significant differences between testing groups, which are indicated as follows: # (black), between control and DMSO treated animals; # (gray), between control and ebselen treated animals; *, between DMSO and ebselen treated animals. **(I):** Clinically relevant change criteria table. (1) Criterion for CRC: A $\geq$ 20 dB shift at one frequency. (2) A $\geq$ 15 dB shift at two adjacent frequencies. (3) A $\geq$ 10 dB shift at three adjacent frequencies. Each ear was analyzed independently. The percentage of ears which met the ABR threshold shift criteria was calculated for each time point (weeks 2, 6, 10, 14, 18). Two-sided Fisher's exact tests were used statistically evaluate differences between testing groups. The effect size represents relative risk (Koopman asymptotic score).

(**Supplementary Figure 1F**). Specific Fisher's LSD post hoc significance values can be seen in **Supplementary Table 1**. The trends observed here closely resemble those seen in amikacin treated mice (Longenecker et al., 2020). Such changes in ratios could be explained by increases in wave III amplitudes or decreases in wave I amplitudes from baseline levels. We found that wave I amplitudes were mainly decreased, especially at higher frequencies (**Supplementary Figures 2, 3**). Additionally, some wave III amplitudes for 40 dB stimuli did increase (**Supplementary Figure 2**).

Such changes electrophysiological changes were not readily explained by damage to cochlear sensory cells. In representative cochlear whole mounts, inner and outer hair cells remained intact from the base to the apex in untreated controls (**Figure 3A**), tobramycin/DMSO treated (**Figure 3B**), and tobramycin/ebselen treated animals (**Figure 3C**). At the region representative of 16 kHz hearing, no observable differences were seen in pre- (CtBP2 green) and post- (GluR2 red) synaptic densities between untreated controls (**Figure 3D**), tobramycin/DMSO treated (**Figure 3E**), and tobramycin/ebselen treated animals (**Figure 3F**). This was true throughout all the cochlea regions we analyzed which spanned all frequencies we examined in this study.

Tobramycin Treatment Can Induce Hyperacusis and Tinnitus-Like Behavior

To investigate if tobramycin treatment resulted in amplified startle responses to loud acoustic stimuli as it did with amikacin treatment (Longenecker et al., 2020), we conducted ASR input/output assessments (**Figures 4, 5**). Following tobramycin treatment startle responses were greatly exaggerated in some mice, examples of which are seen in **Figure 4**. A two-way repeated measures ANOVA showed significance of time after treatment for mouse M94 [$F_{(3.715,467.4)} = 9.624$, $p < 0.001$] and mouse F305 [$F_{(4.061,441.0)} = 34.84$] (**Figures 4A,B**). For these mice, Dunnett's multiple comparison tests revealed that startle responses were significantly elevated at week 2 ($p < 0.001$), week 6 ($p = 0.037$), week 10 ($p < 0.001$), and week 18 ($p = 0.011$) for mouse M94, as well as week 2 ($p < 0.001$) and week 10 ($p < 0.001$) for mouse F305. Such significant elevations in startle were not observed for example mouse F301 (**Figure 4C**). Time after dosing was also a significant factor for Mouse F301 [$F_{(4.526,415.5)} = 12.96$, $p < 0.001$), but startle magnitudes significantly decreased over time, following the normal habituation to the startle stimulus. To tabulate the incidence of hyperacusis-like behavior following tobramycin treatment, the percentage of individual mice that demonstrated statistically significant increases in startle response for each epoch after dosing were evaluated with responder criteria (**Figure 4D**). At the week 2 epoch roughly 40% of mice experienced hyperacusis-like behavior, which fell to less than 10% by week 14. This responder analysis is important because it can elucidate that the symptoms of individual mice, which can be missed by group mean averages as seen in **Figure 5**. Between subject group analysis revealed very little hyperacusis-like behavior, as IO functions for each dosing group were below the baseline (below 0) startle magnitude at most epochs, representative of habituation (**Figure 5**). This was not surprising, because the majority of mice did not show hyperacusis-like behavior (**Figure 4D**). Two-way ANOVAs revealed that significant effect of treatment at week 2 [$F_{(2,367)} = 3.139$, $p = 0.045$], week 6 [$F_{(2, 311)} = 4.758$, $p = 0.009$], and week 10 [$F_{(2, 304)} = 11.11$, $p < 0.001$] (**Figures 5A-C**). Animals treated with tobramycin showed less habituation as a group, because a subset of these animals developed hyperacusis, while control animals did not (**Figure 5**). Šidák's multiple comparison tests revealed that the tobramycin/ebselen treated group maintaining significantly higher levels of startle than the untreated control group at week 6 ($p = 0.007$) and the control group ($p = 0.002$) and DMSO group ($p = 0.003$) at week 10. By week 14 and 18 after the start of dosing, no significant differences were seen between groups with startle responses trending well below baseline startle reactivity (**Figures 5D,E**). To evaluate if increases in hyperacusis-like behavior were significantly different between treatment groups we conducted a Fisher's exact test. Based on relatively similar mean startle response magnitude averages between groups (**Figures 5A-E**), it was unsurprising to see no significant difference between tobramycin/DMSO and tobramycin/ebselen groups (**Figure 5F**). Based on this dataset, ebselen did not play a major role in preventing the development of tobramycin-induced hyperacusis.

To evaluate tobramycin-induced behavioral evidence of tinnitus, we used the GPIAS methodology which has been used to assess drug- and noise- induced tinnitus (**Figure 6**; Longenecker and Galazyuk, 2016; Longenecker et al., 2020). Individual examples of a mice that did and did not develop gap detection deficits following tobramycin treatment demonstrate the variability between mice (**Figures 6A,B**). A repeated measures mixed-effects model showed an effect of time after dosing on gap detection for mouse F305 [$F_{(3.749,263.9)} = 3.859$, $p = 0.006$], but not mouse M089 [$F_{(4.553,321.4)} = 0.5342$, $p = 0.734$]. Fisher's LSD tests revealed frequency specific gap detection deficits (20 kHz) at week 2 ($p = 0.018$) and week 6 ($p = 0.028$) when compared to baseline gap detection for mouse F305 (**Figure 6A**). These sorts of deficits were not observed in example mouse M89 which was also treated with tobramycin (**Figure 6B**), nor mouse M90 which served as an untreated control (**Figure 6C**). To further investigate the overall effect of tobramycin on gap detection we examined the grand mean average of animals that developed tinnitus or those which did not (**Figures 6D,F**). In the tinnitus positive group, a two-way repeated measures ANOVA found an effect of time after tobramycin dosing ($F_{(4.110,164.4)} = 2.943$, $p = 0.021$), but not in the tinnitus negative group ($F_{(4.346,325.9)} = 1.199$, $p = 0.311$), or the untreated controls ($F_{(2.799,27.99)} = 0.8964$, $p = 0.449$). Fisher's LSD tests revealed frequency specific deficits at 8 kHz (week 18: $p = 0.038$), 12.5 kHz (week 14: $p = 0.041$), 16 kHz (week 2: $p = 0.026$), and 20 kHz (week 2: $p = 0.001$, week 6: $p = 0.014$, week 14: $p = 0.048$) in the tinnitus positive group (**Figure 6D**). Interestingly, the tinnitus negative group also demonstrated one significant frequency at 16 kHz (week 6: $p = 0.386$). The incidence of tinnitus-like behavior (**Figure 6G**) demonstrated a similar

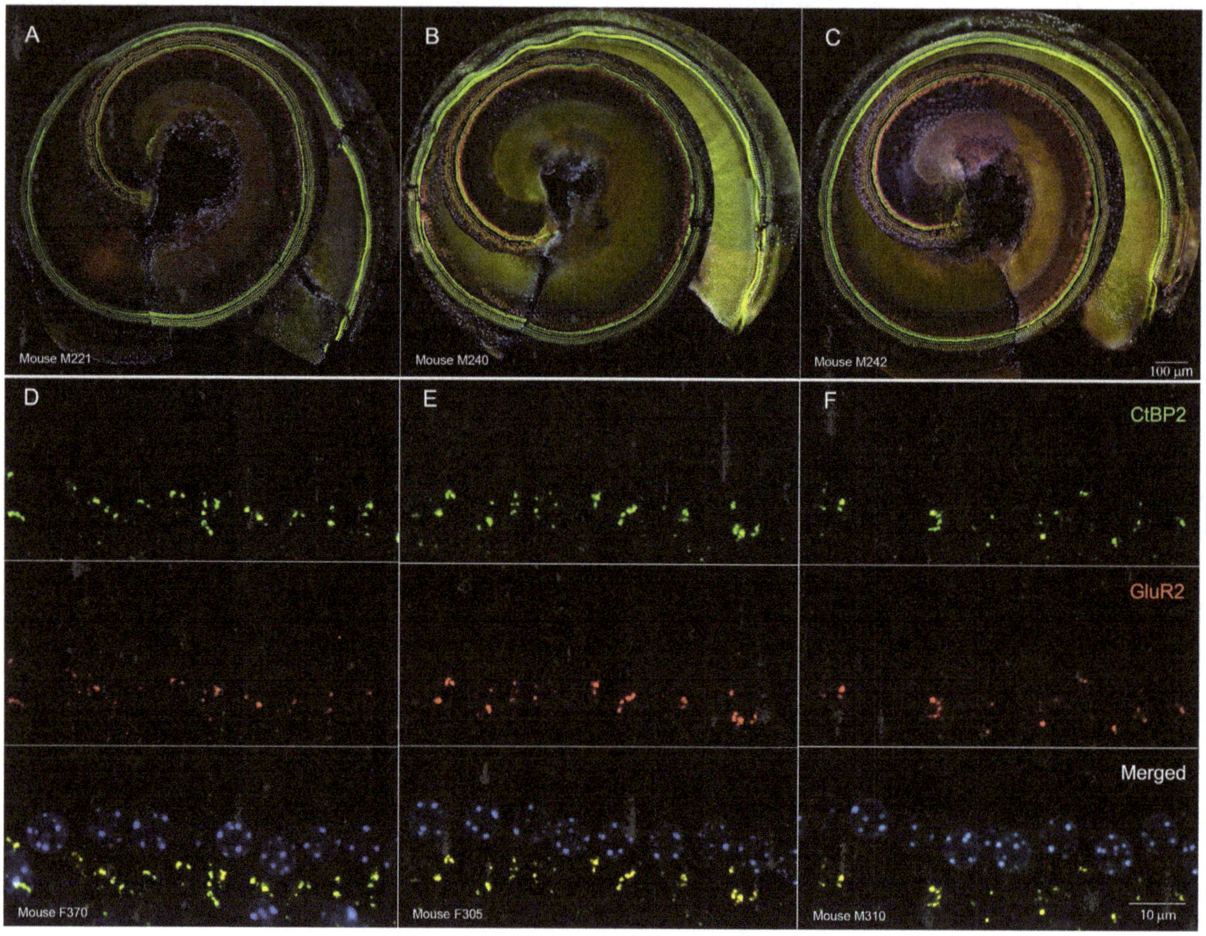

FIGURE 3 | Representative whole mount cochlear images displaying cochlear hair cells for each treatment group (**(A):** untreated control, **(B):** tobramycin/DMSO, **(C):** tobramycin/ebselen [Scale bar = 100 μm]). No observable evidence of tobramycin-induced outer hair cell or inner hair cell loss. Outer hair cells were stained with anti-myosin VIIa antibody (red) and inner hair cells were stained with FITC phalloidin (green). Representative micrographs showing pre and post synaptic densities in the 16 kHz region for each treatment group (**(D):** untreated control, **(E):** tobramycin/DMSO, **(F):** tobramycin/ebselen [Scale bar = 10 μm]). When comparing treatment groups, no observable differences were apparent when examining the immunolabeled presynaptic marker CtBP2 (green), postsynaptic marker GluR2 (red), or the merged images (yellow), which include hair cell nucleus marker DAPI (blue).

pattern as hyperacusis-like behavior (**Figure 4D**), as it was highest at 2 weeks after tobramycin dosing and gradually decreased over time. When examining if ebselen had an effect on preventing tinnitus-like behavior (**Figure 6H**), a Fisher's exact test did not find a significant effect ($p = 0.248$) but was more impactful than in hyperacusis-like behavior (**Figure 5F**).

DISCUSSION

In this study we demonstrated that a 14-day course of tobramycin can lead to hearing deficits, hyperacusis, and tinnitus in CBA/Ca mice, that may be clinically relevant. Ebselen was shown to be effective at preventing hearing loss and demonstrated non-significant evidence of preventing the development of tinnitus or hyperacusis in tobramycin treated mice. These deficits were observed in the absence of obvious cochlear hair cell loss or ribbon synapse degradation. These results are further discussed in context of previous preclinical and clinical studies investigating aminoglycoside-induced auditory dysfunction.

Tobramycin-Induced Temporary Threshold Shifts Can Occur Without Permanent Cochlear Damage

Tobramycin has been known to cause variable magnitudes of temporary and permanent threshold shift following a single course in animal models (Gu et al., 2020; Ogier et al., 2020) and humans (Garinis et al., 2020; Harruff et al., 2020). Here we confirmed that a standard course of tobramycin treatment caused consistent, yet small significant mean threshold shifts of roughly 10-15 dB SPL at 16 kHz in a CBA/Ca animal model (**Figure 2**). After 18 weeks after dosing, these hearing deficits decreased and returned to near baseline levels (**Figures 2D-H**). The responder criteria for hearing loss demonstrated a similar pattern, in which the percentage of mice with a relevant shift

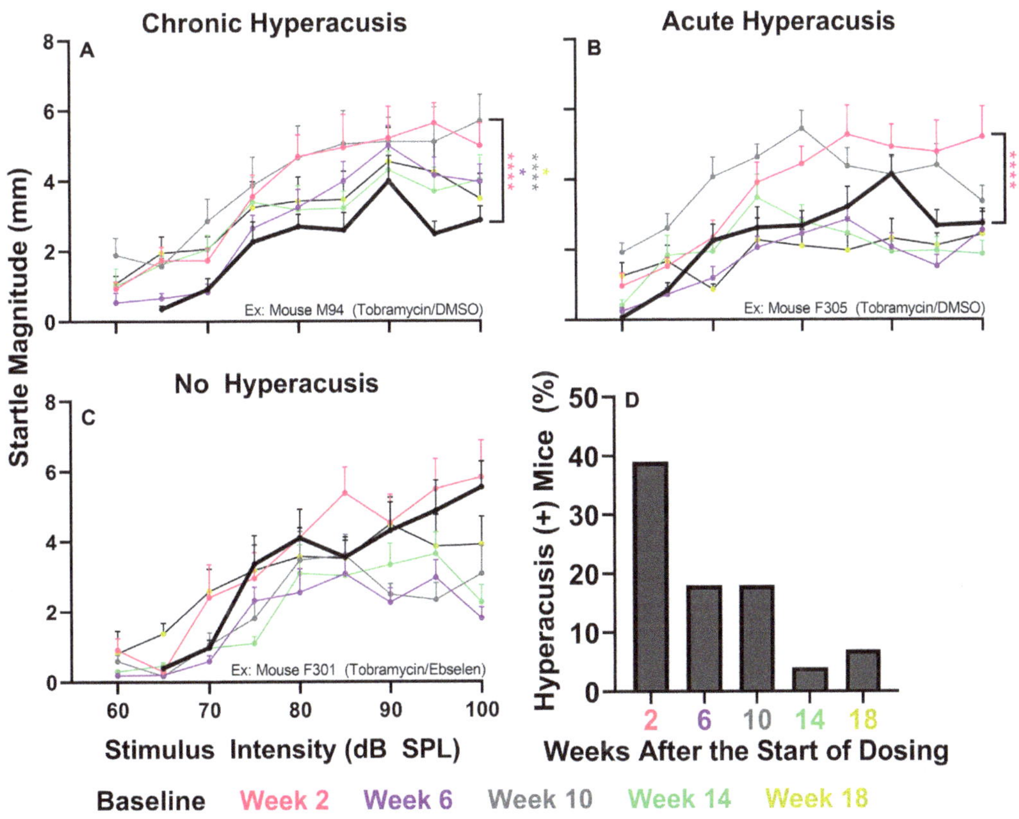

FIGURE 4 | Evaluation of behavioral evidence of hyperacusis for individual animals. IO Startle stimulus/response functions recorded from 3 representative tobramycin-treated mice. **(A):** Example of a tobramycin-treated mouse with chronic hyperacusis, **(B):** Acute hyperacusis, and **(C):** no hyperacusis. Startle response magnitude CMD (mm) as a function of stimulus intensity (60 to 100 dB SPL) represent each specific epoch (color coded) compared to baseline (bolded black line). Data is represented by means and standard errors. *Post hoc* significant differences between specific epochs (color coded) and baseline are indicated as follows: $^{*}p \leq 0.05$; $^{**}p \leq 0.01$; $^{***}p \leq 0.001$; $^{****}p \leq 0.0001$. **(D):** Histogram representing the % of all tobramycin treated mice which showed statistically significant increases in startle IO functions at each epoch after dosing.

decreased over time (**Figure 2I**). When comparing the effect size dosing factors, ebselen demonstrated protection against tobramycin-induced threshold shifts for the first 2 epochs after the start of dosing, but not at later time periods because threshold shifts were non-significant after this point (**Figure 2**). A similar finding was observed with the clinically modified or adopted responder criteria (American Speech-Language-Hearing Association, 1994). This finding was comparable to the effect of ebselen on amikacin treated mice (Longenecker et al., 2020), and provides evidence that ebselen or other otoprotective drugs might work at ameliorating AG-induced hearing loss in clinic (Avci et al., 2016; Fox et al., 2016; Dogan et al., 2017; El-Anwar et al., 2018; Apaydin et al., 2021). However, the threshold shifts seen here were drastically different than those found with a similar tobramycin dosing experiment in Swiss-Webster mice (Gu et al., 2020). While little is reported on the susceptibility of ototoxicity for most strains of mice, the CBA/Ca is well known for its relative resistance to noise- (Davis et al., 2001), and age- (Zheng et al., 1999; Peguero and Tempel, 2015; Liu et al., 2019), related hearing loss. When comparing these studies, it seems the CBA/Ca mouse has more resistant to AG-ototoxicity. However, the commercially available tobramycin used in each experiment could have differed by specific strain. This possibility was highlighted by an important recent finding which demonstrated that specific strains of gentamycin can have differential cochleotoxic effects (O'Sullivan et al., 2020). This could create a major confound in ototoxicity studies due to the variability of strain-induced damage and partially explains the variability of published results in the literature (Ogier et al., 2020). Nevertheless, a future study should investigate a tobramycin ototoxicity/dose response curve for CBA/Ca mice.

Just as we and others have discovered, aminoglycosides are not acutely ototoxic after one course of using non-lethal doses in most species and strains of laboratory animals (Longenecker et al., 2020; Ogier et al., 2020). In fact, cochlear hair cell loss was minimal or absent following one 14-day course of tobramycin (**Figures 3A-C**). It was also shown that spiral ganglion neurons and their synapses remain intact, at least after a recovery period of 16-18 weeks after tobramycin treatment (**Figures 3D-F**) or amikacin treatment (Longenecker et al., 2020). It is possible that immediate or early changes in synapse integrity following tobramycin treatment could explain the temporary auditory dysfunction documented in this study (Liu et al., 2015; Hong et al., 2018). Indeed, potentially relevant but largely

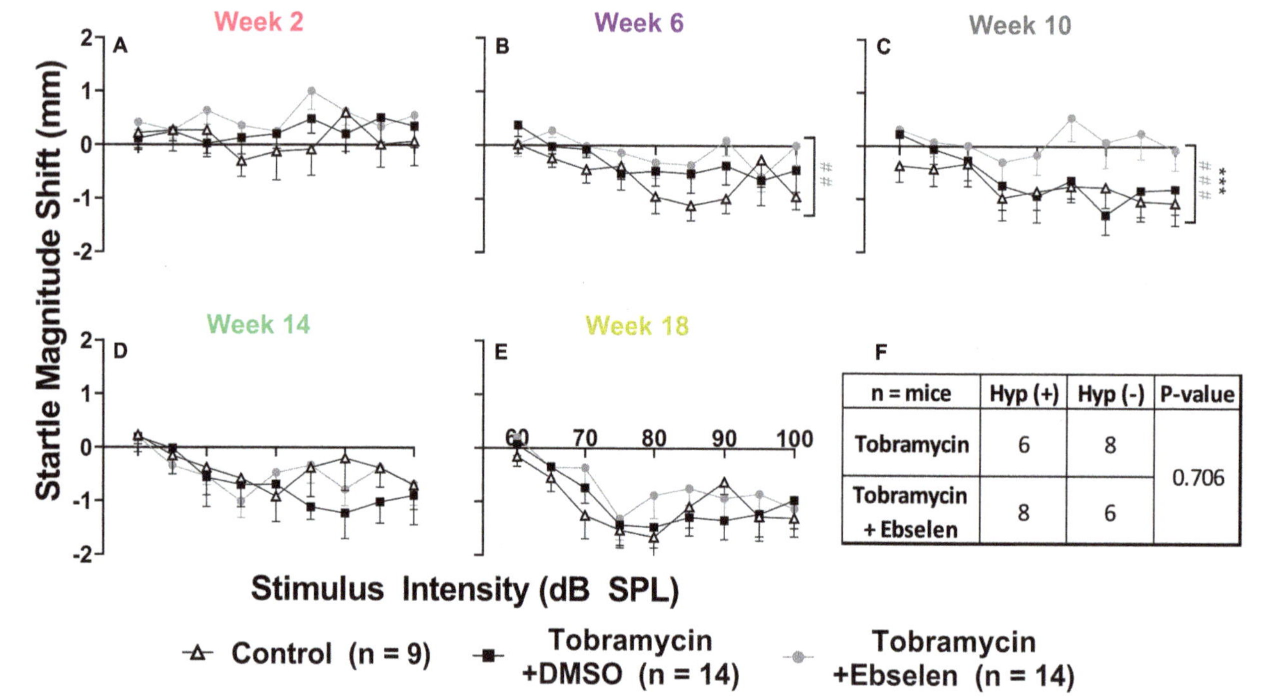

FIGURE 5 | Evaluation of behavioral evidence of hyperacusis by dosing group. Averaged tobramycin-induced IO stimulus/response functions shifts comparing testing groups at different epochs (**(A):** week 2, **(B):** week 6, **(C):** week 10, **(D):** week 14, **(E):** week 18) after the start of treatment. Startle response magnitude CMD (mm) as a function of stimulus intensity (60 to 100 dB SPL) represent each specific epoch minus baseline. The value 0 on the y-axis represents no change from baseline startle reactivity. Data is represented by means and standard errors. Post hoc tests determined significant differences between testing groups, which are indicated as follows: # (black), between control and DMSO treated animals; # (gray), between control and ebselen treated animals; *, between DMSO and ebselen treated animals. **(F):** Contingency table for the development of hyperacusis which shows the number of mice which met or did not meet the criteria for hyperacusis (significant increase in startle IO function at any epoch when compared to baseline). Each animal was analyzed independently. Two-sided Fisher's exact tests were used statistically evaluate differences between tobramycin dosed groups.

non-significant increases in ABR wave III/wave I amplitude ratios (**Supplementary Figure 1**) suggest either central compensation from altered peripheral input (Gold and Bajo, 2014), or direct effects of AGs on the central nervous system (Segal et al., 1999; Abd-Elhakim et al., 2021).

Hyperacusis and Tinnitus Appear After Tobramycin Treatment

The most important finding of this study is that tobramycin can cause behavioral signs of hyperacusis and tinnitus in mice (**Figures 4, 5, 6**). Additionally, these abnormal behaviors occur in the presence of only a mild loss of hearing sensitivity. These new findings are consistent with prior findings that amikacin can cause these behavioral symptoms following a mild threshold shift, although the mechanism will need to be elucidated (Longenecker et al., 2020; **Figure 7**). The largest difference between the two studies was that tobramycin treated mice demonstrated less startle magnitude increases after treatment than amikacin treated mice (**Figure 5** vs. **Figure 6** from Longenecker et al., 2020). This was especially true at the early epochs following treatment (**Figures 5A-C**). Tobramycin led to 50% and amikacin led to 82.3% of mice developing behavioral signs of hyperacusis. In both studies, hyperacusis-like symptoms were highest at epochs tested near the start of dosing and decreased thereafter (**Figure 4D**). The majority of mice treated with amikacin showed drastic increases in startle magnitude in contrast to a minority of mice treated with tobramycin. However, it is important to note that hyperacusis manifested differently between mice. Increased input/output startle functions such as the presented example of tobramycin treated mouse M94 (**Figure 4A**) was more commonly observed in amikacin treated mice (Longenecker et al., 2020). M94 demonstrated consistent hyperacusis throughout the testing period while F305 only experienced hyperacusis at weeks 2 and 10 after the start of dosing followed with clear habituation the rest of the epochs (**Figures 4A,B**). This temporal fluctuation disparity explains the dramatic difference in effect size between these mice which were both treated with tobramycin. Due to the lower incidence and startle magnitude shifts in tobramycin treated animals, it is not surprising that there was a non-significant effect of ebselen in preventing tobramycin-treated hyperacusis (**Figure 5F**). The effect sizes of dosing between epochs remained low throughout the study. The likely explanation of this phenomenon is that hyperacusis can be observed despite the natural response for mice to habituate to the startle reflex over time (**Figures 4B,C, 5**). Long-term habituation of the ASR is a universal phenomenon across multiple species and testing conditions (Davis, 1984) and has been specifically observed

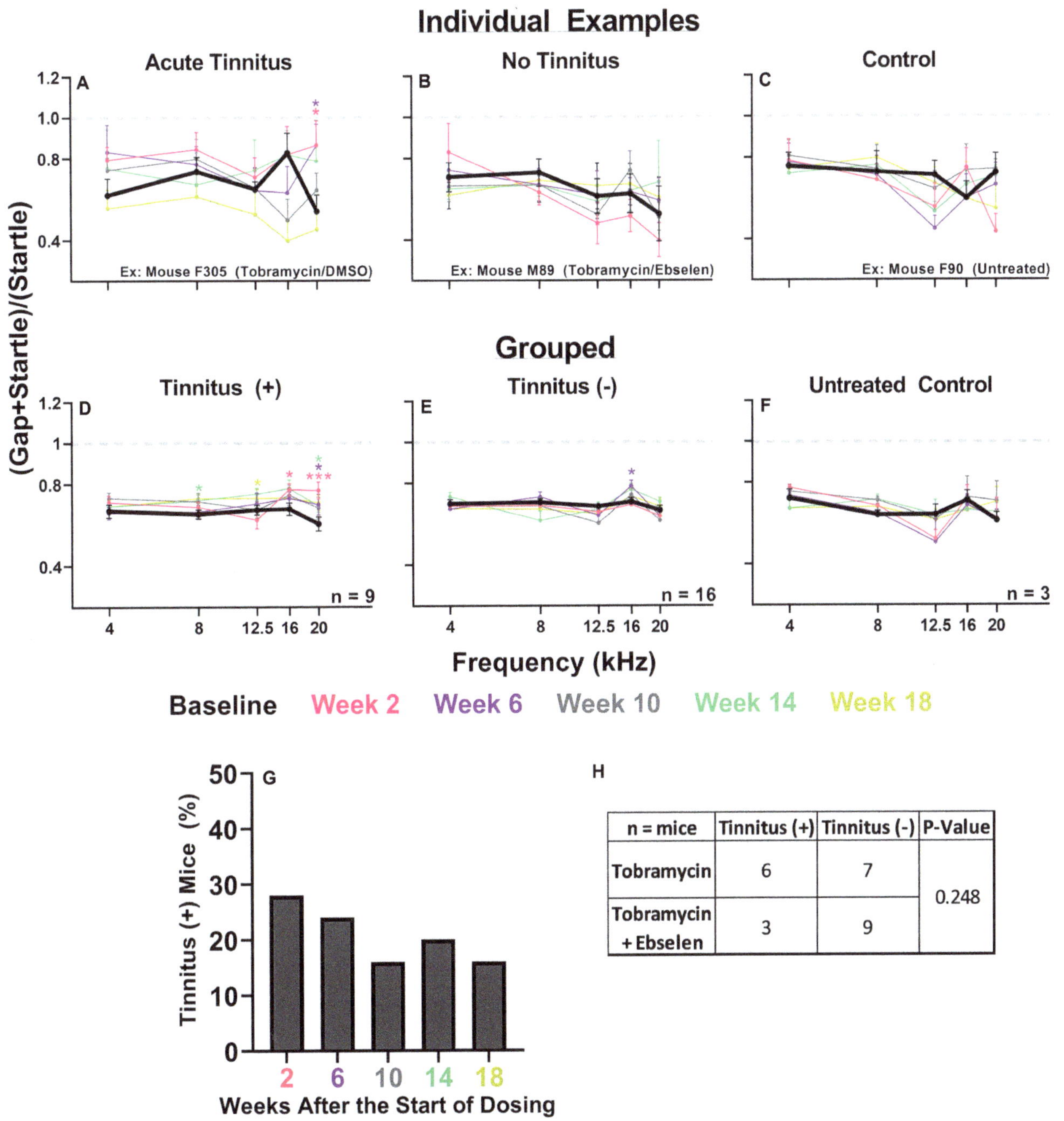

H

n = mice	Tinnitus (+)	Tinnitus (-)	P-Value
Tobramycin	6	7	0.248
Tobramycin + Ebselen	3	9	

FIGURE 6 | Evaluation of behavioral evidence of tinnitus for individual animals and dosing groups. **(A):** Example GPIAS functions for a tobramycin treated mouse with behavioral evidence of acute tinnitus, **(B):** a treated mouse with no tinnitus, and **(C):** an untreated control mouse. **(D):** GPIAS functions for the group mean averages of tinnitus mice, **(E):** tinnitus negative mice, and **(F):** untreated control mice. Tinnitus was defined as a significant GPIAS deficit at 1 or 2 adjacent frequencies at any epoch (color coded) compared to baseline (bolded black line). Data is represented by ratio means and standard errors. Post hoc significant differences between specific epochs (color coded) and baseline are indicated as follows: *$p \leq 0.05$; **$p \leq 0.01$; ***. **(G):** Histogram representing the % of all tobramycin treated mice which showed statistically significant gap detection deficits as described above at each epoch after dosing. **(H):** Contingency table for the development of tinnitus which shows the number of mice which met or did not meet the criteria for tinnitus. Each animal was analyzed independently. Two-sided Fisher's exact tests were used statistically evaluate differences between tobramycin dosed groups.

several strains of mice (Bullock et al., 1997; Pilz et al., 2014; Longenecker et al., 2018). This fact amplifies the importance of the odd behavioral shift towards dramatic increases in startle magnitude seen in some tobramycin (**Figures 4A,B**), and amikacin treated mice (Longenecker et al., 2020). The main reason hyperacusis was not observed in group averages of tobramycin treated mice (**Figure 5**) is because most mice did not develop hyperacusis and habituated to the startle (**Figures 4D, 5F**), which therefore decreased the average startle magnitude (**Figures 5A-E**). Amikacin treatment led to a higher incidence and magnitude of startle response shift, which explains the more elevated treatment group averages previously seen (Longenecker et al., 2020). Taken together, data from these studies suggest that aminoglycosides can dramatically increase startle responses in some animals despite habituation.

Behavioral evidence of tinnitus was also observed in tobramycin treated animals (**Figure 6**), although it is important to note the limitations of the GPIAS method in the context of AG-cochleotoxic experiments which were discussed in detail previously (Longenecker et al., 2020). We found that 9 out of 25 mice (36%) experienced gap detection deficits indicative of tinnitus at some point during the 18 weeks of testing after treatment, and similar to hyperacusis and hearing loss (**Figures 2, 4D**), the incidence decreased over time (**Figure 6G**). AG-induced tinnitus is thought to have an incidence rate between 12 and 37.5% in CF or tuberculosis patients (Daud et al., 2014; Harruff et al., 2020; Sabur et al., 2021). The other interesting point to note is that tobramycin treatment caused consistent gap detection deficits. When tinnitus-positive animals were grouped together, a significant broad-frequency deficit in gap detection was observed at multiple epochs (**Figure 6D**). The greatest deficits were seen at high frequencies (i.e. 20 kHz), which is higher than the frequency with the greatest threshold deficits (16 kHz), a common report following noise exposure in animal studies (Turner et al., 2012; Coomber et al., 2014; Longenecker and Galazyuk, 2016). Importantly, when averaged together, animals determined to be tinnitus negative had a gap detection deficit at 16 kHz at week 6 (**Figure 6E**). This deficit might be due to loss of hearing sensitivity at 16 kHz rather than a tinnitus percept at this frequency (**Figure 2**). Although not statistically significant, ebselen co-treatment trended towards the prevention of the tinnitus-like behaviors (**Figure 6H**).

As discussed above, hyperacusis was found to be more prevalent than tinnitus following tobramycin treatment which is consistent with what has been reported after amikacin treatment (Longenecker et al., 2020). Clinically, the incidence rates of these maladies are correlated, but not 1:1 (Baguley and Hoare, 2018; Cederroth et al., 2020). A major confound is that clinical studies are nearly entirely self-reported and based on patient reported outcomes over the last week or month. Large clinical studies have found a significant positive correlation between tinnitus and hyperacusis (Cederroth et al., 2020; Raj-Koziak et al., 2021). Another study found that hyperacusis percept shows a positive correlation for the persistence of tinnitus (Refat et al., 2021). It is likely that the neural code and anatomy for these maladies have unique but overlapping pathways, which could explain the results from these AG studies (Eggermont, 2021). A recent report demonstrated that hyperacusis was developed in rats to a non-damaging noise exposure of 70 dB SPL (Thomas et al., 2019). This study also showed that hearing sensitivity as assessed by ABR and light and fluorescence cochlear histology are grossly intact after AG treatment, suggesting that hyperacusis can be developed in the absence of significant cochlear cell loss (Thomas et al., 2019; Longenecker et al., 2020). A critical point to make when comparing amikacin and tobramycin studies is that there might be a link between behavior and electrophysiological measures of AG-induced auditory dysfunction. Amikacin treated mice demonstrated significant increases in ABR amplitude wave III/wave I ratios along with higher incidence and magnitude of hyperacusis-like behavior (Longenecker et al., 2020). Here we report lower incidence and magnitude rates of hyperacusis-like behavior which correlated to less significant increases in ABR ratios (**Figure 4** and **Supplementary Figure 1**). Future studies should evaluate if this correlation between behavior and brain physiology reveals an underlying mechanism of tinnitus and/or hyperacusis (**Figure 7**). However, an important validation of this animal work was seen in CF-patients with lifetime histories of AG use (Westman et al., 2021). The Westman et al. (2021), study demonstrated that AG use was correlated with enhanced acoustic reflex growth functions compared to those with less or no AG exposure. The authors speculate that this finding more likely explains a central mechanism of auditory dysfunction, like hyperacusis or tinnitus, rather than cochlear related dysfunctions.

Towards a Mechanistic Understanding of AG-Induced Tinnitus and Hyperacusis

In reviewing data from this tobramycin study, and the prior amikacin study (Longenecker et al., 2020), with the recent human study (Westman et al., 2021), it seems that hyperacusis and tinnitus might be common side-effects of AG treatment. The mechanism(s) to explain these AG-induced symptoms need to be investigated and could be explained in three unique, or more likely, overlapping pathways: peripheral dysfunction (cellular or molecular), central plasticity resulting from peripheral dysfunction, or direct central disfunction (**Figure 7**).

It is thought that all types of cells in the cochlea can be affected by aminoglycosides (Jiang et al., 2017a,b). Hair cells are known to be vulnerable to AGs and many other drugs (**Figure 7(1)**, but at clinically relevant doses, it is unlikely that AGs lead to significant hair cell damage in animals or humans (**Figure 3**; Ogier et al., 2020). Even if hair cell death were observed, the resulting auditory dysfunction would not be fluctuating or diminishing over time (**Figures 2, 4, 6**; Longenecker et al., 2020), as hair cell loss is permanent. Alternatively, cochlear supporting cells, actively phagocytize dying hair cells, and expand into the deficit, and maintain epithelial/ionic integrity (**Figure 7(2)**; Bird et al., 2010; Monzack et al., 2015) as well as release anti-inflammatory proteins (May et al., 2013). These cells need to be studied in more detail to ascertain if they are important in mediating or modulating AG-induced auditory dysfunction. Evidence supporting the hypothesis that SGNs and/or their synapses undergo temporary degradation or remodeling following AG exposure has been observed (**Figure 7(3)**; Liu et al., 2015; Hong et al., 2018). This hypothesis is further supported by data showing decreases in ABR wave I amplitudes following AG treatment, especially at high frequencies (**Supplementary Figures 2, 3**). As mentioned above, when considering the wave III/wave I ratio, a temporary increase was observed (**Supplementary Figure 1**; Longenecker et al., 2020), because

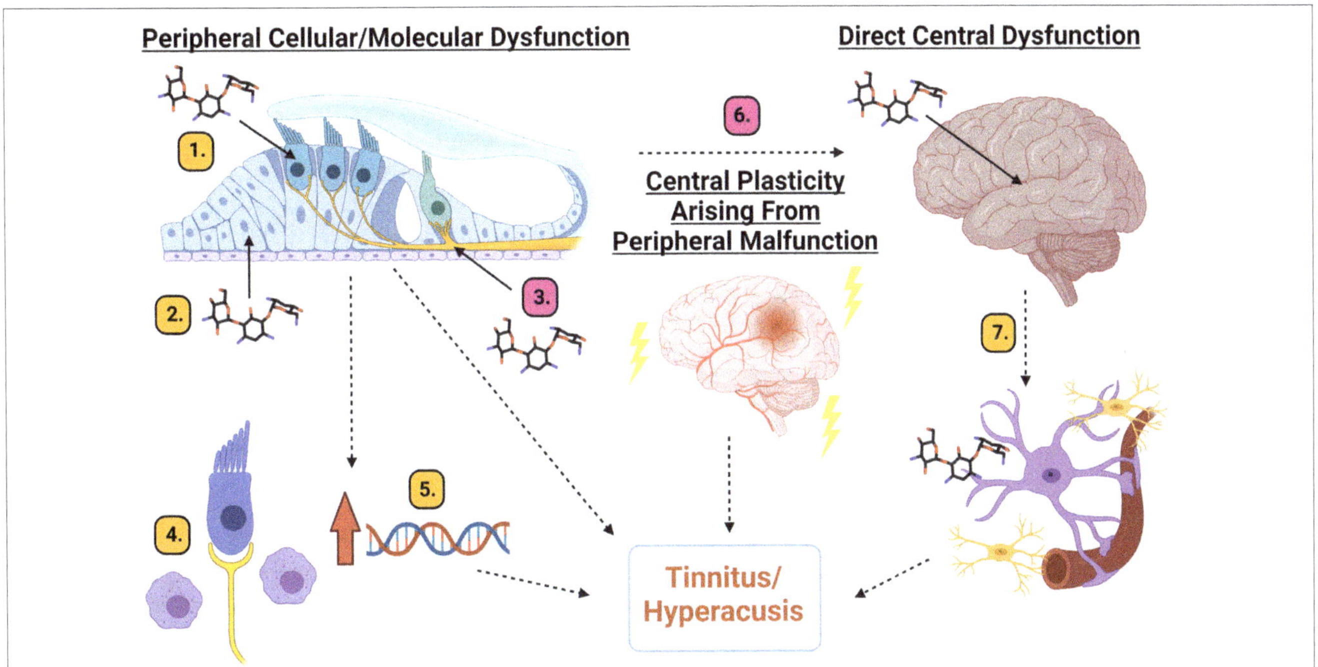

FIGURE 7 | Diagram of potential mechanistic explanations for AG-induced tinnitus and hyperacusis. Peripheral cellular or molecular dysfunction: (1). Hair cell cellular dysfunction. (2). Supporting cell dysfunction. (3). Spiral ganglion neuron/synapse dysfunction. (4). Inflammation induced macrophage activation. (5). Upregulation of genes responsible for inflammation. Central plasticity arising from peripheral malfunction. (6). Changes in the neural code related to maladaptive plastic changes to the auditory system. Direct central dysfunction. (7). Aminoglycoside crossing the blood brain barrier leading to inflammation and cellular/molecular responses from microglia and astrocytes which can result in changes to neural firing patterns. Magenta # mechanisms are partially supported by data from this manuscript and Longenecker et al., 2020. Yellow # mechanisms require further scientific exploration. Created with BioRender.com.

wave III amplitudes increased slightly while wave I decreased. Another likely mechanism for tinnitus and hyperacusis might increase inflammation in the cochlea (Jiang et al., 2017b). It has been shown that AGs cause inflammation in the cochlea and induce macrophage recruitment/activation which may modulate cochleotoxicity (**Figure 7(4)**; Sato et al., 2010; Wood and Zuo, 2017; Hirose and Li, 2019). Lastly, it has been shown that AGs can trigger altered gene expression in several pathways including JNK, NF-κB, stress response, apoptosis, cell cycle control, and DNA repair pathways, or modulate ion channels responsible for signal transduction (**Figure 7(5)**; Tao and Segil, 2015; Jiang et al., 2017b). Transient cochlear inflammation leading to macrophage recruitment and changes in gene expression changes may elicit the upstream dysfunctions marked by the behavioral symptoms of tinnitus and hyperacusis.

Central maladaptive plastic changes in response to peripheral insult has become central dogma in the field of tinnitus (**Figure 7(6)**; Roberts et al., 2010; Langguth et al., 2013; Auerbach et al., 2014; Henton and Tzounopoulos, 2021). Data from animals and humans have found many unique but likely overlapping mechanisms to explain the neural plastic changes related to tinnitus which include: increases in spontaneous (non-sound evoked) firing rate neural activity (Longenecker and Galazyuk, 2011; Berger et al., 2014; Galazyuk et al., 2019); increased incidence of neurons burst firing (Ma et al., 2006; Bauer et al., 2008), increased or decreased neural synchrony (Eggermont and Tass, 2015; Marks et al., 2018), thalamocortical dysrhythmia (De Ridder et al., 2015), altered balance between excitatory and inhibitory neurotransmission (Middleton et al., 2011; Llano et al., 2012; Ma et al., 2020; Zhang et al., 2021), cortical reorganization (Engineer et al., 2011; Jeschke et al., 2021), and neural inflammation (Fuentes-Santamaría et al., 2017; Wang et al., 2019; Deng et al., 2020). The mechanisms of hyperacusis are much less studied but are thought to have similar etiologies as tinnitus (Auerbach et al., 2014). A recent study found that hyperacusis-like behavior correlated to enhanced sound-driven firing rates and reduced first spike-latencies of auditory brainstem neurons (Martel and Shore, 2020). These findings corroborate the mechanistic explanation of hyperacusis observed in models of tobramycin, amikacin, and salicylate, that neural gain increases in the auditory neuroaxis (Supplemental **Figure 1**; Longenecker et al., 2020; Salvi et al., 2021). Central plasticity following any changes to the cochlea are likely, and thus represent a candidate mechanism for explaining the behavioral evidence of tinnitus and hyperacusis seen here (**Figures 4-6**).

To what extent do AGs cross the blood brain barrier and cause direct neural dysfunction (**Figure 7(7)**? Some evidence suggests it is indeed occurring in animals and humans. Recent reviews have described that aminoglycosides such as tobramycin and amikacin are neurotoxic (Grill and Maganti, 2011; Rezaei et al., 2018). Some of the proposed mechanisms for this neurotoxicity include: excitotoxic activation of NMDA receptors within the cochlea, oxidative stress, calcium channels modulation, and localized inflammatory response. Auditory brainstem neurons in a chicken model were shown to decrease in size and then recover after 10 days of gentamicin treatment (Lippe, 1991). A similar set of studies in guinea pigs found that neurotropin-3 could protect spiral ganglion neurons from AG-induced degeneration (Ernfors et al., 1996; Duan et al., 2000). In mice, AG-induced ABR ratio amplitude increases were observed with tobramycin and amikacin (**Figure 4**, **5**, **6**; Longenecker et al., 2020) which suggests a clear trend towards increased neural activity in the auditory brainstem (Auerbach et al., 2014; Roberts and Salvi, 2019). Recent work has shown that brain inflammation can lead to tinnitus-like behavior in animals (Fuentes-Santamaría et al., 2017; Wang et al., 2019; Deng et al., 2020). If so, then ebselen would be a prime candidate for mitigating potential AG-induced inflammation (Kalinec et al., 2017; Jiang et al., 2017b; Wood and Zuo, 2017), as it has been implicated as a powerful anti-inflammatory and neuroprotective therapeutic (Wang et al., 2020). AG-penetration of the blood brain barrier in humans is understudied, however it has been suggested that AGs might be particularly neurotoxic in patients with compromised blood brain barriers (Segal et al., 1999), a condition which has been observed in CF patients (Vaughn et al., 1996).

Future Studies to Evaluate AG-Cochleotoxicity and Otoprotective Strategies

Recent evidence indicates that a single course of IV tobramycin can lead to hearing loss in CF patients (Garinis et al., 2020; Harruff et al., 2020) and that this loss of hearing sensitivity results in poorer speech discrimination (Harruff et al., 2020). More clinical studies need to document and confirm these results. Physiological examinations such as the ABR or middle-ear muscle reflex should also investigate if ABR wave III/wave I amplitude ratios are altered in patients taking AGs as they have been in noise/age related hearing loss investigations (Bharadwaj et al., 2019; Guest et al., 2019; Refat et al., 2021). Preclinical work should investigate the neurotoxic effects of AGs using clinically translatable dosing schedules (Longenecker et al., 2020), to parallel what has been reported in AG treated patients (Segal et al., 1999; Daud et al., 2014; Harruff et al., 2020; Sabur et al., 2021). As discussed above, the CBA/Ca mouse would make a good model for researching this question because of its good hearing sensitivity throughout its lifespan. Furthermore, mice with blood brain barrier vulnerabilities should be tested against CBA/Ca mice to investigate if AGs can cause a higher incidence of hyperacusis and tinnitus. These sorts of studies would benefit from neurological recordings from auditory nuclei as well as brain histology to investigate the direct effects of AGs on neural anatomy and physiology. Additionally, AG strain differences should be examined to see if all strains of common AGs like tobramycin, amikacin, and gentamycin result in differential cochleotoxic effects (O'Sullivan et al., 2020). This could lead to safer AG treatments and prevent many of the permanent side-effects. Future studies should continue to evaluate therapeutic interventions for AG cochleotoxicity. To improve translatability, future experiments should test if ebselen or other anti-inflammatory drugs can provide additional relief from cochleotoxic side-effects with extended dosing beyond the 14 day-AG treatment (Hammill and Campbell, 2018). If so, such pharmaceuticals could prevent or even treat the chronic ototoxic side-effects of AG treatment, especially in CF.

AUTHOR CONTRIBUTIONS

RL, RG, and JK designed research. RL, RG, and JH performed research. RL and RG analyzed data. RL and JK wrote the manuscript. All authors contributed to the article and approved the submitted version.

REFERENCES

Abd-Elhakim, Y. M., Abdel-Motal, S. M., Malhat, S. M., Mostafa, H. I., Moselhy, A. A. A., Beheiry, R. R., et al. (2021). Curcumin mitigates neurotoxic and neurobehavioral changes of gentamicin and sodium salicylate in rats by adjusting oxidative stress and apoptosis. *Life Sci.* 265:118824. doi: 10.1016/j.lfs.2020.118824

American Speech-Language-Hearing Association (1994). Guidelines for the audiologic management of individuals receiving cochleotoxic drug therapy. *ASHA* 36(Suppl. 12), 11–19. doi: 10.1044/policy.GL1994-00003

Apaydin, E., Daǧli, E., Bayrak, S., Kankiliç, E. S., Şahin, H., and Acar, A. (2021). Protective effect of creatine on amikacin-induced ototoxicity. *Braz. J. Otorhinolaryngol.* S1 808-8694, 30155–30155. doi: 10.1016/j.bjorl.2020.09.002

Auerbach, B. D., Rodrigues, P. V., and Salvi, R. J. (2014). Central gain control in tinnitus and hyperacusis. *Front. Neurol.* 5:206. doi: 10.3389/fneur.2014.00206

Avci, D., Erkan, M., Sönmez, M. F., Kökoğlu, K., Güneş, M. S., Gündoğdu, R., et al. (2016). A prospective experimental study on the protective effect on resveratrol against amikacin-induced ototoxicity in rats. *J. Int. Adv. Otol.* 12, 290–297. doi: 10.5152/iao.2016.2617

Baguley, D. M., and Andersson, G. (2007). *Hyperacusis: Mechanisms, Diagnosis, and Therapies.* San Diego, CA: Plural Publishing Inc.

Baguley, D. M., and Hoare, D. J. (2018). Hyperacusis: major research questions. HNO 66, 358–363. doi: 10.1007/s00106-017-0464-3

Bauer, C. A., Turner, J. G., Caspary, D. M., Myers, K. S., and Brozoski, T. J. (2008). Tinnitus and inferior colliculus activity in chinchillas related to three distinct patterns of cochlea trauma. *J. Neurosci. Res.* 86, 2564–2578. doi: 10.1002/jnr.221699

Berger, J. I., Coomber, B., Wells, T. T., Wallace, M. N., and Palmer, A. R. (2014). Changes in the response properties of inferior colliculus neurons relating to tinnitus. *Front. Neurol.* 5:203. doi: 10.3389/fneur.2014.00203

Bharadwaj, H. M., Mai, A. R., Simpson, J. M., Choi, I., Heinz, M. G., and Shinn-Cunningham, B. G. (2019). Non-invasive assays of cochlear synaptopathy – candidates and considerations. *Neuroscience* 407, 53–66. doi: 10.1016/j.neuroscience.2019.02.031

Bird, J. E., Daudet, N., Warchol, M. E., and Gale, J. E. (2010). Supporting cells eliminate dying sensory hair cells to maintain epithelial integrity in the avian inner ear. *J. Neurosci.* 30, 12545–12556. doi: 10.1523/JNEUROSCI.3042-10.2010

Bullock, A. E., Slobe, B. S., Vázquez, V., and Collins, A. C. (1997). Inbred mouse strains differ in the regulation of startle and prepulse inhibition of the startle response. *Behav. Neurosci.* 111, 1353–1360. doi: 10.1037//0735-7044.111.6.1353

Cederroth, C. R., Lugo, A., Edvall, N. K., Lazar, A., Lopez-Escamez, J. A., Bulla, J., et al. (2020). Association between hyperacusis and tinnitus. *J. Clin. Med.* 9:2412. doi: 10.3390/jcm9082412

Coomber, B., Berger, J. I., Kowalkowski, V. L., Shackleton, T. M., Palmer, A. R., and Wallace, M. N. (2014). Neural changes accompanying tinnitus following unilateral acoustic trauma in the guinea pig. *Eur. J. Neurosci.* 40, 2427–2441. doi: 10.1111/ejn.12580

Daud, M. K., Mohamadl, H., Haron, A., and Rahman, N. A. (2014). Ototoxicity screening of patients treated with streptomycin using distortion product otoacoustic emissions. *B-ENT* 10, 53–58.

Davis, M. (1984). "The mammalian startle response," in *Neural Mechanisms of Startle Behavior*, ed. R. C. Eaton (New York, NY: Springer Science & Plenum Press), 287–351.

Davis, R. R., Newlander, J. K., Ling, X. B., Cortopassi, G. A., Krieg, E. F., and Erway, L. C. (2001). Genetic basis for susceptibility to noise-induced hearing loss in mice. *Hear. Res.* 155, 82–90. doi: 10.1016/s0378-5955(01)00250-7

De Ridder, D., Vanneste, S., Langguth, B., and Llinas, R. (2015). Thalamocortical dysrhythmia: a theoretical update in tinnitus. *Front. Neurol.* 6:124. doi: 10.3389/fneur.2015.00124

Deng, D., Wang, W., and Bao, S. (2020). Diffusible tumor necrosis factor-alpha (TNF-α) promotes noise-induced parvalbumin-positive (PV+) neuron loss and auditory processing impairments. *Front. Neurosci.* 14:573047. doi: 10.3389/fnins.2020.573047

Dogan, M., Polat, H., Yasar, M., Bayram, A., Karatas, D., Hira, I., et al. (2017). Protective role of misoprostol in prevention of gentamicin ototoxicity. *Int. J. Pediatr. Otorhinolaryngol.* 96, 140–144. doi: 10.1016/j.ijporl.2017.03.023

Duan, M., Agerman, K., Enfors, P., and Canlon, B. (2000). Complementary roles of neurotrophin 3 and a N-methyl-D-aspartate antagonist in the protection of noise and aminoglycoside-induced ototoxicity. *Proc. Natl. Acad. Sci. U.S.A.* 97, 7597–7602. doi: 10.1073/pnas.97.13.7597

Eggermont, J. J. (2021). Separate auditory pathways for the induction and maintenance of tinnitus and hyperacusis. *Prog. Brain Res.* 260, 101–127. doi: 10.1016/bs.pbr.2020.01.006

Eggermont, J. J., and Tass, P. A. (2015). Maladaptive neural synchrony in tinnitus: origin and restoration. *Front. Neurol.* 6:29. doi: 10.3389/fneur.2015.00029

El-Anwar, M. W., Abdelmonem, S., Nada, E., Galhoom, D., and Abdelsameea, A. A. (2018). Protective effect of pentoxifylline on amikacin-induced ototoxicity. *Ear Nose Throat J.* 97, E8–E12. doi: 10.1177/014556131809700802

Elson, E. C., Meier, E., and Oermann, C. M. (2020). The implementation of an aminoglycoside induced ototoxicity algorithm for people with cystic fibrosis. *J. Cyst. Fibros.* 20, 284–287. doi: 10.1016/j.jcf.2020.08.002

Engineer, N. D., Riley, J. R., Seale, J. D., Vrana, W. A., Shetake, J. A., Sudanagunta, S. P., et al. (2011). Reversing pathological neural activity using targeted plasticity. *Nature* 470, 101–104. doi: 10.1038/nature09656

Ernfors, P., Duan, M. L., Elshamy, W. M., and Canlon, B. (1996). Protection of auditory neurons from aminoglycoside toxicity by neurtrophin-3. *Nat. Med.* 2, 463–467. doi: 10.1038/nm0496-463

Flume, P. A., Mogayzel, P. J. Jr., Robinson, K. A., Goss, C. H., Rosenblatt, R. L., Kuhn, R. J., et al. (2009). Cystic fibrosis pulmonary guidelines: treatment of pulmonary exacerbations. *Am. J. Respir. Crit. Care Med.* 180, 802–808. doi: 10.1164/rccm.200812-1845PP

Fox, D. J., Cooper, M. D., Speil, C. A., Roberts, M. H., Yanik, S. C., Meech, R. P., et al. (2016). D-Methionine reduces tobramycin-induced ototoxicity without antimicrobial interference in animal models. *J. Cyst. Fibros.* 15, 518–530. doi: 10.1016/j.jcf.2015.06.005

Fuentes-Santamaría, V., Alvarado, J. C., Melgar-Rojas, P., Gabaldón-Ull, M. C., Miller, J. M., and Juiz, J. M. (2017). The role of glia in the peripheral and central auditory system following noise overexposure: contribution to TNF-α and IL-1β to the pathogenesis of hearing loss. *Front. Neuroanat.* 11:9. doi: 10.3389/fnana.2017.00009

Galazyuk, A. V., Longenecker, R. J., Voytenko, S. V., Kristaponyte, I., and Nelson, G. I. (2019). Residual inhibition: from the putative mechanisms to potential tinnitus treatment. *Hear. Res.* 375, 1–13. doi: 10.1016/j.heares.2019/01.022

Garinis, A., Gleser, M., Johns, A., Larsen, E., and Vachhani, J. (2020). Prospective cohort study of ototoxicity in persons with cystic fibrosis following a single course of intravenous tobramycin. *J. Cyst. Fibros.* 20, 278–283. doi: 10.1016/j.jcf.2020.07.001

Garinis, A. C., Cross, C. P., Srikanth, P., Carroll, K., Feeney, M. P., Keefe, D. H., et al. (2017). The cumulative effects of intravenous antibiotic treatments on hearing in patients with cystic fibrosis. *J. Cyst. Fibros.* 16, 401–409. doi: 10.1016/j.jcf.2017.01.006

Gold, J. R., and Bajo, V. M. (2014). Insult-induced adaptive plasticity of the auditory system. *Front. Neurosci.* 9:110. doi: 10.3389/fnins.2014.00110

Gómez-Nieto, R., Hormigo, S., and López, D. E. (2020). Perpulse inhibition of the auditory startle reflex assessment as hallmark of brainstem sensorimotor gating mechanisms. *Brain Sci.* 10:639. doi: 10.3390/brainsci10090639

Grill, M. F., and Maganti, R. K. (2011). Neurotoxic effects associated with antibiotic use: management considerations. *Br. J. Clin. Phamacol.* 73, 381–393. doi: 10.1111/j.1365-2125.2011.03991.x

Grimsley, C. A., Longenecker, R. J., Rosen, M. J., Young, J. W., Grimsley, J. M., and Galazyuk, A. V. (2015). An improved approach to separating startle data from noise. *J. Neurosci. Methods* 253, 206–217. doi: 10.1016/j.jneumeth.2015.07.001

Gu, R., Longenecker, R. J., Homan, J., and Kil, J. (2020). Ebselen attenuates tobramycin-induced ototoxicity in mice. *J. Cyst. Fibros.* 20, 271–277. doi: 10.1016/j/jcf.2020.02.014

Guest, H., Munro, K. J., Prendergast, G., and Plack, C. J. (2019). Reliability and interrelations of seven proxy measures of cochlear synaptopathy. *Hear. Res.* 375, 34–43. doi: 10.1016/j.heares.2019.01.018

Hammill, T. L., and Campbell, K. C. (2018). Protection for medication-induced hearing loss: the state of the science. *Int. J. Audiol.* 57, 87–95. doi: 10.1080/14992027.2018.1455114

Harruff, E. E., Kil, J., Ortiz, M. G. T., Dorgan, D., Jain, R., Poth, E. A., et al. (2020). Ototoxicity in cystic fibrosis patients receiving intravenous tobramycin for acute pulmonary exacerbation: ototoxicity following tobramycin treatment. *J. Cyst. Fibros.* 20, 288–294. doi: 10.1016/j.jcf.2020.11.020

Henton, A., and Tzounopoulos, T. (2021). What's the buzz? The neuroscience and the treatment of tinnitus. *Physiol. Rev.* 101, 1609–1632. doi: 10.1152/physrev.00029.2020

Hirose, K., and Li, S. Z. (2019). The role of monocytes and macrophages in the dynamic permeability of the blood-perilymph barrier. *Hear. Res.* 374, 49–57. doi: 10.1016/j.heares.2019.01.006

Hong, H., Dowdy, D. W., Dooley, K. E., Francis, H. W., Budhathoki, C., Han, H. R., et al. (2020). Risk of hearing loss among multidrug-resistant tuberculosis patients according to cumulative aminoglycoside dose. *Int. J. Tuberc. Lung Dis.* 24, 65–72. doi: 10.5588/ijtld.19.0062

Hong, J., Chen, Y., Zhang, Y., Li, J., Ren, L., Yang, L., et al. (2018). N-methyl-D-Aspartate receptors involvement in the gentamicin-induced hearing loss and pathological changes of ribbon synapse in the mouse cochlear inner hair cells. *Neural Plast* 2018:3989201. doi: 10.1155/2018/3989201

Huth, M. E., Ricci, A. J., and Cheng, A. G. (2011). Mechanisms of aminoglycoside ototoxicity and targets of hair cell protection. *Int. J. Otolaryngol.* 2011:937861. doi: 10.1155/2011/937861

Jeschke, M., Happel, M. F. K., Tziridis, K., Krauss, P., Schilling, A., Schulze, H., et al. (2021). Acute and long-term circuit-level effects in the auditory cortex after sound trauma. *Front. Neurosci.* 14:598406. doi: 10.3389/fnins.2020.598406

Jiang, M., Karasawa, T., and Steyger, P. S. (2017a). Aminoglycoside-induced cochleotoxicity: a review. *Front. Cell. Neurosci.* 11:308. doi: 10.3389/fncel.2017.00308

Jiang, M., Taghizadeh, F., and Steyger, P. S. (2017b). Potential mechanisms underlying inflammation-enhanced aminoglycoside-induced cochleotoxicity. *Front. Cell. Neurosci.* 11:362. doi: 10.3389/fncel.2017.00362

Kalinec, G. M., Lomberk, G., Urrutia, R. A., and Kalinec, F. (2017). Resolution of cochlear inflammation: novel target for preventing or ameliorating drug-, noise-, and age-related hearing loss. *Front. Cell. Neurosci.* 11:192. doi: 10.3389/fncel.2017.00192

Kil, J., Harruff, E. E., and Longenecker, R. J. (2021). Development of ebselen for the treatment of sensorineural hearing loss and tinnitus. *Hear. Res.* 108209. doi: 10.1016/j.heares.2021.108209 [Epub ahead of print].

Langguth, B., Kreuzer, P. M., Kleinjung, T., and De Ridder, D. (2013). Tinnitus: causes and clinical management. *Lancet Neurol.* 12, 920–930. doi: 10.1016/S1474-4422(13)70160-1

Lippe, W. R. (1991). Reduction and recovery of neuronal size in the cochlear nucleus of the chicken following aminoglycoside intoxication. *Hear. Res.* 51, 193–202. doi: 10.1016/0378-5955(91)90036-9

Liu, H., Li, G., Lu, J., Gao, Y. G., Song, L., Li, G. L., et al. (2019). Cellular differences in the cochlea of CBA and B6 mice may underlie their difference in susceptibility to hearing loss. *Front. Cell. Neurosci.* 13:60. doi: 10.3389/fncel.2019.00060

Liu, K., Chen, D., Guo, W., Yu, N., Wang, X., Ji, F., et al. (2015). Spontaneous and partial repair of ribbon synapse in cochlear inner hair cells after ototoxic withdrawal. *Mol. Neurobiol.* 52, 1680–1689. doi: 10.1007/s12035-014-8951-y

Llano, D. A., Turner, J., and Caspary, D. M. (2012). Diminished cortical inhibition in an aging mouse model of chronic tinnitus. *J. Neurosci.* 32, 16141–16148. doi: 10.1523/JNEUROSCI.2499-12.2012

Longenecker, R. J., and Galazyuk, A. V. (2011). Development of tinnitus in CBA/CaJ mice following sound exposure. *J. Assoc. Res. Otolaryngol.* 12, 647–658. doi: 10.1007/s10162-011-0276-1

Longenecker, R. J., and Galazyuk, A. V. (2012). Methodological optimization of tinnitus assessment using prepulse inhibition of the acoustic startle reflex. *Brain Res.* 1485, 54–62. doi: 10.1016/j.brainres.2012.02.067

Longenecker, R. J., and Galazyuk, A. V. (2016). Variable effects of acoustic trauma on behavioral and neural correlates of tinnitus in individual animals. *Front. Behav. Neurosci.* 10:207. doi: 10.3389/fnbeh.2016.00207

Longenecker, R. J., Gu, R., Homan, J., and Kil, J. (2020). A novel mouse model of aminoglycoside-induced hyperacusis and tinnitus. *Front. Neurosci.* 14:5611185. doi: 10.3389/fnins.2020.561185

Longenecker, R. J., Kristaponyte, I., Nelson, G. L., Young, J. W., and Galazyuk, A. V. (2018). Addressing variability in the acoustic startle reflex for accurate gap detection assessment. *Hear. Res.* 363, 119–135. doi: 10.1016/j.heares.2018.03.013

Ma, L., Ono, M., Qin, L., and Kato, N. (2020). Acoustic trauma induced the alteration of the activity balance of excitatory and inhibitory neurons in the inferior colliculus of mice. *Hear. Res.* 391:107957. doi: 10.1016/j.heares.2020.107957

Ma, W. L. D., Hidaka, H., and May, B. J. (2006). Spontaneous activity in the inferior colliculus of CBA/J mice after manipulations that induce tinnitus. *Hear. Res.* 212, 9–21. doi: 10.1016/j.heares.2005.10.003

Marks, K. L., Martel, D. T., Wu, C., Basura, G. J., Roberts, L. E., Schvartz-Leyzac, K. C., et al. (2018). Auditory-somatosensory bimodal stimulation desynchronizes brain circuitry to reduce tinnitus in guinea pigs and humans. *Sci. Transl. Med.* 10:eaal3175. doi: 10.1126/scitranslmed.aal3175

Martel, D. T., and Shore, S. E. (2020). Ventral cochlear nucleus bushy cells encode hyperacusis in guinea pigs. *Sci. Rep.* 10:20594. doi: 10.1038/s41598-020-77754-z

Martini, A. C., Gomez-Arboledas, A., Forner, S., Rodriguez-Ortiz, C. J., McQuade, A., Danhash, E., et al. (2019). Amyloid-beta impairs TOM1-mediated IL-1R1 signaling. *Proc. Natl. Acad. Sci. U.S.A.* 116, 21198–21206. doi: 10.1073/pnas.1914088116

May, L. A., Kramarenko, I. I., Brandon, C. S., Voelkel-Johnson, C., Roy, S., Truong, K., et al. (2013). Inner ear supporting cells protect hair cells by secreting HSP70. *J. Clin. Invest.* 123, 3577–3587. doi: 10.1172/JCI68480

Middleton, J. W., Kiritani, T., Pedersen, C., Turner, J. G., Shepherd, G. M. G., and Tzounopoulos, T. (2011). Mice with behavioral evidence of tinnitus exhibit dorsal cochlear nucleus hyperactivity because of decreased GABAergic inhibition. *Proc. Natl. Acad. Sci. U.S.A.* 108, 7601–7606. doi: 10.1073/pnas.1100223108

Monzack, E. L., May, L. A., Roy, S., Gale, J. E., and Cunningham, L. L. (2015). Live imaging the phagocytic activity of inner ear supporting cells in response to hair cell death. *Cell Death Differ.* 22, 1995–2005. doi: 10.1038/cdd.2015.48

Ogier, J. M., Lockhart, P. J., and Burt, R. A. (2020). Intravenously delivered aminoglycoside antibiotics, tobramycin and amikacin, are not ototoxic in mice. *Hear. Res.* 386:107870. doi: 10.1016/j.heares.2019.107870

O'Sullivan, M. E., Song, Y., Greenhouse, R., Lin, R., Perez, A., Atkinson, P. J., et al. (2020). Dissociating antibacterial from ototoxic effects of gentamicin C-subtypes. *Proc. Natl. Acad. Sci. U.S.A.* 117, 32423–32432. doi: 10.1073/pnas.2013065117

Peguero, B., and Tempel, B. L. (2015). A chromosome 17 locus engenders frequency-specific non-progressive hearing loss that contributes to age-related hearing loss in mice. *JARO* 16, 459–471. doi: 10.1007/s10162-015-0519-7

Pienkowski, M., Tyler, R. S., Roncancio, E. R., Jun, H. J., Brozoski, T., Dauman, N., et al. (2014). A review of hyperacusis and future directions: part II. Measurement, mechanisms, and treatment. *Am. J. Audiol.* 23, 420–436. doi: 10.1044/2014_AJA-13-0037

Pilz, P. K. D., Arnold, S. W., Rischawy, A. T., and Plappert, C. F. (2014). Longterm-habituation of the startle response in mice is stimulus modality, but not context specific. *Front. Integr. Neurosci.* 7:103. doi: 10.3389/fnint.2013.00103

Raj-Koziak, D., Gos, E., Kutyba, J., Skarzynski, H., and Sharzynski, P. H. (2021). Decreased sound tolerance in tinnitus patients. *Life* 11:87. doi: 10.3390/life11020087

Refat, F., Wertz, J., Hinrichs, P., Klose, U., Samy, H., Abdelkader, R. M., et al. (2021). Co-occurrence of hyperacusis accelerates with tinnitus burden over time and requires medical care. *Front. Neurol.* 12:627522. doi: 10.3389/fneur.2021.627522

Rezaei, N. J., Bazzazi, A. M., and Alavi, S. A. N. (2018). Neurotoxicity of the antibiotics: a comprehensive study. *Neurol. India* 66, 1732–1740. doi: 10.4103/0028-3886.246258

Roberts, L. E., Eggermont, J. J., Caspary, D. M., Shore, S. E., Melcher, J. R., and Kaltenbach, J. A. (2010). Ringing ears: the neuroscience of tinnitus. *J. Neurosci.* 30, 14972–14979. doi: 10.1523/JNEUROSCI.4028-10.2010

Roberts, L. E., and Salvi, R. (2019). Overview: hearing loss, tinnitus, hyperacusis, and the role of central gain. *Neurosci* 407, 1–7. doi: 10.1016/j.neuroscience.2019.03.021

Sabur, N. F., Brar, M. S., Wu, L., and Brode, S. K. (2021). Low-dose amikacin in the treatment of multidrug-resistant tuberculosis (MDR-TB). *BMC Infect. Dis.* 21:254. doi: 10.1186/s12879-021-05947-6

Salvi, R., Radziwon, K., Manohar, S., Auerbach, B., Ding, D., Liu, X., et al. (2021). Review: neural mechanisms of tinnitus and hyperacusis in acute drug-induced ototoxicity. *Am. J. Audiol.* 1–15. doi: 10.1044/2020_AJA-20-00023 [Epub ahead of print].

Sato, E., Shick, H. E., Ransohoff, R. M., and Hirose, K. (2010). Expression of fractalkine receptor CX3CR1 on cochlear macrophages influences survival of hair cells following ototoxic injury. *JARO* 11, 223–234. doi: 10.1007/s10162-009-0198-3

Segal, J. A., Harris, B. D., Kustova, Y., Basile, A., and Skolnick, P. (1999). Aminoglycoside neurotoxicity involves NMDA receptor activation. *Brain Res.* 815, 270–277. doi: 10.1016/s0006-8993(98)01123-8

Sharpley, A. L., Williams, C., Holder, A. A., Godlewska, B. R., Singh, N., Shanyinde, M., et al. (2020). A phase 2a randomized, double-blind, placebo-controlled, parallel-group, add-on clinical trial of ebselen (SPI-1005) as a novel treatment for mania or hypomania. *Psychopharmacology (Berl.)* 237, 3773–3782. doi: 10.1007/s00213-020-05654-1

Shore, S. E., and Wu, C. (2019). Mechanisms of noise-induced tinnitus: insights from cellular studies. *Neuron* 103, 8–20. doi: 10.1016/j.neuron.2019.05.008

Smith, S., Rowbotham, N. J., and Regan, K. H. (2018). Inhaled anti-pseudomonal antibiotics for long-term therapy in cystic fibrosis. *Cochrane Database of Syst. Rev.* 3:CD001021. doi: 10.1002/14651858.CD001021.pub3

Staecker, H. (2021). Re-evaluating aminoglycoside ototoxicity. *J. Cyst. Fibros.* 20:5. doi: 10.1016/j.jcf.2021.01.003

Tao, L., and Segil, N. (2015). Early transcriptional response to aminoglycoside antibiotic suggests alternate pathways leading to apoptosis in sensory hair cells in the mouse inner ear. *Front. Cell. Neurosci.* 9:190. doi: 10.3389/fncel.2015.00190

Thomas, M. E., Guercio, G. D., Drudik, K. M., and de Villers-Sidani, E. (2019). Evidence of hyperacusis in adult rats following non-traumatic sound exposure. *Front. Syst. Neurosci.* 13:55. doi: 10.3389/fnsys.2019.00055

Turner, J., Larsen, D., Hughes, L., Moechars, D., and Shore, S. (2012). Time course of tinnitus development following noise exposure. *J. Neurosci. Res.* 90, 1480–1488. doi: 10.1002/jnr.22827

Vaughn, B. V., Ali, I. I., Olivier, K. N., Lackner, R. P., Robertson, K. R., Messenheimer, J. A., et al. (1996). Seizures in lung transplant recipients. *Epilepsia* 37, 1175–1179. doi: 10.1111/j.1528-1157.1996.tb00549.x

Wang, J., Wang, P., Dong, C., Zhao, Y., Zhou, J., Yuan, C., et al. (2020). Mechanisms of ebselen as a therapeutic and its pharmacology applications. *Future Med. Chem.* 12, 2141–2160. doi: 10.4155/fmc-2019-0218

Wang, W., Zhang, L. S., Zinsmaier, A. K., Patterson, G., Leptich, E. J., Shoemaker, S. L., et al. (2019). Neuroinflammation mediates noise-induced synaptic imbalance and tinnitus in rodent models. *PLoS Biol.* 17:e3000307. doi: 10.1371/journal.pbio.3000307

Westman, M. R., Putterman, D. B., Garinis, A. C., Hunter, A. C., and Freeney, M. P. (2021). Wideband acoustic reflex growth in adults with cystic fibrosis. *Am. J. Audiol.* 1–9. doi: 10.1044/2020_AJA-20-00117 [Epub ahead of print].

Wood, M. B., and Zuo, J. (2017). The contribution of immune infiltrates to ototoxicity and cochlear hair cell loss. *Front. Cell. Neurosci.* 11:106. doi: 10.3389/fncel.2017.00106

Zhang, L., Wu, C., Martel, D. T., West, M., Sutton, M. A., and Shore, S. E. (2021). Noise exposure alters glutamatergic and GABAergic synaptic connectivity in the hippocampus and its relevance to tinnitus. *Neural Plast.* 2021:8833087. doi: 10.1155/2021/8833087

Zheng, Q. Y., Johnson, K. R., and Erway, L. C. (1999). Assessment of hearing in 80 inbred strains of mice by ABR threshold analysis. *Hear. Res.* 130, 94–107. doi: 10.1016/s0378-5955(99)00003-9

Hearing Loss and Cognition among Older Adults in a Han Chinese Cohort

Fuxin Ren[1†], Jianfen Luo[2,3†], Wen Ma[4], Qian Xin[5], Lei Xu[2,3], Zhaomin Fan[2,3], Yu Ai[2,3], Bin Zhao[1], Fei Gao[1] and Haibo Wang[2,3*]*

[1] Shandong Medical Imaging Research Institute, Shandong University, Jinan, China, [2] Department of Otolaryngology-Head and Neck Surgery, Shandong Provincial ENT Hospital, Shandong University, Jinan, China, [3] Shandong Provincial Key Laboratory of Otology, Jinan, China, [4] Department of Otolaryngology, Jinan Central Hospital, Shandong University, Jinan, China, [5] The Second Hospital of Shandong University, Jinan, China

***Correspondence:**
Fei Gao
feigao6262@163.com
Haibo Wang
whboto11@163.com

† These authors have contributed equally to this work

Presbycusis (PC) is associated with cognitive decline and incident dementia. Speech reception thresholds (SRT) are used to assess speech detection, which points toward a central component of PC. However, to the best of our knowledge, no previous study has reported the relationship between SRT and cognitive function in older adults in a Han Chinese cohort. Therefore, in this study, we investigate the association of hearing loss, indexed using pure tone average (PTA) and SRT, with cognitive function in a Han Chinese cohort using a standardized neurocognitive battery. Subjects (aged ≥60 years) with no history of psychiatric or neurological diseases were recruited. All subjects underwent a battery of neuropsychological and auditory tests. According to the PTA of the better ear, the subjects were further divided into PC and normal PTA (NP) groups. Regression analyses were performed to examine the relationship between cognitive function and hearing loss in the PC and NP groups and all subjects when controlling for age, sex, education level, diabetes, smoking, and hypertension. Cognitive function was significantly associated with PTA and SRT in all subjects. In all subjects, the correlations between non-verbal cognitive scores and SRT were stronger than those between non-verbal cognitive scores and PTA, whereas the correlations between verbal cognitive scores and PTA were stronger than those between verbal cognitive scores and SRT. Moreover, the correlations between PTA or SRT and cognitive function in the PC group were in principle stronger than those in the NP group. Our findings indicate that cognitive function is significantly associated with PTA and SRT in older adults in a Han Chinese cohort. Therefore, SRT could be an important auditory test for exploring cognitive decline in PC and could complement PTA.

Keywords: presbycusis, hearing loss, cognition, older adults, speech reception thresholds

INTRODUCTION

Age-related hearing loss, also known as presbycusis (PC), is among the most common chronic diseases in older adults. The prevalence of PC increases with age, and it has been reported that 30–35% of adults between the ages of 65–75 years and 40–50% of adults over the age of 75 years suffer from PC (Nash et al., 2011). The World Health Organization's World Health Statistics report indicated that the average life expectancy in China has increased significantly in recent years (2018). Age-related hearing loss is becoming a major sensory deficit among older adults in China (Luo et al., 2013). Recently, many audiological studies have suggested that PC is associated with cognitive impairment and incident dementia (Gates and Mills, 2005; Lin, 2011; Lin et al., 2011a,b,c; Jayakody et al., 2018). For instance, one cross-sectional study reported that hearing loss of older American adults is independently associated with lower scores on the symbol digit modalities test (SDMT) (Lin, 2011). In addition, reduced cognitive functioning was associated with age-related hearing loss in older European adults (Quaranta et al., 2014). However, to date, there has been a paucity of studies exploring the association between hearing loss and cognitive function in a Han Chinese cohort.

Presbycusis is usually characterized by progressive hearing loss at high frequencies, which are particularly important for speech recognition. Previous studies have shown that PC represents deteriorated function of both the auditory periphery and the central auditory system (Ouda et al., 2015). Hypofunction of the inner ear is the main reason for the peripheral component of PC (Schuknecht and Gacek, 1993). Moreover, poor speech discrimination and deteriorated temporal sound processing reflect a possible central component of PC (Mazelova et al., 2003). However, research into the association between hearing loss and cognitive function has focused solely on hearing as measured by pure tone thresholds, which assess the function of the auditory periphery. Speech reception thresholds (SRT) are used to assess speech detection, which could reflect a central component of PC. To our knowledge, to date there has been a paucity of studies exploring the relationship between SRT and cognitive function in older adults.

Therefore, in the present study, we investigated the association of hearing loss with cognitive function in a Han Chinese cohort using a standardized neurocognitive battery. Hearing loss was assessed using pure tone thresholds and SRT. We hypothesized that cognitive decline would be associated with both pure tone thresholds and SRT.

MATERIALS AND METHODS

Subjects

The study was approved by the Shandong University institutional review board, and each participant provided informed consent. Subjects aged ≥60 years were recruited from the local community. No one had a history of psychiatric or neurological illness. All subjects were Han Chinese.

Assessment of Auditory Function

First, optimal middle ear conditions were confirmed using tympanometry performed with a GSI Tympstar. Then, the air conduction thresholds were measured through pure tone audiometry at the frequencies from 125, 250, 500, 1000, 2000, 4000, and 8000 Hz using a clinical audiometer (GSI AudioStar Pro). The speech-frequency pure-tone average (PTA) for each side of ears was obtained by calculating the average of hearing thresholds at 500, 1000, 2000, and 4000 Hz in air conduction (1). Hearing loss was defined as PTA >25 decibels hearing level (dB HL) for the better ear (World Health Organization [WHO], 2018), and the subjects were further divided into PC and normal PTA (NP) groups. The exclusion criteria in the study were as follows: (1) asymmetric hearing loss, conductive hearing loss and tinnitus; (2) other causes of sensorineural hearing loss different from PC; (3) previous history of hearing aid use, noise exposure, otologic surgery, head trauma and ototoxic drug therapy.

Speech reception thresholds was performed with a clinical audiometer (GSI AudioStar Pro) and equipped with TDH-50P headphones in quiet conditions. First, according to the value of PTA, an initial sound intensity is groped to ensure that the subject is able to exactly recognize 5 spondee words under this intensity. If the subject cannot recognize, the software will increase the initial sound intensity. The software then automatically controls sound intensity: the sound intensity reduces by 5 dB for every five words played. The test is stopped when the subject is unable to exactly recognize five spondee words. Finally, the number of exact recognized words are counted in the whole descending process, then the software subtracts the number of exact recognized words from initial sound intensity and adds a correction factor (2.5 dB), which is the subject's speech recognition threshold.

Assessment of Cognitive Function

First, the subjects' general cognitive function was tested using the Montreal Cognitive Assessment (MoCA) (Galea and Woodward, 2005; Nasreddine et al., 2005). Then, the subjects' verbal learning and memory, attention, psychomotor speed and executive control were tested using the Auditory Verbal Learning Test (AVLT, Chinese version) (Zhao et al., 2012), the Stroop color word interference test (Savitz and Jansen, 2003), the SDMT (Van Schependom et al., 2014), and the trail-making test (TMT) (Sanchez-Cubillo et al., 2009), respectively. The TMT is made up of two parts. In TMT-A part, the subjects were required to draw lines sequentially connecting 25 encircled numbers, that were distributed on a piece of paper in ascending order (from 1 to 25), as soon as possible. Culturally, most Chinese older adults are less familiar with Arabic numerals than Westerners, therefore, a Chinese version of the TMT-B was applied in our study (Lu et al., 2006; Wei et al., 2018). In TMT-B part, the subjects were required to draw a line alternating between squares and circles while connecting the numbers on a page of the same size in ascending order (from 1 to 25) as soon as possible. Cognitive tests in our study were divided into two categories: verbal tests and non-verbal tests. Verbal tests include MoCA, AVLT and Stroop, which means that verbal communication is required in the test. Non-verbal tests include SDMT, TMT-A, and TMT-B, which means that verbal communication is not required in the test. Finally, the subjects' anxiety and depression status were assessed using the hospital anxiety and depression scale (HADS) (Zigmond and Snaith, 1983). The overall testing time was about 60 min in a fixed order.

Statistical Analysis

The two-tailed t-test was used to assess group differences in continuous variables, and the chi-square test was used to assess group differences in gender-specific, diabetes, smoking and hypertension. Partial correlation analyses were used to explore the correlations between cognitive function and PTA or SRT in the PC and NP groups and all subjects, controlling for age, sex, education level, diabetes, smoking and hypertension. Stepwise Multiple Linear Regression analyses were then performed in the PC group, NP group and all subjects. PTA/SRT, age, sex, education level, diabetes, smoking, and hypertension are independent variables, and cognition measures are dependent variables. P-values of less than 0.05 were accepted as significant.

RESULTS

Demographic and Clinical Characteristics

The demographic and clinical characteristics of the study population are listed in **Table 1**. Eighty subjects aged 60–78 years (40 males/40 females, mean age: 65.78 ± 3.96 years) were screened for inclusion in this study. Thirty-five subjects were assigned to the NP group, and forty-five subjects were assigned to the PC group.

Presbycusis and NP groups did not differ significantly in age, sex or education. Compared to the NP group, the patients with

TABLE 1 | Subjects' demographic and clinical data.

Characteristics	All subjects (n = 80)	PC group (n = 45)	NP group (n = 35)	P-value PC vs. NP	Cohen's d PC vs. NP
Gender (male/female)	40/40	23/22	17/18	0.822	–
Age (years)	65.78 ± 3.96	66.29 ± 4.37	65.11 ± 3.30	0.190	0.30
Education (years)	11.50 ± 2.61	11.42 ± 2.35	11.60 ± 2.94	0.771	−0.07
Diabetes (yes/no)	7/73	4/41	3/32	0.960	–
Smoking (yes/no)	21/59	12/33	9/26	0.923	–
Hypertension(yes/no)	39/41	22/23	17/18	0.978	–
Anxiety	3.26 ± 2.40	3.38 ± 2.59	3.11 ± 2.15	0.629	0.11
Depression	3.38 ± 2.83	3.62 ± 3.43	3.06 ± 1.78	0.344	0.20
PTA (dB/HL)	25.97 ± 13.92	35.97 ± 10.18	13.11 ± 3.67	**<0.001**	**2.98**
SRT (dB/HL)	25.93 ± 13.99	35.43 ± 11.16	13.70 ± 4.49	**<0.001**	**2.48**
MoCA	25.68 ± 2.23	25.24 ± 2.79	26.23 ± 0.97	**0.032**	**−0.51**
AVLT	56.63 ± 8.63	55.58 ± 7.90	57.97 ± 9.44	0.232	−0.27
Stroop (s)	131.50 ± 16.20	135.13 ± 16.66	126.83 ± 14.52	**0.022**	**0.53**
SDMT	39.50 ± 15.12	34.71 ± 12.81	45.66 ± 15.80	**0.001**	**−0.76**
TMT-A (s)	48.86 ± 16.91	52.60 ± 16.89	44.06 ± 15.91	**0.024**	**0.53**
TMT-B (s)	140.48 ± 83.65	150.44 ± 85.40	127.66 ± 80.75	0.229	0.27

The data are presented as means ± standard deviations. Values in bold are statistically significant. Cohen's d is an effect size used to indicate the standardized difference between two means. PTA, pure tone average; SRT, speech reception threshold; PC, presbycusis; NP, normal PTA; MoCA, montreal cognitive assessment; AVLT, auditory verbal learning test; SDMT, symbol digit modalities test; TMT, trail-making test; levels of anxiety and depression were assessed according to the hospital anxiety and depression scale (HADS).

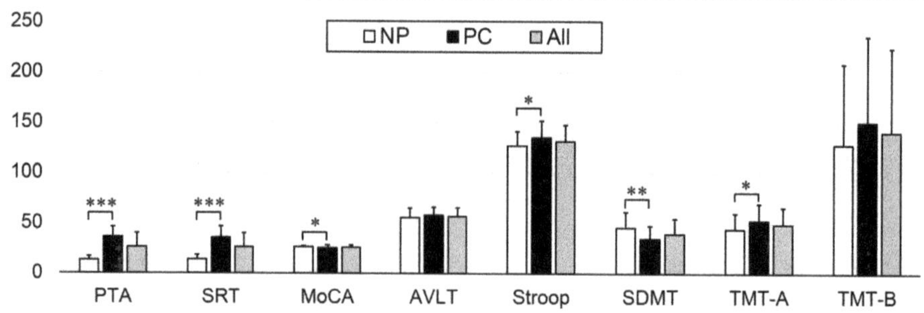

FIGURE 1 | Differences in the neuropsychological and auditory tests between the Normal PTA (NP) group and Presbycusis (PC) group. Compared to the NP group, the patients with PC performed worse on the MoCA, Stroop, SDMT, and TMT-A tests (p < 0.05). The PTA and SRT were significantly higher in the patients with PC than in the NP group (p < 0.001). Statistical significance was set as *p < 0.05, **p < 0.01, and ***p < 0.001.

PC performed worse on the MoCA, Stroop, SDMT, and TMT-A tests ($p < 0.05$) (**Table 1** and **Figure 1**). The correlations between cognitive outcomes in all subjects, NP and PC group were shown in **Supplementary Table S1**. The PTA and SRT were significantly higher in the patients with PC than in the NP group (PTA, $p < 0.001$; SRT, $p < 0.001$) (**Table 1** and **Figure 1**). All subjects had a type A curve on tympanometry, which indicate normal middle ear function. The hearing thresholds of the left and right ears of all subjects are shown in **Figure 2**. Partial correlation analyses (controlling for age, sex, education level, diabetes, smoking and hypertension) revealed that SRT was positively correlated with PAT in all subjects ($r = 0.945$, $p < 0.001$), in the NP group ($r = 0.472$, $p = 0.013$) and in the PC group ($r = 0.897$, $p < 0.001$), as seen in **Supplementary Figure S1**.

Correlations Between Hearing Loss and Cognitive Function (Table 2)

In all subjects, Pearson correlation analyses revealed that PTA (**Figure 3**) was positively correlated with Stroop ($r = 0.311$, $p = 0.008$), TMT-A ($r = 0.414$, $p < 0.001$), and TMT-B ($r = 0.271$, $p = 0.021$) and negatively correlated with the MoCA ($r = -0.323$, $p = 0.006$), AVLT ($r = -0.262$, $p = 0.026$), and SDMT ($r = -0.489$, $p < 0.001$). SRT (**Figure 4**) was positively correlated with Stroop ($r = 0.298$, $p = 0.011$), TMT-A ($r = 0.427$, $p < 0.001$), and TMT-B ($r = 0.318$, $p = 0.007$), and negatively correlated with the MoCA ($r = -0.297$, $p = 0.011$), AVLT ($r = -0.246$, $p = 0.037$), and SDMT ($r = -0.497$, $p < 0.001$).

In the NP group, Pearson correlation analyses revealed that PTA (**Figure 5**) was positively correlated with Stroop ($r = 0.401$,

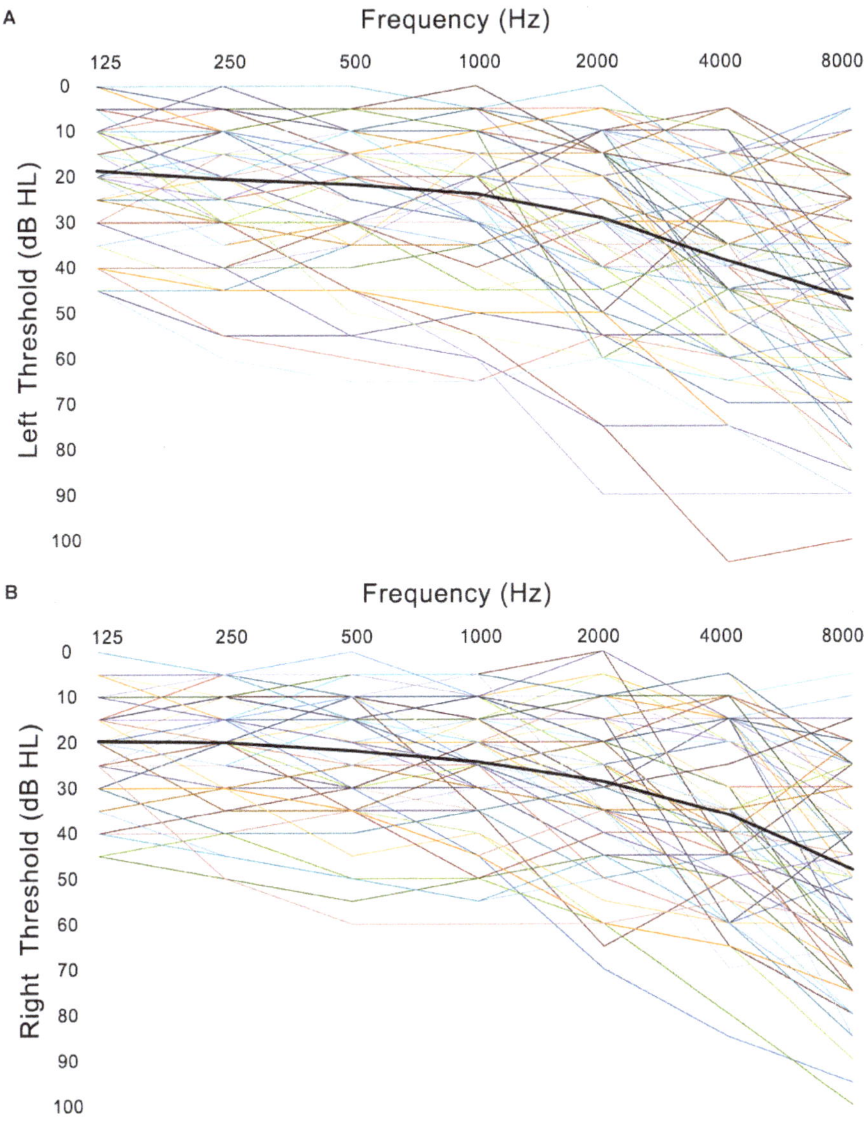

FIGURE 2 | Left **(A)** and right **(B)** ear pure-tone thresholds (dB HL) are plotted for each subject's left and right ear as a function of frequency (Hz) with the mean thresholds across participants and ears (black line).

TABLE 2 | Correlations between audiological (PTA/SRT) and cognitive outcomes (verbal/non-verbal tests).

		Verbal tests			Non-verbal tests		
		MoCA	**AVLT**	**Stroop**	**SDMT**	**TMT-A**	**TMT-B**
All subjects							
PTA	r	**−0.323**	**−0.262**	**0.311**	**−0.489**	**0.414**	**0.271**
	p	**0.006**	**0.026**	**0.008**	**<0.001**	**<0.001**	**0.021**
SRT	r	**−0.297**	**−0.246**	**0.298**	**−0.497**	**0.427**	**0.318**
	p	**0.011**	**0.037**	**0.011**	**<0.001**	**<0.001**	**0.007**
PC group							
PTA	r	**−0.376**	**−0.536**	0.205	**−0.532**	**0.572**	**0.494**
	p	**0.022**	**<0.001**	0.223	**<0.001**	**<0.001**	**0.002**
SRT	r	**−0.373**	**−0.574**	0.245	**−0.594**	**0.652**	**0.528**
	p	**0.023**	**<0.001**	0.143	**<0.001**	**<0.001**	**<0.001**
NP group							
PTA	r	0.245	−0.379	**0.401**	**−0.430**	0.318	0.091
	p	0.219	0.051	**0.038**	**0.025**	0.106	0.652
SRT	r	**0.457**	−0.276	0.297	−0.336	0.175	0.291
	p	**0.017**	0.164	0.132	0.087	0.383	0.141

Partial correlation analyses were used and controlled for age, sex, education level, diabetes, smoking, and hypertension. Bold values indicates a statistically significant difference with a p-value less than 0.05. PTA, pure tone average; SRT, speech reception threshold; PC, presbycusis; NP, normal PTA; MoCA, montreal cognitive assessment; AVLT, auditory verbal learning test; SDMT, symbol digit modalities test; TMT, trail-making test.

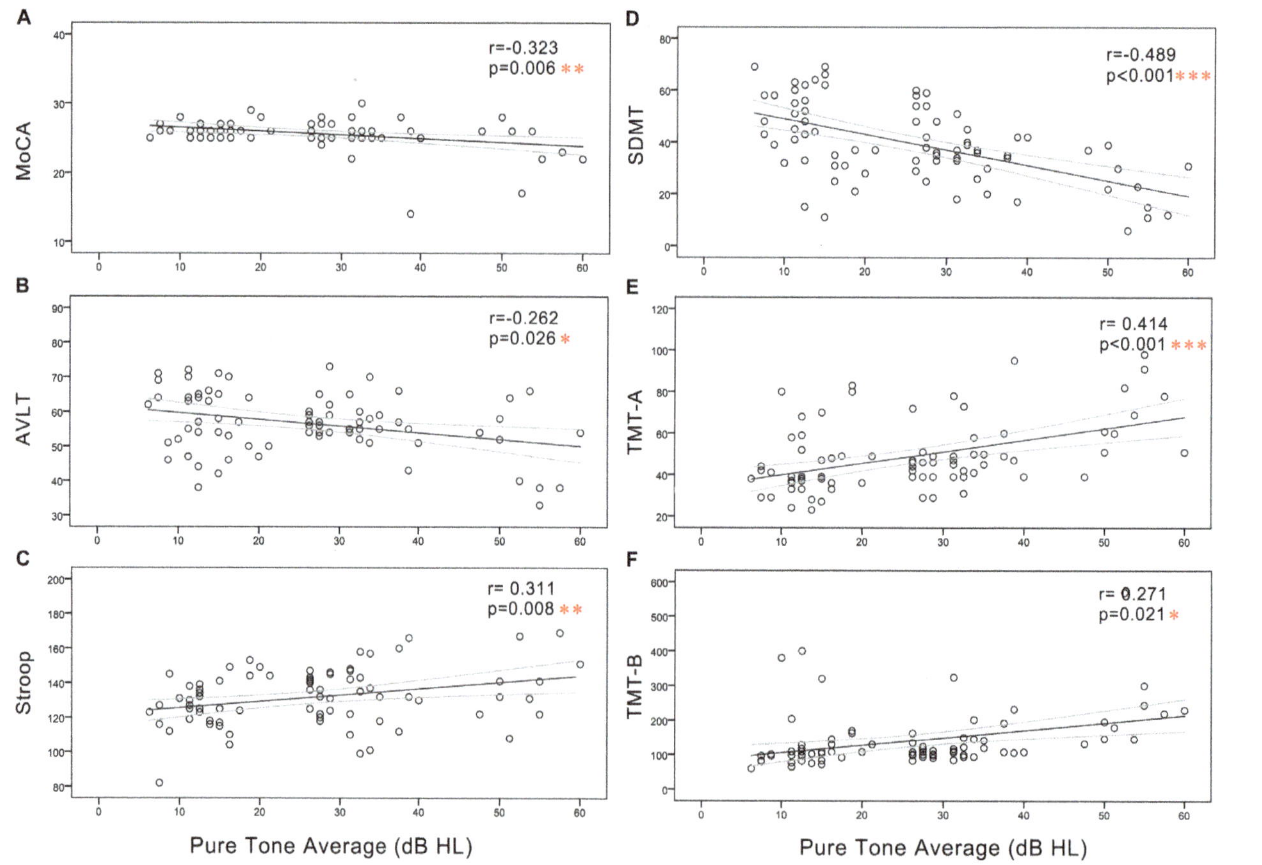

FIGURE 3 | Scatter plots displaying the correlations between PTA and cognitive function in all subjects. Partial correlation analyses (controlling for age, sex, education level, diabetes, smoking, and hypertension) revealed that PTA was positively correlated with **(C)** Stroop (r = 0.311, p = 0.008), **(E)** TMT-A (r = 0.414, p < 0.001), and **(F)** TMT-B (r = 0.271, p = 0.021) and negatively correlated with the **(A)** MoCA (r = −0.323, p = 0.006), **(B)** AVLT (r = −0.262, p = 0.026), and **(D)** SDMT (r = −0.489, p < 0.001). Gray curves: 95% confidence interval of the line of best fit.

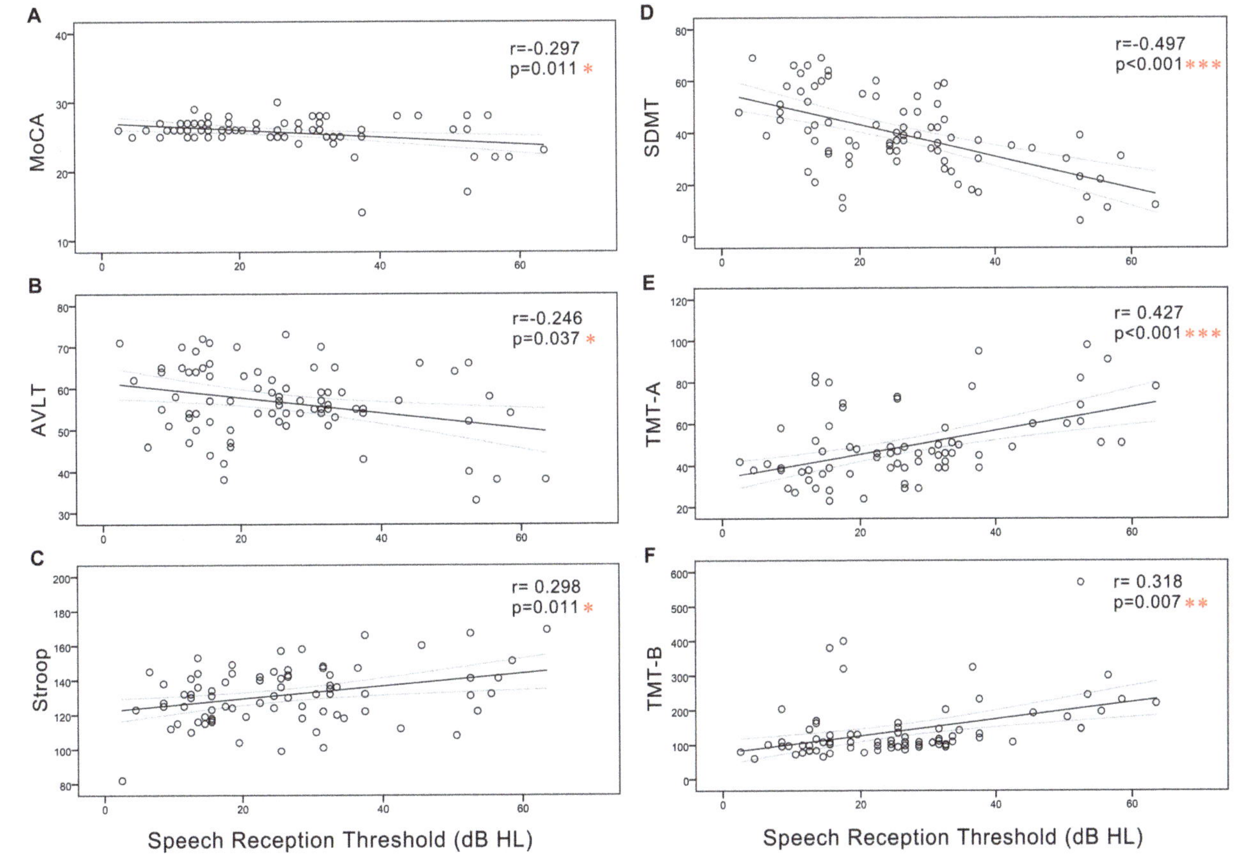

FIGURE 4 | Scatter plots displaying the correlations between SRT and cognitive function in all subjects. Partial correlation analyses (controlling for age, sex, education level, diabetes, smoking, and hypertension) revealed that SRT was positively correlated with **(C)** Stroop ($r = 0.298$, $p = 0.011$), **(E)** TMT-A ($r = 0.427$, $p < 0.001$), and **(F)** TMT-B ($r = 0.318$, $p = 0.007$) and negatively correlated with the **(A)** MoCA ($r = -0.297$, $p = 0.011$), **(B)** AVLT ($r = -0.246$, $p = 0.037$), and **(D)** SDMT ($r = -0.497$, $p < 0.001$). Gray curves: 95% confidence interval of the line of best fit.

$p = 0.038$) and negatively correlated with SDMT ($r = -0.430$, $p = 0.025$). SRT (**Figure 6**) was negatively correlated with SDMT ($r = -0.361$, $p = 0.033$).

In the PC group, Pearson correlation analyses revealed that PTA (**Figure 5**) was positively correlated with TMT-A ($r = 0.572$, $p < 0.001$), TMT-B ($r = 0.494$, $p < 0.001$), and negatively correlated with MoCA ($r = -0.376$, $p = 0.022$), AVLT ($r = -0.536$, $p < 0.001$), and SDMT ($r = -0.532$, $p < 0.001$). SRT (**Figure 6**) was positively correlated with TMT-A ($r = 0.585$, $p < 0.001$) and TMT-B ($r = 0.602$, $p < 0.001$) and negatively correlated with MoCA ($r = -0.300$, $p = 0.046$), AVLT ($r = -0.408$, $p = 0.005$), and SDMT ($r = -0.622$, $p < 0.001$).

Regression Analyses Between Hearing Loss and Cognitive Function (Table 3)

Stepwise Multiple Linear Regression Models were established in all subjects. However, some regression models in NP group and PC group could not be established, so were marked as N/A, presumably because of the small sample size of NP group and PC group.

In all subjects, PTA was found to be significant predictors of MoCA ($\beta = -0.050$, $R^2 = 0.345$, $p = 0.001$), AVLT ($\beta = -0.186$, $R^2 = 0.143$, $p = 0.005$), Stroop ($\beta = 0.348$, $R^2 = 0.219$, $p = 0.004$), SDMT ($\beta = -0.532$, $R^2 = 0.322$, $p < 0.001$), TMT-A ($\beta = 0.561$, $R^2 = 0.203$, $p < 0.001$), and TMT-B ($\beta = 1.611$, $R^2 = 0.220$, $p = 0.013$). SRT was found to be significant predictors of MoCA ($\beta = -0.047$, $R^2 = 0.336$, $p = 0.002$), AVLT ($\beta = -0.180$, $R^2 = 0.138$, $p = 0.007$), Stroop ($\beta = 0.324$, $R^2 = 0.206$, $p = 0.007$), SDMT ($\beta = -0.612$, $R^2 = 0.312$, $p < 0.001$), TMT-A ($\beta = 0.571$, $R^2 = 0.213$, $p < 0.001$), and TMT-B ($\beta = 1.851$, $R^2 = 0.219$, $p = 0.005$).

In the PC group, PTA was found to be significant predictors of MoCA ($\beta = -0.096$, $R^2 = 0.414$, $p = 0.004$), AVLT ($\beta = -0.362$, $R^2 = 0.343$, $p < 0.001$), SDMT ($\beta = -0.617$, $R^2 = 0.459$, $p < 0.001$), TMT-A ($\beta = 0.988$, $R^2 = 0.382$, $p < 0.001$), and TMT-B ($\beta = 4.029$, $R^2 = 0.364$, $p = 0.040$). SRT was found to be significant predictors of MoCA ($\beta = -0.085$, $R^2 = 0.434$, $p = 0.005$), AVLT ($\beta = -0.311$, $R^2 = 0.347$, $p = 0.001$), SDMT ($\beta = -0.607$, $R^2 = 0.507$, $p < 0.001$), TMT-A ($\beta = 0.870$, $R^2 = 0.505$, $p < 0.001$), and TMT-B ($\beta = 4.606$, $R^2 = 0.362$, $p < 0.001$).

In the NP group, PTA was found to be significant predictors of Stroop ($\beta = 1.557$, $R^2 = 0.129$, $p = 0.019$) and SDMT ($\beta = -1.687$, $R^2 = 0.128$, $p = 0.020$). SRT was found to be significant predictors of SDMT ($\beta = -1.268$, $R^2 = 0.104$, $p = 0.033$).

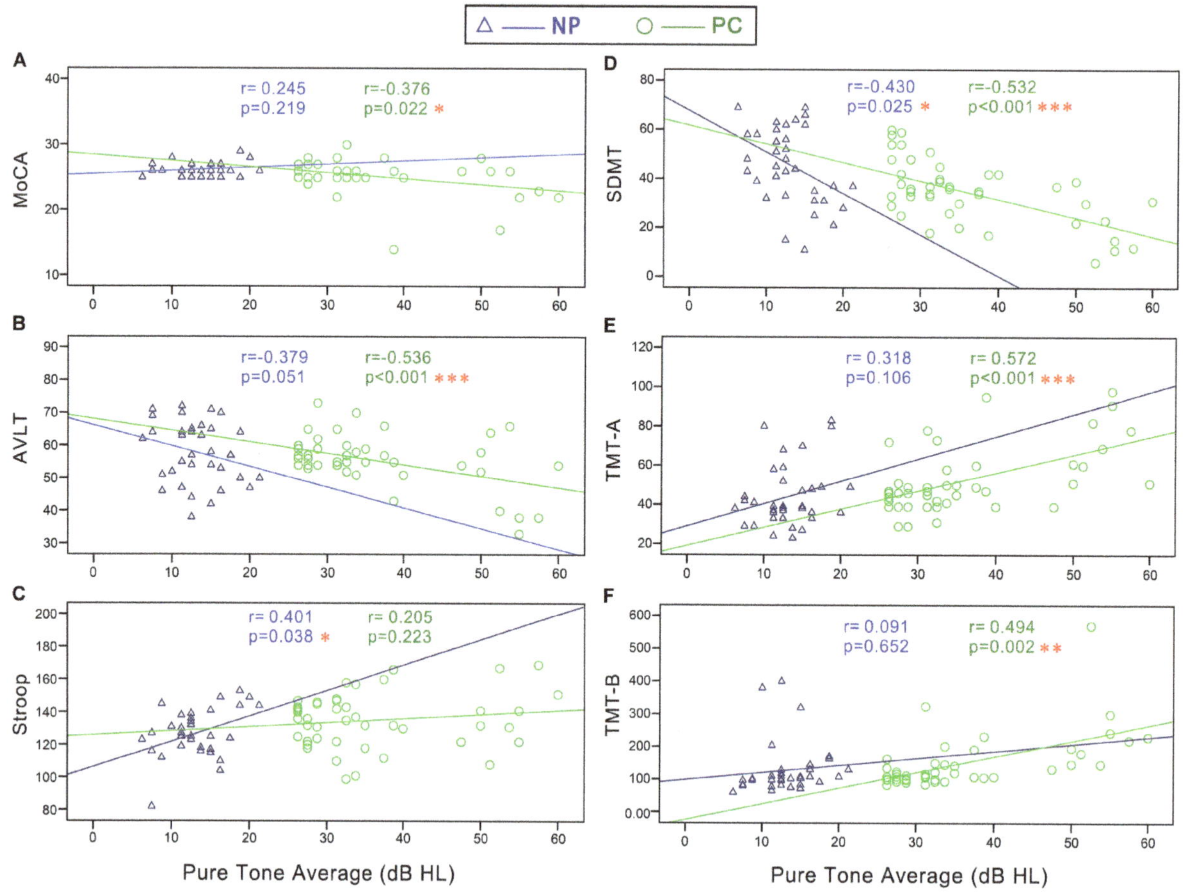

FIGURE 5 | Scatter plots displaying the correlations between PTA and cognitive function in the Normal PTA (NP) group and Presbycusis (PC) group. In the NP group, partial correlation analyses (controlling for age, sex, education level, diabetes, smoking, and hypertension) revealed that PTA was positively correlated with **(C)** Stroop ($r = 0.401$, $p = 0.038$) and negatively correlated with **(D)** SDMT ($r = -0.430$, $p = 0.025$). In the PC group, partial correlation analyses revealed that PTA was positively correlated with **(E)** TMT-A ($r = 0.572$, $p < 0.001$), and **(F)** TMT-B ($r = 0.494$, $p < 0.001$), and negatively correlated with **(A)** MoCA ($r = -0.376$, $p = 0.022$), **(B)** AVLT ($r = -0.536$, $p < 0.001$), and **(D)** SDMT ($r = -0.532$, $p < 0.001$).

DISCUSSION

The results for older adults in a Han Chinese cohort showed that cognitive function was significantly associated with PTA and SRT. In all subjects, the correlations between non-verbal cognitive scores and SRT were stronger than those between non-verbal cognitive scores and PTA, whereas, the correlations between verbal cognitive scores and PTA were stronger than those between verbal cognitive scores and SRT. Moreover, the correlations between PTA or SRT and cognitive function in the PC group were in principle stronger than those in the NP group. Additionally, there was no significant correlation between SRT and cognitive function in the NP group. To the best of our knowledge, this is the first study to elucidate the relationship between SRT and cognitive function in older adults in a Han Chinese cohort.

Previous studies of older American and Australian adults have reported significant relationships between peripheral hearing loss and global cognitive status (Lin et al., 2011a; Gopinath et al., 2012), executive function (Lin, 2011) and psychomotor speed (Lin et al., 2011a). Consistent with these findings, our study indicated, among older adults in a Han Chinese cohort, peripheral hearing, indexed by the four-frequency PTA in the better hearing ear, was significantly related to global cognitive status (MoCA) and multiple domains of cognitive performance, such as psychomotor speed (SDMT), executive function (TMT-A and TMT-B), attention (Stroop) and verbal learning and memory (AVLT). Our results were robust in analyses that accounted for confounders such as age, sex and education level. The strong connection between hearing loss and cognitive decline has been explained by a hypothesis of cognitive resource depletion in older adults (Wayne and Johnsrude, 2015). The hypothesis suggests that hearing loss can lead to increased cognitive resources for understanding acoustically degraded speech. In one functional magnetic resonance imaging study, patients with PC showed greater blood oxygen level-dependent activation responses to acoustic stimuli in the temporal lobes, demonstrating compensatory recruitment of the cortical regions involved in cognitive functions (Ouda et al., 2015). Furthermore, our results demonstrated that the correlations between multiple

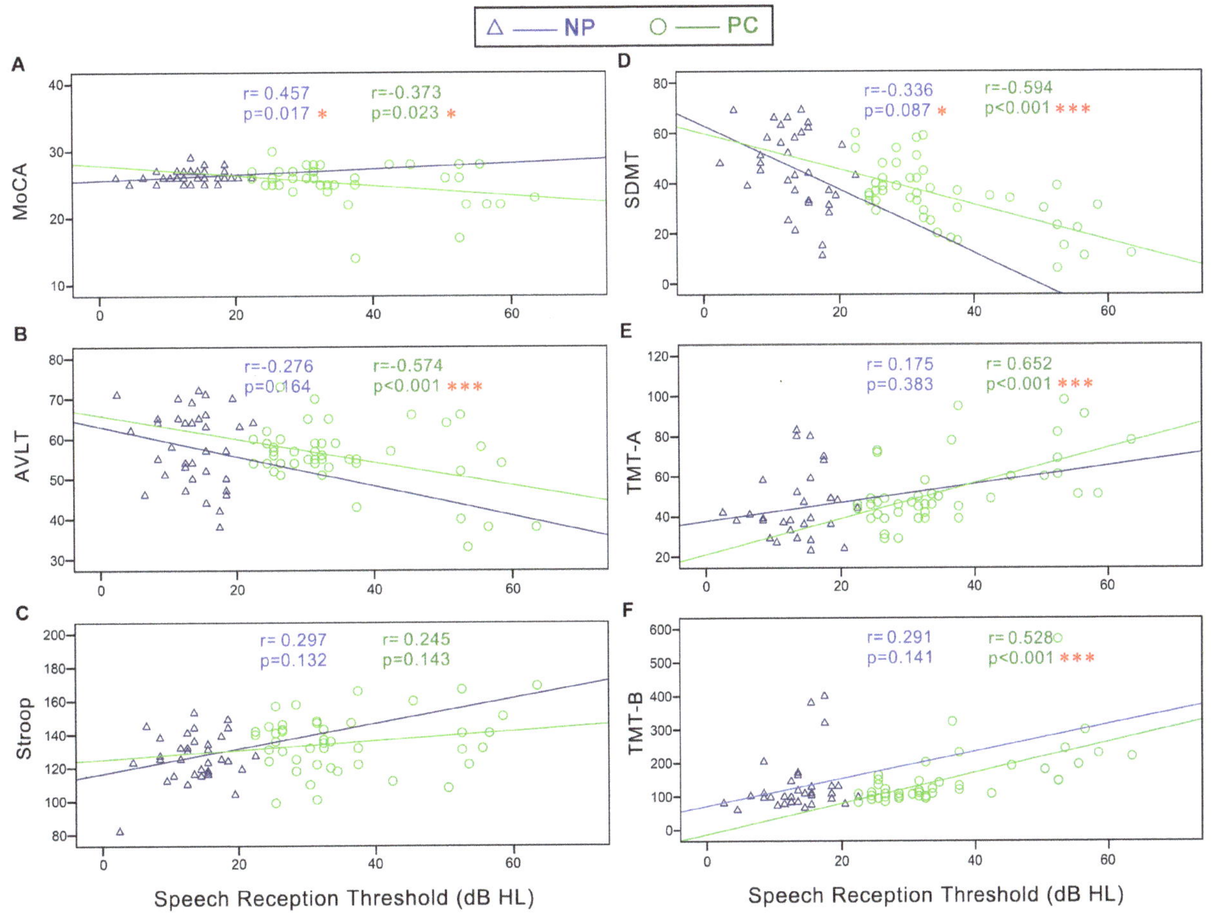

FIGURE 6 | Scatter plots displaying the correlations between SRT and cognitive function in the Normal PTA (NP) group and Presbycusis (PC) group. In the NP group, partial correlation analyses (controlling for age, sex, education level, diabetes, smoking, and hypertension) revealed that SRT was negatively correlated with **(D)** SDMT ($r = -0.361$, $p = 0.033$). In the PC group, Pearson correlation analyses revealed that SRT was positively correlated with **(E)** TMT-A ($r = 0.585$, $p < 0.001$) and **(F)** TMT-B ($r = 0.602$, $p < 0.001$) and negatively correlated with **(A)** MoCA ($r = -0.300$, $p = 0.046$), **(B)** AVLT ($r = -0.408$, $p = 0.005$) and **(D)** SDMT ($r = -0.622$, $p < 0.001$). There were no correlation between SRT and Stroop **(C)** in the NP or PC group.

domains of cognitive performance (e.g., SDMT and TMT) and hearing loss were stronger than those between global cognitive status (e.g., the MoCA) and hearing loss. Tests of multiple domains of cognitive performance are more challenging than the MoCA. Hearing loss could result in a smaller pool of cognitive resources being available for complex cognitive processes, such as psychomotor speed and executive control (Kahneman, 1973).

Pure tone average is considered to be a measure of the auditory periphery because the detection of pure tones relies on cochlear transduction and neuronal afferents to brainstem nuclei, without requiring significant higher auditory cortical processing (Pickles, 1988). It has long been accepted that PC has two components: one that represents aging of the auditory periphery, particularly the inner ear, and another related to aging of the central auditory system. Therefore, in terms of the association between hearing loss and cognitive function, we should take into account the state of both the peripheral hearing and the central auditory system. SRT is used to assess speech detection, and the SRT findings point to a central component of PC. In our study, cognitive function was significantly associated with SRT among older adults. Moreover, in all subjects, the correlations between non-verbal cognitive scores and SRT were stronger than those between non-verbal cognitive scores and PTA, whereas, the correlations between verbal cognitive scores and PTA were stronger than those between verbal cognitive scores and SRT. Therefore, our findings indicated that SRT could be an important auditory test for exploring cognitive decline in PC and could complement PTA. In addition, degraded verbal communication associated with hearing loss may confound cognitive testing. Therefore, non-verbal tests, such as the SDMT and TMT, which do not rely heavily on the presentation of verbal information, were also used in our study; furthermore, mild-moderate hearing loss minimally impairs face-to-face communication in quiet environments, particularly in the setting of testing by experienced examiners (Gordon-Salant, 2005).

Only one study has reported the relationship between SRT and cognitive function in older people (Nkyekyer et al., 2019). In that study, several cognitive domains were associated with SRT, but

TABLE 3 | Stepwise multiple linear regression models (cognitive measures as dependent variables).

Cognitive	Model I(PTA et al.* as independent variables)				Model II(SRT et al.* as independent variables)			
measures	β (95% CI)	R^2	t	p	β (95% CI)	R^2	t	p
All subjects								
MoCA	−0.050 (−0.079 – −0.021)	0.345	−3.393	0.001	−0.047 (−0.076 – −0.018)	0.336	−3.212	0.002
AVLT	−0.186 (−0.315 – −0.057)	0.143	−2.878	0.005	−0.180 (−0.308 – −0.052)	0.138	−2.792	0.007
Stroop SDMT	0.348 (0.117–0.578)	0.219	2.998	0.004	0.324 (0.091 – 0.557)	0.206	2.771	0.007
	−0.532 (−0.742 – −0.322)	0.322	−5.054	< 0.001	−0.612 (−0.813 – −0.411)	0.312	−6.067	< 0.001
TMT-A	0.561 (0.318 – 0.804)	0.203	4.599	< 0.001	0.571 (0.330 – 0.811)	0.213	4.728	< 0.001
TMT-B	1.611 (0.351 – 2.871)	0.220	2.545	0.013	1.851 (0.589 – 3.113)	0.219	2.920	0.005
PC group								
MoCA	−0.096 (−0.160 – −0.033)	0.414	−3.048	0.004	−0.085 (−0.144 – −0.027)	0.434	−2.936	0.005
AVLT	−0.362 (−0.554 – −0.171)	0.343	−3.816	< 0.001	−0.311 (−0.489 – −0.132)	0.347	−3.509	0.001
Stroop SDMT	N/A	N/A	0.919	0.364	N/A	N/A	1.423	0.162
	−0.617 (−0.917 – −0.317)	0.459	−4.154	< 0.001	−0.607 (−0.892 – −0.322)	0.507	−4.303	< 0.001
TMT-A	0.988 (0.588 – 1.388)	0.382	4.999	< 0.001	0.870 (0.529 – 1.210)	0.505	5.160	< 0.001
TMT-B	4.029 (0.260 – 10.341)	0.364	2.122	0.040	4.606 (2.726 – 6.485)	0.362	4.942	< 0.001
NP group								
MoCA	N/A	N/A	0.924	0.392	N/A	N/A	1.489	0.146
AVLT	N/A	N/A	1.098	0.280	N/A	N/A	0.874	0.389
Stroop SDMT	1.557 (0.268 – 2.847)	0.129	2.458	0.019	N/A	N/A	N/A	N/A
	−1.687 (−3.090 – −0.283)	0.128	−2.445	0.020	−1.268 (−2.430 – −0.106)	0.104	−2.221	0.033
TMT-A	N/A	N/A	N/A	N/A	N/A	N/A	N/A	N/A
TMT-B	N/A	N/A	N/A	N/A	N/A	N/A	N/A	N/A

** Other independent variables include age, sex, education level, diabetes, smoking, and hypertension. PTA, pure tone average; SRT, speech reception threshold; PC, presbycusis; NP, normal PTA; MoCA, montreal cognitive assessment; AVLT, auditory verbal learning test; SDMT, symbol digit modalities test; TMT, trail-making test; levels of anxiety and depression were assessed according to the hospital anxiety and depression scale (HADS); N/A, not available (regression model could not be established).*

only the Stroop measure was associated with PTA. In our study, the sample size is larger than that study, and subjects were further divided into presbycusis and normal PTA groups. Moreover, a Han Chinese cohort and a different set of cognition measures were assessed in our study, and we controlled age, sex, education level and other risk factors for cognitive decline in investigating the correlations between cognition and PTA/SRT.

Despite a growing body of literature documenting significant relationships between peripheral hearing and cognition (Gordon-Salant and Fitzgibbons, 1997; Pichora-Fuller and Singh, 2006; Akeroyd, 2008; Lin, 2011; Grassi and Borella, 2013), a few studies have reported negative results (Gates et al., 2002; Idrizbegovic et al., 2011). For example, one study reported no relationship between peripheral hearing and changes in global mental status over 4 years, after adjusting for covariates (Lin et al., 2004). To determine the extent to which the inclusion of many subjects with NP diffused the effects of peripheral hearing loss on measures of cognition, we repeated our correlation analyses within the NP and PC groups. The correlations between PTA or SRT and cognitive function in the PC group were stronger than those in the NP group. Additionally, there was no significant correlation between SRT and cognitive function in the NP group. This suggests that the significant relationship found between hearing and cognition was mainly driven by the older adults with PC. Therefore, some negative results may be attributed to the inclusion of a sample of older adults with NP.

There are several limitations to the present study. First, as this was a cross-sectional study, although correlations between cognitive impairment and hearing loss were found in older adults, the causation is still unknown. Second, the sample size in the study was relatively small. Third, PTA was only measured at four frequencies in the better ear, and it is likely that many subjects would have had high-frequency sensorineural hearing loss that was not captured in our study due to the limited range of frequencies tested.

CONCLUSION

Our findings indicate that cognitive function is significantly associated with PTA and SRT in older adults in a Han Chinese cohort. Moreover, the correlations between PTA or SRT and cognitive function in the PC group were in principle stronger than those in the NP group. Based on these findings, we argue that SRT could be an important auditory test for exploring cognitive decline in PC and could complement PTA.

AUTHOR CONTRIBUTIONS

FG and HW designed the experiments. FR, JL, WM, and LX carried out the experiments. ZF, YA, and BZ analyzed the experimental results. FG and QX assisted. FR and JL wrote the manuscript.

FUNDING

This work was supported by grants from The National Natural Science Foundation of China (Nos. 81601479 and 81670932); The National 973 Basic Research Program of China (No. 2014CB541703); Shandong Provincial Key Research and Development Program of China (No. 2016GSF201090); The Taishan Scholars Project (No. tsqn201812147); Shandong Provincial Natural Science Foundation of China (Nos. ZR2016QZ007 and 2017CXGC1213); Shandong Provincial Medical and Healthy Technology Development Program of China (No. 2017WS610).

REFERENCES

Akeroyd, M. A. (2008). Are individual differences in speech reception related to individual differences in cognitive ability? A survey of twenty experimental studies with normal and hearing-impaired adults. *Int. J. Audiol.* 47(Suppl. 2), S53–S71. doi: 10.1080/14992020802301142

Galea, M., and Woodward, M. (2005). Mini-mental state examination (MMSE). *Aust. J. Physiother.* 51:198. doi: 10.1016/s0004-9514(05)70034-9

Gates, G. A., Beiser, A., Rees, T. S., D'agostino, R. B., and Wolf, P. A. (2002). Central auditory dysfunction may precede the onset of clinical dementia in people with probable Alzheimer's disease. *J. Am. Geriatr. Soc.* 50, 482–488. doi: 10.1046/j.1532-5415.2002.50114.x

Gates, G. A., and Mills, J. H. (2005). Presbycusis. *Lancet* 366, 1111–1120. doi: 10.1016/s0140-6736(05)67423-5

Gopinath, B., Schneider, J., McMahon, C. M., Teber, E., Leeder, S. R., and Mitchell, P. (2012). Severity of age-related hearing loss is associated with impaired activities of daily living. *Age Ageing* 41, 195–200. doi: 10.1093/ageing/afr155

Gordon-Salant, S. (2005). Hearing loss and aging: new research findings and clinical implications. *J. Rehabil. Res. Dev.* 42(4 Suppl. 2), 9–24.

Gordon-Salant, S., and Fitzgibbons, P. J. (1997). Selected cognitive factors and speech recognition performance among young and elderly listeners. *J. Speech Lang. Hear. Res.* 40, 423–431. doi: 10.1044/jslhr.4002.423

Grassi, M., and Borella, E. (2013). The role of auditory abilities in basic mechanisms of cognition in older adults. *Front. Aging Neurosci.* 5:59. doi: 10.3389/fnagi.2013.00059

Idrizbegovic, E., Hederstierna, C., Dahlquist, M., Kampfe Nordstrom, C., Jelic, V., and Rosenhall, U. (2011). Central auditory function in early Alzheimer's disease and in mild cognitive impairment. *Age Ageing* 40, 249–254. doi: 10.1093/ageing/afq168

Jayakody, D. M., Friedland, P. L., Martins, R. N., and Sohrabi, H. R. (2018). Impact of aging on the auditory system and related cognitive functions: a narrative review. *Front. Neurosci.* 12:125. doi: 10.3389/fnins.2018.00125

Kahneman, D. (1973). *Attention and Effort*. Princeton, NJ: Citeseer.

Lin, F. R. (2011). Hearing loss and cognition among older adults in the United States. *J. Gerontol. A Biol. Sci. Med. Sci.* 66, 1131–1136. doi: 10.1093/gerona/glr115

Lin, F. R., Ferrucci, L., Metter, E. J., An, Y., Zonderman, A. B., and Resnick, S. M. (2011a). Hearing loss and cognition in the baltimore longitudinal study of aging. *Neuropsychology* 25, 763–770. doi: 10.1037/a0024238

Lin, F. R., Metter, E. J., O'Brien, R. J., Resnick, S. M., Zonderman, A. B., and Ferrucci, L. (2011b). Hearing loss and incident dementia. *Arch. Neurol.* 68, 214–220. doi: 10.1001/archneurol.2010.362

Lin, F. R., Thorpe, R., Gordon-Salant, S., and Ferrucci, L. (2011c). Hearing loss prevalence and risk factors among older adults in the United States. *J. Gerontol. A Biol. Sci. Med. Sci.* 66, 582–590. doi: 10.1093/gerona/glr002

Lin, M. Y., Gutierrez, P. R., Stone, K. L., Yaffe, K., Ensrud, K. E., Fink, H. A., et al. (2004). Vision impairment and combined vision and hearing impairment predict cognitive and functional decline in older women. *J. Am. Geriatr. Soc.* 52, 1996–2002. doi: 10.1111/j.1532-5415.2004.52554.x

Lu, J., Guo, Q. H., and Hong, Z. (2006). Trail making test used by Chinese elderly patients with mild cognitive impairment and mild Alzheimer dementia. *Chinese J. Clin. Psychol.* 14, 118–121.

Luo, H., Yang, T., Jin, X., Pang, X., Li, J., Chai, Y., et al. (2013). Association of GRM7 variants with different phenotype patterns of age-related hearing impairment in an elderly male han chinese population. *PLoS One* 8:e77153. doi: 10.1371/journal.pone.0077153

Mazelova, J., Popelar, J., and Syka, J. (2003). Auditory function in presbycusis: peripheral vs. central changes. *Exp. Gerontol.* 38, 87–94. doi: 10.1016/s0531-5565(02)00155-9

Nash, S. D., Cruickshanks, K. J., Klein, R., Klein, B. E., Nieto, F. J., Huang, G. H., et al. (2011). The prevalence of hearing impairment and associated risk factors: the beaver dam offspring study. *Arch. Otolaryngol. Head Neck Surg.* 137, 432–439. doi: 10.1001/archoto.2011.15

Nasreddine, Z. S., Phillips, N. A., Bedirian, V., Charbonneau, S., Whitehead, V., Collin, I., et al. (2005). The montreal cognitive assessment, MoCA: a brief screening tool for mild cognitive impairment. *J. Am. Geriatr. Soc.* 53, 695–699. doi: 10.1111/j.1532-5415.2005.53221.x

Nkyekyer, J., Meyer, D., Pipingas, A., and Reed, N. S. (2019). The cognitive and psychosocial effects of auditory training and hearing aids in adults with hearing loss. *Clin. Interv. Aging* 14, 123–135. doi: 10.2147/CIA.S183905

Ouda, L., Profant, O., and Syka, J. (2015). Age-related changes in the central auditory system. *Cell Tissue Res.* 361, 337–358. doi: 10.1007/s00441-014-2107-2

Pichora-Fuller, M. K., and Singh, G. (2006). Effects of age on auditory and cognitive processing: implications for hearing aid fitting and audiologic rehabilitation. *Trends Amplif.* 10, 29–59. doi: 10.1177/108471380601000103

Pickles, J. O. (1988). *An Introduction to the Physiology of Hearing*. London: Academic press.

Quaranta, N., Coppola, F., Casulli, M., Barulli, M. R., Panza, F., Tortelli, R., et al. (2014). The prevalence of peripheral and central hearing impairment and its relation to cognition in older adults. *Audiol. Neurootol.* 19(Suppl. 1), 10–14. doi: 10.1159/000371597

Sanchez-Cubillo, I., Perianez, J., Adrover-Roig, D., Rodriguez-Sanchez, J., Rios-Lago, M., Tirapu, J., et al. (2009). Construct validity of the trail making test: role of task-switching, working memory, inhibition/interference control, and visuomotor abilities. *J. Int. Neuropsychol. Soc.* 15, 438–450. doi: 10.1017/S1355617709090626

Savitz, J. B., and Jansen, P. (2003). The stroop color-word interference test as an indicator of ADHD in poor readers. *J. Genet. Psychol.* 164, 319–333. doi: 10.1080/00221320309597986

Schuknecht, H. F., and Gacek, M. R. (1993). Cochlear pathology in presbycusis. *Ann. Otol. Rhinol. Laryngol.* 102, 1–16. doi: 10.1177/00034894931020s101

Van Schependom, J., D'hooghe, M., Cleynhens, K., D'hooge, M., Haelewyck, M., De Keyser, J., et al. (2014). The symbol D igit M odalities T est as sentinel test for cognitive impairment in multiple sclerosis. *Eur. J. Neurol.* 21:1219-e72. doi: 10.1111/ene.12463

Wayne, R. V., and Johnsrude, I. S. (2015). A review of causal mechanisms underlying the link between age-related hearing loss and cognitive decline. *Ageing Res. Rev.* 23(Pt B), 154–166. doi: 10.1016/j.arr.2015.06.002

Wei, M., Shi, J., Li, T., Ni, J., Zhang, X., Li, Y., et al. (2018). Diagnostic accuracy of the chinese version of the trail-making test for screening cognitive impairment. *J. Am. Geriatr. Soc.* 66, 92–99. doi: 10.1111/jgs.15135

World Health Organization [WHO] (2018). *World Health Statistics*. Geneva: World Health Organization.

Zhao, Q., Lv, Y., Zhou, Y., Hong, Z., and Guo, Q. (2012). Short-term delayed recall of auditory verbal learning test is equivalent to long-term delayed recall for identifying amnestic mild cognitive impairment. *PLoS One* 7:e51157. doi: 10.1371/journal.pone.0051157

Zigmond, A. S., and Snaith, R. P. (1983). The hospital anxiety and depression scale. *Acta Psychiatr. Scand.* 67, 361–370.

11

Cingulate Cortex Atrophy is Associated with Hearing Loss in Presbycusis with Cochlear Amplifier Dysfunction

*Chama Belkhiria[1,2], Rodrigo C. Vergara[1,2], Simón San Martín[1,2], Alexis Leiva[1,2], Bruno Marcenaro[1,2], Melissa Martinez[3], Carolina Delgado[1,3] and Paul H. Delano[1,2,4]**

[1] Department of Neuroscience, Faculty of Medicine, University of Chile, Santiago, Chile, [2] Biomedical Neuroscience Institute, Faculty of Medicine, University of Chile, Santiago, Chile, [3] Department of Neurology and Neurosurgery, Clinical Hospital of the University of Chile, Santiago, Chile, [4] Department of Otolaryngology, Clinical Hospital of the University of Chile, Santiago, Chile

***Correspondence:**
Paul H. Delano
pdelano@med.uchile.cl;
phdelano@gmail.com

Age-related hearing loss is associated with cognitive decline and has been proposed as a risk factor for dementia. However, the mechanisms that relate hearing loss to cognitive decline remain elusive. Here, we propose that the impairment of the cochlear amplifier mechanism is associated with structural brain changes and cognitive impairment. Ninety-six subjects aged over 65 years old (63 female and 33 male) were evaluated using brain magnetic resonance imaging, neuropsychological and audiological assessments, including distortion product otoacoustic emissions as a measure of the cochlear amplifier function. All the analyses were adjusted by age, gender and education. The group with cochlear amplifier dysfunction showed greater brain atrophy in the cingulate cortex and in the parahippocampus. In addition, the atrophy of the cingulate cortex was associated with cognitive impairment in episodic and working memories and in language and visuoconstructive abilities. We conclude that the neural abnormalities observed in presbycusis subjects with cochlear amplifier dysfunction extend beyond core auditory network and are associated with cognitive decline in multiple domains. These results suggest that a cochlear amplifier dysfunction in presbycusis is an important mechanism relating hearing impairments to brain atrophy in the extended network of effortful hearing.

Keywords: presbycusis, neurodegeneration, dementia, cognition, cochlear amplifier

INTRODUCTION

Age-related hearing loss or presbycusis is characterized by bilateral progressive hearing loss and impaired speech understanding, especially in noisy environments (Gates and Mills, 2005). According to recent epidemiological data from the United States more than 50% of people aged over 70 years have presbycusis (Goman and Lin, 2016). In addition, due to population aging, it is expected that by the year 2025 there will be more than one billion people with hearing loss in the world (Sprinzl and Riechelmann, 2010). The increasing number of hearing loss patients is alarming, since epidemiological evidence has shown an association between presbycusis and cognitive decline in elderly people (Lin and Albert, 2014; Thomson et al., 2017). For instance, Lin et al. (2011) have shown that individuals with mild to moderate presbycusis have worse results in executive function and psychomotor processing, while other studies have shown that hearing loss is significantly related to global cognitive decline, which can lead to social isolation and depression (Harrison Bush et al., 2015; Panza et al., 2015). Furthermore, a recent prospective cohort has reported that presbycusis subjects with audiometric hearing thresholds worse than 40 dB are more likely to develop dementia (Deal et al., 2017). In line with this evidence, a Lancet consortium recently proposed a model in which hearing loss is the major potentially preventable risk factor for dementia (Livingston et al., 2017).

Although epidemiological and clinical studies confirm the relationship between hearing loss and cognitive decline, the mechanisms that relate them remain elusive (Lin and Albert, 2014; Wayne and Johnsrude, 2015). The pathological correlate of presbycusis can display different features, including cochlear hair cell loss, stria vascularis atrophy, and auditory-nerve neuron loss (Gates and Mills, 2005). Animal models of presbycusis have shown that in addition to the peripheral auditory damage, aged animals have less GABAergic neurons in the auditory cortex (Martin del Campo et al., 2012). In the same line, several human studies have found brain structural changes in patients with hearing loss, including gray matter volume reduction in the right temporal lobe (Lin et al., 2014; Peelle and Wingfield, 2016) and correlations between hearing impairment and smaller gray matter volume in the auditory cortex (Peelle et al., 2011; Eckert et al., 2012). However, whether the atrophy of specific brain regions and cognitive domains in presbycusis patients are associated with cochlear receptor cell loss is unknown (Shen et al., 2018).

There are two types of receptor cells in the mammalian cochlea: inner hair cells (IHC) and outer hair cells (OHC). While, IHCs are related to sensory transduction of acoustic vibrations, OHCs are responsible for the cochlear amplifier mechanism, which allows high sensitivity and sharp frequency selectivity to low-intensity sounds (Brownell et al., 1985; Robles and Ruggero, 2001; Liberman et al., 2002). In natural hearing, the cochlear amplifier is fundamental for frequency discrimination and speech perception, and can be assessed through otoacoustic emissions (Oghalai, 2004).

Here we hypothesized that a cochlear amplifier dysfunction in presbycusis – an OHC loss – is associated with cognitive decline and structural brain changes in the elderly population. We studied the possible associations between cochlear OHC function (measured by distortion product otoacoustic emissions [DPOAE]), cognitive performance, and brain structure (magnetic resonance imaging, MRI) in a Chilean cohort of elders without dementia (ANDES) and with different levels of hearing loss.

MATERIALS AND METHODS

All procedures were approved by the Ethics Committee of the Clinical Hospital of the University of Chile, permission number: OAIC752/15. All subjects gave written informed consent in accordance with the Declaration of Helsinki.

Subjects

For this cross-sectional prospective study, a total of 142 patients aged $\geq$ 65 years (screened between 2016 and 2018) from Recoleta's primary health public center located in the city of Santiago (Chile) were evaluated for recruitment. According to the inclusion and exclusion criteria of the Auditory and Dementia study (ANDES), 96 subjects were included for neuropsychological, audiological and brain imaging assessments. Inclusion criteria were the following: patients older than 65 years without dementia, which was evaluated by a mini-mental state examination (MMSE) score $\geq$ 24 and preserved functionality measured by the Pfeffer activities questionnaire (Quiroga et al., 2004). Exclusion criteria of recruitment in the study were the following: (i) stroke or other neurological disorders; (ii) dementia; (iii) major psychiatric disorders; (iv) other causes of hearing loss different from presbycusis (e.g., conductive hearing loss); (v) patients using hearing aids and (vi) other causes of significant disability.

Audiological Evaluations

All the audiological evaluations were carried out by an experienced audiologist in a double wall soundproof room located in the Otolaryngology Department of the Clinical Hospital of the University of Chile. Air conduction pure tone audiometric (PTA) hearing thresholds were evaluated at 0.125, 0.25, 0.5, 1, 2, 3, 4, 6 and 8 kHz for each subject in both ears using a clinical audiometer (AC40, Interacoustics®). In addition, in order to rule out conductive hearing loss, bone conduction thresholds were measured at 0.25, 0.5, 1, 2, 3 and 4 kHz. All audiometric data presented in the present work refer to air conduction thresholds. The PTA at 0.5, 1, 2 and 4 kHz were calculated for each subject in both ears. Subjects were classified according to their hearing level: normal hearing ($\leq$20 dB), mild presbycusis (>20 and $\leq$35 dB), and moderate presbycusis (>35 dB) based on the PTA of the better hearing ear. Moderate presbycusis subjects were referred to the Chilean program for hearing aids for elders >65 years.

Distortion Product Otoacoustic Emissions

Otoacoustic emissions are sounds emitted by the OHCs of the inner ear that can be measured through sensitive microphones (Kemp, 1978). DPOAEs are a type of otoacoustic emission, commonly measured in clinical and basic research as a non-invasive tool for assessing the OHC function of the cochlear receptor (Abdala and Visser-Dumont, 2001). In this study, DPOAE (2f1–f2) were measured as a proxy of the cochlear amplifier function, using an ER10C microphone (Etymotic Research®), presenting eight pairs of primary tones (f1 and f2, at 65 and 55 dB SPL, f2/f1 ratio of 1.22) in each ear at eight different 2f1–f2 frequencies: 707, 891, 1122, 1414, 1781, 2244, 2828 and 3563 Hz. **Figure 1A** shows an example of the spectrogram of the microphone signal obtained from the external ear canal of the subjects, in which a 2f1–f2 DPAOE peak can be observed. To consider the presence of a detectable DPOAE, we used an amplitude criterion: the amplitude of a given DPOAE (dB SPL) should be at least 6 dB above noise floor. Using this criterion, we counted the number of detectable DPOAEs per ear, going from 0 to 8: "0" means that the subject had no detectable DPOAE in that ear, and consequently that ear was classified as having cochlear

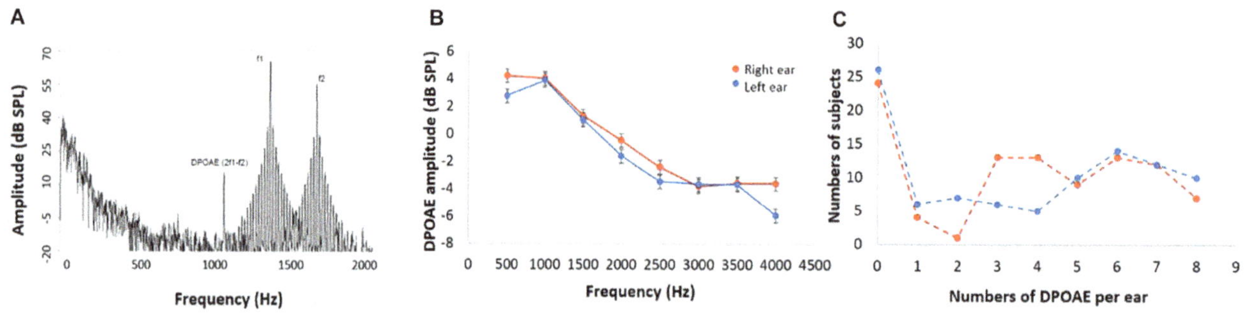

FIGURE 1 | DPOAE measurements. **(A)** Example of the spectrogram of the microphone signal used to obtain the 2f1–f2 DPOAEs in response to f1 and f2 stimuli. DPOAE amplitudes are about 40–50 dB smaller than f1 and f2 primary tones. **(B)** Mean DPOAE amplitudes in response to the eight frequencies for left (blue) and right (red) ears (data shown as mean ± SEM). Notice that low frequency DPOAEs are larger in amplitude than high frequency DPOAEs. **(C)** Frequency histogram of the number of detectable DPOAE per subject for left (blue) and right (red) ears. Note that 24 and 26 subjects had no detectable DPOAEs in right and left ears, respectively.

amplifier dysfunction (see below), while "8" means that the subject had detectable DPOAEs at all tested frequencies in that ear (normal cochlear amplifier function); and "16" means that the subject had detectable DPOAE in all tested frequencies in both ears. In contrast with a method that only measures the amplitude of DPOAE, the procedure of counting the number of detectable DPOAE per ear allowed us to evaluate the cochlear amplifier function in the whole sample (n = 96), without eliminating subjects with no detectable DPOAEs (and no measurable amplitude in dB SPL), which is common in elderly subjects.

Cognitive Assessment

All subjects and their relatives were evaluated by a neurologist during a structured interview and graded according to their cognitive complaints using the clinical dementia rating scale (Morris, 1993). Cognitive performances were assessed by an experienced psychologist in cognitive tests adapted for the Chilean population (Quiroga et al., 2004), including the MMSE for global cognition (Folstein et al., 1975), the Frontal Assessment Battery (FAB) for measuring executive function (Dubois et al., 2000), the Trail Making Test A (TMT A) for processing speed (Army Individual Test Battery, 1944), the Boston Nominating Test for Language (Kaplan, 1978), the Rey–Osterrieth Complex Figure Test for Visuospatial Abilities (Rey, 1959), the Backward Digit Span for Verbal Working Memory, and the total recall of the Free and Cued Selective Reminding Test (FCSRT) to explore verbal episodic memory (Grober et al., 1988). Depression was self-rated by the participants using the Geriatric Depression Scale (GDS), which consists of 15 YES/NO answer questions. Higher scores indicate higher levels of depression, with scores over five indicating significant depressive symptoms (Yesavage et al., 1983). Cognitive training was not performed in this study.

Magnetic Resonance Imaging

Neuroimaging data were acquired by a MAGNETOM Skyra 3-Tesla whole-body MRI Scanner (Siemens Healthcare GmbH®, Erlangen, Germany) equipped with a head volume coil. T1-weighted magnetization-prepared rapid gradient echo (T1-MPRAGE) axial images were collected, and parameters were as follows: time repetition (TR) = 2300 ms, time echo (TE) = 232 ms, matrix = 256 × 256, flip angle = 8°, 26 slices, and voxel size = 0.94 × 0.94 × 0.9 mm^3. T2-weighted turbo spin echo (TSE) (4500 TR ms, 92 TE ms) and fluid attenuated inversion recovery (FLAIR) (8000 TR ms, 94 TE ms, 2500 TI ms) were also collected to inspect structural abnormalities. A total of 440 images were obtained during an acquisition time of 30 min per subject.

Morphometric Analyses

To determine the structural brain changes of controls and presbycusis individuals, we measured the volume and thickness of bilateral cortical regions. FreeSurfer (version 6.0)[1] was used with a single Linux workstation using Centos 6.0 as was suggested by Gronenschild et al. (2012) for T1-weighted images analysis of individual subjects. The FreeSurfer processing involved several stages, as follows: volume registration with the Talairach atlas, bias field correction, initial volumetric labeling, non-linear alignment to the Talairach space, and final volume labeling. We used the "recon-all" function to generate automatic segmentations of cortical and subcortical regions. This command performs regional segmentation and processes gross regional volume in a conformed space (256 × 256 × 256 matrix, with coronal reslicing to 1 mm^3 voxels). The function "recon-all" creates gross brain volume extents for larger-scale regions (i.e., total number of voxels per region): total gray and white matter, subcortical gray matter, brain mask volume, and estimated total intracranial volume.

Additionally, we measured the cortical thickness in native space using FreeSurfer tools. We calculated the cortical thickness of each mesh of vertices by measuring the distance between the point on one surface and the closest conforming point on the opposite surface. Then we measured the average of the two values calculated from each side to the other (Fischl and Dale, 2000). Based on the brain regions that have been previously studied in presbycusis (Lin et al., 2014; Rigters et al., 2017) our regions of interest were the bilateral frontal superior, temporal inferior,

[1] http://surfer.nmr.mgh.harvard.edu

middle and superior gyri, parahippocampus, hippocampus, and amygdala. We also included as regions of interest, cortical areas that have been implicated in the neural networks of degraded speech comprehension: bilateral anterior cingulate cortex (ACC), posterior cingulate cortex (PCC), and precentral and postcentral gyri (Peelle and Wingfield, 2016).

Statistical Analysis

SPSS software version 20.0 was used to perform statistical analysis of demographic data, audiometric measurements, neuropsychological test results and structural MRI data. The ANCOVA method was used to compare cognitive performances and volume and thickness differences between the three tested groups including age, sex, and years of education as covariables. Pearson correlations were performed according to the distribution of data.

We applied general linear models (GLM) to contrast the difference of correlations between the studied groups using PTA as predictor for both volume and thickness. Age, education and sex were adjusted as covariates. The results were corrected for the multiple comparison using a significant alpha value of $p = 0.01$ (Hagler et al., 2006). Regions with significant differences in GLM models were selected based on the results of multiple corrections, and their corresponding brain regions were represented using the scientific notation p-values. The volume and thickness of selected regions were calculated based on the spatially normalized images of each individual in Talairach space (Fischl et al., 2002). In addition, we performed partial correlations including age, sex and education as confound regressors to associate cognitive tests with anterior and PCC volume and thickness.

RESULTS

Demographics Characteristics

The mean age of the recruited subjects (n = 96, 63 female) was 73.6 ± 5.3 years [mean ± standard deviation (SD)] with an average educational level of 9.5 ± 4.2 years of schooling (mean ± SD). The audiometric hearing thresholds were normal in 32 subjects, while 44 and 20 individuals were considered as mild and moderate presbycusis, respectively. None of the 96 subjects used hearing aids at the moment of recruitment. A summary of demographic data, including age, sex, education, hearing level, smoking, and cardiovascular risk factors is presented in **Table 1**.

Cochlear Amplifier Function

Figure 1B shows the mean amplitudes of the DPOAEs measured at eight different frequencies per ear, while **Figure 1C** displays a frequency histogram of the number of detectable DPOAE per ear, showing a bimodal distribution with a peak below two DPOAE per ear, and a broad distribution for more than two detectable DPOAE per ear. According to this bimodal distribution of the number of detectable DPOAE, we decided to split data into two groups: (i) better preserved cochlear amplifier function (≥5 DPOAE in both ears) and (ii) cochlear amplifier dysfunction (<5 DPOAE in both ears). **Figure 2** shows that the number of detectable DPAOE significantly correlates with age and audiometric hearing thresholds, meaning that a lower number of DPOAE is associated with more aged subjects and worse hearing thresholds.

TABLE 1 | Demographic characteristics of the ANDES cohort.

Characteristic	Cohort (n = 96)
Age, mean (SD)	73.62 (5.34)
Sex, n (%)	
Female	63 (65.62)
Education, mean years (SD)	9.53 (4.23)
Hearing loss, mean dB (SD)	25.35 (10.91)
Hearing loss category, n (%)	
Normal (<20 dB)	32 (33.33)
Mild (21–35 dB)	44 (45.83)
Moderate (>35 dB)	20 (20.83)
DPOAEs, mean number (SD)	7.45 (5.35)
Cochlear status, n (%)	
Preserved cochlear amplifier	64 (66.66)
Cochlear amplifier dysfunction	32 (33.33)
Hypertension, n (%)	39 (40.62)
Smoking, n (%)	18 (18.75)
Diabetes, n (%)	25 (26.04)
Hearing aid use, n (%)	0 (0.0)

Next, in addition to the classification based on the cochlear amplifier status, we used the degree of hearing loss (PTA) to divide subjects into three groups: (i) Controls: normal hearing (≤20 dB PTA, better hearing ear) with preserved cochlear amplifier function (≥5 detectable DPOAE) (n = 31); (ii) mild and moderate presbycusis (>20 dB PTA, better hearing ear) with preserved cochlear amplifier (PCF) (n = 33); and (iii) mild and moderate presbycusis (>20 dB PTA, better hearing ear) with cochlear amplifier dysfunction (<5 detectable DPOAE) (CD) (n = 31). One subject could not be classified within these criteria as he presented normal hearing with cochlear amplifier dysfunction and was excluded for further analyses.

Table 2 shows a summary of the audiological and cognitive performance of the three groups (controls, PCF and CD) controlled by age, gender and years of education. There was a significant difference in age between controls and the group of presbycusis with cochlear amplifier dysfunction, while non-significant differences in age and education were found between the two presbycusis groups (PCF and CD). At the cognitive level, the group with presbycusis and cochlear amplifier dysfunction had worse executive function than the other groups.

Structural Brain Changes

Our next step was to evaluate whether structural brain changes were associated with cochlear amplifier dysfunction. Hence, we compared the MRI volumes and thickness of cortical and limbic brain regions in the three groups (controls, PCF and CD) using ANCOVA models adjusted by age, sex and education. Structural volumes were normalized by the total estimated intracranial volume. The ANCOVA models for brain volumes yielded significant differences between the three groups in the precentral

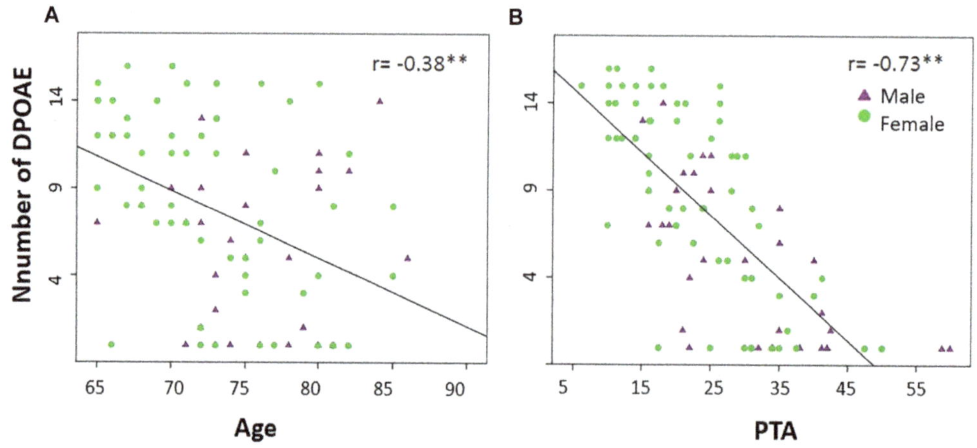

FIGURE 2 | The number of detectable DPOAEs correlates with age and hearing thresholds (PTA). **(A)** A significant negative Spearman correlation was found between age and the number of detectable DPOAE in both ears (**$p < 0.05$, $r = -0.38$). **(B)** A significant negative Spearman correlation was found between the audiometric thresholds of the better hearing ear (PTA) and the number of detectable DPOAE in both ears (**$p < 0.05$, $r = -0.73$). Green circles and purple triangles represent female and male subjects, respectively.

TABLE 2 | Demographic, audiological and cognitive differences between controls and presbycusis groups with and without cochlear amplifier dysfunction.

	Controls (n = 31)	Presbycusis-PCF (n = 33)	Presbycusis-CD (n = 31)	F	p
Age (years)	70.84 ± 4.84	73.78 ± 5.79£	76.12 ± 4.27¥	6.52	0.002*
Education (years)	9.65 ± 3.73	9.39 ± 4.36	9.77 ± 4.46	0.06	0.94
Sex, Female (%)	25 (80.64%)	21 (63.63%)	16 (51.61%)	1.15	0.31
DPOAEs (n)	12.06 ± 3.1	9.18 ± 3£	1.126 ± 2.32¥#	96.02	<0.001*
PTA (dB)	14.16 ± 3.15	25.68 ± 4.86£	36.45 ± 9.13¥#	73.38	<0.001*
Global Cognition (MMSE)	28.06 ± 1.12	28.33 ± 1.24	27.87 ± 1.05	1.46	0.23
Executive functions (FAB)	14.48 ± 1.82	13.70 ± 2.42	12.5 ± 2.43¥#	7.65	<0.001*
Visuospatial capacities (Rey figure)	29.77 ± 5.17	28.56 ± 6.48	30.89 ± 2.59	1.89	0.15
Processing speed (TMT A)	60.74 ± 31.05	57.16 ± 26.90	59.53 ± 18.72	0.19	0.82
Episodic Memory (FCSRT)	44.97 ± 3.43	44.22 ± 3.73	43.03 ± 6.25	1.54	0.22
Nomination (Boston)	25.38 ± 2.94	25.38 ± 2.84	24.33 ± 2.89	1.37	0.25
Working memory(backward digit n°)	3.81 ± 1.07	4.36 ± 1.51	3.48 ± 1.09	0.41	0.66
Depression score (GDS-15)	3.10 ± 2.99	3.07 ± 3.49	3.25 ± 2.68	0.11	0.89

*Data were analyzed using ANCOVA for comparing variables between the three groups corrected by age, sex and education. Mean ± SD values for age, education, sex, DPOAEs, PTA, cognitive tests are shown for controls, presbycusis with preserved cochlear function (PCF) and presbycusis with cochlear amplifier dysfunction (CD) groups. *p < 0.05 for significant ANCOVA. ¥p < 0.05 significantly different when comparing presbycusis with cochlear amplifier dysfunction vs. controls. #p < 0.05 significantly different when comparing presbycusis with CD vs. presbycusis without CD. £p < 0.05 significantly different when comparing presbycusis without CD vs. controls.*

($F(2,89) = 3.92$, $p = 0.02$) and postcentral gyri ($F(2,89) = 3.92$, $p = 0.02$), parahippocampus ($F(2,89) = 4.55$, $p = 0.01$) and amygdala ($F(2,89) = 3.31$, $p = 0.04$). Tukey *post hoc* tests showed significant differences between the CD and controls in the volume of precentral and postcentral gyri and parahippocampus. The only significant difference in brain volume between PCF and CD groups was obtained from parahippocampus (**Table 3**).

Regarding cortical thickness, we found significant differences in the ANCOVA models for ACC ($F(2,89) = 3.04$, $p = 0.04$), PCC $F(2,89) = 4.17$, $p = 0.01$), precentral gyrus ($F(2,89) = 4.00$, $p = 0.02$), postcentral gyrus ($F(2,89) = 6.43$, $p = 0.002$) and parahippocampus ($F(2,89) = 3.3$, $p = 0.04$). Tukey *post hoc* tests showed that the thickness of precentral and postcentral gyri in the CD group were significantly reduced compared to that of the control group, while the thickness of ACC and PCC in the CD group were thinner than those of the PCF group (**Table 3**).

Next, in order to isolate the effect of hearing levels and cochlear amplifier dysfunction on brain structures, we ran GLM analyses. The GLM contrasted the difference of associations between PCF and CD groups using PTA as predictor for both volume and thickness. This method can effectively select voxels that correlate with PTA when contrasting PCF and CD groups. The whole brain analyses of volume and thickness related to cochlear amplifier dysfunction revealed significant correlations between PTA and different brain regions (corrected by age, education and sex, and using a level of significance = $p < 0.01$) shown in red and blue colors in **Figure 3**. These associations were significant for large clusters of voxels in bilateral ACC and

TABLE 3 | Brain volume and thickness differences between the controls and presbycusis groups with and without cochlear amplifier dysfunction.

	Controls *n* = 31	PCF *n* = 33	CD *N* = 31	*F*	*P*
Brain volume regions (cm³)					
Anterior cingulate	2.87 ± 0.4	2.74 ± 0.53	2.69 ± 0.38	1.2	0.3
Posterior cingulate	4.03 ± 0.53	3.98 ± 0.59	3.94 ± 0.47	0.23	0.79
Precentral gyrus	8.01 ± 1.1	7.6 ± 1.0	7.2 ± 1.0¥	3.92	0.02*
Postcentral gyrus	5.1 ± 0.1	4.9 ± 0.7	4.5 ± 0.7¥	3.92	0.02*
Parahippocampus	2.9 ± 0.5	2.9 ± 0.4	2.6 ± 0.4¥#	4.55	0.01*
Frontal superior	13.7 ± 2.2	13.3 ± 1.7	13.1 ± 1.9	0.66	0.51
Temporal inferior	8.8 ± 1.6	8.8 ± 0.8	8.6 ± 1.9	0.25	0.77
Temporal middle	14.4 ± 2.5	14.3 ± 1.8	13.7 ± 2.5	0.89	0.41
Temporal superior	20.4 ± 0.2	20.5 ± 0.2	19.8 ± 0.2	0.59	0.55
Amygdala	2.2 ± 0.3	2.2 ± 0.3	2.01 ± 0.4	3.31	0.04*
Hippocampus	5.5 ± 0.8	5.3 ± 0.7	5.01 ± 0.8	2.41	0.09
Cortical thickness (mm)					
Anterior cingulate	4.81 ± 0.26	4.78 ± 0.33	4.48 ± 0.32¥#	3.04	0.04*
Posterior cingulate	4.99 ± 0.18	4.97 ± 0.25	4.6 ± 0.28¥#	4.17	0.01*
Precentral gyrus	4.97 ± 0.24	4.9 ± 0.24	4.79 ± 0.29¥	4.00	0.02*
Postcentral gyrus	4.08 ± 0.21	3.99 ± 0.18	3.91 ± 0.21¥	6.43	0.002*
Parahippocampus	5.36 ± 0.58	5.33 ± 0.48	5.06 ± 0.57	3.30	0.04*
Frontal superior	4.91 ± 0.18	4.91 ± 0.22	4.86 ± 0.25	0.54	0.58
Temporal inferior	5.51 ± 0.19	5.52 ± 0.26	5.48 ± 0.26	0.23	0.79
Temporal middle	5.32 ± 0.17	5.31 ± 0.21	5.22 ± 0.22	2.07	0.13
Temporal superior	5.33 ± 0.25	5.30 ± 0.25	5.21 ± 0.3	2.08	0.13

*Data were analyzed using ANCOVA for comparing variables between the three groups corrected by age, sex and education. Mean ± SD values for the sum of bilateral brain region thickness and volumes normalized by total estimated intracranial volume. *$p < 0.05$ for significant ANCOVA. ¥$p < 0.05$ significantly different when comparing presbycusis with CD vs. controls. #$p < 0.05$ significantly different when comparing presbycusis with CD vs. presbycusis without CD.*

PCC. Cochlear amplifier dysfunction was also associated with significant negative correlations between PTA and volume and between PTA and thickness in scattered regions of the right superior temporal, right postcentral and left precentral areas. We also found small clusters resulting from positive correlation between PTA and volume in the right superior and middle frontal areas in the CD group (**Figure 3A**). **Figure 4** shows examples of the correlations between PTA and bilateral ACC thickness in CD and PCF groups, illustrating that PTA was negatively correlated with the thickness of bilateral ACC gyri only in the CD group.

Cognitive Performance, Depression Scores and Cingulate Cortices Volume and Thickness

Pearson partial correlation analyses were performed between the bilateral volume and thickness of ACC and PCC and cognitive performance in PCF and CD groups. Age, sex and education were controlled as covariates (**Table 4**). Correlations between cognitive tests and structural measures of ACC and PCC were different between CD and PCF groups. In CD patients, there were significant correlations between episodic memory (total recall in the FCSRT), nomination, verbal working memory tests and volume of the left ACC. On the other hand, processing speed and verbal working memory correlated with the volume of the left PCC, while visuospatial abilities with the right PCC. These results indicate that, in the group with cochlear amplifier dysfunction, the volume of cingulate cortices and cognition performance decreased together. In addition, there was a negative correlation between depression scores and ACC volume in the CD group, indicating that higher depressive symptoms were associated with a decreased ACC volume.

Regarding cortical thickness, we found significant correlations between visuospatial capacities and right ACC, processing speed and left ACC, and nomination with bilateral ACC in the CD group. The visuospatial capacities test also correlated significantly with the thickness of the right PCC in the CD group. Taken together, these results indicate that the more severe the cognitive impairment, the thinner the cortex is in the anterior and posterior cingulate area.

DISCUSSION

In this combined approach, we found that structural brain changes in presbycusis subjects with cochlear amplifier dysfunction extend beyond central auditory pathways, including the cingulo-opercular network which is fundamental for effortful hearing. In addition, these changes were associated with impairments in verbal and non-verbal cognitive domains and depressive symptoms.

Cochlear Amplifier Dysfunction and Hearing Loss

A reduced number of detectable DPOAEs correlated with age, confirming that cochlear damage increases with aging

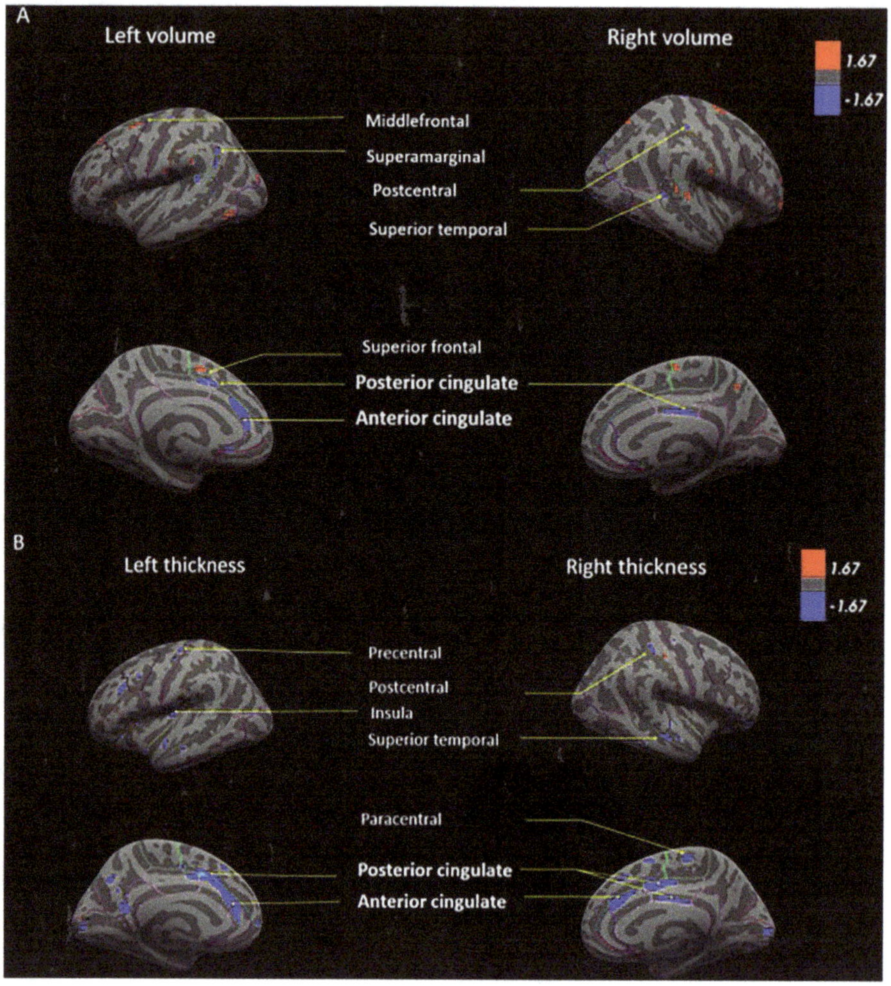

FIGURE 3 | GLM models for brain volume **(A)** and cortical thickness **(B)** correlated with PTA in presbycusis patients. The GLM contrasts the difference of correlations between PCF and CD groups using PTA as predictor for both volume and thickness. Age, education and sex were adjusted as covariates. The color blue shows regions in which individuals with cochlear dysfunction had a higher rate of gray matter decrease compared to those with normal cochlear ($p < 0.01$). The color red shows regions in which individuals with cochlear impairment had a higher rate of gray matter increase compared to those with normal cochlear ($p < 0.01$).

(Abdala and Dhar, 2012; Abdala et al., 2018). In addition, the number of DPOAE and hearing levels were also correlated, which could be explained by the fact that cochlear aging is one of the main causes of presbycusis (Gates and Mills, 2005). However, it is important to highlight that both measures (DPOAE and PTA) are not identical and several differences can be described. DPOAE are objective measures that can be obtained with a microphone positioned in the external ear canal of anesthetized or unconscious subjects, while audiometric thresholds need the voluntary response of individuals. DPOAEs specifically reflect the function of the cochlear amplifier located in the OHCs of the cochlear receptor (Robles et al., 1991), while audiometric thresholds depend on the normal function of the complete auditory pathway.

In our work, according to the bimodal distribution of DPOAE presence, we divided data of presbycusis patients into two groups with different levels of cochlear amplifier function. As the cochlear amplifier is essential for auditory sensitivity, frequency and speech discrimination (Robles and Ruggero, 2001), we hypothesized that the group of patients with loss of OHCs would have more severe neural and cognitive consequences of hearing loss. Indeed, our results showed that the CD group had worse executive functions in comparison with the group with PCF, even after adjusting by age, education, and sex. This finding is in agreement with previous reports showing that executive functions are associated with hearing impairment (Lin et al., 2011), but we extended this association showing that executive functions are more impaired in the group with cochlear amplifier dysfunction.

Cochlear Amplifier Dysfunction and Brain Structure

At the brain structural level, we compared the volume and cortical thickness of regions of interest that were previously reported to be related to hearing loss, but we also included areas

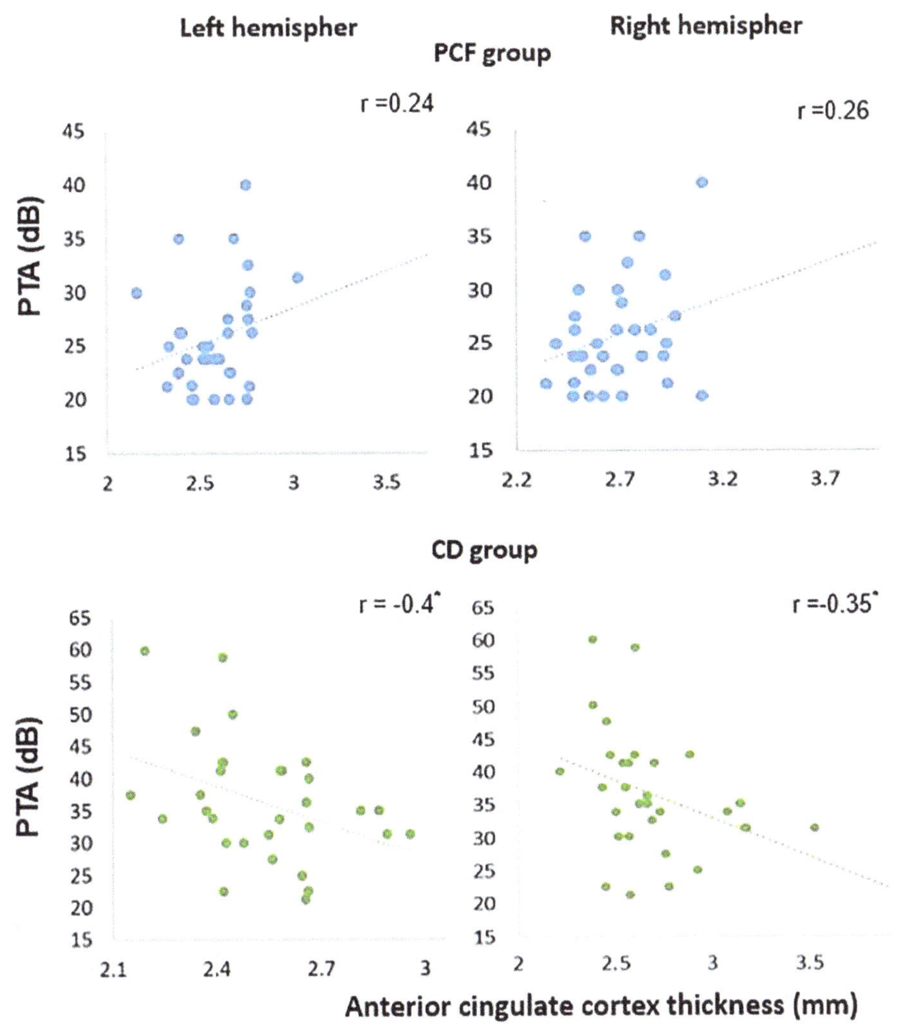

FIGURE 4 | Significant negative correlations between PTA and ACC thickness in presbycusis patients with cochlear amplifier dysfunction. Pearson correlations between PTA and anterior cingulate thickness for PCF (blue) and CD (green) groups.

beyond the temporal lobe, that have been involved in effortful hearing (Peelle and Wingfield, 2016). Our results confirm that hearing impairment was associated to right superior temporal volume decrease (Lin et al., 2014; Rigters et al., 2017), but also to right superior temporal thickness decrease in the CD group. Notably, in the group of patients with CD, hearing loss produced larger effects in the network of effortful hearing, including the ACC, PCC, precentral and postcentral cortices, and the parahippocampus (**Figure 3**). While these findings are in agreement with a study reporting volume decrease in the right ACC in a group of middle-aged hearing loss patients (Husain et al., 2011), our results stress the importance of cochlear amplifier function in the neural structures related to the effortful hearing network in aged people.

Previous studies using functional MRI in presbycusis patients have demonstrated activation of non-auditory cortical regions related to the extended cortical network that supports spoken language processing (Peelle et al., 2011; Sharma and Glick, 2016). The cingulo-opercular cortex is one of the principal components of this network (Peelle and Wingfield, 2016). Increased activation of this area is related to better speech comprehension in normal hearing subjects (Peelle, 2018), and in mild hearing loss patients during passive listening (Campbell and Sharma, 2013).

Our work shows that the atrophy of the ACC is associated with cognitive and emotional deficits in presbycusis patients with cochlear amplifier dysfunction. The ACC is a key structure of cognitive and emotional variables necessary for decision making and social behavior that has also been implicated in pain, negative affect, and autonomic networks (Fornito et al., 2004; Shackman et al., 2011). Interestingly, we found that in the CD group, the reduction of the ACC volume was correlated not only with impairments in tests related to language processing (episodic and verbal working memories and nomination), but also with non-language functions such as visuospatial abilities and processing speed (**Table 4**). The decrease in performance in non-auditory cognitive domains could be explained by an

TABLE 4 | Pearson partial correlation corrected by age, sex, and education between cognitive tests and volume and thickness of anterior and posterior cingulate cortex for PCF and CD groups (*$p < 0.05$).

	ACC volume				ACC thickness				PCC volume				PCC thickness			
	PCF		CD		PCF		CD		PCF		CD		PCF		CD	
Cognitive tests	**r-Left**	**r-Right**	**r-Left**	**r-Right**	**r-Left**	**r-Right**	**r-Left**	**r-Right**	**r-Left**	**r-Right**	**r-Left**	**r-Right**	**r-Left**	**r-Right**	**r-Left**	**r-Right**
Cognitive functions (MMSE)	0.14	0.46*	−0.19	0.00	0.22	0.17	0.03	−0.13	0.05	0.40	−0.10	0.00	0.14	0.14	−0.01	−0.19
Executive functions (FAB)	0.29	0.07	−0.01	0.21	0.14	0.26	0.62	0.13	−0.12	−0.13	−0.01	0.02	−0.03	0.04	−0.11	−0.24
Visuospatial capacities (Rey figure)	0.05	0.41*	0.14	0.30	0.01	0.28	0.15	0.49*	0.32	0.27	0.35	0.54*	0.00	0.02	0.35	0.45*
Processing speed (TMT A)	−0.27	0.01	−0.37	−0.04	−0.22	−0.17	−0.34*	−0.26	−0.40*	−0.21	−0.41*	−0.31	0.02	−0.01	−0.20	−0.11
Episodic Memory (FCSRT)	−0.20	0.19	0.44*	0.31	0.01	0.08	0.34	0.10	−0.26	0.05	0.28	0.22	0.05	0.11	0.08	−0.18
Nomination (Boston)	0.21	0.03	0.47*	0.29	0.03	0.07	0.48*	0.41*	0.19	0.11	0.23	0.31	−0.16	0.03	0.28	0.20
Working memory (backward digit n°)	0.10	−0.14	0.64*	0.40	−0.06	−0.42	0.18	0.07	0.10	0.05	0.45*	0.18	0.12	0.40	−0.35	0.00
Depression score (GDS-15)	0.32	−0.20	−0.53*	−0.01	−0.17	0.36	0.05	0.00	0.17	0.00	−0.12	0.04	0.27	0.35	0.25	−0.09

increased listening effort in the group of CD patients, which needs the recruitment of non-auditory brain areas, decreasing resources for other cognitive functions (Peelle, 2018).

Another possible mechanism to explain the relation between episodic memory and semantic impairment with ACC atrophy in presbycusis could be a functional disconnection between the temporal lobe and the cingulate region (Warrington and Weiskrantz, 1982), as the functional connectivity between the cingulate and temporal areas has been correlated with memory performance in patients with mild cognitive impairment. Furthermore, the cingulate region and the parahippocampus gyrus are key components of the default mode network (Greicius et al., 2003; Raichle, 2015) which were significantly atrophied in the group of presbycusis with cochlear amplifier dysfunction. Taken together, our findings suggest that the relations between the ACC atrophy and episodic memory impairment could reflect an impairment of the Papez circuit in presbycusis patients with cochlear amplifier dysfunction (Tsivilis et al., 2008; Carlesimo et al., 2011).

At the emotional level, several functional neuroimaging studies have found hypoperfusion of the ACC cortex in subjects with major depression (Fitzgerald et al., 2008). Accordingly, we found that the volume of the left ACC was correlated with depressive symptoms in the group with cochlear amplifier dysfunction. However, it is important to highlight that our study only included subjects with mild to moderate depressive symptoms that could be interpreted as "negative affect or sadness" (Mayberg et al., 1999).

In our study the volume and thickness of the right PCC was also significantly correlated with visuospatial abilities in the CD group. This could be explained by role of the right PCC and the right hippocampus in the cortical network associated with spatial abilities, including spatial navigation and egocentric orientation (Hirono et al., 1998; Burles et al., 2018), suggesting that presbycusis could contribute to these spatial deficits.

In addition to the atrophy of the limbic areas in the CD group, we found changes in sensorimotor brain regions. The volume and thickness of the precentral and postcentral gyri were significantly reduced in the group with CD in comparison with the two other groups (**Figure 3**). These results could be explained by aging, as these regions are known to be affected in elderly people with gait disorders. Another possibility is the recruitment of precentral and postcentral gyri for speech perception in situations with degraded acoustic signal as part of the extended network of language processing (Peelle et al., 2010; Peelle and Wingfield, 2016).

Why Is Cochlear Amplifier Dysfunction Associated With Brain Atrophy?

One possible explanation is that the loss of OHC could be a general indicator of accelerated cell death in the nervous system of elderly people (Shen et al., 2018). In this sense, we can speculate that the absence of DPAOE in mild presbycusis patients could be an early risk factor for detecting accelerated neurodegeneration that could lead to cingulate cortex atrophy and executive dysfunction. This hypothesis could be addressed by performing experiments with selective loss of OHC in animal models.

Another speculative mechanism is that the constant activation of the effortful listening network could produce an accelerated neurodegeneration of cingulate neurons caused by glutamate excitotoxicity (Eckert et al., 2009; Adank, 2012; Vaden et al., 2015). This mechanism has been proposed in other neuropsychiatric diseases with ACC atrophy including fibromyalgia (Luerding et al., 2008; Cagnie et al., 2014) and psychotic depression (Bijanki et al., 2014; Zhang et al., 2017). Moreover, the constant activation of the cingulate cortices and other regions of the extended language network in presbycusis patients with cochlear amplifier dysfunction could act as a "secondary injury" that triggers neurodegeneration in a susceptible brain (Sperling et al., 2011).

Limitations of the Study

In our study, we have a relatively reduced number of presbycusis patients with moderate or severe hearing loss. This is partially due to the inclusion criterion that requires subjects to have never used hearing aids before the moment of recruitment. This criterion was planned to eliminate possible neural compensatory plasticity associated to the use of hearing devices, but it hindered the recruitment of moderate to severe presbycusis patients (as most of them had used hearing aids previously). Consequently, the majority of the study's subjects have only mild to moderate presbycusis. Another limitation of the present work is that DPOAE loss, aging and brain changes could be associated with other peripheral and central auditory impairments that might affect cognition. These factors include IHC damage, auditory-nerve fiber loss and central auditory processing abnormalities, which could also be associated with DPOAE loss. Finally, the three groups are not perfectly matched by age and PTA. We control this limitation using these and other variables as covariates when needed. This control has its limitations, however, given our conditions, main conclusions should not be affected (see **Supplementary Materials 1, 2**). Therefore, our results are promising, but more research using DPOAEs as predictor for cognitive and neural decline is needed to evaluate the extent of this relation.

CONCLUSION

In non-demented patients with mild to moderate presbycusis, cochlear amplifier dysfunction was associated with brain atrophy and cognitive decline. We found structural changes in non-auditory brain areas related to the extended language processing network: the anterior and posterior cingulate cortices, sensorimotor areas and the parahippocampus. The dysfunction of this network is related to impairments in cognitive domains beyond auditory processing. Future longitudinal studies should consider measuring DPOAE, as a potentially early biomarker of cognitive decline and structural brain alterations.

AUTHOR CONTRIBUTIONS

CB analyzed the data and wrote the manuscript. RV and SSM analyzed the data. AL, BM, and MM performed the data acquisition. CD and PD performed experimental design and data analysis, and edited the manuscript.

ACKNOWLEDGMENTS

We thank Dr. Luis Robles for reading a previous version of this manuscript.

REFERENCES

Abdala, C., and Dhar, S. (2012). Maturation and aging of the human cochlea: a view through the DPOAE looking glass. *J. Assoc. Res. Otolaryngol.* 13, 403–421. doi: 10.1007/s10162-012-0319-2

Abdala, C., Ortmann, A. J., and Shera, C. A. (2018). Reflection- and distortion-source otoacoustic emissions: evidence for increased irregularity in the human cochlea during aging. *J. Assoc. Res. Otolaryngol.* 19, 493–510. doi: 10.1007/s10162-018-0680-x

Abdala, C., and Visser-Dumont, L. (2001). Distortion product otoacoustic emissions: a tool for hearing assessment and scientific study. *Volta. Rev.* 103, 281–302.

Adank, P. (2012). The neural bases of difficult speech comprehension and speech production: two activation likelihood estimation (ALE) meta-analyses. *Brain Lang.* 122, 42–54. doi: 10.1016/j.bandl.2012.04.014

Army Individual Test Battery (1944). *Manual of Directions and Scoring.* Washington, DC: War Department, Adjunct General's Office.

Bijanki, K. R., Hodis, B., Brumm, M. C., Harlynn, E. L., and McCormick, L. M. (2014). Hippocampal and left subcallosal anterior cingulate atrophy in psychotic depression. *PLoS One* 9:e110770. doi: 10.1371/journal.pone.0110770

Brownell, W. E., Bader, C. R., Bertrand, D., and de Ribaupierre, Y. (1985). Evoked mechanical responses of isolated cochlear outer hair cells. *Science* 227, 194–196. doi: 10.1126/science.3966153

Burles, F., Umiltá, A., McFarlane, L. H., Potocki, K., and Iaria, G. (2018). Ventral-dorsal functional contribution of the posterior cingulate cortex in human spatial orientation: a meta-analysis. *Front. Hum. Neurosci.* 12:190. doi: 10.3389/fnhum.2018.00190

Cagnie, B., Coppieters, I., Denecker, S., Six, J., Danneels, L., and Meeus, M. (2014). Central sensitization in fibromyalgia? A systematic review on structural and functional brain MRI. *Semin. Arthritis Rheum.* 44, 68–75. doi: 10.1016/j.semarthrit.2014.01.001

Campbell, J., and Sharma, A. (2013). Compensatory changes in cortical resource allocation in adults with hearing loss. *Front. Syst. Neurosci.* 7:71. doi: 10.3389/fnsys.2013.00071

Carlesimo, G. A., Lombardi, M. G., and Caltagirone, C. (2011). Vascular thalamic amnesia: a reappraisal. *Neuropsychologia* 49, 777–789. doi: 10.1016/j.neuropsychologia.2011.01.026

Deal, J., Betz, J., Yaffe, K., and Harris, T. (2017). Hearing impairment and incident dementia and cognitive decline in older adults: the health ABC study. *J. Gerontol. A Biol. Sci. Med. Sci.* 72, 703–709. doi: 10.1093/gerona/glw069

Dubois, B., Slachevsky, A., Litvan, I., and Pillon, B. (2000). The FAB: a frontal assessment battery at bedside. *Neurology* 55, 1621–1626. doi: 10.1212/wnl.55.11.1621

Eckert, M., Cute, S., Vaden, K., and Kuchinsky, S. (2012). Auditory cortex signs of age-related hearing loss. *J. Assoc. Res. Otolaryngol.* 13, 703–713. doi: 10.1007/s10162-012-0332-5

Eckert, M. A., Menon, V., Walczak, A., Ahlstrom, J., Denslow, S., Horwitz, A., et al. (2009). At the heart of the ventral attention system: the right anterior insula. *Hum. Brain Mapp.* 30, 2530–2541. doi: 10.1002/hbm.20688

Fischl, B., and Dale, A. M. (2000). Measuring the thickness of the human cerebral cortex from magnetic resonance images. *Proc. Natl. Acad. Sci. U.S.A.* 97, 11050–11055. doi: 10.1073/pnas.200033797

Fischl, B., Salat, D. H., Busa, E., Albert, M., Dieterich, M., Haselgrove, C., et al. (2002). Whole brain segmentation: automated labeling of neuroanatomical structures in the human brain. *Neuron* 33, 341–355.

Fitzgerald, P. B., Laird, A. R., Maller, J., and Daskalakis, Z. J. (2008). A meta-analytic study of changes in brain activation in depression. *Hum. Brain Mapp.* 29, 683–695. doi: 10.1002/hbm.20426

Folstein, M. F., Folstein, S. E., and McHugh, P. R. (1975). Mini-mental state". A practical method for grading the cognitive state of patients for the clinician. *J. Psychiatr. Res.* 12, 189–198.

Fornito, A., Yücel, M., Wood, S., Stuart, G. W., Buchanan, J. A., Proffitt, T., et al. (2004). Individual differences in anterior cingulate/paracingulate morphology are related to executive functions in healthy males. *Cereb. Cortex* 14, 424–431. doi: 10.1093/cercor/bhh004

Gates, G. A., and Mills, J. H. (2005). Presbycusis. *Lancet* 366, 1111–1120.

Goman, A. M., and Lin, F. R. (2016). Prevalence of hearing loss by severity in the United States. *Am. J. Public Health* 106, 1820–1822. doi: 10.2105/AJPH.2016.303299

Greicius, M. D., Krasnow, B., Reiss, A. L., and Menon, V. (2003). Functional connectivity in the resting brain: a network analysis of the default mode hypothesis. *Proc. Natl. Acad. Sci. U.S.A.* 100, 253–258. doi: 10.1073/pnas.0135058100

Grober, E., Buschke, H., Crystal, H., Bang, S., and Dresner, R. (1988). Screening for dementia by memory testing. *Neurology* 38, 900–900. doi: 10.1212/wnl.38.6.900

Gronenschild, E. H., Habets, P., Jacobs, H. I., Mengelers, R., Rozendaal, N., van Os, J., et al. (2012). The effects of freesurfer version, workstation type, and macintosh operating system version on anatomical volume and cortical thickness measurements. *PLoS One* 7:e38234. doi: 10.1371/journal.pone.0038234

Hagler, D. J., Saygin, P., and Sereno, M. I. (2006). Smoothing and cluster thresholding for cortical surface-based group analysis of fMRI data. *Neuroimage* 33, 1093–1103. doi: 10.1016/j.neuroimage.2006.07.036

Harrison Bush, A. L., Lister, J. J., Lin, F. R., Betz, J., and Edwards, J. D. (2015). Peripheral hearing and cognition. *Ear Hear.* 36, 395–407. doi: 10.1097/aud.0000000000000142

Hirono, N., Mori, E., Ishii, K., Ikejiri, Y., Imamura, T., Shimomura, T., et al. (1998). Hypofunction in the posterior cingulate gyrus correlates with disorientation for time and place in Alzheimer's disease. *J. Neurol. Neurosurg. Psychiatry* 64, 552–554. doi: 10.1136/jnnp.64.4.552

Husain, F. T., Medina, R. E., Davis, C. W., Szymko-Bennett, Y., Simonyan, K., Pajor, N. M., et al. (2011). Neuroanatomical changes due to hearing loss and chronic tinnitus: a combined VBM and DTI study. *Brain Res.* 1369, 74–88. doi: 10.1016/j.brainres.2010.10.095

Kaplan, E. (1978). *The Boston Naming Test*. Philadelphia, PA: Lea & Febiger.

Kemp, D. T. (1978). Stimulated acoustic emissions from within the human auditory system. *J. Acoust. Soc. Am.* 64, 1386–1391. doi: 10.1121/1.382104

Liberman, M. C., Gao, J., He, D. Z., Wu, X., Jia, S., and Zuo, J. (2002). Prestin is required for electromotility of the outer hair cell and for the cochlear amplifier. *Nature* 19, 300–304. doi: 10.1038/nature01059

Lin, F. R., Ferrucci, L., An, Y., Goh, J. O., Doshi, J., Metter, E. et al. (2014). Association of hearing impairment with brain volume changes in older adults. *Neuroimage* 15, 84–92. doi: 10.1016/j.neuroimage.2013.12.059

Lin, F., Ferrucci, L., Metter, E., and An, Y. (2011). Hearing loss and cognition in the baltimore longitudinal study of aging. *Neuropsychology* 25, 763–770. doi: 10.1037/a0024238

Lin, F. R., and Albert, M. (2014). Hearing loss and dementia-who is listening? *Aging Ment. Health* 18, 671–673. doi: 10.1080/13607863.2014.915924

Livingston, G., Sommerlad, A., Orgeta, V., Costafreda, S. G., Huntley, J., Ames, D., et al. (2017). The lancet commissions dementia prevention, intervention, and care. *Lancet* 390, 2673–2734.

Luerding, R., Weigand, T., Bogdahn, U., and Schmidt-Wilcke, T. (2008). Working memory performance is correlated with local brain morphology in the medial frontal and anterior cingulate cortex in fibromyalgia patients: structural correlates of pain-cognition interaction. *Brain* 131, 3222–3231. doi: 10.1093/brain/awn229

Martin del Campo, H. N., Measor, K. R., and Razak, K. A. (2012). Parvalbumin immunoreactivity in the auditory cortex of a mouse model of presbycusis. *Hear. Res.* 294, 31–39. doi: 10.1016/j.heares.2012.08.017

Mayberg, H. S., Liotti, M., Brannan, S. K., McGinnis, S., Mahurin, R. K., Jerabek, P. A., et al. (1999). Reciprocal limbic-cortical function and negative mood: converging PET findings in depression and normal sadness. *Am. J. Psychiatry* 156, 675–682.

Morris, J. C. (1993). The clinical dementia rating (CDR): current version and scoring rules. *Neurology* 43, 2412–2414.

Oghalai, J. S. (2004). The cochlear amplifier: augmentation of the traveling wave within the inner ear. *Curr. Opin. Otolaryngol. Head Neck Surg.* 12, 431–438 . doi: 10.1097/01.moo.0000134449.05454.82

Panza, F., Seripa, D., Solfrizzi, V., and Tortelli, R. (2015). Targeting cognitive frailty: clinical and neurobiological roadmap for a single complex phenotype. *J. Alzheimers Dis.* 47, 793–813. doi: 10.3233/JAD-150358

Peelle, J., Troiani, V., and Grossman, M. (2011). Hearing loss in older adults affects neural systems supporting speech comprehension. *J. Neurosci.* 31, 12638–12643. doi: 10.1523/JNEUROSCI.2559-11.2011

Peelle, J. E. (2018). Listening effort: how the cognitive consequences of acoustic challenge are reflected in brain and behavior. *Ear hear.* 39, 204–214. doi: 10.1097/AUD.0000000000000494

Peelle, J. E., Johnsrude, I. S., and Davis, M. H. (2010). Hierarchical processing for speech in human auditory cortex and beyond. *Front. Hum. Neurosci.* 4:51.

Peelle, J. E., and Wingfield, A. (2016). The neural consequences of age-related hearing loss. *Trends Neurosci.* 39, 486–497. doi: 10.1016/j.tins.2016.05.001

Quiroga, P., Albala, C., and Klaasen, G. (2004). Validation of a screening test for age associated cognitive impairment in Chile. *Rev. Med. Chil.* 132, 467–478.

Raichle, M. E. (2015). The brain's default mode network. *Annu. Rev. Neurosci.* 38, 433–447.

Rey, A. (1959). *Test de Copie D'une Figure Complexe*. Paris: Centre de Psychologie Appliquée.

Rigters, S. C., Bos, D., Metselaar, M., Roshchupkin, G. V., Baatenburg de Jong, R. J., Ikram, M. A., et al. (2017). Hearing impairment is associated with smaller brain volume in aging. *Front. Aging Neurosci.* 9:2.

Robles, L., and Ruggero, M. A. (2001). Mechanics of the mammalian cochlea. *Physiol. Rev.* 81, 1305–1352. doi: 10.1152/physrev.2001.81.3.1305

Robles, L., Ruggero, M. A., and Rich, N. C. (1991). Two-tone distortion in the basilar membrane of the cochlea. *Nature* 349, 413–414. doi: 10.1038/349413a0

Shackman, A. J., Salomons, T. V., Slagter, H. A., Fox, A. S., Winter, J. J., and Davidson, R. J. (2011). The integration of negative affect, pain and cognitive control in the cingulate cortex. *Nat. Rev. Neurosci.* 12, 154–167. doi: 10.1038/nrn2994

Sharma, A., and Glick, H. (2016). Cross-modal re-organization in clinical populations with hearing loss. *Brain Sci.* 6:4. doi: 10.3390/brainsci6010004

Shen, Y., Ye, B., Chen, P., Wang, Q., Fan, C., Shu, Y., et al. (2018). Cognitive decline, dementia, alzheimer's disease and presbycusis: examination of the possible molecular mechanism. *Front. Neurosci.* 12:394.

Sperling, R. A., Aisen, P. S., Beckett, L. A., Bennett, D. A., Craft, S., Fagan, A. M., et al. (2011). Toward defining the preclinical stages of Alzheimer's disease: recommendations from the national institute on aging-Alzheimer's association workgroups on diagnostic guidelines for Alzheimer's disease. *Alzheimers Dem.* 7, 280–292.

Sprinzl, G., and Riechelmann, H. (2010). Current trends in treating hearing loss in elderly people: a review of the technology and treatment options–a mini-review. *Gerontology* 56, 351–358. doi: 10.1159/000275062

Thomson, R. S., Auduong, P., Miller, A. T., and Gurgel, R. K. (2017). Hearing loss as a risk factor for dementia: a systematic review. *Laryngosc. Investig. Otolaryngol.* 2, 69–79. doi: 10.1002/lio2.65

Tsivilis, D., Vann, S. D., Denby, C., Roberts, N., Mayes, A. R., Montaldi, D., et al. (2008). A disproportionate role for the fornix and mammillary bodies in recall versus recognition memory. *Nat. Neurosci.* 11, 834–842. doi: 10.1038/nn.2149

Vaden, K. I., Kuchinsky, S. E., Ahlstrom, J. B., Dubno, J. R., Eckert, M. A., and Eckert, M. A. (2015). Cortical activity predicts which older adults recognize speech in noise and when. *J. Neurosci.* 35, 3929–3937. doi: 10.1523/JNEUROSCI.2908-14.2015

Warrington, E. K., and Weiskrantz, L. (1982). Amnesia: a disconnection syndrome? *Neuropsychologia* 20, 233–248. doi: 10.1016/0028-3932(82)90099-9

Wayne, R., and Johnsrude, I. (2015). A review of causal mechanisms underlying the link between age-related hearing loss and cognitive decline. *Ageing Res. Rev.* 23, 154–166. doi: 10.1016/j.arr.2015.06.002

Yesavage, J. A., Brink, T. L., Rose, T. L., Lum, O., Huang, V., Adey, M., et al. (1983). Development and validation of a geriatric depression screening scale: a preliminary report. *J. Psychiatr. Res.* 17, 37–49. doi: 10.1016/0022-3956(82)90033-4

Zhang, J., Guo, Z., Liu, X., Jia, X., Li, J., Li, Y., et al. (2017). Abnormal functional connectivity of the posterior cingulate cortex is associated with depressive symptoms in patients with Alzheimer's disease. *Neuropsychiatr. Dis. Treat.* 13, 2589–2598. doi: 10.2147/ndt.s146077

12

The Effect of Cochlear Implants on Cognitive Function in Older Adults: Initial Baseline and 18-Month Follow up Results for a Prospective International Longitudinal Study

Julia Sarant[1], David Harris[2], Peter Busby[1], Paul Maruff[3], Adrian Schembri[3], Richard Dowell[1] and Robert Briggs[4]*

[1] Department of Audiology and Speech Pathology, The University of Melbourne, Melbourne, VIC, Australia, [2] Department of Economics, The University of Melbourne, Melbourne, VIC, Australia, [3] Cogstate Ltd., Melbourne, VIC, Australia, [4] The Royal Victorian Eye and Ear Hospital, Melbourne, VIC, Australia

****Correspondence:***
Julia Sarant
jsarant@unimelb.edu.au

In older adults, hearing loss is independently associated with an increased rate of cognitive decline, and has been identified to be a modifiable risk factor for dementia. The mechanism underlying the cognitive decline associated with hearing loss is not understood, but it is known that the greater the hearing loss, the faster the rate of decline. It is unknown whether remediation of hearing loss with hearing devices can delay cognitive decline. This 5-year international longitudinal study is investigating the impact of cochlear implants on cognitive function in older people with severe-profound hearing loss, and whether remediation of hearing loss could delay the onset of cognitive impairment. This is the first study to examine the major primary risk factors associated with dementia in the same cohort. Participants were assessed before cochlear implantation and 18 months later using an identical battery including a visually presented cognitive assessment tool (Cogstate battery) that is highly sensitive to small changes in cognition and suitable for use with people with hearing loss. Hearing and speech perception ability were assessed in sound-treated conditions by an audiologist, and a range of questionnaire tools was administered to assess self-perceived ease of listening, quality of life, physical activity, diet, social and emotional loneliness, isolation, anxiety, and depression. A detailed medical health history was taken. Pre-operatively, despite the small initial sample size ($n = 59$), increased hearing loss and age predicted significantly poorer executive function and visual attention, while tertiary education predicted better executive function. Better self-reported quality of life was correlated with better visual learning performance, and engaging in frequent vigorous physical activity was correlated with poorer visual learning performance. At 18 months, for the first 20 participants, significant benefits of cochlear implants were seen in terms of speech perception, communication ability, and quality of life. Multiple linear regression modeling showed executive function improved significantly for non-tertiary educated males, while cognitive function remained stable for other participants. Further follow-up at 18 month intervals with a larger sample will reveal the effects of cochlear implant intervention on all outcomes, and whether this can delay cognitive decline.

Keywords: cognitive decline, hearing loss, cochlear implants, executive function, visual attention, education, age, speech perception

INTRODUCTION

The prevalence of hearing loss increases with age. In people aged over 65 years it is 30–60%, and increases to 70–90% in people aged over 85 years (Cruickshanks et al., 1998; Sindhusake et al., 2001; Amieva et al., 2015). In older adults (i.e., >65 years) the negative impact of hearing loss on quality of life is substantial, with population norms showing that any form of hearing disability results in poorer physical and mental health outcomes. People with a greater degree of hearing loss are the most affected (Hogan et al., 2009; World Health Organization [WHO], 2009; Swan, 2010). A study of the impact of hearing loss on physical health in older people found that hearing loss was rated the third most problematic condition, after chronic pain and restricted physical activity (Hogan et al., 2009). Hearing loss also causes poorer quality of life, with social, emotional and communication difficulties of increasing magnitude the greater the degree of the hearing loss (Bryant and Sonerson, 2006; Hogan et al., 2009). Communication difficulties often lead to communication breakdown and resulting social and emotional isolation (Wilson et al., 1998) and loneliness (Heine and Browning, 2002; Arlinger, 2003). Social isolation is a form of chronic stress that has been shown to cause depression, poorer cognitive function and poorer overall quality of life (Gopinath et al., 2009; World Health Organization [WHO], 2009; Huang et al., 2010). The World Health Organization has identified three characteristics to define healthy aging: participation in society, physical and mental health, and security. Hearing loss in many cases prevents people from achieving the first two of these characteristics.

Cognitive impairment and dementia in older people with or without hearing loss are also common. Age-related cognitive impairment can progress with time leading to functional disability and loss of independence, both of which increase the burden of caregiving for families and often necessitate institutionalization. After age 65 years, the risk of cognitive impairment is doubled every 5 years, with 3–12% of people aged 70–80 years affected, and 25–35% of people older than 85 years affected (Chen et al., 2009). Cognitive impairment has also been associated with decreases in sensory acuity, particularly as a consequence of hearing loss (Mulrow et al., 1990b). In 2010, there were 35.5 million people worldwide living with cognitive impairment or dementia. By 2030, that number is predicted to increase to 65.7 million, and by 2050 to over 131 million (Wimo and Prince, 2010; Prince et al., 2015). Although some recent reports estimate a slight reduction in the expected incidence of dementia for younger generations (Matthews et al., 2013), this may be balanced by increasing survival, and given the predicted exponential rise in dementia rates over the next few decades, it is expected that the cost of caring for those affected will escalate considerably. Cognitive impairment and dementia will therefore be a significant health problem in the future. In 2009, the global cost of cognitive impairment was estimated at USD422 billion (Wimo et al., 2010), in 2015 USD818 billion, and in 2050 is expected to be USD2 trillion (Prince et al., 2015). Understanding the pathways that lead to cognitive impairment and identifying factors that affect this process in older people is therefore an urgent public health priority.

Hearing loss has recently been shown to be associated independently with the rate of cognitive decline for older adults. A recent large-scale population-based study reported that people with hearing loss had a 30–40% accelerated rate of cognitive decline, and a 24% increased risk for incident cognitive impairment over a 6-year period, compared with people who had normal hearing (Lin et al., 2011). The rate of cognitive decline increased with the severity of hearing loss, with every 10 dB of hearing loss associated with faster decline. The first meta-analysis in 2015 of the link between hearing loss and cognitive decline concluded that cognition was significantly poorer in people with untreated hearing loss, with the magnitude of cognitive deficit associated with the degree of hearing loss (Taljaard et al., 2016). The Lancet Commission has recently identified hearing loss as a modifiable risk factor for dementia, contributing 9% of the risk for incident dementia (Livingston et al., 2017). In a systematic review of the impact of cochlear implantation on cognition, a significant difference in cognitive function was also found between people whose hearing loss was ameliorated by cochlear implants and those whose loss remained untreated, however, this conclusion was based on only three studies that included devices that would now be considered obsolete. It was concluded that "further research is required to understand whether hearing impairment is a cause of cognitive deficits. . .and whether hearing intervention mitigates any effects on cognitive function" given significant methodological limitations in the studies conducted to date.

It is possible that associations between hearing loss and poorer cognitive function could reflect degeneration of a common neuropathologic origin, i.e., both are caused by the degenerative/aging process. A further hypothesis is that for older people with a significant hearing loss, communication difficulties, and the resulting isolation from others and consequent loneliness contribute to cognitive decline. Neuroanatomic (Lindenberger and Baltes, 1994) and epidemiological studies provide support for this theory (Fratiglioni et al., 2000; Bennett et al., 2006), with strong reported associations between loneliness and cognitive decline. Having a limited social network has been found to increase the risk of dementia by 60% (Barnes et al., 2004), while a further study reported having a high level of social engagement reduced cognitive decline by 91% (Cacciatore et al., 1999). Hearing loss has also been found to be associated strongly with depression (Mulrow et al., 1990a; Chia et al., 2007), and depression in turn with cognitive impairment (Forsell et al., 1994), depression even being considered a risk factor for cognitive impairment (Jorm, 2000). As concluded in a recent review of the possible mechanisms of the hearing-cognition relationship (Fulton et al., 2015), these appear to be multiple, and include neuropathic degeneration, sensory degradation/deprivation, increased cognitive load, social isolation and depression, and over diagnosis (as a result of the use of cognitive assessment tools inappropriate for people with hearing loss).

There is some evidence that treatment of hearing loss with hearing aids can significantly reduce depression, anxiety, and loneliness for people with hearing loss, and may improve cognitive function (Dawes et al., 2015; Deal et al., 2015). There is also some evidence that use of cochlear implants can improve quality of life and/or cognitive function, although most of the studies have been short term (Francis et al., 2002; Vermeire et al., 2005; Mosnier et al., 2015, 2018; Manrique-Huarte et al., 2016; Jayakody et al., 2017b; Maharani et al., 2018). However, studies that have examined the effect of treatment of hearing loss on cognition in older adults to date have had numerous and significant methodological limitations that limit the applicability of the findings. For example, many rely on small samples (e.g., Jayakody et al., 2017b; $n = 16$) or use a retrospective design (e.g., Manrique-Huarte et al., 2016). Audiological data on hearing loss was often not obtained, or this was done via self-report, which is known to be highly inaccurate (Gallacher et al., 2012; Mick, 2018). Change in hearing was often not assessed over time, and information about frequency of hearing aid use or benefit was also not collected (Maharani et al., 2018). Further, a number of other factors likely to influence outcomes, such as social participation, mood, exercise, quality of life, diet, hearing aid use, and speech perception, were often not considered. For many studies, as is current standard practice (Dupuis et al., 2015), the assessment of cognitive function was conducted using screening tools for dementia which are not sensitive and are usually administered using verbal instructions, such as the Mini Mental State Examination (Amieva et al., 2015; Mosnier et al., 2015, 2018). However, the use of verbal instructions disadvantages people even with mild-moderate hearing loss, and is therefore likely lead to an overestimation of cognitive deficit (Murphy et al., 2006; Dupuis et al., 2015). The use of such tools also provides no specific information about changes in cognitive function or rates of change over time, and likely underestimates cognitive function for people with hearing loss. These methodological limitations make it difficult to determine whether there is a relationship between rate of hearing loss decline and rate of cognitive decline in the samples in these studies. Further, the effects of degree of hearing loss, device benefit or amount of hearing aid use also could not be established. Therefore, although it is known that faster cognitive decline is associated with greater degrees of hearing loss, the effects of treatment of hearing loss on cognitive function in adults have not yet been investigated in a well-designed study that accurately assesses both hearing loss and cognition and controls for the factors associated with decline in both hearing loss and cognition. As concluded in the 2015 meta-analysis of hearing loss and cognitive decline (Miller et al., 2015), "further research is required to understand. . .whether hearing intervention mitigates any effects on cognitive function."

Other factors that are reported to influence the incidence of cognitive decline include sex and education. Although many studies and a meta-analysis of eight European population-based studies have suggested that females are at higher risk of dementia (e.g., Gao et al., 1998; Andersen et al., 1999; Roberts et al., 2012; Chene et al., 2015), many others have reported no difference in incidence (e.g., Prencipe et al., 1996; Ruitenberg et al., 2001; Katz et al., 2012). It is therefore still unclear whether females have a higher risk than males of developing dementia (Rocca et al., 2014). Given the contradictory nature of the published evidence to date, and reported differences in the incidence of cognitive decline according to clinical subtype and sex (e.g., amnestic and non-amnestic mild cognitive impairment), it has been recommended that risk factors for cognitive decline should be investigated separately for males and females (Roberts et al., 2012). Conversely, lower education is widely accepted as one of the most established risk factors for dementia, and therefore is an important predictive factor for cognitive outcomes, although the exact mechanisms through which education is protective of cognitive function are still unknown (Cobb et al., 1995; Ott et al., 1995; Prencipe et al., 1996; Livingston et al., 2017).

The current multi-center study follows cognitive function over time in a prospectively recruited cohort of older recipients of cochlear implants in Australia and New Zealand. The study addresses the methodological limitations of previous studies in conducting rigorous audiological hearing assessments at baseline (prior to implantation) and at all follow-up 18-month intervals. Other factors likely to influence outcomes, such as social isolation and loneliness, mood, exercise, quality of life, diet, and device use are assessed so that their effects of cognitive outcomes can be taken into account. Cognitive ability is measured using a computerized non-auditory tool to avoid the use of verbal instructions, and device use and outcomes (speech perception and ease of listening) are also assessed in order to determine the degree of treatment benefit. Outcomes for this population of older people with the most significant degree of hearing loss will be compared in the future with those of a healthy aging comparison group of older Australians with typical hearing for their age; data collection to enable this is ongoing. The first aim of this study is to investigate the relationship between degree of hearing loss and the extent of cognitive impairment at baseline. The second aim is to examine the effect on cognition of cochlear implantation. The third aim is to determine the extent to which cochlear implantation is associated with changes in quality of life. This study will provide important and world-first rigorous evidence that will inform future policy and clinical practice on the management of older adults around the world with hearing loss. It is critically important to investigate whether treatment of hearing loss with cochlear implants could delay the onset of cognitive impairment in this population of older adults who are most affected by hearing loss.

MATERIALS AND METHODS

Participants

Fifty-nine adults aged 61–89 years, with severe-profound hearing loss (mean better ear PTA 76 dB) and no previously diagnosed or suspected cognitive impairment participated in this study. They had sufficient English to be able to give informed consent, comprehend test instructions and complete questionnaires. The participants were all patients of the Royal Victorian Eye and Ear Hospital Cochlear Implant Clinic, and had been identified as suitable to proceed with cochlear implantation at the time of recruitment. **Table 1** shows participant audiometric and demographic information. Participants received either the CI512, CI522, or CI532 Cochlear Nucleus implants (contour array, slim straight, or slim contour). All participants used the ACE speech processing strategy (Skinner et al., 2002), along with either the Cochlear Nucleus 6 or Nucleus 7 speech processor.

Procedures

This study was carried out in accordance with the recommendations of the Australian National Health and Medical Research Council guidelines for ethical research conduct. The protocol was approved by the Royal Victorian Eye and Ear Hospital (reference no. 15/1217H). All participants gave written informed consent in accordance with the Declaration of Helsinki. All participants completed a pre-operative (baseline) assessment battery comprising audiometry, speech perception testing, cognitive screening and assessment, and health, quality of life, lifestyle and ease of listening questionnaires. Participants who were assessed at the 18-month post-operative point completed an identical assessment battery, and in addition reported on their device use, data for which was also obtained through the data logging function of their speech processor.

TABLE 1 | Demographic and audiometric characteristics of the study sample (N = 59).

	All	Male	Female	p^*
Number	59	36	23	
Age (Mean)	72.3	72.4	72.1	
Age (SD)	6.8	7.5	5.6	
Pre-op PTA better ear (Mean)	76.2	71.4	83.7	**0.011**
Pre-op PTA better ear (SD)	18.7	18.4	16.8	
Pre-op worse ear (Mean)	98.4	96.6	101.2	0.255
Pre-op worse ear (SD)	15.8	16.9	13.7	
Retired (%)	79.3	74.3	87	0.227
Diabetes (%)	12.1	8.6	17.4	0.354
Past smoker (%)	44.8	45.7	43.5	0.87
Cardiac conditions (%)	70.7	71.4	69.6	0.882
Depression (%)	13.8	11.4	17.4	0.544
Anxiety (%)	19	11.4	30.4	0.099
Vigorous activity (%)	31.5	35.5	26.1	0.466
Highest education level				
High school (%)	58.6	51.4	69.6	0.17
Undergraduate (%)	13.8	11.4	17.4	0.544
Postgraduate (%)	27.6	37.1	13	0.032

*PTA, pure tone average threshold. *p-value for test for difference of means between male and female. All bolded values are significant at the 5% level.*

Audiological Assessment

All participants were assessed pre-operatively by an audiologist in a sound-treated booth, as part of the RVEEH standard pre-operative cochlear implant workup, and again 18 months later by the research team. Audiometric assessment included air and bone conduction thresholds, speech discrimination assessment, and tympanometry. Speech perception ability was assessed in the best aided condition (using hearing aids where possible) using both word and sentence level materials. Consonant-vowel-consonant (CVC) monosyllabic words (50 word lists; scored for words and phonemes correct) were presented at 65 dBSPL in quiet in the left ear, right ear and binaurally. Speech Reception Threshold testing (SRT) was conducted using 20 Bamford-Kowal-Bench-like sentence lists in four-talker babble background noise. The test sentence was presented at 65 dBSPL, while the noise level was adaptive, i.e., the level of noise presented was altered depending on the score for each sentence, with the final measure reflecting the signal-to-noise ratio at which 50% of the key words were identified. Both the target sentence and background noise were presented one meter in front of the participant via a single speaker in the free field. Correctly repeated target words were scored for each sentence, and the mean performance score in signal to noise ratio in decibels was used to calculate the participants' ability to perceive speech in noise for the right ear, left ear and binaurally. The non-test ear was masked in the unilateral listening conditions using white noise set at 30 dB above the average of the 1 and 2 kHz thresholds.

Cognitive Assessment

Cognitive screening was conducted for all participants using the Mini Mental State Examination (MMSE; Folstein et al., 1975), a screening test for dementia. In accordance with the latest NICE (2011) guidelines, a cut-off score of 24/30 was used to identify people with cognitive impairment.

Cognitive function was assessed using the Cogstate Brief Battery and the Cogstate Groton Maze Learning Test (GMLT) of executive function (CSBB; Westerman et al., 2001; Collie et al., 2003; Falleti et al., 2006; Maruff et al., 2009) by trained staff both pre-operatively, and 18 months post-operatively. The CSBB is a computerized test battery that has been developed for repeated assessment of cognitive performance. The battery is relatively quick to administer (30 min), highly reliable (test-retest reliability for each measure ranges between 0.84 and 0.94), and facilitates minimal practice effects (Falleti et al., 2006). The CSBB includes tests of visual learning, working memory, attention, and psychomotor function. It can detect decline in cognitive function that is not apparent over even a 6-month period (Lim et al., 2013). This tool is ideal for use with people with hearing loss, as it is visually presented. Both the speed and accuracy of responses are recorded (Falleti et al., 2006; Maruff et al., 2009).

The GMLT assesses executive function, and takes 7 min to administer on average. Using a maze learning paradigm, the total number of errors made when attempting to learn the same hidden pathway across five trials presented consecutively is calculated. Lower scores indicate better performance.

The Detection (DET) Task assesses psychomotor function and takes 3 min to administer on average. The participant must respond "yes" when a card in the center of the screen turns over until 25 correct responses are obtained, or the maximum time limit (2 min) has been reached (whichever occurs first). Performance speed (milliseconds) taken to complete the task is recorded. Lower scores indicate better performance.

The Identification (IDN) Task assesses visual attention and takes 3 min to administer on average. A choice reaction paradigm in which the participant must answer "yes" or "no" to the question "Is the card red?" when a playing card in the center of the screen turns over is used. Performance speed (milliseconds) to complete the task is recorded. Lower scores indicate better performance.

The One Card Learning (OCL) Task assesses visual learning and takes 6 min to administer on average. A pattern separation paradigm in which the participant must answer "yes" or "no" to the question "Have you seen this card before in this test?" when a playing card in the center of the screen turns over is used. The test measures performance accuracy. Higher scores indicate better performance.

The One Back (ONB) Task assesses working memory and takes 4 min to administer on average. Working memory is assessed using an n-back paradigm in which the participant must answer "yes" or "no" to the question "Is the previous card the same?" when a playing card in the center of the screen turns over. Both the speed and accuracy of performance are measured. Lower scores indicate better performance.

Composite scores were also calculated (Processing speed and Memory composite) using normalized *Z* scores (Falleti et al., 2006; Maruff et al., 2009).

Medical Health History

A detailed health history, including medical history was taken, (including family history of mental and other neurological illnesses), along with a personal health history, including smoking, current and past alcohol use, illicit drug and medication use.

Quality of Life Measures

Anxiety and Depression

The Hospital Anxiety and Depression Scale (HADS; Zigmond and Snaith, 1983) measures levels of depressive and anxiety symptoms. This tool generates ordinal data, and was designed for use with people who have physical health problems. For anxiety, specificity is 0.78, with a sensitivity of 0.9, and for depression, 0.79 and 0.83, respectively.

HUI-3 Quality of Life

Health status and health-related quality of life (HRQOL) for all participants was assessed using the Health Utilities Index-3 Quality of Life Questionnaire (HUI-3; Horsman et al., 2003), as one means of measuring CI benefit. The HUI-3 measures vision, hearing, speech, ambulation, dexterity, emotion, cognition, and pain. It has been a reliable, responsive and valid measure in a number of clinical studies. Utility scores provide an overall assessment of the HRQOL of patients.

Ease of Listening/Subjective Device Benefit

Ease of listening and difficulties in everyday communication situations were measured using the Abbreviated Profile of Hearing Aid Benefit (APHAB; Cox and Alexander, 1995), a questionnaire designed to measure self-reported auditory disability in everyday living. The scale covers hearing speech in a variety of competing contexts and different everyday sounds across four subscales: Ease of Communication, Reverberation, Background Noise, and Aversiveness of sounds. Higher scores indicate better performance, with the exception of Aversiveness, where a higher score indicates increased aversiveness.

Health and Lifestyle

Two questionnaires were used to assess health and lifestyle.

The International Physical Activity Questionnaire (IPAQ; long form, 31 items; Craig et al., 2003) monitors population levels of physical activity and inactivity in adults. It has four domains: (1) during transportation, (2) at work, (3) during household and gardening tasks, and (4) during leisure time, including exercise and sport participation.

The Bayer Activities of Daily Living Scale (Hindmarch et al., 1998) was used to assess difficulties in the performance of everyday activities. The 25-item scale was completed by a caregiver or person familiar with the participant. The items in the scale are sensitive to cognitive impairment, are simple in concept, and reflect a wide range of domains. Lower scores indicate less difficulty.

Loneliness and Social Participation

The Lubben Social Network Scale (LSNS; Lubben, 1988) is a brief instrument designed to gauge social isolation in older adults by measuring perceived support received from family and friends. It typically takes 5–10 min to complete and comprises an equally weighted number of items used to measure size, closeness and frequency of a respondent's social network.

The Loneliness Scale (de Jong-Gierveld and Kamphuls, 1985) is an 11-item scale designed to measure subjective feelings of loneliness as well as feelings of social isolation. Participants rate each item as either O ("I often feel this way"), S ("I sometimes feel this way"), R ("I rarely feel this way"), N ("I never feel this way"). Typically, scale reliability in the 0.80–0.90 range is observed.

Device Use Compliance

In evaluating treatment effects, it is important to measure compliance with device use. All participants who were assessed at the 18-month post-operative point completed a brief questionnaire about their use of their CI, including how many hours per day they used it.

Statistical Analysis

Summary statistics and correlations are calculated to describe the characteristics of the participants at baseline and the pairwise relationships between the various outcomes. Given the published evidence that cognition in adults is dependent on age, sex, and education level, baseline relationships between cognition, hearing, age, sex, and education were quantified using regression. For a cognition score Y (which could be one of GML, IDN, OCL, ONB, or OCL), the regression has the form:

$$Y = \beta_0 + \beta_1 \text{ BPTA} + \beta_2 \text{ Age} + \beta_3 \text{ Female} + \beta_4 \text{ UGrad} + \beta_5 \text{ PGrad} + U \quad (1)$$

where BPTA is the PTA hearing loss in the better ear measured in units of 10 dB, Age is age in years, Female = 1 for a female participant and 0 otherwise, UGrad = 1 if years of education is 13–15 years and 0 otherwise, and PGrad = 1 if years of education is 16 years or greater and 0 otherwise. U represents the regression error. The interpretation of β_1 is that an increase of 10 dB in better ear hearing loss corresponds to a change of β_1 in the mean of Y, controlling for age, sex, and educational level.

Average changes from baseline to 18 months in cognition, quality of life, loneliness and social participation, physical activity, and ease of listening were calculated and tested for significance. Changes in the key cognitive and quality of life outcomes were also analyzed in more detail in terms of age, sex and education using the regression:

$$DY = \gamma_0 \text{ Male} + \gamma_1 \text{ Female} + \gamma_2 \text{ Higher Ed.} + \gamma_3 \text{ Age70} + U \quad (2)$$

where DY is the change in outcome Y (any cognitive or HUI score) from baseline to 18 months, Male and Female are 0/1 indicators as described above, and Higher Ed. is the combination of the UGrad and PGrad indicators in Eq. (1) (the combination being necessary because of the smaller sample size of 18 month observations available), and Age 70 is age in years above or below 70. For example, the average of DY for females of age 70 with fewer than 13 years education would be given by γ_1.

RESULTS

Baseline

A summary of the baseline characteristics of the participants (overall, and by sex) is presented in **Table 1**. Average better ear hearing loss was greater for females (83.7 dB) than for males (71.4 dB), a difference that was statistically significant ($p = 0.011$).

Pairwise correlations between cognition scores and other measurements are presented in **Table 2**. There was a positive correlation ($r = 0.280$) between baseline better ear hearing loss and the GMLT where greater hearing loss was associated with poorer executive function. The APHAB Global score, Ease of Communication score, Reverberation score and Aversiveness score were all negatively associated with GMLT scores - better APHAB scores were associated with better executive function. Although only three participants had anxiety at baseline, greater anxiety was also positively correlated with poorer executive function ($r = 0.31$). Only one participant had results consistent with depression. Better self-reported quality of life (HUI-3) was also moderately positively correlated with improved visual learning performance (0.40), and engaging in frequent vigorous physical activity was moderately correlated with poorer visual learning performance (−0.30).

Table 3 presents results of regression models for the primary outcome scores for the five aspects of cognition as functions of hearing, age, sex, and education level. The table shows coefficient estimates (standard errors in brackets) for Eq. (1) for each of the five cognition outcomes, along with R^2 and the mean and standard deviation of each outcome. The results show a statistically significant increase (i.e., deterioration) in the mean GMLT scores of 5.663 points for every 10 dB increase in hearing loss (PTA) in the better ear, controlling for age, sex, and education. The magnitude of this change was 9.2% of the mean GML outcome. Also, the mean GMLT score was 19.915 points lower (i.e., better) for participants with at least 16 years of education, a difference of 32.5% of the overall mean. The regression explains 34.1% of the variation in GMLT scores. The regression for ONB contains two marginally statistically significant but practically non-significant coefficients.

18 Months Post Switch-On

Table 4 presents means for the outcomes at baseline and at 18 months, with the mean differences and p-values included.

Device Use and Benefit

Device use questionnaire responses indicated that participants were using their device on average 14 h per day, with a range of 6.5 h per day (one participant only) up to 16 h per day. All except one participant showed an improvement in speech perception scores in both quiet and noise at 18 months post switch-on. In quiet, the mean CVC word score increased from 9.4 to 66.3% correct, and the mean CVC phoneme score increased from 27.4 to 82.4%. In noise, for those who were able to do SRT testing pre-operatively, the mean SRT score decreased from 16.0 to 6.2, demonstrating an improved ability, on average, to perceive speech in background noise. Considered jointly, these changes in speech perception were highly statistically significant ($p < 0.0001$).

All APHAB scores except for Aversiveness significantly improved from baseline to 18 months. In particular, the Global score improved from an average of 15.19 at baseline to 44.66 after 18 months, almost tripling the baseline average score on this scale of self-reported listening disability in everyday life. The changes in the mean APHAB scores were highly statistically significant ($p < 0.0001$).

The mean difficulty score on the Bayer conversation scale improved substantially, from 5.22 to 2.83, with a reduction in difficulty of 54%.

Cognition

Of the cognition scores, the improvement of greatest magnitude was in the GMLT score (18% of baseline mean).

The key cognitive outcomes were analyzed in more detail using regressions of the form of Eq. (2), with results given in **Table 5**. For executive function (GMLT) the average score for males without higher education (i.e., Higher Ed. = 0) changed by −21.949 points ($p = 0.010$), relative to the overall baseline mean of 61.368, indicating an improvement

TABLE 2 | Pairwise correlations.

	GML	IDN	OCL	ONB	DET	PS	MC	BPTA
Past smoking years	−0.03	−0.19	−0.07	−0.02	0.08	0.02	−0.03	−0.01
Memory complaints score	−0.19	−0.19	0.11	−0.30	−0.12	0.16	0.27	−0.04
HUI3 – total scores	−0.19	0.14	0.40	0	−0.05	−0.11	0.24	0.01
HUI3 hearing disability score	−0.12	0.19	0.11	0.12	−0.02	−0.15	−0.03	−0.08
IPAQ activity – total score	0.04	0.03	−0.23	0.08	0.02	−0.04	−0.25	−0.09
IPAQ activity – walking	0.06	−0.02	−0.15	0.11	−0.14	0.08	−0.23	−0.14
IPAQ activity – moderate	0.11	0.15	−0.12	0.06	0.17	−0.16	−0.12	0.09
IPAQ activity – vigorous	−0.12	−0.15	−0.30	0	−0.08	0.08	−0.27	−0.26
IPAQ activity – sitting	−0.05	−0.20	0	−0.23	−0.05	0.13	0.17	0.05
LSNS Loneliness Scale – total score	0.16	−0.11	0.11	0.14	0.07	0.04	0.01	0.03
Lubben Loneliness Scale – total score	0.03	0.24	−0.06	0.14	0	−0.12	−0.13	0.18
Bayer conversation score	−0.12	0.09	−0.10	−0.13	−0.10	0.03	0.03	0.13
Bayer telephone score	0.15	0.10	0.01	0.07	0	−0.06	−0.02	0.02
APHAB, Global score	−0.52	0.09	0.08	0.06	−0.10	−0.03	−0.01	−0.08
APHAB, Ease of communication	−0.53	0.19	0.17	0	−0.12	−0.04	0.12	0.02
APHAB, Background noise	0.39	0.08	−0.09	0.12	0.03	−0.11	−0.20	−0.08
APHAB, Aversiveness	−0.35	0.15	0.16	0.03	−0.05	−0.05	0.11	−0.07
Speech perception – CVC word score, CI ear	−0.27	−0.09	−0.11	0.06	0.04	−0.01	−0.14	−0.75
Speech perception – CVC phoneme score, CI ear	−0.32	−0.09	−0.12	0.04	0.01	0	−0.14	−0.74
Speech perception in noise – SRT score, CI ear	0.26	0.18	0.04	−0.09	0	−0.07	0.11	0.66
Depression	−0.03	−0.09	−0.07	0.02	−0.14	0.13	−0.07	−0.24
Anxiety	0.31	−0.01	−0.05	0.06	−0.12	0.04	−0.12	0.07
Better ear PTA (pre-op)	0.28	0.17	0.07	−0.04	0.01	−0.07	0.1	

PS, processing speed composite score; MC, memory composite score; BPTA, better ear pure tone average hearing threshold.

TABLE 3 | Regressions for baseline cognitive scores.

	GML	IDN	OCL	ONB	DET
Intercept	10.401	2.694*	0.963*	2.917*	2.563*
	(15.631)	(0.040)	(0.067)	(0.049)	(0.045)
BPTA	**5.663***	0.006	0.002	−0.002	0.002
	(1.976)	(0.005)	(0.008)	(0.006)	(0.006)
Age	0.998	0.003	−0.003	**0.003***	0.003
	(0.545)	(0.001)	(0.002)	(0.002)	(0.002)
Female	−1.384	−0.018	0.051	−0.009	−0.03
	(7.746)	(0.019)	(0.032)	(0.024)	(0.022)
Undergraduate Ed.	8.579	0.027	−0.045	**0.072***	0.003
	(10.071)	(0.026)	(0.043)	(0.032)	(0.029)
Postgraduate Ed.	**−19.915***	−0.02	0.008	−0.027	−0.035
	(8.528)	(0.020)	(0.034)	(0.025)	(0.024)
R^2	0.341	0.151	0.116	0.2	0.153
Outcome					
Mean	61.368	2.766	0.946	2.945	2.591
SD	29.251	0.066	0.112	0.084	0.076

**Significant at 5% level. Specification: see Eq. (1). BPTA, better ear pure tone average hearing threshold; Age, age in years; Female, 1 if participant was female, 0 otherwise; Undergraduate Ed, 1 if participant had 13–15 years of education, 0 otherwise; Postgraduate Ed, 1 if participant had more than 15 years of education, 0 otherwise. All bolded values are significant at the 5% level.*

in average executive function. The average GMLT score for males with higher education (i.e., Higher Ed. = 1) changed by −21.949 + 18.768 = −3.181, but this change was not statistically significant. The average GMLT score for females also improved, changing by −11.883 points, but this difference was not statistically significant. There was only one female with higher education so separate results by education for females are not available from this sample. The overall implication is that the average executive function (GMLT) score improved by a statistically and practically significant amount for males with at most 12 years of education, but apart from these less educated males the average GMLT scores were not (statistically) different in this sample.

Quality of Life/Mood

As shown in **Table 4**, the mean HUI-3 quality of life scores (total and hearing disability) both improved from baseline to 18 months. The regression results in **Table 5** show that the HUI-3 outcomes for females had statistically significant improvements at 18 months post switch-on. For females, the mean HUI-3 total score increased by 0.141 ($p = 0.041$) relative to the female mean baseline score of 0.466, and the mean HUI-3 hearing disability score increased by 0.338 ($p = 0.005$) relative to the overall mean of 0.274. Significant improvements were not found for males, whose baseline means of 0.596 for the HUI-3 total score and 0.427 for the HUI-3 hearing disability score were higher than for the females (albeit only significant at the 10% level for the total score). These results show that average quality of life for the female participants was improving, with their scores "catching up" to those for the males. The Age variable was statistically significant in the regression for the HUI-3 hearing disability score, implying that older participants showed larger mean improvements in this aspect of quality of life.

TABLE 4 | Mean outcomes at baseline and 18 months (N = 20).

	Baseline	18 months	*p*-value*
Hearing – Objective measures			0.000
Speech perception – CVC word score %	9.4	66.3	
Speech perception – CVC phoneme score %	27.4	82.4	
Speech perception – SRT	16.0	6.2	
Hearing – Subjective measures			0.000
APHAB Global	15.19	44.66	
APHAB Ease of communication	18.41	52.49	
APHAB Reverberation	12.76	42.27	
APHAB Background noise	14.41	39.23	
APHAB Aversiveness	−22.12	−16.02	
Cognition			
GML	59.17	48.26	
IDN	2.77	2.79	
OCL	0.94	0.93	
ONB	2.95	2.95	
DET	2.61	2.64	
HUI3 total	0.56	0.67	
HUI3 hearing disability	0.38	0.67	
Activity – total	4541.17	5984.76	
Loneliness total	2.64	1.39	
Lubben total	45.36	44.77	
Bayer conversation	5.22	2.83	
Bayer telephone	6.13	5.57	
Depression	2.22	1.96	
Anxiety	4.00	3.13	

**p-values are from joint tests of equality of means for the multiple outcomes.*

At 18 months after cochlear implantation, the number of participants with anxiety had reduced from one to three, and one participant remained depressed.

DISCUSSION

Baseline Outcomes

Hearing Loss and Cognition

At baseline, regression modeling (controlling for age, sex, and education) predicted significantly poorer executive function with greater hearing loss, with marginal effects modeling predicting that for every 10 dB increase in hearing loss, there would be a corresponding decline in executive function of over 9% of the mean outcome on this measure. As mentioned earlier, a relationship between age-related hearing loss and cognitive function has been reported in several studies of older adults (see Miller et al., 2015) and in a recent systematic review and meta-analysis of both cross-sectional and longitudinal cohort studies (n = 15) (Loughrey et al., 2018). Executive function was also reported to be significantly poorer with increasing hearing loss in another recent study of 119 potential CI recipients aged 45–85 years with bilaterally symmetrical mild-profound hearing loss (Jayakody et al., 2017a).

The current study and that of Jayakody et al. (2017a) found that of all the cognitive domains assessed at baseline (i.e., prior to cochlear implantation), executive function was most

TABLE 5 | Regressions for baseline – 18 months changes.

	GML	IDN	OCL	ONB	DET	HUI-3 total	HUI-3 hearing
Male	**−21.949***	0.013	−0.019	0.012	−0.01	0.015	0.136
	(7.548)	(0.017)	(0.033)	(0.031)	(0.055)	(0.068)	(0.111)
Female	−11.883	−0.002	−0.044	−0.037	**0.116***	**0.141***	**0.338***
	(6.906)	(0.017)	(0.031)	(0.029)	(0.052)	(0.064)	(0.105)
Higher Ed.	**18.768***	0.013	0.015	−0.008	−0.002	0.072	0.066
	(8.591)	(0.021)	(0.039)	(0.037)	(0.065)	(0.080)	(0.132)
Age 70	0.846	**0.005***	0.004	0.000	0.001	0.01	**0.027***
	(0.733)	(0.002)	(0.003)	(0.003)	(0.005)	(0.007)	(0.011)
R^2	0.379	0.488	0.129	0.109	0.267	0.471	0.683
n	20	23	23	23	23	23	23

**Significant at 5% level. Specification: see Eq. (2). Male, 1 if participant was male, 0 otherwise; Female, 1 if participant was female, 0 otherwise; Higher Ed., 1 if participant had more than 12 years of education, 0 otherwise; Age 70, difference of age in years from 70. All bolded values are significant at the 5% level.*

affected by hearing loss. Cortical auditory evoked potential and neuroimaging studies have shown increases in P2 latency and amplitude and decreased activation of the temporal cortex, even in the early stages of mild-moderate hearing loss, and it has been theorized that short-term memory and executive functions are recruited to assist with the perception of speech in the presence of hearing loss and the associated shrinking of the auditory cortex, thus preserving these functions while others are lost due to reallocation of cognitive resources (Campbell and Sharma, 2013).

A meta-analysis by Loughrey et al. (2018), which included 14 studies that had measured aspects of executive function as well as attention and working memory, concluded that hearing loss was associated less with decline in executive function and impacted more on delayed and semantic memory, although in many studies of older adults, performance on the tests of semantic memory are used as indices of executive function. The differences in findings between the current study and those of the meta-analysis could be due to the types of tests used to assess executive function. Whereas the Cogstate battery utilizes a visual and non-linguistic method of presentation suitable for use with adults with severe-profound hearing loss, has no measurable practice effects, and very high sensitivity and reliability, no details of the tests used in the studies included in the meta-analysis were provided, with the exception of one screening tool. In addition, information about whether the tasks were verbal or non-verbal was not presented. If verbal executive function tasks were used, there could be issues of confounding due to the inter-relationship between verbal language and executive function, as well as that between hearing loss and comprehension of instructions. Further, while the GMLT from the Cogstate Battery comprehensively assesses multiple aspects of executive function, many of the tests used in the 14 studies covered limited aspects of executive function (e.g., attention only), or used measures of global cognitive function. The latter are insensitive in the absence of significant cognitive impairment and are clearly unsuitable for administration with people with hearing loss (such as the MMSE), which in this study was used only as a screening tool to exclude participants at baseline with clear dementia.

Education and Cognition

Lower education has long been identified as a risk factor for dementia, and is thought to contribute to vulnerability to cognitive decline because it results in lower cognitive reserve. Cognitive reserve enables more highly educated people to maintain cognitive function in the presence of brain pathology (Anstey and Christensen, 2000; Livingston et al., 2017). Low educational attainment has been identified as one of the strongest modifiable risk factors for cognitive decline, estimated using relative risks from meta-analyses to contribute over 19% of the population-attributable risk (PAR) of Alzheimer's disease worldwide (Norton et al., 2014). The fact that education is protective of cognitive function was evident in the baseline finding of this study that executive function was significantly better for participants with at least 16 years of education.

Exercise and Cognition

Inactivity has also been identified as a modifiable risk factor for dementia, and was recently the highest estimated PAR in the United States (21%), Europe (20.3%), and the United Kingdom (21.8%) (Norton et al., 2014). Despite this, the literature examining the relationship between exercise and cognition reports mixed findings. Some studies have reported that exercise is effective in maintaining cognitive function and should be considered as a non-pharmaceutical intervention for the prevention of cognitive decline and neurodegenerative diseases (Bherer et al., 2013; Mandolesi et al., 2018). It is thought that a beneficial effect on cognition is due to the effects of exercise on vascular function and on increasing the size of the prefrontal and hippocampal areas of the brain, promoting better working memory (Brown et al., 2010; Davenport et al., 2012; Erickson et al., 2012). However, there is also evidence suggesting that exercise does not appear to promote any improvement in cognitive function in older people either with or without cognitive impairment (Sink et al., 2015; Young et al., 2015). In the current study, vigorous physical activity was correlated with poorer visual learning performance at baseline. This is only one correlation, however, there is some emerging evidence in the recent literature of negative effects of physical over-exertion on cognition in older people, with a recent study suggesting that moderate intensity exercise programs may even increase the rate of cognitive decline in people with dementia (Lamb et al., 2018). As suggested in a systematic review by van Uffelen et al. (2008), further high quality trials of the effect of physical activity on cognition in older adults are required, as the current literature suffers from a lack of high quality studies, with large variability in study populations, exercise protocols, and outcome measures. The current study will continue to monitor the effects of physical activity on cognition over time.

18 Months Post Switch-On

Device Use and Benefit

As discussed earlier, a limitation of many studies of the effect of treatment of hearing loss with a hearing device is the lack of follow up and information regarding device use and the effectiveness of the devices, without which it is not possible to examine the relationships between the treatment and its effects. In the current study, average CI usage of 14 h per day was reported, along with significant mean improvements in speech perception in both quiet and noise at 18 months post switch-on. Only one participant did not improve in their speech perception ability post cochlear implantation. Study participants also reported a threefold decrease in listening disability in their everyday lives, and there was a statistically significant improvement in their ability to conduct conversations. These benefits are similar to those reported in the only other longitudinal study of cognition in older adults after cochlear implantation (Mosnier et al., 2015, 2018).

Cognition Outcomes

At 18 months post switch-on, there was no significant decline in group mean performance on any cognitive test, apart from a trivial (less than 1% of the baseline mean) negative change in the average visual attention (IDN) score. However, the mean executive function (GMLT) score increased by 18% of the baseline mean score, although this improvement was not statistically significant at the 5% level, (p = 0.097) in this small sample. Further exploration of this result using regressions showed that males who did not have higher education had significantly improved executive function (GMLT) by almost one third of the baseline mean score. The average executive function (GMLT) score for males with higher education and also for females (only one female had higher education, so this factor was not examined separately for females) did not change significantly, although there was a non-significant improvement in average score in both groups.

While cochlear implants have been shown to significantly improve speech perception (Dowell, 2012; Lazard et al., 2012; Blamey et al., 2013), mood, social isolation, function and quality of life in adults (Francis et al., 2002; Mo, 2005), until 2015 there were no studies in the English literature that prospectively examined the effect of CIs on cognitive function in older adults (Miller et al., 2015). Since then, three studies have evaluated cognitive function in CI recipients. The first two studies evaluated the same group of patients aged 65 and older at baseline at two postoperative intervals (N = 94 and 70, respectively). A battery of tests to evaluate episodic memory, visuospatial abilities, attention span, processing speed, mental flexibility and executive function was used pre-operatively, at 6 and 12 months post-operatively (Mosnier et al., 2015), and again 7 years after cochlear implantation (Mosnier et al., 2018). Cognitive scores were not treated as continuous data, but were instead categorized as normal or abnormal, with the number of normal/abnormal test outcomes documented for each participant. At 1 year post cochlear implantation, group mean scores had improved across all cognitive domains for 80% of the participants with the poorest pre-operative scores, while for patients with normal cognitive pre-operative performance, scores for memory, attention and executive function did not change significantly. It was not possible to evaluate change in verbal fluency scores, as the stimulus words were changed at each test session to avoid practice effects. The degree of improvement in cognitive performance for the poorest participants in the Mosnier et al. (2015) study at 1 year after implantation appears greater than that observed in the current study at 18 months post-switch-on. However, at baseline in the Mosnier study, many of the participants were functioning at a lower level cognitively than those in the current study. Half of the participants in the Mosnier et al. (2015) study had mild cognitive impairment at baseline, and 14% did not achieve a score in the normal range on the MMSE, whereas 100% of the participants in the current study did. It should be noted that executive function in the Mosnier study was measured using the Trail Making Tests (versions A and B), which have only poor (version A; 0.53) to moderate (version B; 0.67) test-re-test reliability, and are subject to significant practice effects over time periods of less than a year (participants in the first study were tested at 6-month intervals after cochlear implantation). These factors may have affected the cognitive results obtained in these studies. Further, the use of written test instructions for tests that were designed to be presented verbally in order to avoid over-diagnosis of cognitive impairment due to participants misunderstanding instructions may also have affected the results. For several of the cognitive tests used, changing the modality of test administration changes the cognitive task, and may confound the test results.

The third study (Jayakody et al., 2017b) evaluated 16 CI recipients 1 year after cochlear implantation using a non-verbal computer-based assessment battery (CANTAB; Cambridge Cognition Ltd., 2012). As in the current study, participants showed significantly improved speech perception in quiet (performance in noise was not measured) and performed significantly better on working memory, attention and processing speed, and some measures of executive function. Depression, anxiety and stress scores also significantly decreased. Other risk factors for cognitive decline were not measured or controlled for, the statistical analysis comprising *t*-tests and correlation analyses.

Quality of Life

Unsurprisingly, the benefits to audition and speech perception conferred by a CI were accompanied by significantly improved HUI-3 HRQOL outcomes for overall self-rated HRQOL and also for hearing disability for females at 18 months post switch-on. HRQOL did not improve significantly for males, but their baseline HRQOL scores were already higher than those for females. Given females are often more sociable than males, it is possible that the females in this sample were more affected by the social limitations of having a severe-profound hearing loss than the males, and this may have contributed to their lower self-reported QOL. Significant improvements in these domains have been reported previously in many studies of cochlear implant recipients, both male and female (e.g., Cohen et al., 2004; Damen et al., 2007). The significant association between better QOL and better executive function observed at baseline was sustained post-operatively, and higher QOL was also significantly correlated with better psychomotor function and also with a greater CogState composite Processing Speed score. It was also interesting to see that older participants reported larger reductions in their hearing disability after receiving a CI, although there is no obvious reason for this.

Mosnier et al. (2015) also reported significant improvements in QOL at 6 months post implantation on all six subdomains of the Nijmegen Cochlear Implant Questionnaire (Hinderink et al., 2000; NCIQ). In longer-term follow up, there was no significant change in scores on any sub-domains between 6 months and 7 years after cochlear implantation however (Mosnier et al., 2018). Although higher QOL was correlated with higher speech perception scores 1 year after implantation, the effect of QOL on cognitive outcomes was not investigated.

Strengths and Limitations of This Study

Currently, the number of participants in this study is small, particularly in the group assessed 18 months after cochlear implantation, but this will grow over time as recruitment and further follow-up continues. The study has several significant advantages over previous studies of the effects of hearing devices on cognition in older adults, in particular the use of the Cogstate cognitive assessment battery, which is one of few suitable for people with severe-profound hearing loss, is comprehensive, not susceptible to practice effects, highly reliable and sensitive to change in function. Further strengths of the study are repeated audiometric assessment of hearing loss, documentation of device use (both objectively and subjectively), and assessment of many other risk factors for cognitive decline (e.g., biomarkers [the APOE 4 allele], social isolation, loneliness, education, mood, activity, quality of life, diet, and medical health), most of which were not included in the studies of Mosnier and colleagues, or in many other studies, and which will facilitate the analysis of the interactions of these factors and the device on cognitive outcomes. The inclusion of this comparison group will enable rates of cognitive decline to be compared between the cochlear implant recipients with older adults in the general community, and to determine whether long term cognitive function is related to the CI treatment of hearing loss or to a natural trajectory of decline in cognitive function in older adults.

CONCLUSION

Despite the fact that these are initial results based on a small sample size, increased hearing loss and age were found to predict significantly poorer executive function and visual attention prior to cochlear implantation, while tertiary education predicted better executive function. Eighteen months after cochlear implantation, in addition to the expected benefits to speech perception, communication and QOL, significant improvements in executive function were observed for non-tertiary educated males, while cognitive function did not decline for the other participants. Long-term data collected at 18 month intervals with a larger sample of CI recipients and compared with that of the comparison group of healthy aging adults without severe-profound hearing loss will enable the effects of treatment of hearing loss with CIs on all outcomes to be evaluated, and whether this intervention can delay or even partially reverse the onset of cognitive decline.

AUTHOR CONTRIBUTIONS

JS, DH, PM, and PB contributed to the conception and design of the study. PB and JS designed the database. PB programmed the database and extracted the data. DH performed the statistical analysis and wrote the section "Results." JS wrote the first draft of the manuscript and subsequent revisions. All authors contributed to the manuscript revision, and read and approved the submitted version. JS and DH revised the submitted version.

ACKNOWLEDGMENTS

We would like to thank Cogstate Ltd., for their support and assistance with the project. We thank the clinicians of the Cochlear Implant Clinic, Royal Victorian Eye and Ear Hospital, and in particular Sylvia Tari and Alexandra Rousett for their support and effort with the recruitment. We also thank research assistants Lisa Bennett and Manasi Canagasabey for their invaluable work on data collection and participant management. We are very grateful to the participants and their families for their time and commitment.

REFERENCES

Amieva, H., Ouvrard, C., Giulioli, C., Meillon, C., Rullier, L., and Dartigues, J.-F. (2015). Self-reported hearing loss, hearing aids, and cognitive decline in elderly adults: a 25-year study. *J. Am. Geriatr. Soc.* 63, 2099–2104. doi: 10.1111/jgs.13649

Andersen, K. E., Launer, L. J., Dewey, M. E., Letenneur, L., Ott, A., Copeland, J. R. M., et al. (1999). Gender differences in the incidence of AD and vascular dementia: The EURODEM Studies. EURODEM Incidence Research Group. *Neurology* 53, 1992–1997. doi: 10.1212/WNL.53.9.1992

Anstey, K., and Christensen, H. (2000). Education, activity, health, blood pressure and apolipoprotein E as predictors of cognitive change in old age: a review. *Gerontology* 46, 163–177. doi: 10.1159/000022153

Arlinger, S. (2003). Negative consequences of uncorrected hearing loss - a review. *Int. J. Audiol.* 42(Suppl. 2), 17–20. doi: 10.3109/14992020309074639

Barnes, L. L., Mendes De Leon, C. F., Wilson, R. S., Bienias, J. L., and Evans, D. A. (2004). Social resources and cognitive decline in a population of older African Americans and whites. *Neurology* 63, 2322–2326. doi: 10.1212/01.wnl.0000147473.04043.b3

Bennett, D. A., Schneider, J. A., Tang, Y., Arnold, S. E., and Wilson, R. S. (2006). The effect of social networks on the relation between Alzheimer's disease pathology and level of cognitive function in old people: a longitudinal cohort study. *Lancet Neurol.* 5, 406–412. doi: 10.1016/s1474-4422(06)70417-3

Bherer, L., Erickson, K., and Liu Ambrose, T. (2013). A review of the effects of physical activity and exercise on cognitive and brain functions in older adults. *J. Aging Res.* 2013:657508. doi: 10.1155/2013/657508

Blamey, P., Artieres, F., Başkent, D., Bergeron, F., Beynon, A., Burke, E., et al. (2013). Factors affecting auditory performance of postlinguistically deaf adults using cochlear implants: an update with 2251 patients. *Audiol. Neurotol.* 18, 36–47. doi: 10.1159/000343189

Brown, A. D., Mcmorris, C. A., Longman, R. S., Leigh, R., Hill, M. D., Friedenreich, C. M., et al. (2010). Effects of cardiorespiratory fitness and cerebral blood flow on cognitive outcomes in older women. *Neurobiol. Aging* 31, 2047–2057. doi: 10.1016/j.neurobiolaging.2008.11.002

Bryant, J., and Sonerson, A. (2006). Gauging the cost of aging. *Finance Dev.* 43, 48–50.

Cacciatore, F., Napoli, C., Abete, P., Marciano, E., Triassi, M., and Rengo, F. (1999). Quality of life determinants and hearing function in an elderly population: Osservatorio Geriatrico Campano Study Group. *Gerontology* 45, 323–328. doi: 10.1159/000022113

Cambridge Cognition Ltd. (2012). *CANTAB Eclipse Test Administration Guide.* Bottisham, CA: Cambridge Cognition Ltd.

Campbell, J., and Sharma, A. (2013). Compensatory changes in cortical resource allocation in adults with hearing loss. *Front. Syst. Neurosci.* 7:71. doi: 10.3389/fnsys.2013.00071

Chen, J.-H., Lin, K.-P., and Chen, Y.-C. (2009). Risk factors for dementia. *J. Formos. Med. Assoc.* 108, 754–764. doi: 10.1016/S0929-6646(09)60402-2

Chene, G., Beiser, A., Au, R., Preis, S. R., Wolf, P. A., Dufouil, C., et al. (2015). Gender and incidence of dementia in the Framingham Heart Study from mid-adult life. *Alzheimers Dement.* 11, 310–320. doi: 10.1016/j.jalz.2013.10.005

Chia, E.-M., Wang, J. J., Rochtina, E., Cumming, R. R., Newall, P., and Mitchell, P. (2007). Hearing impairment and health-related quality of life: the Blue Mountains Hearing Study. *Ear Hear.* 28, 187–195. doi: 10.1097/aud.0b013e31803126b6

Cobb, J. L., Wolf, P. A., Au, R., White, R., and D'Agostino, R. B. (1995). The effect of education on the incidence of dementia and Alzheimer's disease in the Framingham Study. *Neurology* 45, 1707–1712. doi: 10.1212/wnl.45.9.1707

Cohen, S. M., Labadie, R. F., Dietrich, M., and Haynes, D. (2004). Quality of life in hearing-impaired adults: the role of cochlear implants and hearing aids. *Otolaryngol. Head Neck Surg.* 131, 413–422. doi: 10.1016/j.otohns.2004.03.026

Collie, A., Maruff, P., Makdissi, M., McCrory, P., McStephen, M., and Darby, D. (2003). CogSport: reliability and correlation with conventional cognitive tests used in postconcussion medical evaluations. *Clin. J. Sport Med.* 13, 28–32. doi: 10.1097/00042752-200301000-00006

Cox, R. M., and Alexander, G. C. (1995). The abbreviated profile of hearing aid benefit. *Ear Hear.* 16, 176–186. doi: 10.1097/00003446-199504000-00005

Craig, C. L., Marshall, A. L., Sjostrom, M., Bauman, A. E., Booth, M. L., Ainsworth, B. E., et al. (2003). International Physical Activity Questionnaire: 12 county reliability and validity. *Med. Sci. Sports Exerc.* 35, 1381–1395.

Cruickshanks, K. J., Wiley, T. L., Tweed, T. S., Klein, B. E. K., Klein, R., Mares-Perlman, J. A., et al. (1998). Prevalence of hearing loss in older adults in Beaver Dam, Wisconsin: the epidemiology of hearing loss study. *Am. J. Epidemiol.* 148, 879–886. doi: 10.1093/oxfordjournals.aje.a009713

Damen, G. W., Beynon, A., Krabbe, P. F., Mulder, J. J., and Mylanus, E. A. (2007). Cochlear implantation and quality of life in postlingually deaf adults: long-term follow-up. *Otolaryngol. Head Neck Surg.* 136, 597–604. doi: 10.1016/j.otohns.2006.11.044

Davenport, M., Hogan, D., Eskes, G., Longman, R. S., and Poulin, M. (2012). Cerebrovascular reserve: the link between fitness and cognitive function? *Exerc. Sport Sci. Rev.* 40, 153–158. doi: 10.1097/JES.0b013e3182553430

Dawes, P., Emsley, R., Cruickshanks, K., Moore, D., Fortnum, H., Edmondson Jones, M., et al. (2015). Hearing loss and cognition: the role of hearing aids, social isolation and depression. *PLoS One* 10:e0119616. doi: 10.1371/journal.pone.0119616

de Jong-Gierveld, J., and Kamphuls, F. (1985). The development of a Rasch-Type loneliness scale. *Appl. Psychol. Meas.* 9, 289–299. doi: 10.1177/014662168500900307

Deal, J., Sharrett, A. R., Albert, M., Coresh, J., Mosley, T., Knopman, D., et al. (2015). Hearing impairment and cognitive decline: a pilot study conducted within the atherosclerosis risk in communities neurocognitive study. *Am. J. Epidemiol.* 181, 680–690. doi: 10.1093/aje/kwu333

Dowell, R. C. (2012). "Evidence about the effectiveness of cochlear implants for adults," in *Evidence Based Practice in Audiology: Evaluating Interventions for Children and Adults with Hearing Impairment*, eds L. W. Wong and L. H. Hickson (San Diego, CA: Plural Publishing), 141–166.

Dupuis, K., Pichora-Fuller, M. K., Chasteen, A. L., Marchuk, V., Singh, G., and Smith, S. L. (2015). Effects of hearing and vision impairments on the Montreal cognitive assessment. *Aging Neuropsychol. Cogn.* 22, 413–437. doi: 10.1080/13825585.2014.968084

Erickson, K., Weinstein, A., and Lopez, O. (2012). Physical activity, brain plasticity, and Alzheimer's disease. *Arch. Med. Res.* 43, 615–621. doi: 10.1016/j.arcmed.2012.09.008

Falleti, M. G., Maruff, P., Collie, A., and Darby, D. G. (2006). Practice effects associated with the repeated assessment of cognitive function using the CogState Battery at 10-minute, one week and one month test-retest intervals. *J. Clin. Exp. Neuropsychol.* 28, 1095–1112. doi: 10.1080/13803390500205718

Folstein, M. F., Folstein, S. E., and Mchugh, P. R. (1975). "Mini-mental state": a practical method for grading the cognitive state of patients for the clinician. *J. Psychiatr. Res.* 12, 189–198.

Forsell, Y., Jorm, A. F., and Winblad, B. (1994). Association of age, sex, cognitive dysfunction, and disability with major depressive symptoms in an elderly sample. *Am. J. Psychiatry* 151, 1600–1604. doi: 10.1176/ajp.151.11.1600

Francis, H. W., Chee, N., Yeagle, J., Cheng, A., and Niparko, J. K. (2002). Impact of cochlear implants on the functional health status of older adults. *Laryngoscope* 112, 1482–1488. doi: 10.1097/00005537-200208000-00028

Fratiglioni, L., Wang, H.-X., Ericsson, K., Maytan, M., and Winblad, B. (2000). Influence of social network on occurrence of dementia: a community-based longitudinal study. *Lancet* 355, 1315–1319. doi: 10.1016/s0140-6736(00)02113-9

Fulton, S. E., Lister, J. J., Bush, A. L. H., Edwards, J. D., and Andel, R. (2015). Mechanisms of the hearing–cognition relationship. *Semin. Hear.* 36, 140–149. doi: 10.1055/s-0035-1555117

Gallacher, J., Ilubaera, V., Ben Shlomo, Y., Bayer, A., Fish, M., Babisch, W., et al. (2012). Auditory threshold, phonologic demand, and incident dementia. *Neurology* 79, 1583–1590. doi: 10.1212/WNL.0b013e31826e263d

Gao, S., Hendrie, H. C., Hall, K. S., and Hui, S. (1998). The relationships between age, sex, and the incidence of dementia and Alzheimer disease. *Arch. Gen. Psychiatry* 55, 809–815.

Gopinath, B., Wang, J. J., Schneider, J., Burlutsky, G., Snowdon, J., Mcmahon, C. M., et al. (2009). Depressive symptoms in older adults with hearing impairments: the Blue Mountains Study. *J. Am. Geriatr. Soc.* 57, 1306–1308. doi: 10.1111/j.1532-5415.2009.02317.x

Heine, C., and Browning, C. J. (2002). Communication and psychosocial consequences of sensory loss in older adults: overview and rehabilitation directions. *Disabil. Rehabil.* 24, 763–773. doi: 10.1080/09638280210129162

Hinderink, J., Krabbe, P. F. M., and Van Den Broek, P. (2000). Development and application of a health-related quality-of-life instrument for adults with cochlear implants: the Nijmegen Cochlear Implant Questionnaire. *Otolaryngol. Head Neck Surg.* 123, 756–765. doi: 10.1067/mhn.2000.108203

Hindmarch, I., Lehfeld, H., De Jongh, P., and Erzigkeit, H. (1998). The Bayer activities of daily living scale (B-ADL). *Dement. Geriatr. Cogn. Disord.* 9, 20–26. doi: 10.1159/000051195

Hogan, A., O'loughlin, K., Miller, P., and Kendig, H. (2009). The health impact of a hearing disability on older people in Australia. *J. Aging Health* 21, 1098–1111. doi: 10.1177/0898264309347821

Horsman, J., Furlong, W., Feeny, D., and Torrance, G. (2003). The Health Utilities Index (HUI®): concepts, measurement, properties and applications. *Health Qual. Life Outcomes* 1:54.

Huang, C.-Q., Dong, B.-R., Lu, Z.-C., Yue, J.-R., and Liu, Q.-X. (2010). Chronic diseases and risk for depression in old age: a meta-analysis of published literature. *Ageing Res. Rev.* 9, 131–141. doi: 10.1016/j.arr.2009.05.005

Jayakody, D. M. P., Friedland, P., Eikelboom, R. H., Martins, R., Atlas, M., and Sohrabi, H. (2017a). A novel study on the association between untreated hearing loss and cognitive functions of older adults: baseline non-verbal cognitive assessment results. *Clin. Otolaryngol.* 43, 182–191. doi: 10.1111/coa.12937

Jayakody, D. M. P., Friedland, P., Nel, E., Martins, R., Atlas, M., and Sohrabi, H. (2017b). Impact of cochlear implantation on cognitive functions of older adults. *Otol. Neurotol.* 38, e289–e295. doi: 10.1097/mao.0000000000001502

Jorm, A. F. (2000). Is depression a risk factor for dementia or cognitive decline? *Gerontology* 46, 219–227. doi: 10.1159/000022163

Katz, M. J., Lipton, R. B., Hall, C. B., Zimmerman, M. E., Sanders, A. E., Verghese, J., et al. (2012). Age-specific and sex-specific prevalence and incidence of mild cognitive impairment, dementia, and Alzheimer dementia in blacks and whites: a report from the Einstein Aging Study. *Alzheimer Dis. Assoc. Disord.* 26, 335–343. doi: 10.1097/WAD.0b013e31823dbcfc

Lamb, S. E., Sheehan, B., Atherton, N., Nichols, V., Collins, H., Mistry, D., et al. (2018). Dementia and physical activity (DAPA) trial of moderate to high intensity exercise training for people with dementia: randomised controlled trial. *BMJ* 361:k1675. doi: 10.1136/bmj.k1675

Lazard, D. S., Vincent, C., Venail, F., Heyning, P. V. D., Truy, E., Sterkers, O., et al. (2012). Pre-, per- and postoperative factors affecting performance of postlinguistically deaf adults using cochlear implants: a new conceptual model over time. *PLoS One* 7:e48739. doi: 10.1371/journal.pone.0048739

Lim, Y. Y., Pietrzak, R. H., Ellis, K., Jaeger, J., Harrington, K., Ashwood, T., et al. (2013). Rapid decline in episodic memory in healthy older adults with high amyloid-B. *J. Alzheimers Dis.* 33, 675–679. doi: 10.3233/JAD-2012-121516

Lin, F. R., Ferrucci, L., Metter, E. J., An, Y., Zonderman, A. B., and Resnick, S. M. (2011). Hearing loss and cognition in the Baltimore Longitudinal Study of Aging. *Neuropsychology* 25, 763–770. doi: 10.1037/a0024238

Lindenberger, U., and Baltes, P. B. (1994). Sensory functioning and intelligence in old age: a strong connection. *Psychol. Aging* 9, 339–355. doi: 10.1037//0882-7974.9.3.339

Livingston, G., Sommerlad, A., Orgeta, V., Costafreda, S. G., Huntley, J., Ames, D., et al. (2017). Dementia prevention, intervention, and care. *Lancet* 390, 2673–2734.

Loughrey, D. G., Kelly, M. E., Kelley, G. A., Brennan, S., and Lawlor, B. A. (2018). Association of age-related hearing loss with cognitive function, cognitive impairment, and dementia: a systematic review and meta-analysis. *JAMA Otolaryngol. Head Neck Surg.* 144, 115–126. doi: 10.1001/jamaoto.2017.2513

Lubben, J. (1988). Assessing social networks among elderly populations. *Fam. Commun. Health* 11, 42–52. doi: 10.1097/00003727-198811000-00008

Maharani, A., Dawes, P., Nazroo, J., Tampubolon, G., and Pendleton, N. (2018). Longitudinal relationship between hearing aid use and cognitive function in older Americans. *J. Am. Geriatr. Soc.* 66, 1130–1136. doi: 10.1111/jgs.15363

Mandolesi, L., Polverino, A., Montuori, S., Foti, F., Ferraioli, G., Sorrentino, P., et al. (2018). Effects of physical exercise on cognitive functioning and wellbeing: biological and psychological benefits. *Front. Psychol.* 9:509. doi: 10.3389/fpsyg.2018.00509

Manrique-Huarte, R., Calavia, D., Huarte Irujo, A., Girón, L., and Manrique-Rodríguez, M. (2016). Treatment for hearing loss among the elderly: auditory outcomes and impact on quality of life. *Audiol. Neurotol.* 21(Suppl. 1), 29–35. doi: 10.1159/000448352

Maruff, P., Thomas, E., Cysique, L., Brew, B., Collie, A., Snyder, P., et al. (2009). Validity of the CogState brief battery: relationship to standardized tests and sensitivity to cognitive impairment in mild traumatic brain injury, schizophrenia, and AIDS dementia complex. *Arch. Clin. Neuropsychol.* 24, 165–178. doi: 10.1093/arclin/acp010

Matthews, F. E., Arthur, A., Barnes, L. E., Bond, J., Jagger, C., Robinson, L., et al. (2013). A two-decade comparison of prevalence of dementia in individuals aged 65 years and older from three geographical areas of England: results of the Cognitive Function and Ageing Study I and II. *Lancet* 382, 1405–1412. doi: 10.1016/S0140-6736(13)61570-6

Mick, P. (2018). Associations between sensory loss and social networks, participation, support, and loneliness: analysis of the Canadian Longitudinal Study on Aging. *Can. Fam. Physician* 64, e33–e41.

Miller, G., Miller, C., Marrone, N., Howe, C., Fain, M., and Jacob, A. (2015). The impact of cochlear implantation on cognition in older adults: a systematic review of clinical evidence. *BMC Geriatr.* 15:16. doi: 10.1186/s12877-015-0014-3

Mo, B. (2005). Cochlear implants and quality of life: a prospective study. *Ear Hear.* 26, 186–194. doi: 10.1097/00003446-200504000-00006

Mosnier, I., Bebear, J., Marx, M., Fraysse, B., Truy, E., Lina-Granade, G., et al. (2015). Improvement of cognitive function after cochlear implantation in elderly patients. *JAMA Otolaryngol. Head Neck Surg.* 141, 442–450. doi: 10.1001/jamaoto.2015.129

Mosnier, I., Vanier, A., Bonnard, D., Lina Granade, G., Truy, E., Bordure, P., et al. (2018). Long-term cognitive prognosis of profoundly deaf older adults after hearing rehabilitation using cochlear implants. *J. Am. Geriatr. Soc.* 66, 1553–1561. doi: 10.1111/jgs.15445

Mulrow, C. D., Aguilar, C., Endicott, J. E., Tuley, M. R., Velez, R., Charlip, W. S., et al. (1990a). Quality-of-life changes and hearing impairment: a randomized trial. *Ann. Intern. Med.* 113, 188–194.

Mulrow, C. D., Aguilar, C., Endicott, J. E., Velez, R., Tuley, M. R., Charlip, W. S., et al. (1990b). Association between hearing impairment and the quality of life of elderly individuals. *J. Am. Geriatr. Soc.* 38, 45–50. doi: 10.1111/j.1532-5415.1990.tb01595.x

Murphy, D. R., Daneman, M., and Schneider, B. A. (2006). Why do older adults have difficulty following conversations? *Psychol. Aging* 21, 49–61. doi: 10.1037/0882-7974.21.1.49

Norton, S., Matthews, F., Barnes, D., Yaffe, K., and Brayne, C. (2014). Potential for primary prevention of Alzheimer's disease: an analysis of population-based data. *Lancet Neurol.* 13, 788–794. doi: 10.1016/S1474-4422(14)70136-X

Ott, A., Breteler, M. M. B., van Harskamp, F., Claus, J. J., van der Cammen, T. J. M., Grobbee, D. E., et al. (1995). Prevalence of Alzheimer's disease and vascular dementia: association with education. The Rotterdam study. *BMJ* 310, 970–973. doi: 10.1136/bmj.310.6985.970

Prencipe, M., Casini, A. R., Ferretti, C., Lattanzio, M. T., Fiorelli, M., and Culasso, F. (1996). Prevalence of dementia in an elderly rural population: effects of age, sex, and education. *J. Neurol. Neurosurg. Psyshiatry* 60, 628–633. doi: 10.1136/jnnp.60.6.628

Prince, M., Wimo, A., Guerchet, M., Ali, G., Wu, Y., and Prina, M. (2015). *The Global Impact of Dementia: an Analysis of Prevalence, Incidence, Cost and Trends.* London: Alzheimer's Disease International, 1–82.

Roberts, R. O., Geda, Y. E., Knopman, D. S., Cha, R. H., Pankratz, V. S., Boeve, B. F., et al. (2012). The incidence of MCI differs by subtype and is higher in men. *Neurology* 78, 342–351. doi: 10.1212/WNL.0b013e3182452862

Rocca, W. A., Mielke, M. M., Vemuri, P., and Miller, V. M. (2014). Sex and gender differences in the causes of dementia: a narrative review. *Maturitas* 79, 196–201. doi: 10.1016/j.maturitas.2014.05.008

Ruitenberg, A., Ott, A., van Swieten, J. C., Hofman, A., and Breteler, M. B. (2001). Incidence of dementia: does gender make a difference? *Neurobiol. Aging* 22, 575–580. doi: 10.1016/s0197-4580(01)00231-7

Sindhusake, D., Mitchell, P., Smith, W., Golding, M., Newall, P., Hartley, D., et al. (2001). Validation of self-reported hearing loss. The Blue Mountains Hearing Study. *Int. J. Epidemiol.* 30, 1371–1378. doi: 10.1093/ije/30.6.1371

Sink, K., Espeland, M., Castro, C., Church, T., Cohen, R., Dodson, J., et al. (2015). Effect of a 24-month physical activity intervention vs health education on cognitive outcomes in sedentary older adults. *JAMA* 314, 781–790. doi: 10.1001/jama.2015.9617

Skinner, M. W., Arndt, P. L., and Staller, S. J. (2002). Nucleus 24 advanced encoder conversion study: performance versus preference. *Ear Hear.* 23, 2S–17S. doi: 10.1097/00003446-200202001-00002

Swan, W. (2010). *Australia to 2050: Future Challenges*, ed. D. O. T. Treasury (Canberra: Australian Government).

Taljaard, D. S., Olaithe, M., Brennan-Jones, C. G., Eikelboom, R. H., and Bucks, R. S. (2016). The relationship between hearing impairment and cognitive function: a meta-analysis in adults. *Clin. Otolaryngol.* 41, 718–729. doi: 10.1111/coa.12607

van Uffelen, J. G. Z., Chin Paw, A. M. J., Hopman Rock, M., and Van Mechelen, W. (2008). The effects of exercise on cognition in older adults with and without cognitive decline: a systematic review. *Clin. J. Sport Med.* 18, 486–500. doi: 10.1097/JSM.0b013e3181845f0b

Vermeire, K., Brokx, J. P., Wuyts, F. L., Cochet, E., Hofkens, A., and Van De Heyning, P. H. (2005). Quality-of-life benefit from cochlear implantation in the elderly. *Otol. Neurotol.* 26, 188–195. doi: 10.1097/00129492-200503000-00010

Westerman, R., Darby, D. G., Maruff, P., and Collie, A. (2001). Computer-assisted cognitive function assessment of pilots. *AustDefence Force Health* 2, 29–36.

Wilson, D., Walsh, P. G., Sanchez, L., and Read, P. (1998). *Hearing Impairment in an Australian Population.* Adelaide, SA: Centre for Population Studies in Epidemiology.

Wimo, A., and Prince, M. (2010). *World Alzheimer Report 2010: The Global Economic Impact of Dementia.* London: Alzheimer's Disease International.

Wimo, A., Winblad, B., and Jönsson, L. (2010). The worldwide societal costs of dementia: estimates for 2009. *Alzheimers Dement.* 6, 98–103. doi: 10.1016/j.jalz.2010.01.010

World Health Organization [WHO] (2009). *Ageing.*

Young, J., Angevaren, M., Rusted, J., and Tabet, N. (2015). Aerobic exercise to improve cognitive function in older people without known cognitive impairment. *Cochrane Database Syst. Rev.* 4:CD005381.

Zigmond, A. S., and Snaith, R. P. (1983). The hospital anxiety and depression scale. *Acta Psychiatr. Scand.* 67, 361–370.

13

Kif15 is Required in the Development of Auditory System using Zebrafish as a Model

Shimei Zheng[1†], Dongmei Tang[2,3†], Xin Wang[4†], Chang Liu[2,3], Na Zuo[1], Renchun Yan[1], Cheng Wu[1], Jun Ma[1], Chuanxi Wang[1], Hongfei Xu[5], Yingzi He[2,3], Dong Liu[4*] and Shaofeng Liu[1*]*

[1] Department of Otolaryngology-Head and Neck Surgery, Yijishan Hospital of Wannan Medical College, Wuhu, China, [2] State Key Laboratory of Medical Neurobiology and MOE Frontiers Center for Brain Science, ENT Institute and Department of Otorhinolaryngology, Eye & ENT Hospital, Fudan University, Shanghai, China, [3] NHC Key Laboratory of Hearing Medicine, Fudan University, Shanghai, China, [4] Nantong Laboratory of Development and Diseases, School of Life Sciences, Co-innovation Center of Neuroregeneration, Key Laboratory of Neuroregeneration of Jiangsu and MOE, Nantong University, Nantong, China, [5] Department of Forensic Medicine, Soochow University, Suzhou, China

***Correspondence:**
Yingzi He
yingzihe09611@126.com
Dong Liu
liudongtom@gmail.com;
tom@ntu.edu.cn
Shaofeng Liu
liusf_cn@163.com

†These authors have contributed equally to this work

Kif15, a kinesin family member, is powerful in the formation of bipolar spindles. There is emerging evidence indicating that Kif15 plays vital roles in influencing the growth of axons and interference with the progression of the tumor. However, the function of Kif15 in the auditory organs remains unknown. The Western blotting test was used to examine the effect of Kif15 downregulation by specific morpholino targeting Kif15 (Kif15-MO). The development of the inner ear and posterior lateral line (PLL) system in zebrafish was under continuous observation from spawns to 96 h postfertilization (hpf) to investigate the potential role of Kif15 in the auditory and vestibular system. We uncovered that Kif15 inhibition induced otic organ deformities in zebrafish, including malformed semicircular canals, abnormal number and location of otoliths, and reduced number of hair cells (HCs) both in utricle and saccule. Furthermore, a remarkable reduction in the number of PLL neuromasts was also explored in Kif15-MO morphants compared to the normal larvae. We also detected notably reduced activity in locomotion after Kif15 was knocked down. Additionally, we performed rescue experiments with co-injection of Kif15 mRNA and found that the Kif15 splicing MO-induced deformities in otic vesicle and PLL of zebrafish were successfully rescued, and the severely reduced locomotor activity caused by Kif15-MO was partially rescued compared to the control-MO (Con-MO) embryos. Our findings uncover that Kif15 is essential in the early development of auditory and vestibular organs using zebrafish as models.

Keywords: Kif15, morpholino knockdown, auditory organs, development, zebrafish

INTRODUCTION

Kif15 (also called Kinesin-12), a pivotal member of the kinesin family, is essential for the production of bipolar spindles (Sturgill and Ohi, 2013). Recent studies have revealed that some kinesin family members are exploited for the invention of antimitotic drugs especially used in cancer therapy (Milic et al., 2018). Among those, Eg5 (Kif11 or Kinesin-5) and Kif15 are most highlighted. Eg5 is fundamental for spindle assembly while Kif15 is non-essential in the establishment of spindle bipolarity when Eg5 is in full activity. However, Kif15 becomes essential in the maintenance of spindle bipolarity when Eg5 is partially inhibited (Tanenbaum et al., 2009). Kif15 is also demonstrated involved in developing neurons, influencing axonal growth, navigation, and branching. For example, using morpholino (MO) injection strategy or CRISPR/Cas9-based knockout technology, the axons grow faster and longer when the Kif15 level is reduced compared to the Kif15 wild type (Liu et al., 2010; Dong et al., 2019). More and more studies show that Kif15 plays a pretty important role in the occurrence and development of some cancers (Gao et al., 2020a,b; Kitagawa et al., 2020; Ma et al., 2020). Moreover, previous studies have demonstrated that Kif15 also plays a pretty important role in mitosis, meiosis, spermiogenesis, cell growth, and differentiation (Ma et al., 2017; Malaby et al., 2019; Yu et al., 2019). Increasingly, the functions of Kif15 in distinct models have gained more attention. As reported by Mei Liu's laboratory, Kif15 is detected from two-cell stage, mainly concentrated in the central nervous system from 14 to 30 hpf and also distributed in organs such as brain, eyes, ears, fin, and olfactory bulbs in zebrafish (Xu et al., 2014). However, the role of Kif15 in ears has not been explored.

In recent years, zebrafish has become a popular experimental model in the study of auditory system development and inner ear hair cell (HC) regeneration for advantages in the transparent body, short growth period, large oviposition, direct observation, and easier regulation (Blanco-Sánchez et al., 2017; He et al., 2017; Tang et al., 2019, 2021). The mechanosensory organs of zebrafish are composed of the otic vesicle, anterior lateral line in the cephalic region, and posterior lateral line (PLL; Kimmel et al., 1995). Different from the mammals, zebrafish is devoid of the cochlea, and the main components of zebrafish otic vesicle are three pairs of semicircular canals, two pairs of sensory patches named utricle and saccule (Kimmel et al., 1995; Whitfield et al., 2002; Geng et al., 2013). Otoliths composed of calcium carbonate crystalline are overlain on the two maculae; thus, utricle and saccule are called otolith organs (Whitfield et al., 2002; Lundberg et al., 2015; Kalka et al., 2019). The PLL neuromasts (NMs) consist of HCs in the center and supporting cells and mantle cells in the periphery; these HCs share similar structure and function with those in the mammalian inner ear (Whitfield et al., 2002; Nicolson, 2017).

In this study, we first investigated the function of Kif15 in the development of zebrafish otic vesicle and PLL using splicing- and translation-blocking MO targeting Kif15. Our findings uncover the pivotal role of Kinesin superfamily member Kif15 in the development of hearing organs for the purpose of hearing research.

MATERIALS AND METHODS

Zebrafish Maintenance and Operation

The embryos of zebrafish were obtained from *Tg(cldnb:lynGFP)*^{zf106} line, *Tg(brn3c:mGFP)*^{s356t} line, and AB wild type. Spawns were maintained in embryo medium at 28.5°C according to the standard recipe. Hours/days postfertilization (hpf/dpf) was used to take a record of marking embryos' different developmental stages. Embryos lived in E3 water which add 0.03‰ 1-phenyl-2-thiourea (PTU; Sigma–Aldrich, St Louis, MO, United States) at the stage of 14 hpf, in the result of avoiding pigment formation. The Institutional Animal Care and Use Committee of Fudan University approved all the animal experiments.

Morpholino Injections

Two endogenous blocking strategies were used for inhibiting the expression of Kif15 (Kif15-MO), and the precise sequences were shown as follows:

> Splicing-blocking: 5′-ATGTATTAAAAACCTCACCTGG CTG-3′;
> Translation-blocking: 5′-CATGATTCATTACTATATTTC CTCT-3′.

A total final concentration of 0.3 mM was injected into the yolk sacs of zebrafish embryos at the one- to two-cell stage for Kif15 knockdown. As a control, the parallel embryos were injected with the standard control-MO (Con-MO), sequenced in 5′-CCTCTTACCTCAGTTACAATTTATA-3′ to avoid errors due to injections.

Imaging

The live zebrafish were anesthetized in 0.02% MS-222 (ethyl 3-aminobenzoate methanesulfonate; Sigma–Aldrich, Inc., Saint Louis, MO, United States) for 3 min and then placed on the glass slide with E3 water under the corresponding microscope. The images were taken with a stereomicroscope or an inverted fluorescence microscope.

Zebrafish Locomotion Assay

After treatment, larvae were moved into wells of a 48-well plate (1 fish/well) to monitor their swimming behavior. Zebrafish behavior was monitored by a digital video tracking system (DVTS, Noldus Information Technology, United States). Each larva was allowed to habituate to the test environment of the system for 30 min before the start of the data acquisition. Notably, 10 acoustic/vibrational stimuli (Danio Vision intensity setting 6) with a 20-s interstimulus interval were set and applied. The total swimming distance of the larvae that responded to this stimulus was recorded. Swimming behavior studies were repeated at least three times.

Western Blotting Analysis

Zebrafish embryos at 48 hpf after removal of yolk sac were immersed in precooled radioimmunoprecipitation assay (RIPA) lysis buffer plus cocktail and phenylmethanesulfonyl fluoride (PMSF) for schizolysis. To know the exact concentrations of the extracted proteins, we chose a BCA Protein Kit (Beyotime Institute Biotechnology, China) with the supernatant of the RIPA lysate after dissolving the samples. After electrophoresis on SDS–PAGE, the separated proteins were transferred onto poly(vinylidene fluoride) (PVDF) membranes (Immobilon-P;

Millipore, Bedford, United States). Before incubation with the primary antibodies, the membranes were blocked with 5% skim milk for 2 h at room temperature. Anti-Kif15 (1:400 dilution, Proteintech, Shanghai, China) and anti-glyceraldehyde 3-phosphate dehydrogenase (anti-GAPDH; 1: 2000) were incubated with the membranes for a whole night at 4°C. Corresponding proteins were combined with Goat Anti-Mouse/Anti-Rabbit immunoglobulin G [IgG; (H + L)] HRP (1:2000 dilution, Abways Technology, Shanghai, China) after being incubated for 2 h. Using an ECL Kit (Millipore, United States), such protein bands could be colored and detected by an Azure C280 imager. The membranes need to be washed thoroughly with Tris-buffered saline with Tween 20 (TBST) before each incubation step. All experiments were strictly from three repeats. GAPDH served as the internal reference.

Statistical Analysis

GraphPad Prism (version, 8.0) supports whole statistical analyses. Comparisons between every two groups were demonstrated with a *t*-test (two-tailed), while multiple comparisons were illustrated using one-way ANOVA. Statistics were all displayed as mean ± standard error of the mean (SEM), with p-value < 0.05 identified as statistical significance.

RESULTS

Knockdown of Kif15 Inhibits the Normal Formation of Vestibular Apparatus

The role of Kif15 during inner ear development was investigated by the knockdown of Kif15 through the injection of Kif15 splicing MO to the zebrafish embryos at one- or two-cell stages. We used the Western blotting analysis to test the efficacy of Kif15 downregulation, and we detected a substantial transcript reduction of Kif15 in the zebrafish larvae after Kif15-MO injection compared to the controls injected with Con-MO (**Figures 1A,B**). We chose 48, 72, and 96 hpf in chronology to observe the morphology changes in the inner

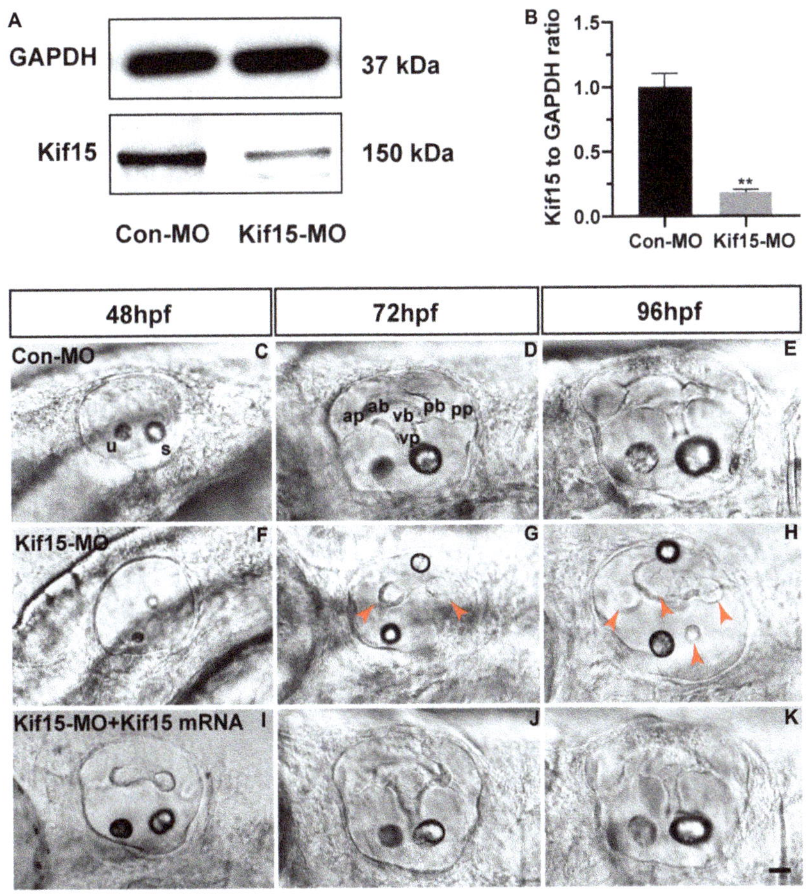

FIGURE 1 | Knockdown of Kif15 with splicing-blocking method inhibits the normal formation of vestibular. **(A,B)** The protein level of Kif15 is severely decreased in Kif15-morpholino (MO)-injected embryos both in the band intensity **(A)** and in the semiquantitative analysis **(B)**, in comparison with control embryos. Data are recorded as mean ± SEM. $^{**}p < 0.01$. **(C–H)** Kif15-MO suppresses the normal development of semicircular canals. The abnormal manifestations are observed at 48 hpf **(C,F)**, 72 hpf **(D,G)**, and 96 hpf **(E,H)**, respectively. ap, anterior protrusion; ab, anterior bulge; vb, ventral bulge; vp, ventral protrusion; pb, posterior bulge; pp, posterior protrusion; u, utricle; and s, saccule. Red arrowheads show the abnormal fusion of anterior and posterior protrusions. **(I–K)** Co-injection using Kif15-MO and Kif15 mRNA successfully rescues the phenotypes of semicircular canals and otoliths at 48 hpf **(I)**, 72 hpf **(J)**, and 96 hpf **(K)**, respectively. Scale bar is 20 μm.

ear of zebrafish after Kif15-MO injection (**Figures 1C–H**). At 72 and 96 hpf, the essential structures of three pairs of semicircular canals (i.e., anterior, posterior, and lateral) were clearly discernible as labeled in **Figure 1D**, including anterior (a-), posterior (p-), and ventral (v-) protrusions and bulges. However, the normal structures of semicircular canals disappeared and were replaced by short and fused protuberances in Kif15-MO morphants (**Figures 1F–H**). To verify the role of Kif15 on zebrafish semicircular canal development, we performed a rescue experiment by the co-injection of Kif15 mRNA together with Kif15 splicing MO, and we found a successful rescue in the phenotype of otic vesicle (**Figures 1I–K**). Our observation implied that the inhibition of Kif15 by specific MO completely ruined the normal development of semicircular canals in the inner ear of zebrafish.

Kif15 Inhibition Induces Malformed Otolith Organs in Zebrafish

The morphology of otoliths in control and Kif15-MO-injected embryos was detected with a white optical microscope in the bright field at 48 hpf (**Figures 2A–E**). Kif15 splicing MO-injected embryos exhibited various abnormalities containing increased number of otoliths (35.5%), decreased number of otoliths (4.3%), and two abnormal otoliths (15.4%) (**Figures 2B–E,G**). Among them, the two abnormal otolith deformities involved situations such as the abnormal size of two otoliths (**Figure 2C**), the abnormal arranged position of two otoliths (**Figure 2D**), and the combined disordered form. The proportion of normal otolith phenotype in the Kif15-MO group is only 44.9% in contrast to 87.5% in controls (**Figure 2G**). On the contrary, there is almost no abnormality in the number of otoliths in the Con-MO injection group (**Figure 2G**). We also detected successful rescue in the phenotype of otoliths after co-injecting Kif15 mRNA and Kif15 splicing MO compared to that in Kif15-MO morphants (**Figures 2F,G**).

Both Utricular and Saccular HCs Decreased Severely After Kif15 Knockdown

Using *Tg(brn3c:mGFP)*^{s356t} line, the HCs that insert into the otoliths were identifiable and labeled by green fluorescence, named utricular (anterior to left) and saccular (posterior to right) HCs, respectively (**Figures 3A,D,G**). After Kif15 knockdown with splicing MO, two smaller sizes of otoliths were examined, and the numbers of both utricular and saccular HCs in otic vesicles were reduced significantly compared to the controls (**Figures 3B,E,H**). However, the decreased number of HCs in both utricle and saccule after Kif15 knocking down could be completely rescued by co-injection with Kif15 mRNA (**Figures 3C,F,I**). The quantitative analysis further showed that the number of utricular HCs in Kif15 morphants was significantly decreased at 48 hpf compared to that in Con-MO-injected larvae, while a remarkably increased number of utricular HCs were found in Kif15-MO + Kif15 mRNA group (**Figure 3J**). Similarly,

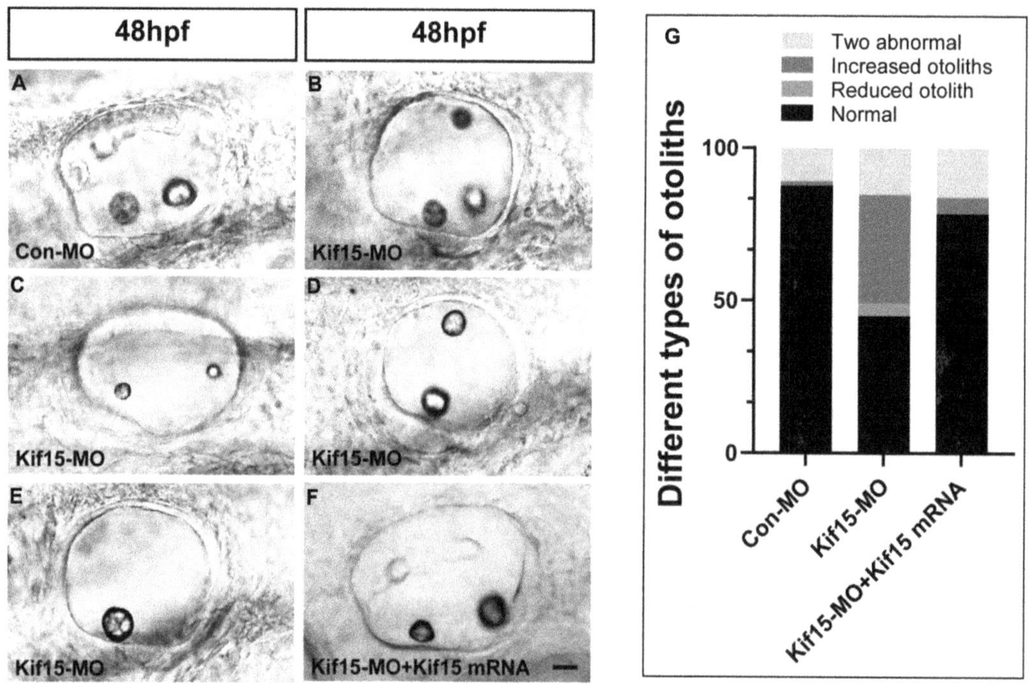

FIGURE 2 | Knockdown of Kif15 disturbs the normal development of otolith organs. **(A–E)** Kif15 inhibition causes abnormal phenotypes of otoliths, including multiplication **(B)** and reduction **(E)** in number, and two abnormal otoliths **(C,D)** at 48 hpf. **(F)** Co-injection Kif15 mRNA with Kif15-MO successfully rescues the phenotypes of otolith organs at 48 hpf. **(G)** Different types of abnormal otoliths and the corresponding proportion analysis in Kif15-MO-injected embryos (n = 234), untreated controls (n = 136), and Kif15-MO + Kif15 mRNA group (n = 111). Scale bar is 20 μm.

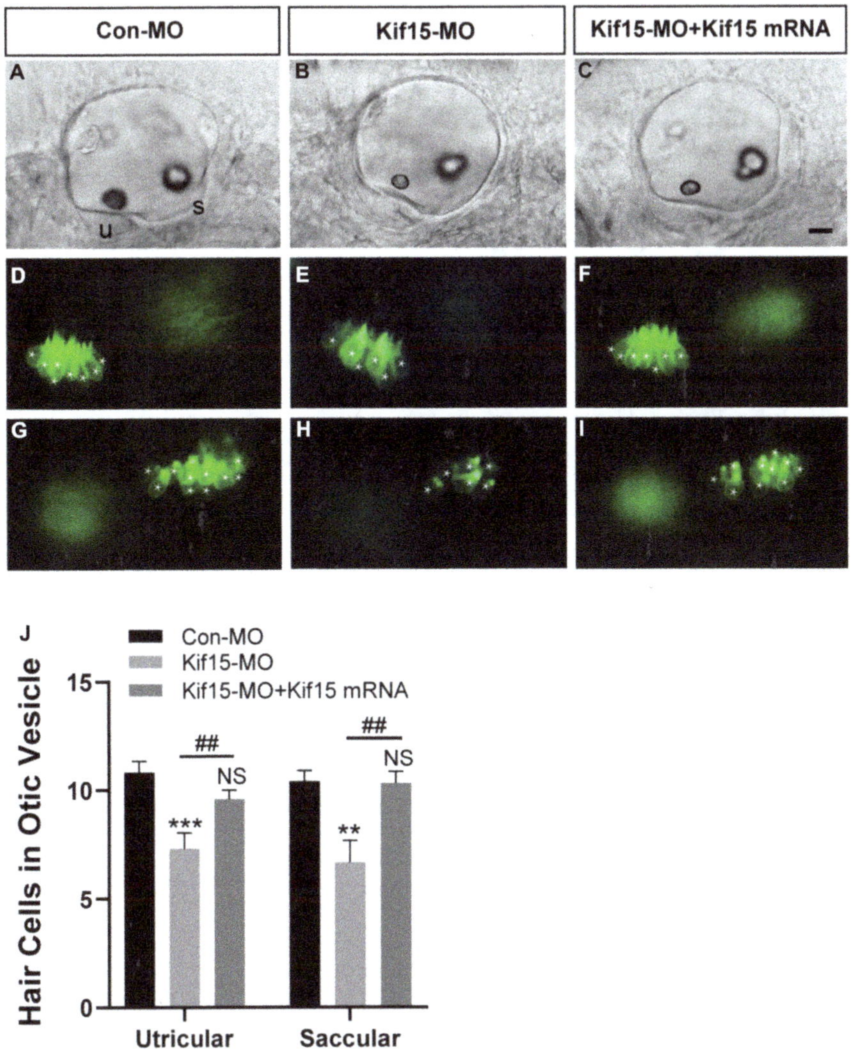

FIGURE 3 | Kif15 inhibition results in decreased hair cells (HCs) in the inner ear. **(A–C)** The gross morphology of otic vesicle in different groups at 48 hpf using the white light field microscope. u, utricle; s, saccule. Scale bar is 20 μm. **(D–F)** Representative images of utricular HCs in different groups at 48 hpf. **(G–I)** Representative images of saccular HCs in different groups at 48 hpf. White star labels the HC. **(J)** Quantification of the number of HCs in utricle and saccule in control-MO (Con-MO) group ($n = 22$), Kif15-deficient morphants ($n = 22$), and Kif15-MO + Kif15 mRNA group. Data are recorded as mean ± SEM. $^{**}p < 0.01$, $^{***}p < 0.001$ vs. Con-MO group; $^{\#\#}p < 0.01$ vs. Kif15-MO group; NS, no significance.

HCs in saccule also severely reduced in Kif15-MO-injected morphants but markedly increased in Kif15-MO + Kif15 mRNA co-injected embryos (**Figure 3J**).

Kif15-MO Leads to Decreased Number of Neuromasts in Posterior Lateral Line System of Zebrafish

Then, the function of Kif15 during the development of the PLL system was investigated. The transgenic zebrafish *Tg(cldnb:lynGFP)*^{zf106} was used to visualize NMs in green fluorescence (Haas and Gilmour, 2006). The NMs manifested in severely reduced number and disordered arrangement along the trunk of zebrafish after Kif15-MO injection at 48 hpf, a time point when PLL primordium finishes migration (**Figures 4A–C**). Co-injecting Kif15 mRNA and splicing MO notably increased the number of NMs in comparison with that in Kif15-MO morphants (**Figure 4D**). The quantitative analysis showed that the number of PLL NMs in Kif15 morphants was significantly decreased compared to that displayed in Con-MO-injected larvae at 48 hpf (**Figure 4E**). The number of PLL NMs in the Kif15-MO + Kif15 mRNA group was remarkably larger than that in Kif15-MO morphants but a little smaller than that in Con-MO embryos, indicating a successful but not complete rescue in the number of NMs by Kif15 mRNA (**Figure 4E**). The diagrammatic sketch demonstrating changes in the number and arrangement of NMs along the trunk and tail of zebrafish was presented after injection with Kif15-MO (**Figure 4F**). The result provided substantial evidence that Kif15 is critical to zebrafish in auditory system development.

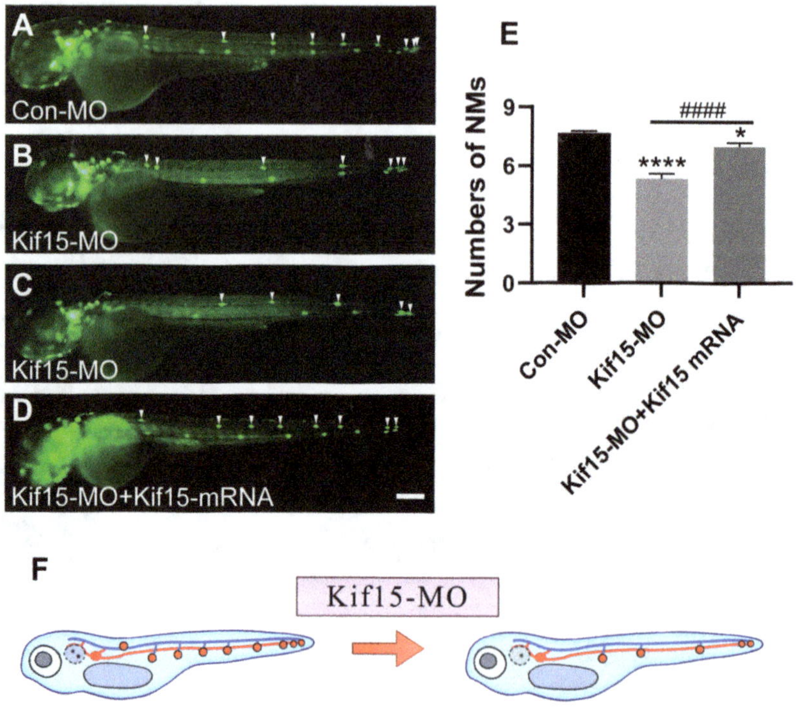

FIGURE 4 | Kif15 knocking down leads to abnormal posterior lateral line (PLL) development, which is represented by a decrease in the number of neuromasts (NMs). **(A–D)** Kif15 inhibition induces the reduction of NMs in zebrafish PLL, while co-injection of Kif15 mRNA with Kif15-MO successfully rescues the decreased number of NMs compared to the Con-MO-treated controls. The PLL NMs are indicated by white arrowheads. Scale bar is 200 μm. **(E)** Statistical analysis in quantification of PLL NMs in Con-MO-injected controls, Kif15-MO-injected embryos, and Kif15-MO + Kif15 mRNA group (n = 50 in the three groups). Data are recorded as mean ± SEM. $^{*}p < 0.05$, $^{****}p < 0.0001$ vs. Con-MO group; $^{\#\#\#\#}p < 0.0001$ vs. Kif15-MO group. **(F)** Simple and intuitive schematic diagram of changes in PLL development after Kif15 knockdown by MO.

Kif15 Transcript Knockdown Disrupts the Normal Locomotor Activity of Zebrafish

According to the brief review of the literature in the background that sensory organs of zebrafish including otoliths, semicircular canals, and PLL NMs can detect sound and water movement stimuli and move in directionality, we wondered if the locomotor behavior of zebrafish was disturbed in Kif15-MO embryos. The locomotion assay was conducted to detect the locomotor behavior of zebrafish after Kif15 inhibition with splicing MO since behavioral change is a comprehensive indicator to show the impact of environmental factors on the organisms. The locomotor traces were recorded during the light-dark photoperiod stimulation with a 20-s interstimulus interval, and we detected a severe reduction in locomotor traces compared to that in the controls (**Figure 5A**). However, a significant increase in locomotor traces was found after performing the rescue experiment with co-injected Kif15 mRNA compared to that in Kif15-MO morphants (**Figure 5A**). Data analysis on the distance moved from the original point in different groups showed that the Kif15-MO injection caused a significant reduction in the distance of locomotion in comparison with the parallel controls. There was also a significant difference in distance of movement between Kif15-MO + Kif15 mRNA and Con-MO groups, indicating a partial rescue effect of Kif15 mRNA in the locomotor behavior (**Figure 5B**). The results were indicative that behavioral dysfunction also existed in addition to morphological deformity after Kif15 inhibition.

DISCUSSION

Kif15 has been previously reported to be widely involved in the progression of several malignancies, such as hepatocellular carcinoma (HCC), and gastric, breast, colorectal, and prostate cancer by regulating cell cycle, migration, and invasion (Li et al., 2020; Zeng et al., 2020; Qureshi et al., 2021). The previous study detected high expression of Kinesin-12 (Kif15) in the otic vesicle of zebrafish (Xu et al., 2014), indicating a potential role of Kif15 in the embryonic development of the inner ear. However, to our knowledge, there are no reports considering the effect of Kif15 on the auditory system. In this study, we first explored the role of Kif15 in the developing hearing organ of zebrafish using the knocking down strategy by Kif15-MO injection.

An MO knockdown approach is a popular tool in studying the function of objective genes (Moulton and Yan, 2008; Stainier et al., 2017); however, the known off-target effect by MOs limits the application of MO to some extent (Gerety and Wilkinson, 2011). In this study, we chose splicing-blocking MO for Kif15 knockdown, and the efficacy of Kif15 inhibition in transcript level was examined by the Western blotting experiment

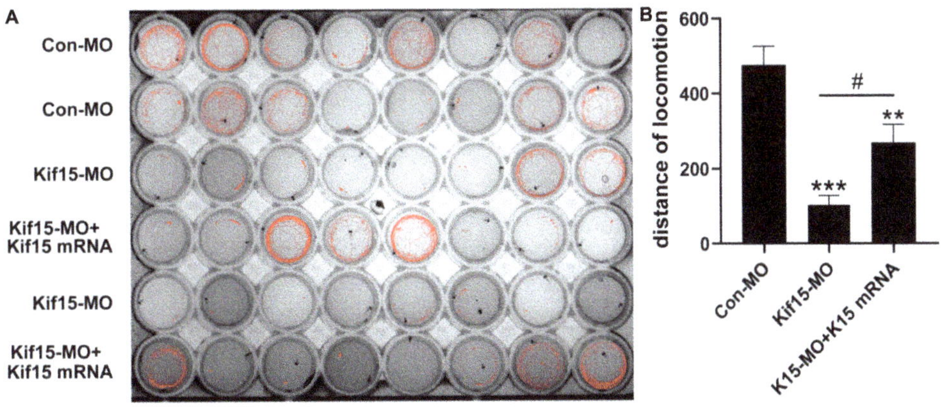

FIGURE 5 | The activity and behavior of zebrafish are abnormal after knocking down Kif15. **(A)** The locomotion assay of zebrafish in Con-MO ($n = 32$), Kif15-MO ($n = 31$), and Kif15-MO + Kif15 mRNA ($n = 30$) injected larvae in traced locomotion curve. **(B)** The moved distance from the original point is analyzed and compared among different groups. The unit of the Y-axis is mm. Data are recorded as mean ± SEM. $^{**}p < 0.01$, $^{***}p < 0.001$ vs. Con-MO group; $^{\#}p < 0.05$ vs. Kif15-MO group.

with anti-Kif15 antibody. We found that the formations of otolith organs, semicircular canals, and PLL NMs were all remarkably deformed in the structure after the inhibition of Kif15. Besides, the further rescue experiments with Kif15 mRNA demonstrated successful rescue of the phenotypical deformities caused by Kif15-MO. To confirm our findings by Kif15 splicing MO, we performed an experiment using the translation-blocking MO strategy for Kif15. As shown in **Supplementary Figure 1**, the expression of Kif15 was significantly decreased in Kif15 translation MO morphants compared to the Con-MO group (**Supplementary Figures 1A,B**). Additionally, malformed otoliths and semicircular canals, together with the reduced number of PLL NMs, were also found in Kif15 translation MO morphants (**Supplementary Figures 1C,D**), which were consistent with the findings in Kif15 splicing MO morphants. Therefore, our findings uncovered that Kif15 is essential in the maintenance of the normal structures and functions of auditory organs of zebrafish, and Kif15-MO with splicing- and translation-blocking strategy was potent for the regulation of Kif15.

As previously reported, the knockdown of Kif15 inhibits cell proliferation, promotes cell apoptosis, and causes cell cycle arrest in glioma cells (Wang et al., 2020). Another study reveals that the inhibition of Kif15 in human HCC xenograft models delays the invasive and proliferative ability of tumors *via* increasing intracellular reactive oxygen species (ROS) levels (Li et al., 2020). In this study, Kif15-MO induced remarkable inhibition of the HC differentiation in both utricle and saccule. Since the proliferative behavior is active in the early development of zebrafish inner ear and lateral line system, we speculated that the reduced number of NMs in PLL and decreased HCs in otic vesicle might be related to the suppression of cell proliferation or increased apoptosis by Kif15 knockdown. Moreover, we detected abnormal locomotion in the Kif15-MO morphants, and the reduced locomotor distance could be partially rescued by co-injection with Kif15 mRNA, indicating a potential role of Kif15 in zebrafish mechanosensory organ function. However, Kif15 is also known to influence neuronal development so it is possible that these defects are simply locomotor defects unrelated to the response to the vibrational stimulus (Xu et al., 2014; Dong et al., 2019). Therefore, in future study, we will use alternative approaches such as prepulse assay to test if abnormal locomotion by Kif15 knockdown is due to ear defects. Altogether, we explored that Kif15 plays an important role during the development of the auditory and vestibular system of zebrafish.

AUTHOR CONTRIBUTIONS

YH, DL, and SL: conceptualization, methodology, writing—review and editing, and project administration. SZ, DT, CL, XW, NZ, RY, CWu, HX, JM, and CWa: methodology and formal analysis. SZ, DT, and XW: validation, investigation, and formal analysis. All authors read and approved the final manuscript.

SUPPLEMENTARY MATERIAL

Supplementary Figure 1 | Knockdown of Kif15 with the translation-blocking method inhibits the normal development of zebrafish. **(A,B)** The protein level of Kif15 is severely decreased in Kif15-MO (translation-blocking)-injected embryos both in the band intensity **(A)** and in the semiquantitative analysis **(B)**, compared to the control embryos. Data are recorded as mean ± SEM. $^{***}p < 0.001$. **(C)** Kif15-MO (translation-blocking) disturbs the normal development of otic vesicles. The abnormal manifestations in both otolith organs and semicircular canals are observed at 48, 72, and 96 hpf, respectively. Scale bar is 20 μm. **(D)** A reduced number of NMs in zebrafish PLL is detected in Kif15 morphants (translation-blocking). Scale bar is 200 μm, $n = 10$.

REFERENCES

Blanco-Sánchez, B., Clément, A., Phillips, J. B., and Westerfield, M. (2017). Zebrafish models of human eye and inner ear diseases. *Methods Cell. Biol.* 138, 415–467. doi: 10.1016/bs.mcb.2016.10.006

Dong, Z., Wu, S., Zhu, C., Wang, X., Li, Y., Chen, X., et al. (2019). Clustered Regularly Interspaced Short Palindromic Repeats (CRISPR)/Cas9-mediated kif15 mutations accelerate axonal outgrowth during neuronal development and regeneration in zebrafish. *Traffic* 20, 71–81. doi: 10.1111/tra.12621

Gao, L., Zhang, W., Zhang, J., Liu, J., Sun, F., Liu, H., et al. (2020a). KIF15-mediated stabilization of AR and AR-V7 contributes to enzalutamide resistance in prostate cancer. *Cancer Res.* 81, 1026-1039

Gao, X., Zhu, L., Lu, X., Wang, Y., Li, R., and Jiang, G. (2020b). KIF15 contributes to cell proliferation and migration in breast cancer. *Hum Cell* 33, 1218–1228. doi: 10.1007/s13577-020-00392-0

Geng, F. S., Abbas, L., Baxendale, S., Holdsworth, C. J., Swanson, A. G., Slanchev, K., et al. (2013). Semicircular canal morphogenesis in the zebrafish inner ear requires the function of gpr126 (lauscher), an adhesion class G protein-coupled receptor gene. *Development* 140, 4362–4374. doi: 10.1242/dev.098061

Gerety, S. S., and Wilkinson, D. G. (2011). Morpholino artifacts provide pitfalls and reveal a novel role for pro-apoptotic genes in hindbrain boundary development. *Dev. Biol.* 350, 279–289. doi: 10.1016/j.ydbio.2010.11.030

Haas, P., and Gilmour, D. (2006). Chemokine signaling mediates self-organizing tissue migration in the zebrafish lateral line. *Dev. Cell.* 10, 673–680. doi: 10.1016/j.devcel.2006.02.019

He, Y., Bao, B., and Li, H. (2017). Using zebrafish as a model to study the role of epigenetics in hearing loss. *Expert Opin. Drug Discov.* 12, 967–975. doi: 10.1080/17460441.2017.1340270

Kalka, M., Markiewicz, N., Ptak, M., Sone, E. D., Ożyhar, A., Dobryszycki, P., et al. (2019). *In vivo* and *in vitro* analysis of starmaker activity in zebrafish otolith biomineralization. *FASEB J.* 33, 6877–6886. doi: 10.1096/fj.201802268R

Kimmel, C. B., Ballard, W. W., Kimmel, S. R., Ullmann, B., and Schilling, T. F. (1995). Stages of embryonic development of the zebrafish. *Dev. Dyn.* 203, 253–310. doi: 10.1002/aja.1002030302

Kitagawa, A., Masuda, T., Takahashi, J., Tobo, T., Noda, M., Kuroda, Y., et al. (2020). KIF15 Expression in Tumor-associated Monocytes Is a Prognostic Biomarker in Hepatocellular Carcinoma. *Cancer Genomics Proteomics* 17, 141–149. doi: 10.21873/cgp.20174

Li, Q., Qiu, J., Yang, H., Sun, G., Hu, Y., Zhu, D., et al. (2020). Kinesin family member 15 promotes cancer stem cell phenotype and malignancy via reactive oxygen species imbalance in hepatocellular carcinoma. *Cancer Lett.* 482, 112–125. doi: 10.1016/j.canlet.2019.11.008

Liu, M., Nadar, V. C., Kozielski, F., Kozlowska, M., Yu, W., and Baas, P. W. (2010). Kinesin-12, a mitotic microtubule-associated motor protein, impacts axonal growth, navigation, and branching. *J. Neurosci.* 30, 14896–14906. doi: 10.1523/JNEUROSCI.3739-10.2010

Lundberg, Y. W., Xu, Y., Thiessen, K. D., and Kramer, K. L. (2015). Mechanisms of otoconia and otolith development. *Dev. Dyn.* 244, 239–253.

Ma, D. D., Wang, D. H., and Yang, W. X. (2017). Kinesins in spermatogenesis. *Biol. Reprod.* 96, 267–276. doi: 10.1095/biolreprod.116.144113

Ma, Y., Zhan, S., Lu, H., Wang, R., Xu, Y., Zhang, G., et al. (2020). B7-H3 regulates KIF15-activated ERK1/2 pathway and contributes to radioresistance in colorectal cancer. *Cell Death Dis.* 11, 824. doi: 10.1038/s41419-020-03041-4

Malaby, H. L. H., Dumas, M. E., Ohi, R., and Stumpff, J. (2019). Kinesin-binding protein ensures accurate chromosome segregation by buffering KIF18A and KIF15. *J. Cell Biol.* 218, 1218–1234. doi: 10.1083/jcb.201806195

Milic, B., Chakraborty, A., Han, K., Bassik, M. C., and Block, S. M. (2018). KIF15 nanomechanics and kinesin inhibitors, with implications for cancer chemotherapeutics. *Proc. Natl. Acad. Sci.U.S.A.* 115, E4613–E4622. doi: 10.1073/pnas.1801242115

Moulton, J. D., and Yan, Y.-L. (2008). Using Morpholinos to control gene expression. *Curr. Proto. Mol. Biol.* 26, 2681–2626. doi: 10.1002/0471142727.mb2608s83

Nicolson, T. (2017). The genetics of hair-cell function in zebrafish. *J. Neurogenet.* 31, 102–112. doi: 10.1080/01677063.2017.1342246

Qureshi, Z., Ahmad, M., Yang, W. X., and Tan, F. Q. (2021). Kinesin 12 (KIF15) contributes to the development and tumorigenicity of prostate cancer. *Biochem. Biophys. Res. Commun.* 576, 7–14. doi: 10.1016/j.bbrc.2021.08.072

Stainier, D. Y. R., Raz, E., Lawson, N. D., Ekker, S. C., Burdine, R. D., Eisen, J. S., et al. (2017). Guidelines for morpholino use in zebrafish. *PLoS. Genet.* 13:e1007000. doi: 10.1371/journal.pgen.1007000

Sturgill, E. G., and Ohi, R. (2013). Kinesin-12 differentially affects spindle assembly depending on its microtubule substrate. *Curr. Biol.* 23, 1280–1290. doi: 10.1016/j.cub.2013.05.043

Tanenbaum, M. E., Macùrek, L., Janssen, A., Geers, E. F., Alvarez-Fernández, M., and Medema, R. H. (2009). Kif15 cooperates with eg5 to promote bipolar spindle assembly. *Curr. Biol.* 19, 1703–1711. doi: 10.1016/j.cub.2009.08.027

Tang, D., He, Y., Li, W., and Li, H. (2019). Wnt/β-catenin interacts with the FGF pathway to promote proliferation and regenerative cell proliferation in the zebrafish lateral line neuromast. *Exp. Mol. Med.* 51, 1–16. doi: 10.1038/s12276-019-0247-x

Tang, D., Lu, Y., Zuo, N., Yan, R., Wu, C., Wu, L., et al. (2021). The H3K27 demethylase controls the lateral line embryogenesis of zebrafish. *Cell Biol. Toxicol.*[Online ahead of print].doi: 10.1007/s10565-021-09669-y

Wang, Q., Han, B., Huang, W., Qi, C., and Liu, F. (2020). Identification of KIF15 as a potential therapeutic target and prognostic factor for glioma. *Oncol. Rep.* 43, 1035–1044. doi: 10.3892/or.2020.7510

Whitfield, T. T., Riley, B. B., Chiang, M. Y., and Phillips, B. (2002). Development of the zebrafish inner ear. *Dev. Dyn.* 223, 427–458. doi: 10.1002/dvdy.10073

Xu, M., Liu, D., Dong, Z., Wang, X., Wang, X., Liu, Y., et al. (2014). Kinesin-12 influences axonal growth during zebrafish neural development. *Cytoskeleton* 71, 555–563. doi: 10.1002/cm.21193

Yu, X., He, X., Heindl, L. M., Song, X., Fan, J., and Jia, R. (2019). KIF15 plays a role in promoting the tumorigenicity of melanoma. *Exp. Eye Res.* 185:107598. doi: 10.1016/j.exer.2019.02.014

Zeng, H., Li, T., Zhai, D., Bi, J., Kuang, X., Lu, S., et al. (2020). ZNF367-induced transcriptional activation of KIF15 accelerates the progression of breast cancer. *Int. J. Biol. Sci.* 16, 2084–2093. doi: 10.7150/ijbs.44204

14

The Peripheral Hearing and Central Auditory Processing Skills of Individuals with Subjective Memory Complaints

Dona M. P. Jayakody[1,2], Holly K. Menegola[1], Jessica M. Yiannos[1,3], Jack Goodman-Simpson[1], Peter L. Friedland[4,5], Kevin Taddei[6], Simon M. Laws[7,8], Michael Weinborn[6,9], Ralph N. Martins[6,10] and Hamid R. Sohrabi[6,10,11]**

[1] Ear Science Institute Australia, Subiaco, WA, Australia, [2] Ear Sciences Centre Faculty of Health and Medical Sciences, The University of Western Australia, Crawley, WA, Australia, [3] School of Human Sciences, The University of Western Australia, Crawley, WA, Australia, [4] Department of Otolaryngology Head Neck Skull Base Surgery, Sir Charles Gairdner Hospital, Nedlands, WA, Australia, [5] School of Medicine, University Notre Dame, Fremantle, WA, Australia, [6] School of Medical and Health Sciences, Edith Cowan University, Joondalup, WA, Australia, [7] Collaborative Genomics Group, School of Medical and Health Sciences, Edith Cowan University, Joondalup, WA, Australia, [8] School of Pharmacy and Biomedical Sciences, Faculty of Health Sciences, Curtin Health Innovation Research Institute, Curtin University, Bentley, WA, Australia, [9] School of Psychological Science, The University of Western Australia, Nedlands, WA, Australia, [10] Department of Biomedical Sciences, Faculty of Medicine and Health Sciences, Macquarie University, Sydney, NSW, Australia, [11] Centre for Healthy Ageing, School of Psychology and Exercise Science, Murdoch University, Murdoch, WA, Australia

***Correspondence:**
Dona M. P. Jayakody
dona.jayakody@earscience.org.au
Hamid R. Sohrabi
Hamid.Sohrabi@murdoch.edu.au

Purpose: This study examined the central auditory processing (CAP) assessment results of adults between 45 and 85 years of age with probable pre-clinical Alzheimer's disease – i.e., individuals with subjective memory complaints (SMCs) as compared to those who were not reporting significant levels of memory complaints (non-SMCs). It was hypothesized that the SMC group would perform significantly poorer on tests of central auditory skills compared to participants with non-SMCs (control group).

Methods: A total of 95 participants were recruited from the larger Western Australia Memory Study and were classified as SMCs ($N = 61$; 20 males and 41 females, mean age 71.47 ±7.18 years) and non-SMCs ($N = 34$; 10 males, 24 females, mean age 68.85 ±7.69 years). All participants completed a peripheral hearing assessment, a CAP assessment battery including Dichotic Digits, Duration Pattern Test, Dichotic Sentence Identification, Synthetic Sentence Identification with Ipsilateral Competing Message (SSI-ICM) and the Quick-Speech-in-Noise, and a cognitive screening assessment.

Results: The SMCs group performed significantly poorer than the control group on SSI-ICM −10 and −20 dB signal-to-noise conditions. No significant differences were found between the two groups on the peripheral hearing threshold measurements and other CAP assessments.

Conclusions: The results suggest that individuals with SMCs perform poorly on specific CAP assessments in comparison to the controls. The poor CAP in SMC individuals may result in a higher cost to their finite pool of cognitive resources. The CAP results provide yet another biomarker that supports the hypothesis that SMCs may be a primary indication of neuropathological changes in the brain. Longitudinal follow up of individuals with SMCs, and decreased CAP abilities should inform whether this group is at higher risk of developing dementia as compared to non-SMCs and those SMC individuals without CAP difficulties.

Keywords: hearing loss, central auditory processing, dementia, subjective memory complaints, *APOE*-ε4

INTRODUCTION

With over 47 million individuals living with dementia worldwide in 2015, this syndrome is considered a growing global epidemic in older adults (Prince et al., 2015). According to the World Alzheimer Report, the number of people with a dementia diagnosis will rise to 74.7 million in 2030 and 132 million by 2050 (Prince et al., 2015). Alzheimer's disease (AD) is the most common cause of dementia in older adults accounting for 60–80% of all-cause dementia (Lambert et al., 2014).

The neuropathological changes associated with AD, including the deposition of amyloid plaques and neurofibrillary tangles, start 20–30 years before the clinical diagnosis (Serrano-Pozo et al., 2011). The National Institute of Aging-Alzheimer's Association Work Groups on diagnostic guidelines suggest that the course of AD can be divided into three subsequent stages: (1) the pre-clinical stage of AD (no impairment in cognition on standard assessments and biomarker evidence for AD), (2) mild cognitive impairment (MCI) due to AD (impairment on memory or other domains of cognition on a standard assessment and biomarker evidence for AD), and (3) dementia due to AD (dementia and biomarker evidence for AD plus subtle cognitive decline) (Jack et al., 2011; McKhann et al., 2011; Sperling et al., 2011; Albert et al., 2013). Current evidence suggests that the self-reported decline in memory or other cognitive functions in the presence of normal performance on neuropsychological measures is associated with an increased risk for future cognitive decline and AD dementia (Glodzik-Sobanska et al., 2007; Wang et al., 2011; Scheef et al., 2012).

With no cure or effective treatment currently insight, it is critical to identify those factors that may prevent or delay cognitive decline and dementia in older adults. Of the potentially modifiable risk factors, untreated hearing loss contributes up to 8% of the modifiable risk factors in mid-life (Livingston et al., 2020). Age-related hearing loss (ARHL) or presbycusis is a multifactorial disorder affecting hearing acuity that varies from mild to profound and results from lifetime insults to the auditory system (Gates and Mills, 2005). Prevalence data indicates that 63% of adults aged 70 years and older have a >25 dBHL speech frequency (4 PTA average of 0.5, 1, 2, and 4 kHz) hearing loss in their better ear (Lin et al., 2011b). Evidence from both cross-sectional (Jayakody et al., 2017) and longitudinal (Lin et al., 2011a; Deal et al., 2016) studies confirmed an increase in the risk of cognitive impairment and incident dementia among older adults with ARHL (Lin et al., 2011a; Deal et al., 2016). In an 11-year longitudinal study, baseline peripheral hearing loss was associated with the increased risk of incident AD (1.27 times per 10 dB hearing loss).

Central auditory processing (CAP) impairment refers to auditory perceptual difficulties that cannot be explained by impairment in peripheral hearing but refers to the impairment in the central auditory pathway affecting speech understanding such as neural transmission, feature extraction and detecting small gaps in the speech which is crucial in speech discrimination, integrating and separating binaural auditory information (Humes et al., 2012; Musiek and Chermak, 2013; Fortunato et al., 2016). A typical hearing complaint of older adults is their inability to understand speech, especially in the presence of background noise (CHABA, 1988). Together, peripheral hearing loss, cognitive decline, aging, and diminished CAP skills (i.e., decline in speech-in-noise processing, dichotic processing and temporal processing skills, or a combination of all these abilities) contribute to the poor speech understanding skills of older adults (Humes et al., 2012; Musiek and Chermak, 2013).

Results from several longitudinal studies suggest that central hearing or CAP skills, in the absence of a severe peripheral hearing loss, are associated with high incidences of cognitive decline and AD dementia (Gates et al., 2002, 2008, 2011) and may precede cognitive impairments and dementia diagnosis by three to 12 years (Gates et al., 1996). These studies have demonstrated that individuals with CAP dysfunction were at a significantly higher risk for incident dementia with hazard ratios ranging from 9.9 (95% CI, 3.6–26.7) to 23.3 (95% CI, 6.6–82.7) (Gates et al., 1996, 2011). Central auditory processing impairment is now considered the primary auditory impairment associated with an increased risk of AD (Panza et al., 2018).

A few studies have previously investigated the CAP skills in individuals diagnosed with MCI (Idrizbegovic et al., 2013; Edwards et al., 2017) and dementia (Gates et al., 2011; Golden et al., 2015; Quaranta et al., 2015). However, to date, no study has investigated the CAP skills in individuals with subjective memory complaints (SMCs). The SMCs include self-reported concerns about one's memory, which is a major component of subjective cognitive decline (SCD) and is considered a risk factor for future dementia due to AD (Choe et al., 2018). Investigating whether SMC individuals have poor CAP skills compared to those with non-SMCs would provide a unique opportunity to identify people at high risk of developing dementia or who are probably at pre-clinical phases of AD and dementia, years before clinical diagnosis (Jessen et al., 2014; Rönnlund et al., 2015).

The primary aim of our study was to measure the peripheral and central hearing of participants with SMCs and non-SMCs. We hypothesized that participants in the SMC group would perform significantly poorer on tests of peripheral and central hearing assessment compared to non-SMC participants.

Many studies have explored the contribution of genetic factors to ARHL (Karlsson et al., 1997; Gates et al., 1999; Friedman et al., 2009), and to AD (Poorkaj et al., 1998; Cai et al., 2015; Hardy, 2017). However, there is no conclusive evidence on whether cognitive impairment/dementia and ARHL share a common genetic etiology. Kurniawan et al. (2012) reported that apolipoprotein E (*APOE*) ε4 allele, a major genetic risk factor for AD, is strongly associated with poorer hearing thresholds, whereas, Mener et al. (2016) reported that participants with two *APOE* ε4 alleles had better hearing thresholds at 1.0 kHz ($\beta = -8.56$, $p = 0.021$) compared to those with no *APOE* ε4 alleles. However, whether *APOE* ε4 allele status is associated with impaired peripheral hearing sensitivity and CAP skills is yet to be investigated. Therefore, we also investigated the association between peripheral and central auditory functions and cognitive functions, and the impact of *APOE* ε4 carriage as the primary genetic risk factor for late-onset AD. We hypothesized that the *APOE* ε4 carriers would perform significantly poorer than the non-carries on central and peripheral hearing assessments.

METHODS

Study Design: Prospective Study

Participants were recruited from the Western Australia Memory Study (WAMS), a longitudinal study into aging and dementia. The ethics approval for this study was received from the Ramsay Health Care WA| SA Human Research Ethics Committee (previously, the Hollywood Private Hospital Ethics Committee, Western Australia). All procedures were undertaken per this approval. The participants completed an informed consent form prior to taking part in the study. The hearing assessments were conducted by a trained researcher under the supervision of a qualified audiologist, and the cognitive assessments were performed by a qualified psychometric rater trained and certified by the study neuropsychologists.

Participants

A total of 95 individuals who have been speaking Australian English for 10 years or longer, aged between 45–85 years, in a general state of good health and with a 4PTA (average of better ear hearing thresholds at 0.5, 1, 2, and 4 kHz) of less than 40 dBHL were recruited for the study. None of the participants used hearing aids. All participants were recruited from the WAMS (Sohrabi et al., 2012).

MATERIALS AND PROCEDURE

The assessment materials included measures of cognition, psychological status, and peripheral and central hearing.

Demographic information: All participants completed a demographic questionnaire that was asking for information on age, sex, education, and family history of stroke, dementia, diabetes, smoking, and high blood pressure.

Hearing Assessment

The hearing assessment consisted of two components: peripheral and central.

Peripheral Hearing Assessment

The hearing assessment included an otoscopic examination and pure-tone audiometric testing. The pure-tone audiometric assessment was conducted using a KUDUwave 5000, Type 2 clinical audiometer (Emoyo, Johannesburg, South Africa). Bilateral air-conduction thresholds between 0.5 and 8 kHz and bone-conduction thresholds between 0.5 and 4 kHz were obtained through standard audiometric assessment in a sound-attenuating booth that meets the standard for audiometric testing. This task took approximately 20 min to complete.

Central Auditory Processing Assessment

The CAP functions were assessed using a battery of five central auditory tests to identify the central auditory deficits. The assessments were presented at 65 dBHL, for participants who had 4PTA $>$ 25 dBHL. For those who had 4PTA $<$ 25 dBHL, test materials were presented at 4PTA + 20 dB.

The following CAP tests were administered.

Dichotic Digits Test

Dichotic Digits Test (DDT; Musiek et al., 1991) is a test of binaural integration. The participants were instructed that "you will hear two numbers in each of your ears. Listen carefully and repeat all the numbers you hear. The order doesn't matter. If you are unsure of the numbers, please guess." The participant was presented with one practice presentation and 25 assessed presentations. Each digit repeated back was marked as correct or incorrect. The ears were scored separately, and the order in which the participant repeated the digits back did not matter. Scores above 90% in each ear are considered within the normal limits for adults with normal hearing sensitivity and under the age of 65 years. For adults over the age of 65 years or with a hearing loss, the cut-off is 82% (Musiek, 1983).

Dichotic Sentence Identification

Dichotic Sentence Identification (DSI; Fifer et al., 1983) is a test of binaural separation. During the DSI, the participant was presented with 20 sentence pairs from a printed list of six sentences. In each sentence pair, the participant was presented with one of the six sentences in each ear; the sentences always differed in each ear. The 20 sentence pairs were presented in two blocks of 10; in the first block, the participant was asked to attend to the sentence being presented to their right ear and then indicate the sentence number that corresponded to the sentence presented in their directed ear. In the second block, the participants were asked to attend to their left ear and complete the same task. Each trial was marked as correct or incorrect and then each ear was scored as a percentage correct.

Duration Pattern Test

In the Duration Pattern Test (DPT; Musiek, 1994), participants were presented with 1 kHz tones in sequences of three, where each tone could have a duration of either 250 ms (short) or 500 ms (long) with 300 ms intervals between the tones in the sequence of three tones (Musiek and Chermak, 1994). The participants were asked to linguistically label each of the tone durations as either short (S) or long (L) in each series, for example, "short, long, long." There were six possible combinations of the three tones (SSL, LLS, LSL, SLS, LSS, SLL). Each three-item sequence of the tones had to be identified with the lengths in the correct order to be scored as correct. The participant was presented with three practice presentations and then with 30 assessed presentations, with 15 in each ear. Percent correct scores for each ear were recorded.

Synthetic Sentence Identification with Ipsilateral Competing Message

In the Synthetic Sentence Identification with Ipsilateral Competing Message (SSI-ICM; Speaks et al., 1967; Orchik and Burgess, 1977) test, the participant selected which nonsense sentence out of 10 was being presented against a competing narrative in the same ear. The competing narrative was a passage about Davy Crockett presented by the same presenter, ipsilateral to the target sentence (Jerger and Jerger, 1974; **Supplementary Material 1**). Studies have shown both hearing loss and age can affect SSI-ICM scores (Gates et al., 2008), therefore, the lists were presented at 65 dBHL for those who had 4PTA > 25 dBHL. For those who had 4PTA < 25 dBHL, test materials were presented at 4PTA + 20 dB. Four sets of ten sentences were presented at + 10 dB speech-to-noise ratio (SNR), 0 dB SNR, −10 dB SNR, and −20 dB SNR conditions. The target sentences presented at 10 dB above the competing narrative in the + 10 dB SNR condition, 10dB below the competing narrative in the −10dB condition and 20 dB below the competing narrative in the −20 dB condition. The target sentence and competing narrative were presented at the same level in the 0 dB SNR condition.

Percent correct score was calculated for each test condition and each ear separately.

Quick Speech-in-Noise

In the Quick Speech-in-Noise (QuickSIN; Killion et al., 2004) test, the participant was presented with two practice sentences and two pre-recorded test lists in each ear; each list is comprised of six sentences with five target words in each. The multi-talker babble increased by 5 dB per sentence between 40 and 65 dBHL, creating varying conditions between a 25 dB speech-to-noise ratio and a 0 dB SNR for the final sentence. The participant was asked to repeat the sentence back to the assessor and was scored one point for each word they correctly repeated. The total score was then subtracted from 25.5 to calculate the signal-to-noise ratio loss (Killion et al., 2004). Examples are provided in **Supplementary Material 2.**

Cognitive Assessment

The WAMS is a longitudinal study of community-dwelling older adults in Perth Western Australia, specifically enriched for recruiting individuals with SMCs. All participants complete a comprehensive neuropsychological assessment, including self and informant scales and questionnaires. The WAMS assessment battery takes up to 3 h and has various measures assessing global cognition, verbal and visual episodic memory, attention, executive functions, language, orientation, visuospatial skill, and so on. In addition, the participants provide blood samples and undergo brain imaging. Self-reports and informant-reports surveys and questioners are collected for the psychological, cognitive, and personality characteristics of the WAMS participants. As this paper is focused on the relationship between hearing loss and SMCs, we have not reported on the neuropsychological measures. Further information on the neuropsychological measures used as part of WAMS can be found in Sohrabi et al. (2019).

To assess the participants' general cognitive abilities and screen for potential cognitive impairment, the WAMS utilizes the Montreal Cognitive Assessment (MoCA) (Nasreddine et al., 2005). Only participants with a MoCA cut-off score of ≥23 were considered cognitively normal and recruited for this study (Rossetti et al., 2011). For those participants with borderline or concerning results, the full neurocognitive battery, as well as the clinical data, are examined by the study Lead Neuropsychs (HRS and MW) to ensure that such results are appropriately communicated with participants and their medical doctors. Of note, the endpoint for participation in the WAMS is a diagnosis of MCI, AD, or other types of dementia.

In this study, participants were divided into two groups: a control (non-SMC), and a high-risk group (SMC) based on completing a self-reported survey, namely the Memory Assessment Clinics Questionnaire (MAC-Q; Crook et al., 1992). The MAC-Q is a self-report questionnaire designed to capture concerns about memory decline. The first five questions assess age-related decline in memory on daily activities and the last question asks about overall memory decline. Participants in the current study were asked to rate all six items on a 5-point Likert scale ranging from "Much better now" to "Much poorer now," compared to when they were at high school or college. The total score on the MAC-Q ranges from 7 to 35, and higher scores indicate more complaints about one's memory abilities. Participants were considered SMCs if they scored ≥25 on the MAC-Q (Crook et al., 1992).

Genotyping

In this study, the *APOE* ε4 allele was determined using TaqMan® genotyping assays (rs7412, assay ID: C____904973_10; rs429358, assay ID: C___3084793_20) from DNA extracted from 5ml of a whole blood sample using QIAamp DNA Blood Maxi Kits (Qiagen, Hilden, Germany). TaqMan® genotyping assays were performed on a QuantStudio 12K Flex™ Real-Time-PCR systems (Applied Biosystems, Foster City, CA) using the TaqMan® GTXpress™ Master Mix (Life Technologies) as per manufacturer instructions. *APOE* ε4 carriers included participants with at least one ε4 allele (i.e., ε2/ε4, ε3/ε4, ε4/ε4) and non-carriers included no copies of the ε4 allele (ε2/ε2, ε2/ε3, ε3/ε3).

Statistical Analysis

Data were recorded in Excel and statistically analyzed using IBM SPSS Statistics, Version 25.0 (IBM Corp, Armonk, NY). Analyses of Co-Variance (ANCOVA) were run for each ear in each test to test the hypotheses that SMC participants perform significantly poorer than non-SMC participants in tests of peripheral and central hearing. Age was considered a covariate and adjustments for multiple comparisons were made using Bonferroni corrections. The participants of this study cohort had a wide age range and (50–85 years). Also, age is the primary risk factor for both ARHL and cognitive impairment in older adults (Glisky, 2007). In addition, SMCs increases in frequency (number of times given individual complaints) and prevalence as a factor of age (Koivisto et al., 1995; Coley et al., 2008). Therefore, adjusting for age was required to be able to disentangle the effect of age on the relationship between hearing loss and SMCs. Assumptions for linearity, homogeneity and homoscedasticity were met for each test and there were no outliers in the data, as assessed by no cases with standardized residuals greater than ±3 standard deviations. Data are reported as unadjusted mean ± standard deviation unless otherwise stated.

To investigate the relationship between SMC and age, gender, better ear 4PTA and CAP tests, we have conducted binomial logistic regression with the presence of SMCs as the dependent variables and age, gender, better ear 4PTA and CAP tests as independent variables.

RESULTS

Demographic details of the participants are reported in **Table 1**. Of the 95 participants who were selected for the study, 61 participants (20 males and 41 females, mean age 71.47 ±7.18 years) had MAC-Q scores ≥25, hence, categorized as SMC. Thirty-four participants (10 males, 24 females, mean age 68.85 ±7.69 years) had MAC-Q scores < 25, hence categorized as non-SMC. Mean and SD values for both SMC and non-SMC groups for all the CAP tests are reported in **Table 2**. There was no significant interaural asymmetry observed in any of the participants. CAPS test protocols suggest assessing each ear separately and the scores were calculated for each ear as well. Hence, rather than averaging scores of right and left ear, we analyzed results for each ear which is a routine way of analyzing hearing assessment results.

Analysis of Co-variance results of the SMC and non-SMC participants revealed no significant difference between peripheral left and right ear 4PTA and 2 HF PTA (high frequency average of 6 and 8 kHz) of the SMC and non-SMC participant groups (**Table 3**). Both groups of participants had their 4PTA mean hearing thresholds within normal limits (<25 dBHL). The SMC group performed significantly poorer than the non-SMC group on SSI-ICM −10 dB SNR [right ear, F (1, 89) = 6.59, p = 0.012; left ear F (1, 89) = 7.87, p = 0.006) and −20 dB SNR (right ear F (1, 87) = 13.85, p < 0.001; and left ear F (1,88) = 20.06, p < 0.001] conditions. No significant differences were found between participant groups for the other CAP measures i.e., Quick-SIN, DDT, DSI, and DPT tasks (**Table 3**).

TABLE 1 | Demographic data of the participants.

Parameters	Total N (%)/Mean (SD)
Sex	
Female	65 (68.4%)
Male	30 (31.6%)
Apolipoprotein E (*APOE*) ε4 carriers	26 (27.4%)
Subjective memory complainers (SMCs)	61 (64.1%)

Results of the binomial logistic regression failed to reveal any significant association between 4PTA and SMC. However, SSI-ICM −20 and −10 dB SNR conditions were statistically significant. For SSI-ICM left ear −20dB SNR condition the model explained 24.8% of the total variance, sensitivity was 79.6% and the specificity was 57.6% and the positive predictive value was 75.43%. For SSI-ICM right ear −20 dB SNR condition the model explained 33.1% of the total variance, sensitivity was 74.5% and the specificity was 54.5% and the positive predictive value was 73.21%. Results of the binomial logistic regression analysis are reported in **Supplementary Table 3**.

AD Genetic Risk Factor and Hearing

Of the 95 participants tested 26 were *APOE* ε4 carriers (10 males, 16 females; mean age 68.85 ±8.33 years), and 69 were non-carriers (20 males, 49 females; mean age 71.17 ±7.03 years). No significant difference was observed between carriers and non-carriers on better and poorer ear 4PTA scores or better and poorer ear 2HF PTA average. The performance of carriers and non-carriers on all central auditory test measures were not significantly different (**Table 4**). Of the total cohort, 20 were SMC and positive for *APOE* ε4 carriage. However, when compared with the remaining 75 participants, there was no significant difference between the two groups on any of the hearing tests.

DISCUSSION

A significant difference between the SMC and non-SMC groups was observed on tests of SSI-ICM −10 and −20 dB SNR conditions. Of note, mean values of right and left ear 4PTA results of both groups were not significantly different. The hearing thresholds of left ear, right ear, and better ear 4PTA for both groups were approximately 25 dB. Therefore, we conclude that the SSI-ICM results were not influenced by the peripheral hearing loss.

Central auditory processing difficulties are known to place additional demands and strain on an individual's cognitive processing capacity (Bellis and Jorgensen, 2014). This is due to the requirement for additional "upstream" resources to facilitate auditory perception and other higher-order central auditory processes (Bellis and Jorgensen, 2014). This study's findings suggest that while there may be a decline in some CAP skills in individuals with SMCs, this deficit may only become visible when the CAP system is significantly challenged, and cognitive resources are exhausted or depleted, such as in the SSI-ICM −10 or −20 SNR subtests. Moreover, speech processing is one of the most challenging and cognitively demanding CAP tasks that rely on several auditory processing skills, including auditory attention, temporal resolution, temporal patterning, and auditory closure (Chermak and Lee, 2005). Speech processing becomes even more difficult and cognitively complex when the speech

TABLE 2 | Mean and standard deviation scores of central auditory processing tests for both participant groups.

Task	SMC			Non-SMC		
	N	Mean	SD	N	Mean	SD
Age	61	71.47	7.18	34	68.85	7.70
Years of Formal Education	61	13.59	2.62	34	14.74	2.80
Right Ear 4PTA (0.5,1,2, and 4 kHz average) dBHL	59	25.57	15.02	34	22.72	12.24
Left Ear 4PTA (0.5,1,2, and 4 kHz average) dBHL	59	25.41	12.85	34	23.09	10.74
Better Ear 4PTA (0.5,1,2, and 4 kHz average) dBHL	59	23.01	12.25	34	19.93	9.87
Right ear 2 HF PTA average (6 and 8 kHz) dBHL	59	33.90	21.19	34	30.93	20.27
Left Ear 2 HF PTA average (6 and 8 kHz) dBHL	59	37.77	19.75	34	35.59	19.46
Better ear 2 HF PTA average (6 and 8 kHz) dBHL	59	31.13	19.68	34	28.24	19.32
Dichotic Digits Test (DDT) Right Ear-Percent correct score	59	86.07	13.52	33	85.08	14.37
Dichotic Digits Test (DDT) Left Ear-Percent correct score	59	80.83	13.45	33	81.65	13.39
Quick Speech in Noise Test (QuickSIN) Right Ear-dBSNR	60	5.96	4.45	33	5.43	4.01
Quick Speech in Noise Test (QuickSIN) Left Ear-dBSNR	60	5.91	4.49	33	5.69	4.45
Duration Pattern Test (DPT) Right Ear-Percent correct score	60	89.44	18.33	33	95.33	7.79
Duration Pattern Test (DPT)- Left Ear-Percent correct score	60	90.29	17.43	33	93.52	13.61
Dichotic Speech Identification Test-Right Ear-Percent correct score	60	97.33	7.78	33	97.77	5.71
Dichotic Speech Identification Test-Left Ear-Percent correct score	60	93.22	16.86	32	96.02	6.76
Synthetic Sentence Identification-Ipsilateral Competing Message (SSI-ICM) Right Ear−20 dBSNR condition-Percent correct score	56	23.21	21.67	33	42.12	19.33
Synthetic Sentence Identification-Ipsilateral Competing Message (SSI-ICM) Left Ear−20 dBSNR condition- Percent correct score	57	29.47	24.16	33	53.91	21.14
Synthetic Sentence Identification-Ipsilateral Competing Message (SSI-ICM) Right Ear−10 dBSNR condition-Percent correct score	58	53.97	22.08	33	67.58	17.32
Synthetic Sentence Identification-Ipsilateral Competing Message (SSI-ICM) Left Ear−10 dBSNR condition- Percent correct score	58	54.14	21.36	33	68.18	17.22
Synthetic Sentence Identification-Ipsilateral Competing Message (SSI-ICM) Right Ear 0 dBSNR condition-Percent correct score	59	87.93	17.30	33	90.61	13.91
Synthetic Sentence Identification-Ipsilateral Competing Message (SSI-ICM) Left Ear 0 dBSNR condition-Percent correct score	59	93.05	13.93	33	94.24	10.01
Synthetic Sentence Identification-Ipsilateral Competing Message (SSI-ICM) Right Ear + 10 dBSNR condition-Percent correct score	59	98.47	8.05	34	99.41	2.39
Synthetic Sentence Identification-Ipsilateral Competing Message (SSI-ICM) Left Ear + 10 dBSNR condition-Percent correct score	59	98.14	8.20	34	99.71	1.72
The Montreal Cognitive Assessment(MOCA) Total Score – out of 30	61	26.75	2.08	34	26.56	2.58
Memory Complaint Questionnaire (MAC-Q) Total Score-out of 35	61	27.33	3.03	34	23.50	3.83

signal is distorted by other competing messages, meaning apt auditory attention is also required to discriminate and accurately understand what is being said (Gates et al., 2010).

The SSI-ICM test appears to be sensitive to the decline of CAP skills in MCI populations and accurately predicts the future clinical diagnosis of AD (Gates et al., 2008 and 2010; Edwards et al., 2017). Gates et al. (2008) found that individuals with a diagnosis of MCI performed significantly poorer on the 0 dB SNR condition of the SSI-ICM compared to a control group. The −10 and −20 dB SNR conditions of the SSI-ICM were not assessed in the Gates et al. (2008) study. However, given the known progression of the neuropathology and differences in cognition between MCI and SMC groups, it can be assumed that a more difficult task, where the signal is more distorted and therefore requires more cognitive resources, is necessary to differentiate between SMC and control groups as compared to other groups.

TABLE 3 | Analysis of Co-variance results of the subjective memory complainers and non-memory complainers.

Parameter	*F*	*P* value	Partial η^2	Observed power
Better ear 4PTA average (0.5,1,2, and 4 kHz)	*F* (1,91) = 0.60	0.43	0	0.12
Right ear 4PTA average (0.5,1,2, and 4 kHz)	*F* (1,91) = 0.34	0.56	0	0.08
Left ear 4 PTAaverage (0.5,1,2, and 4 kHz)	*F* (1,91) = 0.16	0.69	0	0.06
Better ear 2 HF PTA average (6 and 8 kHz)	*F* (1,91) = 0.09	0.75	0	0.06
Right ear 2 HF PTA average (6 and 8 kHz)	*F* (1,91) = 0.14	0.7	0	0.06
Left ear 2 HF PTA average (6 and 8 kHz)	*F* (1,91) = 0.00	0.97	0	0.05
Dichotic Digits Test (DDT) Right Ear	*F* (1,90) = 1.45	0.23	0.01	0.22
Dichotic Digits Test (DDT) Left Ear	*F* (1,90) = 2.82	0.59	0	0.08
Duration Pattern Test (DPT) Right Ear	*F* (1,91) = 3.40	0.06	0.03	0.44
Duration Pattern Test (DPT) Left Ear	*F* (1,91) = 0.99	0.32	0.01	0.16
QuickSpeech in Noise Test (QuickSin) Right Ear	*F* (1,91) = 0.01	0.9	0.01	0.05
QuickSpeech in Noise Test (QuickSin) Left Ear	*F* (1,91) = 0.38	0.53	0	0.09
Dichotic Speech Identification Test (DSI) Right Ear	*F* (1,91) = 0.01	0.89	0	0.05
Dichotic Speech Identification Test (DSI) Left Ear	*F* (1,90) = 0.10	0.75	0	0.06
Synthetic Sentence Identification-Ipsilateral Competing Message (SSI-ICM) −20 dBSNR Right Ear	*F* (1,87) = 13.85	0.001*	0.13	0.95
Synthetic Sentence Identification-Ipsilateral Competing Message (SSI-ICM) −20 dBSNR Left Ear	*F* (1,88) = 20.06	0.001*	0.19	0.99
Synthetic Sentence Identification-Ipsilateral Competing Message (SSI-ICM) −10 dBSNR Right Ear	*F* (1,89) = 6.59	0.012*	0.06	0.71
Synthetic Sentence Identification-Ipsilateral Competing Message (SSI-ICM) −10 dBSNR Left Ear	*F* (1,89) = 7.87	0.006*	0.08	0.79
Synthetic Sentence Identification-Ipsilateral Competing Message (SSI-ICM) 0 dBSNR Right Ear	*F* (1,90) = 0.00	0.97	0	0.05
Synthetic Sentence Identification-Ipsilateral Competing Message (SSI-ICM) 0 dBSNR Left Ear	*F* (1,90) = 0.01	0.91	0	0.05
Synthetic Sentence Identification-Ipsilateral Competing Message (SSI-ICM) + 10 dBSNR Right Ear	*F* (1,91) = 0.02	0.87	0.02	0.05
Synthetic Sentence Identification-Ipsilateral Competing Message (SSI-ICM) + 10 dBSNR Left Ear	*F* (1,91) = 0.38	0.53	0	0.09

P < 0.05 marked with an asterisk (*). Age has been considered as a co-variate in the analysis.

TABLE 4 | Analysis of Co-variance results for the *APOE* e4 carriers and non-carriers.

Parameter	*F*	*P* value	Partial η^2	Observed power
Better ear 4PTA average (0.5,1,2, and 4 kHz)	*F* (1,91) = 0.22	0.63	0.00	0.02
Poor ear 4PTA average (0.5,1,2, and 4 kHz)	*F* (1,91) = 0.38	0.53	0.00	0.09
Right ear 4PTA average (0.5,1,2, and 4 kHz)	*F* (1,91) = 0.73	0.39	0.00	0.13
Left ear 4 PTA average (0.5,1,2, and 4 kHz)	*F* (1,91) = 0.02	0.87	0.00	0.05
Dichotic Digits Test (DDT) Right Ear	*F* (1,90) = 0.55	0.48	0.01	0.11
Dichotic Digits Test (DDT) Left Ear	*F* (1,90) = 3.92	0.51	0.04	0.50
Duration Pattern Test (DPT) Right Ear	*F* (1,91) = 0.35	0.55	0.00	0.09
Duration Pattern Test (DPT) left ear	*F* (1,91) = 0.17	0.89	0.00	0.05
QuickSpeech in Noise Test (QuickSin) Right Ear	*F* (1,91) = 0.29	0.59	0.00	0.08
QuickSpeech in Noise Test (QuickSin) Left Ear	*F* (1,91) = 0.06	0.80	0.00	0.05
Dichotic Speech Identification Test (DSI) Right Ear	*F* (1,91) = 0.34	0.56	0.00	0.08
Dichotic Speech Identification Test (DSI) Left Ear	*F* (1,91) = 1.54	0.21	0.01	0.23
Synthetic Sentence Identification-Ipsilateral Competing Message (SSI-ICM) −20 dBSNR Right Ear	*F* (1,87) = 1.05	0.31	0.01	0.17
Synthetic Sentence Identification-Ipsilateral Competing Message (SSI-ICM) −20 dBSNR Left Ear	*F* (1,88) = 0.00	0.94	0.00	0.05
Synthetic Sentence Identification-Ipsilateral Competing Message (SSI-ICM) −10 dBSNR Right Ear	*F* (1,89) = 1.13	0.28	0.01	0.14
Synthetic Sentence Identification-Ipsilateral Competing Message (SSI-ICM) −10 dBSNR Left Ear	*F* (1,89) = 0.03	0.85	0.00	0.05
Synthetic Sentence Identification-Ipsilateral Competing Message (SSI-ICM) 0 dBSNR Right Ear	*F* (1,90) = 0.26	0.61	0.00	0.08
Synthetic Sentence Identification-Ipsilateral Competing Message (SSI-ICM) 0 dBSNR Left Ear	*F* (1,90) = 0.20	0.65	0.00	0.07
Synthetic Sentence Identification-Ipsilateral Competing Message (SSI-ICM) + 10 dBSNR Right Ear	*F* (1,91) = 0.00	0.92	0.00	0.05
Synthetic Sentence Identification-Ipsilateral Competing Message (SSI-ICM) + 10 dBSNR Left Ear	*F* (1,91) = 0.13	0.71	0.00	0.06

Age has been considered a co-variate in this analysis.

To understand why the SMC group performed poorly in the SSI-ICM task, we need to understand the nature of this task. The human auditory system perceptually segregates the competing acoustic stimuli into different streams in a process known as auditory scene analysis (Bregman, 1990). The auditory scene analysis makes use of the spatial, spectral and supra-segmental composition, as well as temporal information to segregate the foreground from background information (Bregman, 1990). It does this by matching the incoming acoustic information to previously stored auditory "templates," mediated by attentional mechanisms (Carlyon et al., 2001; Billig et al., 2013). Synthetic Sentence Identification with Ipsilateral Competing Message is a test of auditory closure that helps fill in the missing information in the presence of a competing signal (Speaks et al., 1967). Synthetic sentences are third-order approximations of English sentences. These sentences contain seven semantically meaningless words. They are designed to reduce the listener's reliance on linguistic skills while preserving the syntax and temporal features of the English language (Jerger and Jerger, 1974). The SSI-ICM test sentences were presented at different signal to noise ratios in the same ear making the task more challenging at higher signal-to-noise ratios. The −10 and −20 dB SNR condition of the SSI-ICM was considered the most challenging test of speech processing used. The competing message was 10 dB louder than the target signal/sentence in −10 dB SNR, and 20 dB louder than the target signal in −20 dB SNR conditions, which results in a more distorted signal in comparison to the Quick-SIN and 0 and +10 dB SNR conditions of the SSI-ICM.

Consequently, the SMC group performed significantly poorer than the control group only in a subset of CAP tests, despite there being no significant difference between the peripheral hearing thresholds of the two groups. This is not surprising, as a more distorted speech signal requires greater processing for speech understanding, which then subsequently places increased strain on the higher-order auditory processing skills and consequently requires more cognitive resources (Bellis and Jorgensen, 2014). To recognize speech in challenging situations, proficient listeners rely either on high predictability or clarity of the speech (Bradlow and Alexander, 2007). The SSI-ICM target sentences are semantically and syntactically unrelated; hence predictability is poor. Medwetsky (1994, 2011), reported that the spatial location of the sound sources and fundamental frequency differences in talkers allows the speakers to segregate the acoustic signals into meaningful units. In the absence of both spatial and fundamental frequency difference cues, short sentences with 5–6 word length can still be recalled to a certain extent (Medwetsky, 1994). In this study SSI-ICM sentences contained seven words in each sentence list, hence the listeners could not rely on spatial cues or talker gender differences to segregate the information into different acoustic streams, making the task extremely difficult.

Several neural networks are required to work synchronously to facilitate speech recognition. For example, the lateral prefrontal cortex is involved in the organization and execution of behavior, speech and reasoning (Fuster, 2001), the posterior portion of Broca's area plays a vital role in processing phonological working memory information (Gelfand and Bookheimer, 2003), primary and associated auditory cortices with stream segregation during auditory scene analysis (Deike et al., 2004, 2010; Gutschalk et al., 2007), posterior superior temporal gyrus and planum temporale with the detailed perceptual representation of segregated objects (Schönwiesner et al., 2007), parietal cortex in mapping sensory inputs to motor actions (Cusack, 2005; Cohen, 2009) and mid-ventrolateral prefrontal cortex driving the top-down attentional processes (Schönwiesner et al., 2007).

Tuwaig et al. (2017) reported an association between poor SSI-ICM scores (−10 dB SNR) and atrophy in the right Heschl's gyrus cortical thickness and thinner right parahippocampal and entorhinal cortices, bilateral precuneus, occipital cortex, left inferior parietal lobule, inferior and mid temporal gyri on structural magnetic resonance imaging (MRI), after adjusting for age, gender, education, pure-tone hearing, and *APOE* ε4 status. Heschl's gyrus is involved in the temporal processing of the auditory signal (Zatorre and Belin, 2001). The inferior parietal lobe plays a vital role in auditory working memory: integration of sensory-motor information and monitoring and updating the location of the sound source (Alain et al., 2008). Changes in the cortical thickness of inferior parietal cortices are observed early in the neurodegeneration from normal to MCI, and neurodegeneration of parahippocampal/entorhinal regions is seen in progression from MCI to AD (Devanand et al., 2012). Neuroimaging studies that examined the biomarkers of early AD (accumulation of global Aβ and tau burdens) in SMC individuals have found an increased accumulation of early tauopathy in the entorhinal cortex (Buckley et al., 2017) as well as an increase in global Aβ burden (Rodda et al., 2010; Amariglio et al., 2012); both are considered neuropathological hallmarks of AD (Braak and Braak, 1997). Attending to a challenging task such as SSI-ICM requires the optimal functioning of neural networks. Hence, we propose that neuropathological impairment associated with SMC may have impeded their ability in segregating foreground from background information under higher signal-to-noise ratios reflecting in poor performances in the SSI-ICM task.

Furthermore, if numerous cognitive processes and auditory processing skills are required for the SSI-ICM, this suggests the task is highly taxing on an individual's finite pool of cognitive resources. In this study perhaps individuals with SMC could compensate for impaired CAP skills by drawing on more upstream cognitive resources until the task became too demanding and the cognitive resources are exhausted, creating significant differences between the SMCs and control group. Therefore, given the numerous cortical areas and cognitive processes involved in attending to the SSI-ICM task, it can be expected that this task would be sensitive to the effects of potential neurodegeneration in SMC populations.

In our study, the SMC group did not perform significantly poorer than the non-SMCs in the peripheral hearing assessment. Both participant groups performed within the normal range for the global cognitive functions, yet SMCs performed poorly in some of the CAP functions. Two prominent theories have been proposed to explain the interaction between peripheral hearing and CAP in older adults: the central effects of biological aging (CEBA) and central effects of peripheral pathology (CEPP; Willott, 1996). Central effects of biological aging hypothesis is that changes in central hearing occur due to the anatomical and physiological changes that occur in the central nervous system as a result of aging without any peripheral deficits. Evidence from animal studies that have reported age-related pathophysiological changes in the central auditory pathway without any peripheral impairment (Walton et al., 1998; Ouda and Syka, 2012) seems to support this hypothesis. The CEPP hypothesis argues that the pathophysiological changes in the central auditory pathway occur as a result of peripheral hearing impairment (Willott, 1996). Increase in the cognitive load resulting from peripheral hearing loss (CHABA, 1988; Lindenberger and Baltes, 1994) or longstanding hearing loss could lead to impaired cognitive functions (CHABA, 1988; Lindenberger and Baltes, 1994; Schneider and Pichora-Fuller, 2000; Lin et al., 2011b, 2013; Humes et al., 2012). As there was no significant difference between the peripheral hearing thresholds of the SMC and non-SMC groups, our study supports the CEBA theory; therefore, we conclude that CAP deficits that we have seen may indicate early signs of neurodegeneration.

Similar to previous findings (O'Grady et al., 2007; Tuwaig et al., 2017), we also failed to observe any significant difference between *APOE* ε4 carriers and non-carriers on peripheral hearing thresholds. However, in the Leiden 85-plus Study (Kurniawan et al., 2012), participants with the *APOE* ε4/ε4 genotype had more than moderately-severe levels of hearing loss (n = 6; mean 56.1 dBHL) and participants with the *APOE* ε3/ε4 or ε2/ε4 genotype showed moderate levels of (n = 89, mean 51.0 dBHL) while those without the *APOE*-ε4 allele (n = 340) had the poorest levels of hearing loss (48.9 dBHL). In our study, the recruited participants had 4PTA [4-frequency pure-tone average 500, 1000, 2000, and 4000 Hz) hearing thresholds within approximately 25 dBHL but were significantly younger than the Kurniawan et al. (2012) study, furthermore, the number of carriers was not large enough to confirm whether such differences would exist in higher levels of hearing losses. However, the mechanism underlying these observations should be explored in a larger sample size.

This study was considered a cross-sectional pilot study and consequently was limited in its interpretation and relatively small sample size. Ideally, the CAP skills of more participants should be examined longitudinally to note any deterioration in participants' cognition and/or CAP skills. Our study also did not have access to brain imaging that could have been informative in substantiating the presence or absence of neurodegenerative processes (if any) in their earlier stages.

In summary, the results of this study are cautiously promising and have established a potential diagnostic opportunity in identifying probable pre-clinical AD that may assist in delaying or arresting the cognitive decline in older adults. However, these results should be validated and replicated in larger groups over a more extended period. Furthermore, future research can combine these two measures (CAP and SMC) to examine the predictive value of each one as well as the increased accuracy when they are used together. While SSI and SMC are independent, the added benefit of using these two in identifying individuals at higher risk of dementia is another potential research that can inform the field.

AUTHOR CONTRIBUTIONS

DJ: study design and manuscript preparation. HM, JG-S, and JY: hearing data collection. KT, SL, and MW: genetic assessment. RM and HS: cognitive assessment. All authors provided interpretation of the results and reviewed the manuscript.

ACKNOWLEDGMENTS

This study was supported by the Australian Alzheimer's Research Foundation and the Ear Science Institute, Australia.

REFERENCES

Alain, C., He, Y., and Grady, C. (2008). The contribution of the inferior parietal lobe to auditory spatial working memory. *J. Cogn. Neurosci.* 20, 285–295. doi: 10.1162/jocn.2008.20014

Albert, M. S., Dekosky, S. T., Dickson, D., Dubois, B., Feldman, H. H., Fox, N. C., et al. (2013). The Diagnosis of Mild Cognitive Impairment due to Alzheimer's Disease: recommendations from the National Institute on Aging-Alzheimer's Association Workgroups on Diagnostic Guidelines for Alzheimer's disease. *FOCUS* 11, 96–106. doi: 10.1176/appi.focus.11.1.96

Amariglio, R. E., Becker, J. A., Carmasin, J., Wadsworth, L. P., Lorius, N., Sullivan, C., et al. (2012). Subjective cognitive complaints and amyloid burden in cognitively normal older individuals. *Neuropsychologia* 50, 2880–2886. doi: 10.1016/j.neuropsychologia.2012.08.011

Bellis, T. J., and Jorgensen, L. E. (2014). "Aging of the auditory system and differential diagnosis of central auditory processing disorders in older listeners," in *Handbook of Central Auditory Processing Disorders*, Vol. I, eds E. F. Musiek and G. D. Chermak (San Diego, CA: Plural Publishing Inc), 598–642.

Billig, A. J., Davis, M. H., Deeks, J. M., Monstrey, J., and Carlyon, R. P. (2013). Lexical Influences on Auditory Streaming. *Curr. Biol.* 23, 1585–1589. doi: 10.1016/j.cub.2013.06.042

Braak, H., and Braak, E. (1997). Frequency of Stages of Alzheimer-Related Lesions in Different Age Categories. *Neurobiol. Aging* 18, 351–357. doi: 10.1016/S0197-4580(97)00056-0

Bradlow, A. R., and Alexander, J. A. (2007). Semantic and phonetic enhancements for speech-in-noise recognition by native and non-native listeners. *J. Acoust. Soc. Am.* 121, 2339–2349. doi: 10.1121/1.2642103

Bregman, A. S. (1990). *Auditory Scene Analysis: The Perceptual Organization of Sound.* Cambridge, MA: MIT Press.

Buckley, R. F., Hanseeuw, B., Schultz, A. P., Vannini, P., Aghjayan, S. L., Properzi, M. J., et al. (2017). Region-Specific Association of Subjective Cognitive Decline With Tauopathy Independent of Global β-Amyloid Burden. *JAMA Neurol.* 74, 1455–1463. doi: 10.1001/jamaneurol.2017.2216

Cai, Y., An, S. S., and Kim, S. (2015). Mutations in presenilin 2 and its implications in Alzheimer's disease and other dementia-associated disorders. *Clin. Intervent. Aging* 10, 1163–1172. doi: 10.2147/CIA.S85808

Carlyon, R. P., Cusack, R., Foxton, J. M., and Robertson, I. H. (2001). Effects of attention and unilateral neglect on auditory stream segregation. *J. Exp. Psychol. Hum. Percept. Perform.* 27, 115–127. doi: 10.1037//0096-1523.27.1.11510.1016/j.cub.2013.06.042

CHABA (1988). Speech Understanding and Aging. Working Group on Speech Understanding and Aging. Committee on Hearing, Bioacoustics, and Biomechanics, Commission on Behavioral and Social Sciences and Education, National Research Council. *J. Acoust. Soc. Am.* 83, 859–895. doi: 10.1121/1.395965

Chermak, G. D., and Lee, J. (2005). Comparison of children's performance on four tests of temporal resolution. *J. Am. Acad. Audiol.* 16, 554–563.

Choe, N., Ousset, P. J., Andrieu, S., Mathiex-Fortunet, H., Vellas, B., and GuidAge Study Group. (2018). Memory complaints to the general practitioner: data from the GuidAge study. *J. Nutr. Health Aging* 12, S66–S72.

Cohen, Y. E. (2009). Multimodal activity in the parietal cortex. *Hear. Res.* 258, 100–105. doi: 10.1016/j.heares.2009.01.011

Coley, N., Ousset, P. J., Andrieu, S., Mathiex-Fortunet, H., Vellas, B., The, et al. (2008). Memory complaints to the general practitioner: data from the GuidAge study. *J. Nutr. Health Aging* 12, S66–S72. doi: 10.1007/BF02982590

Crook, T. H., Feher, E. P., and Larrabee, G. J. (1992). Assessment of Memory Complaint in Age-Associated Memory Impairment: the MAC-Q. *Int. Psychogeriatr.* 4, 165–176. doi: 10.1017/S1041610292000991

Cusack, R. (2005). The Intraparietal Sulcus and Perceptual Organization. *J. Cogn. Neurosci.* 17, 641–651. doi: 10.1162/0898929053467541

Deal, J. A., Betz, J., Yaffe, K., Harris, T., Purchase-Helzner, E., Satterfield, S., et al. (2016). Hearing impairment and incident dementia and cognitive decline in older adults: the Health ABC Study. *J. Gerontol. Ser. A Biol. Sci. Med. Sci.* 72, 703–709. doi: 10.1093/gerona/glw069

Deike, S., Gaschler-Markefski, B., Brechmann, A., and Scheich, H. (2004). Auditory stream segregation relying on timbre involves left auditory cortex. *NeuroReport* 15, 1511–1514. doi: 10.1097/01.wnr.0000132919.12990.34

Deike, S., Scheich, H., and Brechmann, A. (2010). Active stream segregation specifically involves the left human auditory cortex. *Hear. Res.* 265, 30–37. doi: 10.1016/j.heares.2010.03.005

Devanand, D. P., Bansal, R., Liu, J., Hao, X., Pradhaban, G., and Peterson, B. S. (2012). MRI hippocampal and entorhinal cortex mapping in predicting conversion to Alzheimer's disease. *NeuroImage* 60, 1622–1629. doi: 10.1016/j.neuroimage.2012.01.075

Edwards, J. D., Lister, J. J., Elias, M. N., Tetlow, A. M., Sardina, A. L., Sadeq, N. A., et al. (2017). Auditory Processing of Older Adults With Probable Mild Cognitive Impairment. *J. Speech Lang. Hear. Res.* 60, 1427–1435.

Fifer, R. C., Jerger, J. F., Berlin, C. I., Tobey, E. A., and Campbell, J. C. (1983). Development of a dichotic sentence identification test for hearing-impaired adults. *Ear Hear.* 4, 300–305.

Fortunato, S., Forli, F., Guglielmi, V., De Corso, E., Paludetti, G., Berrettini, S., et al. (2016). A review of new insights on the association between hearing loss and cognitive decline in ageing. *Acta Otorhinolaryngol. Ital.* 36, 155–166. doi: 10.14639/0392-100x-993

Friedman, R. A., Van Laer, L., Huentelman, M. J., Sheth, S. S., Van Eyken, E., Corneveaux, J. J., et al. (2009). GRM7 variants confer susceptibility to age-related hearing impairment. *Hum. Mol. Genet.* 18, 785–796. doi: 10.1093/hmg/ddn402

Fuster, J. M. (2001). *The Prefrontal Cortex—An Update: Time Is of the Essence Neuron*, Vol. 30. Amsterdam: Elsevier Inc, 319–333.

Gates, G. A., Anderson, M. L., Feeney, M. P., McCurry, S. M., and Larson, E. B. (2008). Central auditory dysfunction in older persons with memory impairment or Alzheimer's dementia. *Arch. Otolaryngol. Head Neck Surg.* 134, 771–777.

Gates, G. A., Anderson, M. L., McCurry, S. M., Feeney, M. P., and Larson, E. B. (2011). Central auditory dysfunction as a harbinger of Alzheimer's dementia. (Clinical report). *Arch. Otolaryngol. Head Neck Surg.* 137:390.

Gates, G. A., Beiser, A., Rees, T. S., D' Agostino, R. B., Wolf, P. A., Gates, G. A., et al. (2002). Central Auditory Dysfunction May Precede the Onset of Clinical Dementia in People with Probable Alzheimer's Disease. *J. Am. Geriatr. Soc.* 50, 482–488. doi: 10.1046/j.1532-5415.2002.50114.x

Gates, G. A., Cobb, J. L., Linn, R. T., Rees, T., Wolf, P. A., and D'Agostino, R. B. (1996). Central auditory dysfunction, cognitive dysfunction, and dementia in older people. *Arch. Otolaryngol. Head Neck Surg.* 122, 161–167.

Gates, G. A., Couropmitree, N. N., and Myers, R. H. (1999). Genetic Associations in Age-Related Hearing Thresholds. *Arch. Otolaryngol. Head Neck Surg.* 125, 654.

Gates, G. A., Gibbons, L. E., McCurry, S. M., Crane, P. K., Feeney, M. P., and Larson, E. B. (2010). Executive dysfunction and presbycusis in older persons with and without memory loss and dementia. *Cogn. Behav. Neurol.* 23, 218. doi: 10.1097/WNN.0b013e3181d748d7

Gates, G. A., and Mills, J. H. (2005). Presbycusis. *Lancet* 366, 1111–1120.

Gelfand, J. R., and Bookheimer, S. Y. (2003). Dissociating Neural Mechanisms of Temporal Sequencing and Processing Phonemes. *Neuron* 38, 831–842. doi: 10.1016/S0896-6273(03)00285-X

Glisky, E. L. (2007). *Changes in Cognitive Function in Human Aging Brain Aging: Models, Methods, and Mechanisms.* Boca Raton, FL: CRC Press, 3–20.

Glodzik-Sobanska, L., Reisberg, B., De Santi, S., Babb, J. S., Pirraglia, E., Rich, K. E., et al. (2007). Subjective memory complaints: presence, severity and future outcome in normal older subjects. *Dement. Geriatr. Cogn. Disord.* 24, 177–184. doi: 10.1159/000105604

Golden, H. L., Nicholas, J. M., Yong, K. X. X., Downey, L. E., Schott, J. M., Mummery, C. J., et al. (2015). Auditory spatial processing in Alzheimer's disease. *Brain* 138, 189–202. doi: 10.1093/brain/awu337

Gutschalk, A., Oxenham, A. J., Micheyl, C., Wilson, E. C., and Melcher, J. R. (2007). Human Cortical Activity during Streaming without Spectral Cues Suggests a General Neural Substrate for Auditory Stream Segregation. *J. Neurosci.* 27, 13074–13081. doi: 10.1523/JNEUROSCI.2299-07.2007

Hardy, J. (2017). The discovery of Alzheimer-causing mutations in the APP gene and the formulation of the "amyloid cascade hypothesis". *FEBS J.* 284, 1040–1044. doi: 10.1111/febs.14004

Humes, L. E., Dubno, J. R., Gordon-Salant, S., Lister, J. J., Cacace, A. T., Cruickshanks, K. J., et al. (2012). Central presbycusis: a review and evaluation of the evidence. *J. Am. Acad. Audiol.* 23, 635–666. doi: 10.3766/jaaa.23.8.5

Idrizbegovic, E., Hederstierna, C., Dahlquist, M., and Rosenhall, U. (2013). Short-term longitudinal study of central auditory function in Alzheimer's disease and mild cognitive impairment. *Dement. Geriatr. Cogn. Dis. Extra* 3, 468–471. doi: 10.1159/000355371

Jack, C. R., Albert, M. S., Knopman, D. S., McKhann, G. M., Sperling, R. A., Carrillo, M. C., et al. (2011). Introduction to the recommendations from the National Institute on Aging-Alzheimer's Association workgroups on diagnostic guidelines for Alzheimer's disease. *Alzheimer's Dement.* 7, 257–262. doi: 10.1016/j.jalz.2011.03.004

Jayakody, D. M. P., Friedland, P. L., Eikelboom, R. H., Martins, R. N., and Sohrabi, H. R. (2017). A novel study on the association between untreated hearing loss and cognitive functions of older adults: baseline non-verbal cognitive assessment results. *Clin. Otolaryngol.* 43, 182–191. doi: 10.1111/coa.12937

Jerger, J., and Jerger, S. (1974). Auditory findings in brain stem disorders. *Arch. Otolaryngol.* 99, 342–350. doi: 10.1001/archotol.1974.00780030354006

Jessen, F., Amariglio, R. E., van Boxtel, M., Breteler, M., Ceccaldi, M., Chételat, G., et al. (2014). A conceptual framework for research on subjective cognitive decline in pre-clinical Alzheimer's disease. *Alzheimer's Dement.* 10, 844–852. doi: 10.1016/j.jalz.2014.01.001

Karlsson, K. K., Harris, J. R., and Svartengren, M. (1997). Description and primary results from an audiometric study of male twins. *Ear Hear.* 18, 114. doi: 10.1097/00003446-199704000-00003

Killion, M. C., Niquette, P. A., Gudmundsen, G. I., Revit, L. J., and Banerjee, S. (2004). Development of a quick speech-in-noise test for measuring signal-to-noise ratio loss in normal-hearing and hearing-impaired listeners. *J. Acous. Soc. Am.* 16, 2395–2405.

Koivisto, K., Reinikainen, K. J., Hänninen, T., Vanhanen, M., Helkala, E. L., Mykkänen, L., et al., (1995). Prevalence of age-associated memory impairment in a randomly selected population from eastern Finland. *Neurology* 45, 741–747.

Kurniawan, C., Westendorp, R. G., de Craen, A. J., Gussekloo, J., de Laat, J., and van Exel, E. (2012). Gene dose of apolipoprotein E and age-related hearing loss. *Neurobiol. Aging* 33, 2230.e2237-2230.e2212. doi: 10.1016/j.neurobiolaging.2012.04.001

Lambert, M. A., Bickel, H., Prince, M., Fratiglioni, L., Von Strauss, E., Frydecka, D., et al. (2014). Estimating the burden of early-onset dementia; systematic review of disease prevalence. *Eur. J. Neurol.* 21, 563–569.

Lin, F. R., Metter, E. J., O'Brien, R. J., Resnick, S. M., Zonderman, A. B., and Ferrucci, L. (2011a). Hearing loss and incident dementia. *Arch. Neurol.* 68, 214–220. doi: 10.1001/archneurol.2010.362

Lin, F. R., Thorpe, R., Gordon-Salant, S., and Ferrucci, L. (2011b). Hearing Loss Prevalence and Risk Factors Among Older Adults in the United States. *J. Gerontol. Ser. A* 66A, 582–590. doi: 10.1093/gerona/glr002

Lin, F. R., Yaffe, K., Xia, J., Xue, Q.-L., Harris, T. B., Purchase-Helzner, E., et al. (2013). Hearing loss and cognitive decline in older adults. *JAMA Int. Med.* 173, 293–299.

Lindenberger, U., and Baltes, P. B. (1994). Sensory Functioning and Intelligence in Old Age: a Strong Connection. *Psychol. Aging* 9, 339–355.

Livingston, G., Huntley, J., Sommerlad, A., Ames, D., Ballard, C., Banerjee, S., et al. (2020). Dementia prevention, intervention, and care: 2020 report of the Lancet Commission. *Lancet* 396, 413–446. doi: 10.1016/S0140-6736(20)30367-6

McKhann, G. M., Knopman, D. S., Chertkow, H., Hyman, B. T., Jack, C. R., Kawas, C. H., et al. (2011). The diagnosis of dementia due to Alzheimer's disease: recommendations from the National Institute on Aging-Alzheimer's Association workgroups on diagnostic guidelines for Alzheimer's disease. *Alzheimer's Dement.* 7, 263–269. doi: 10.1016/j.jalz.2011.03.005

Medwetsky, L. (1994). *The Importance of Spatial and Talker Cues in Competing Sentence Recall.* Unpublished Doctoral thesis, City University of New York, New York, NY.

Medwetsky, L. (2011). Spoken language processing model: bridging auditory and language processing to guide assessment and intervention. *Lang. Speech Hear. Serv. Sch.* 42, 286–296. doi: 10.1044/0161-1461(2011/10-0036)

Mener, D. J., Betz, J., Yaffe, K., Harris, T. B., Helzner, E. P., Satterfield, S., et al. (2016). Apolipoprotein E Allele and Hearing Thresholds in Older Adults. *Am. J. Alzheimers Dis. Other Dement.* 31, 34–39. doi: 10.1177/1533317514537549

Musiek, E. F. (1983). Assessment of Central Auditory Dysfunction: the Dichotic Digit Test Revisited. *Ear Hear.* 4, 79–83. doi: 10.1097/00003446-198303000-00002

Musiek, F. E. (1994). Frequency (pitch) and duration pattern tests. *J. Am. Acad. Audiol.* 5, 265–268.

Musiek, F. E., and Chermak, G. D. (1994). Three commonly asked questions about central auditory processing disorders: assessment. *Am. J. Audiol.* 3, 23–27. doi: 10.1044/1059-0889.0303.23

Musiek, F. E., and Chermak, G. D. (2013). *Handbook of Central Auditory Processing Disorder Volume 1 Auditory Neuroscience and Diagnosis*, 2nd Edn, Vol. 1. San Diego, CA: Plural Publishing, Inc.

Musiek, F. E., Gollegly, K. M., Kibbe, K. S., and Verkest-Lenz, S. B. (1991). Proposed screening test for central auditory disorders: follow up on the dichotic digits test. *Test Otol. Neurotol.* 12, 109–113.

Nasreddine, Z. S., Phillips, N. A., Bedirian, V., Charbonneau, S., Whitehead, V., Collin, I., et al. (2005). The Montreal Cognitive Assessment, MoCA: a brief screening tool for mild cognitive impairment. *J. Am. Geriatr. Soc.* 53, 695–699. doi: 10.1111/j.1532-5415.2005.53221.x

O'Grady, G., Boyles, A. L., Speer, M., DeRuyter, F., Strittmatter, W., and Worley, G. (2007). Apolipoprotein E alleles and sensorineural hearing loss. *Int. J. Audiol.* 46, 183–186. doi: 10.1080/14992020601145294

Orchik, D. J., and Burgess, J. (1977). Synthetic sentence identification as a function of the age of the listener. *Ear Hear.* 3, 42–46.

Ouda, L., and Syka, J. (2012). Immunocytochemical profiles of inferior colliculus neurons in the rat and their changes with aging. *Front. Neural Circ.* 6:68. doi: 10.3389/fncir.2012.00068

Panza, F., Lozupone, M., Sardone, R., Battista, P., Piccininni, M., Dibello, V., et al. (2018). Sensorial frailty: age-related hearing loss and the risk of cognitive impairment and dementia in later life. *Ther. Adv. Chronic Dis.* 10:2040622318811000.

Poorkaj, P., Sharma, V., Anderson, L., Nemens, E., Alonso, M. E., Orr, H., et al. (1998). Missense mutations in the chromosome 14 familial Alzheimer's disease presenilin 1 gene. *Hum. Mutat.* 11, 216–221. doi: 10.1002/(sici)1098-1004199811:3<216::aid-humu6<3.0.co;2-f

Prince, M., Wimo, A., Guerchet, M., Ali, G. C., Wu, Y. T., and Prina, M. (2015). *World Alzheimer's Report 2015—the Global Impact of Dementia: An Analysis of Prevalence, Incidence, Cost and Trends.* London: Alzheimer's Disease International.

Quaranta, N., Coppola, F., Casulli, M., Barulli, O., Lanza, F., Tortelli, R., et al. (2015). The prevalence of peripheral and central hearing impairment and its relation to cognition in older adults. *Audiol. Neurootol.* 19, 10–14. doi: 10.1159/000371597

Rodda, J., Okello, A., Edison, P., Dannhauser, T., Brooks, D. J., and Walker, Z. (2010). (11)C-PIB PET in subjective cognitive impairment. *Eur. Psychiatry* 25, 123–125. doi: 10.1016/j.eurpsy.2009.07.011

Rönnlund, M., Sundström, A., Adolfsson, R., Nilsson, L.-G., Rönnlund, M., Sundström, A., et al. (2015). Subjective memory impairment in older adults predicts future dementia independent of baseline memory performance: Evidence from the Betula prospective cohort study. *Alzheimers Dement.* 11, 1385–1392. doi: 10.1016/j.jalz.2014.11.006

Rossetti, H. C., Lacritz, L. H., Cullum, C. M., and Weiner, M. F. (2011). Normative data for the Montreal Cognitive Assessment (MoCA) in a population-based sample. *Neurology* 77, 1272–1275.

Scheef, T. L., Spottke, J. A., Daerr, H. M., Joe, H. A., Striepens, H. N., Kölsch, H. H., et al. (2012). Glucose metabolism, gray matter structure, and memory decline in subjective memory impairment. *Neurology* 79, 1332–1339. doi: 10.1212/WNL.0b013e31826c1a8d

Schneider, B. A., and Pichora-Fuller, M. K. (2000). *Implications of Perceptual Deterioration for Cognitive Aging Research The Handbook of Aging and Cognition*, 2nd Edn. Mahwah, NJ: Lawrence Erlbaum Associates Publishers, 155–219.

Schönwiesner, M., Novitski, N., Pakarinen, S., Carlson, S., Tervaniemi, M., and Näätänen, R. (2007). Heschl's Gyrus, Posterior Superior Temporal Gyrus, and Mid-Ventrolateral Prefrontal Cortex Have Different Roles in the Detection of Acoustic Changes. *J. Neurophysiol.* 97, 2075–2082. doi: 10.1152/jn.01083.2006

Serrano-Pozo, A., Frosch, M. P., Masliah, E., and Hyman, B. T. (2011). Neuropathological alterations in Alzheimer's disease. *Cold Spring Harb. Perspect. Med.* 1:a006189. doi: 10.1101/cshperspect.a006189

Sohrabi, H. R., Bates, K. A., Weinborn, M. G., Johnston, A. N. B., Bahramian, A., Taddei, K., et al. (2012). Olfactory discrimination predicts cognitive decline among community-dwelling older adults. *Transl. Psychiatry* 2:e118.

Sohrabi, H. R., Weinborn, M., Laske, C., Bates, K. A., Christensen, D., Taddei, K., et al. (2019). Subjective memory complaints predict baseline but not future cognitive function over three years: results from the Western Australia Memory Study. *Int. Psychogeriatr.* 31, 513–525.

Speaks, C., Karmen, J. L., and Benitez, L. (1967). Effect of a competing message on synthetic sentence identification. *J. Speech Hear. Res.* 10, 390–395. doi: 10.1044/jshr.1002.390

Sperling, R. A., Aisen, P. S., Beckett, L. A., Bennett, D. A., Craft, S., Fagan, A. M., et al. (2011). Toward defining the pre-clinical stages of Alzheimer's disease: recommendations from the National Institute on Aging-Alzheimer's Association workgroups on diagnostic guidelines for Alzheimer's disease. *Alzheimer's Dement.* 7, 280–292. doi: 10.1016/j.jalz.2011.03.003

Tuwaig, M., Savard, M., Jutras, B., Poirier, J., Collins, D. L., Rosa-Neto, P., et al. (2017). Deficit in central auditory processing as a biomarker of pre-clinical Alzheimer's disease. *J. Alzheimer's Dis.* 60, 1589–1600. doi: 10.3233/JAD-170545

Walton, J. P., Frisina, R. D., and O'Neill, W. E. (1998). Age-related alteration in the processing of temporal sound features in the auditory midbrain of the CBA mouse. *J. Neurosci.* 18, 2764–2776. doi: 10.1523/JNEUROSCI.18-07-02764.1998

Wang, Y., West, J. D., Flashman, L. A., Wishart, H. A., Santulli, R. B., Rabin, L. A., et al. (2011). Selective changes in white matter integrity in MCI and older adults with cognitive complaints. *BBA Mol. Basis Dis.* 1822:2. doi: 10.1016/j.bbadis.2011.08.002

Willott, J. F. (1996). Anatomic and physiologic aging: a behavioral neuroscience perspective. *J. Am. Acad. Audiol.* 7, 141–151.

Zatorre, R. J., and Belin, P. (2001). Spectral and temporal processing in human auditory cortex. *Cereb. Cortex*11, 946–953. doi: 10.1093/cercor/11.10.946

15

Disruption of *Hars2* in Cochlear Hair Cells Causes Progressive Mitochondrial Dysfunction and Hearing Loss in Mice

Pengcheng Xu[1,2,3†], *Longhao Wang*[1,2,3†], *Hu Peng*[4], *Huihui Liu*[1,2,3], *Hongchao Liu*[1,2,3], *Qingyue Yuan*[1,2,3], *Yun Lin*[1,2,3], *Jun Xu*[1,2,3], *Xiuhong Pang*[5*], *Hao Wu*[1,2,3*] and *Tao Yang*[1,2,3*]

[1] Department of Otolaryngology-Head and Neck Surgery, Shanghai Ninth People's Hospital, Shanghai Jiao Tong University School of Medicine, Shanghai, China, [2] Ear Institute, Shanghai Jiao Tong University School of Medicine, Shanghai, China, [3] Shanghai Key Laboratory of Translational Medicine on Ear and Nose Diseases, Shanghai, China, [4] Department of Otolaryngology-Head and Neck Surgery, Changzheng Hospital, Second Military Medical University, Shanghai, China, [5] Department of Otolaryngology-Head and Neck Surgery, Taizhou People's Hospital, The Fifth Affiliated Hospital of Nantong University, Taizhou, China

***Correspondence:**
Tao Yang
yangtfxl@sina.com
Hao Wu
wuhao@shsmu.edu.cn
Xiuhong Pang
pxhzxy@163.com

† These authors have contributed equally to this work

Mutations in a number of genes encoding mitochondrial aminoacyl-tRNA synthetases lead to non-syndromic and/or syndromic sensorineural hearing loss in humans, while their cellular and physiological pathology in cochlea has rarely been investigated *in vivo*. In this study, we showed that histidyl-tRNA synthetase HARS2, whose deficiency is associated with Perrault syndrome 2 (PRLTS2), is robustly expressed in postnatal mouse cochlea including the outer and inner hair cells. Targeted knockout of *Hars2* in mouse hair cells resulted in delayed onset (P30), rapidly progressive hearing loss similar to the PRLTS2 hearing phenotype. Significant hair cell loss was observed starting from P45 following elevated reactive oxygen species (ROS) level and activated mitochondrial apoptotic pathway. Despite of normal ribbon synapse formation, whole-cell patch clamp of the inner hair cells revealed reduced calcium influx and compromised sustained synaptic exocytosis prior to the hair cell loss at P30, consistent with the decreased supra-threshold wave I amplitudes of the auditory brainstem response. Starting from P14, increasing proportion of morphologically abnormal mitochondria was observed by transmission electron microscope, exhibiting swelling, deformation, loss of cristae and emergence of large intrinsic vacuoles that are associated with mitochondrial dysfunction. Though the mitochondrial abnormalities are more prominent in inner hair cells, it is the outer hair cells suffering more severe cell loss. Taken together, our results suggest that conditional knockout of *Hars2* in mouse cochlear hair cells leads to accumulating mitochondrial dysfunction and ROS stress, triggers progressive hearing loss highlighted by hair cell synaptopathy and apoptosis, and is differentially perceived by inner and outer hair cells.

Keywords: *HARS2*, mitochondrial, apoptosis, hair cells, hearing loss

INTRODUCTION

Hearing loss is the most common sensory disorder affecting approximately 6.1% of the world population (Davis and Hoffman, 2019), which can be caused by excessive noise exposure (Guo L. et al., 2021), ototoxic drugs (He et al., 2017; Li et al., 2018; Liu et al., 2019c, 2021; Zhong et al., 2020), aging (Cheng et al., 2019; Zhou et al., 2020; He et al., 2021), genetic factors (Qian et al., 2020;

Cheng et al., 2021; Fu et al., 2021a; Lv et al., 2021; Zhang S. et al., 2021), and infections (Han et al., 2020; He et al., 2020; Zhang Y. et al., 2021). To date, more than 100 genes have been identified associating with genetic hearing loss (Hereditary Hearing Loss Homepage; https://hereditaryhearingloss.org/, updated in September 2021), which contribute to more than 50% of congenital hearing loss as well as a significant portion of pediatric-onset hearing loss (Sheffield and Smith, 2019). Autosomal recessive mutations in a number of genes encoding Aminoacyl-tRNA synthetases (ARSs), including *HARS2* (Perrault syndrome 2), *LARS2* (Perrault syndrome 4), *NARS2* (DFNB94), *IARS2* (Cataracts, growth hormone deficiency, sensory neuropathy, sensorineural hearing loss, and skeletal dysplasia), *PARS2* (Developmental and epileptic encephalopathy 75 including deafness), and *KARS* (DFNB89) may lead to a variety of syndromic and non-syndromic hearing loss (Konovalova and Tyynismaa, 2013; Oprescu et al., 2017; Wang et al., 2020). ARSs are a group of nuclear-encoded enzymes that ensure correct translation of the genetic code by conjugating each of the 20 amino acids to their cognate tRNA molecule in the cytoplasm and mitochondria (Oprescu et al., 2017). Deficiency of ARSs, especially the mitochondrial ARSs (mtARSs) often affect tissues with high metabolic demands such as the brain, muscle, and inner ear (Fine et al., 2019). Clinical features associated with mutations in mtARS-encoding genes typically include encephalopathy, leukodystrophy, cardiomyopathy, ovarian dysgenesis, and deafness (Figuccia et al., 2021).

Characterized by enzyme kinetic assays, yeast complementation assays and studies of patient-derived cell cultures, most of the mtARS mutations have been shown to disrupt its aminoacylation activity (Oprescu et al., 2017; Figuccia et al., 2021). Previous study on a *Dars2* conditional knockout mouse showed that DARS2 depletion in heart and skeletal muscle causes severe dysfunction of mitochondrial protein synthesis in both tissues, which activates various stress responses predominantly in the cardiomyocytes (Dogan et al., 2014). In another *Dars2* neuron-specific knockout mouse, the immune and cell stress pathways have been shown to be initiated prior to behavioral dysfunction and cerebral deficits (Nemeth et al., 2020). Studies in zebrafish and rat have shown that inhibition of WARS2 leads to cardiac angiogenesis defects and impaired heart function (Wang et al., 2016). A mouse line harboring hypomorphic p.V117L mutation in *Wars2* displays various pathologies including progressive hearing loss, adipose dysfunction and hypertrophic cardiomyopathy (Agnew et al., 2018). The homozygous mutant mice have been shown to gradually lose their outer hair cells and spiral ganglion neurons, but the cellular pathogenesis associated with the hearing loss has not been studied in depth.

Numerous studies have shown that mitochondrial dysfunction is an important step toward a broad spectrum of sensorineural hearing loss associated with noise, ototoxic-drug, and aging (Fischel-Ghodsian et al., 2004; Zhang L. et al., 2021). For example, it has been reported that noise exposure leads to mitochondrial swollen and cristae disruption in outer hair cells and stria vascularis in guinea pig and rat (Spoendlin, 1971; Yu et al., 2014), administration of gentamicin induces opening of the mitochondrial permeability transition pore and reduction of mitochondrial membrane potential (Dehne et al., 2002), and accumulation of mitochondrial DNA common deletion contributes to development of age-related hearing loss (Du et al., 2012; Natarajan et al., 2020). As a major source of reactive oxygen species (ROS) production, mitochondrial dysfunction often leads to ROS formation and accumulation after noise (Wu et al., 2020) or ototoxic drug exposure (Fu et al., 2021b), and ultimately lead to death of hair cells and spiral ganglion neurons (Bock and Tait, 2020).

Though mutations in many mtARS-encoding genes are associated with sensorineural hearing loss, their cellular and physiological pathology in inner ear has rarely been investigated *in vivo*. In this study, we established a hair cell specific knockout mouse model for the mitochondrial histidyl-tRNA synthetase encoding gene *Hars2*, whose recessive mutations lead to decreased levels of aminoacylated $tRNA^{His}$ and sensorineural hearing loss with female ovarian dysgenesis (Perrault syndrome 2) in humans (Pierce et al., 2011), and whose overexpression restores mitochondrial dysfunction caused by a deafness-associated m.12201T > C mutation in $tRNA^{His}$ (Gong et al., 2020). Morphological and electrophysiological studies of this conditional knockout (CKO) mouse model furthered our understanding of the pathogenic mechanism underlying the mtARS-associated hearing loss.

MATERIALS AND METHODS

Generation and Genotyping of the *Hars2* Conditional Knockout Mice

The $Hars2^{Loxp/+}$ mice were generated using the CRISPR/Cas9 system (GemPharmatech, China). Briefly, Cas9 mRNA, single guide RNAs and donor were co-injected into the zygotes, directing Cas9 endonuclease cleavage and Loxp site insertion in intron 1 and intron 8 of mouse *Har2* (NM_080636.2, **Figure 1C**). As the $Hars2^{Loxp/Loxp}$; $ACTB^{Cre/+}$ full-body knockout (KO) mice die perinatally, the $Hars2^{Loxp/Loxp}$;$Gfi1^{Cre/+}$ mice (*Hars2* CKO mice) were used to specifically knockout *Hars2* in hair cells (Yang et al., 2010; He et al., 2019). Considering the $Gfi1^{Cre/+}$ mice have been previously reported to have early-onset, progressive hearing loss (Matern et al., 2017), we used littermates of the *Hars2* CKO and wild-type (WT) control mice under the same $Gfi1^{Cre/+}$ background. All animal procedures were approved by the Committee of Laboratory Animals of the Ninth People's Hospital, Shanghai Jiao Tong University School of Medicine. All efforts were practiced to minimize the number of animals used and to prevent their suffering.

For genotyping of the *Hars2* CKO mice, DNA was extracted from mouse tails and PCR amplified using the primers listed in **Supplementary Table 1**. The PCR products of 351, 256, and 672 bp represent the *Hars2* CKO, wild-type, and $Gfi1^{Cre}$ alleles, respectively (**Figure 1D**).

Auditory Brainstem Response

Auditory brainstem response (ABR) analysis was performed in anesthetized mice at P21, P30, P45, and P60. Following a

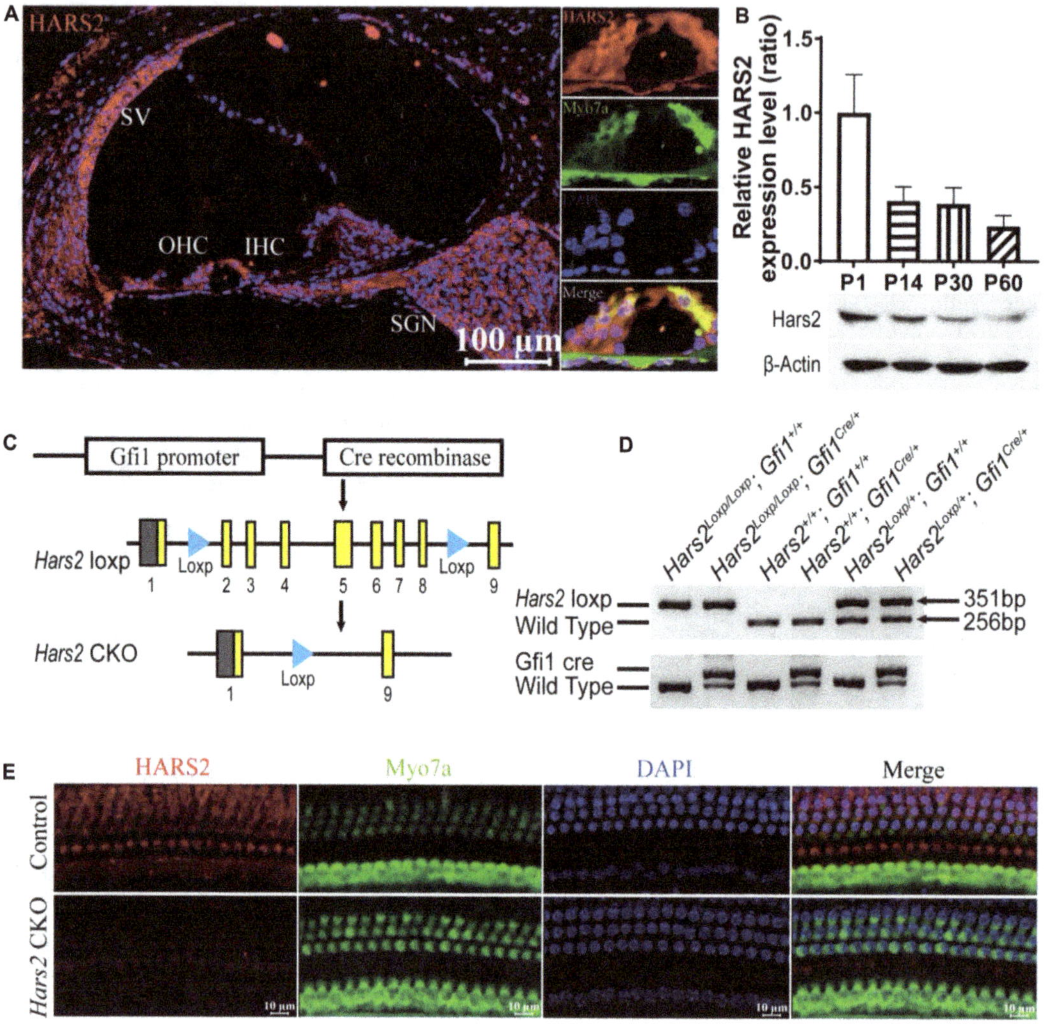

FIGURE 1 | Cochlear expression of HARS2 in the wild-type and *Hars2* CKO mice. **(A)** Immunofluorescence staining of HARS2 in cochlea (left) and organ of corti (right) of the wild-type mice at P30 using anti-HARS2 (red) and anti-Myo7a (green, labeling hair cells) antibodies and DAPI (blue). Scale bar = 100 µm. OHC, outer hair cell; IHC, inner hair cell; SGN, spiral ganglion neuron; SV, stria vascularis. **(B)** Relative protein expression levels of HARS2 at different ages by Western blotting, which was normalized by endogenous β-actin expression. **(C)** Generation of the hair cell-specific *Hars2* CKO mice with the Loxp sites inserted into intron 1 and 8 of mouse *Hars2* and crossed with the $Gfi1^{Cre}$. **(D)** Verification of targeted genomic deletion of the *Hars2*-Loxp allele by PCR amplification. **(E)** Immunofluorescence staining of HARS2 in the cochleae of P30 control and *Hars2* CKO mice, showing the successful knockout of *Hars2* in hair cells. Scale bars = 10 µm.

previously described protocol with minor modification (Zheng et al., 1999; Liu et al., 2019a), hearing thresholds at sound frequencies 4, 5.6, 8, 11.3, 16, 22.6, and 32 kHz were assessed in TDT system 3 (Tucker-Davies Technologies, United States). Briefly, Animals were deeply anesthetized with an intraperitoneal injection of 0.01 g/ml pentobarbital sodium (100 mg/kg), and body temperature was kept on 37°C in the recording process using a Homeothermic Monitoring System (Harvard Apparatus) in a soundproof chamber. ABR was recorded with three subcutaneously implanted stainless needle electrodes. The active electrode was positioned at the vertex, the reference at the right mastoid region, and the ground at the left shoulder. Before ABR analysis was conducted, mice with normal external auditory canal and tympanic membrane were examined using an otoscope. Pure tone bursts were produced by the RZ6 workstation (Tucker-Davis Technologies, United States). Free-field acoustic stimulation was performed through an MF1 speaker (Tucker-Davis Technologies, United States), located 10 cm from the vertex. The evoked potentials were filtered with a bandpass filter from 100 to 3000 Hz and averaged 400 times. For each analyzed frequency, the sound level was reduced from 90 to 0 dB SPL in 5 dB steps. ABR thresholds were determined by minimal stimulus level that evoked any visible recording of waveforms at each frequency. If the hearing threshold could not be measured at 90 dB SPL, the result was noted as threshold of 100 dB SPL for statistical analysis. All amplitudes and latencies of ABR peak I were measured and analyzed using BioSigRZ software (Tucker-Davis Technologies, United States) as previously described (Scimemi et al., 2014; McKay et al., 2015). Amplitude was calculated from the average value of $\triangle V$ on both sides of peak I, and latency referred to the time from the beginning of the stimulus signal to peak I.

Immunofluorescence Staining and Confocal Imaging

After animals were deeply anesthetized and sacrificed, cochleae were quickly harvested from dissected temporal bones in cold 4% paraformaldehyde (PFA). A small hole was punctured at the top of cochlea and then 4% PFA was slowly perfused through the small hole, oval window and round window. The cochleae were kept in this fixation overnight at 4°C. The next day, after decalcified in 10% EDTA for 2–24 h at room temperature according to postnatal age, the organ of corti was dissected and cut into three turns (apex, middle, and base) for immunofluorescent staining (Akil and Lustig, 2013). For frozen cochlear sections, after making sure the cochleae were soft enough after decalcification, the samples were dehydrated through the 15% and 30% sucrose solution successively for 24 h, immerged into the OCT compound (Sakura Finetek United States, Inc., 4583) and hardened at −20°C. Slices with thickness of 10 μm were cut through the modiolus by a freezing microtome (Leica Biosystems Inc., CM3050S). Slices containing 3–4 organs of corti were collected on glass slides.

For immunofluorescent staining, all samples were first permeabilized with 1% Triton X-100 for 1 h and immersed in blocking solution containing 10% goat serum, 1% bovine serum albumin, and 1% Triton X-100 in PBS (pH 7.2) for 2 h at room temperature. The samples were then incubated with primary antibodies including mouse monoclonal anti-Myo7a (Developmental Studies Hybridoma Bank, MYO7A 138-1), rabbit polyclonal anti-Myo7a (Thermo Fisher Scientific, PA1-936), rabbit polyclonal anti-HARS2 (Abcam, 46545), mouse monoclonal anti-3-nitrotyrosine (3-NT) (Sigma-Aldrich, N5538), rabbit polyclonal anti-4-hydroxynonenal (4-HNE) (Abcam, 46545), and mouse monoclonal anti-CtBP2 (BD Biosciences, 612044) at 1:200 dilution at 4°C overnight. Next day, after three 10-min washing with PBS, the samples were incubated with appropriate secondary antibodies at 1:400 dilution for 2 h at room temperature in darkness, which include Alexa Fluor 488-conjugated goat anti-mouse (CST, 4408S), Alexa Fluor 594-conjugated goat anti-rabbit (CST, 8889S), and Alexa Fluor 488-conjugated goat anti-rabbit (Thermo Fisher Scientific, A32731). According to immunofluorescence staining requirement, the samples were incubated with Alexa-Fluor 647-phalloidin (Thermo Fisher Scientific, A22287) for 1 h at room temperature in darkness. After three final washes with PBS, all immunolabeling samples were mounted on a slide with anti-fade reagent (Invitrogen, P10144). Immunofluorescence images were captured by Zeiss LSM 880 laser confocal microscope (Carl Zeiss Microscopy, Germany).

Semi-Quantification of the Immunofluorescence Images

Immunofluorescence images for 3-NT and 4-HNE were semi-quantified from original confocal images as previously described (Wu et al., 2020). Briefly, samples were processed in parallel under identical immunofluorescence staining conditions, and confocal microscope images were acquired with the same parameter settings. Using the ImageJ software (NIH, United States), the immunofluorescence images of hair cells were converted into 16-bit grayscale images for further measurement. After subtraction of the background intensity, the averaged grayscale intensity per cell was analyzed. For each repetition, the relative grayscale value was determined by normalizing the ratio to controls.

Transmission Electron Microscopy

Cochleae were quickly immersed and dissected in 2.5% glutaraldehyde (Sigma-Aldrich, G7651) in phosphate buffer (PB) solution. After fixed with 2.5% glutaraldehyde at 4°C overnight, the basilar membranes were fixed with 1% osmium tetroxide for 2 h at room temperature. The samples were dehydrated through an ethanol and acetone gradient and gradually embedded in Epon-812 (Sigma-Aldrich, 45345). Ultrathin sections were made by a diamond knife on a PowerTome-PC ultramicrotome (RMC, United States) and then placed on copper mesh, sequentially post-stained with uranyl acetate and lead citrate. The samples were imaged with a JEM-1230 transmission electron microscope (JEOL, Japan).

qPCR Analysis

Cochleae RNA extraction and qPCR analysis were performed as previous described (Vikhe Patil et al., 2015). Briefly, total RNA was extracted from sensory epithelia (without spiral ganglion neurons) of three mice for each genotype group using the TRIzol reagent (Invitrogen, 15596018). cDNA was reverse transcribed by applying RevertAid First Strand cDNA synthesis Kit (Invitrogen, K1622). The primers are listed in **Supplementary Table 1**. The qPCR was performed on a Roche 480II Real Time PCR System (Roche, United States) using the QuantiNova SYBR Green PCR Kit (QIAGEN, 208052). The mRNA relative expression levels were normalized to the endogenous control *Gapdh*. Each reaction was performed at least in triplicate, and the results were analyzed using the $2^{--\Delta\Delta CT}$ method (Schmittgen and Livak, 2008).

Western Blotting Analysis

Five mice (10 cochleae) were sacrificed for each genotype group. The cochleae were rapidly dissected in ice-cold PBS. Tissues of sensory epithelia (without spiral ganglion neurons) were gathered in tubes and mixed with ice-cold RIPA lysis buffer plus protease inhibitor cocktail and phosphatase inhibitors. The samples were homogenized and centrifuged at 10000 × *g* at 4°C for 20 min. The supernatants were collected and the protein concentration was measured using the BCA Protein Assay Kit (Beyotime, P0010). With 5 × SDS sample loading buffer added, the samples were boiled for 5 min and centrifuged at 3000 × *g* for 1 min. A total of 20 μg of each protein sample was separated by polyacrylamide gel electrophoresis (PAGE) and transferred onto a Polyvinylidene Fluoride (PVDF) membrane. The membranes were blocked with 5% non-fat milk for 2 h at room temperature and then incubated overnight at 4°C with the primary antibodies including anti-cleaved caspase-3 Rabbit mAb (CST, 9664) at 1:700, anti-Bcl2 Rabbit mAb (CST, 3498) at 1:700, anti-Cytochrome C Rabbit mAb (CST, 11940) at 1:700, anti-cleaved caspase-9 (CST, 9509) at 1:700, and anti-HARS2 (proteintech, 11301-1-AP) at 1:1000.

The membranes were washed three times in TBS with Tween 20 buffer and then incubated with secondary antibody conjugated with horseradish peroxidase for 2 h at room temperature. The immunoreactive bands were detected using a Tanon-4600 Chemiluminescent Imaging System (Tanon, China). The ImageJ software was used to calculate the relative density of probe protein. For HARS2 protein expression analysis, the relative protein expression was determined by normalizing the ratio to P1 HARS2 protein expression.

Whole-Cell Patch Clamp Recordings

The apical turn of the basilar membrane of the mouse cochlea was micro dissected in the extracellular solution. Whole-cell Patch clamp recordings were performed using the EPC10/2 amplifier (HEKA Electronics, Germany) with the Patchmaster software (HEKA Electronics, Germany) as described in our previous studies (Lin et al., 2019; Liu et al., 2019a; Zhao et al., 2020). Current-voltage relationships of Ca^{2+} influx in inner hair cells (IHCs) were obtained from current responses to ramp depolarization from -90 to 60 mV, and fitted to the following equation:

$$I(V) = (V - V_{rev}) \times \frac{G_{max}}{1 + \exp\left(-(V - V_{half})/K_{slope}\right)}$$

where V is the command membrane potential, V_{rev} is the reversal potential, G_{max} is the maximum conductance, V_{half} is the half activation potential, and the K_{slope} is steepness of voltage dependence in current activation.

Inner hair cell capacitance measurement (C_m) were performed with the lock-in feature and the "Sine + DC" method in the software Patchmaster (Liu et al., 2019b). Briefly, a 1 kHz sine wave and 70 mV peak-to-peak magnitude was superposed on the IHC holding potential of −90 mV. The averaged capacitances change before and after the depolarization were calculated to monitor exocytosis from IHCs: $\Delta C_m = C_m$ (response) − C_m (baseline). Ca^{2+} current charge (Q_{ca}) was calculated by taking the integral of the leak-subtracted current during depolarization.

In situ Apoptosis Staining

Hair cell apoptosis in the cochlea was evaluated using a terminal deoxynucleotidyl transferase-mediated deoxyuridine triphosphate nick-end labeling (TUNEL) staining kit (*in situ* cell death detection kit, Roche). After hair cells were labeled with anti-Myo7a antibody, the cochlear tissues were incubated with freshly prepared TUNEL working solution at 37°C for 1 h in a humidified chamber away from light. After rinsing in PBS three times, Nuclei were counterstained with a 4′, 6-diamidino-2-phenylindole (DAPI) staining solution (Beyotime, P0131). Nuclei of TUNEL positive cells intensely labeled by green were identified as apoptotic cells. Images were captured on a Zeiss LSM 880 laser confocal scanning microscopy (Carl Zeiss Microscopy, Germany).

Date Processing and Statistical Analysis

Imaging data processing and statistical analyses were carried out with GraphPad Prism 8.0 and Adobe Illustrator CC 2018. A two-tailed, unpaired Student's *t*-test with Welch's correction was used for comparisons between the *Hars2* CKO and control mice. For multiple comparison which involves sound level, frequency and cochlear turn, statistical analysis was performed using two-way ANOVA followed by Bonferroni *post-hoc* test. Data were expressed as mean ± SEM. For all statistical analysis, values were considered statistically significant when $P < 0.05$. In Figures, NS represents $P > 0.05$, * represents $P < 0.05$, ** represents $P < 0.01$, *** represents $P < 0.001$.

RESULTS

HARS2 Is Robustly Expressed in Postnatal Mouse Cochlea

To explore the role of HARS2 in hearing function, we first examined the expression pattern of HARS2 in the mouse cochlea. As shown in **Figure 1A**, cryosection immunostaining of the P30 WT mice indicated that HARS2 is widely expressed in the cochlea including inner (IHC) and outer hair cells (OHC), spiral ganglia neurons, stria vascularis, and supporting cells. Western blot analysis in cochleae of different postnatal ages showed that the expression of HARS2 is highest at P1 and gradually decreases at P14, P30, and P60 (**Figure 1B**).

The *Hars2* Conditional Knockout Mice Have Rapidly Progressive Hearing Loss

The $Hars2^{Loxp/Loxp}$;$ACTB^{Cre}$ full-body KO mice died perinatally, hindering further investigation of *Hars2* in auditory function. To overcome this obstacle, we generated a $Hars2^{Loxp/Loxp}$; $Gfi1^{Cre}$ CKO mouse line (**Figures 1C,D**). The specifical knockout of *Hars2* in cochlear hair cells was confirmed by immunofluorescence staining (**Figure 1E**). The *Hars2* CKO mice has apparently normal development. ABR thresholds of the *Hars2* CKO mice were initially indistinguishable from that of the littermate $Hars2^{+/+}$; $Gfi1^{Cre}$ controls at P21 (**Figure 2A**), but gradually elevated at P30 and P45 and rapidly reached profoundly deaf before P60 (**Figures 2B–D**). At P30 but not P21, the *Hars2* CKO mice also showed decreased supra-threshold amplitude and prolonged latency of the ABR wave I at sound frequencies 8, 16, and 22.6 kHz (**Figures 2E,F** and **Supplementary Figure 1**), which indicates abnormal IHC synaptic transmission, synchronization and auditory nerve conduction (McKay et al., 2015).

The *Hars2* Conditional Knockout Mice Have Progressive Hair Cell Loss

Immunostaining of the cochlear hair cells showed that the *Hars2* CKO mice have normal OHC and IHC numbers as the wild-type at P21 and P30 (**Figures 3A,B**). At P45, mild hair cell loss, more notable in OHCs than IHCs, can be observed at the basal turns of the *Hars2* CKO cochleae (**Figure 3C**). The hair cell loss proceeds rapidly and extends from the basal turn to the middle and apical. At P60, most OHCs of the *Hars2* CKO mice are lost, especially in the middle and basal turns, while the IHC loss is relatively less severe (**Figure 3D**).

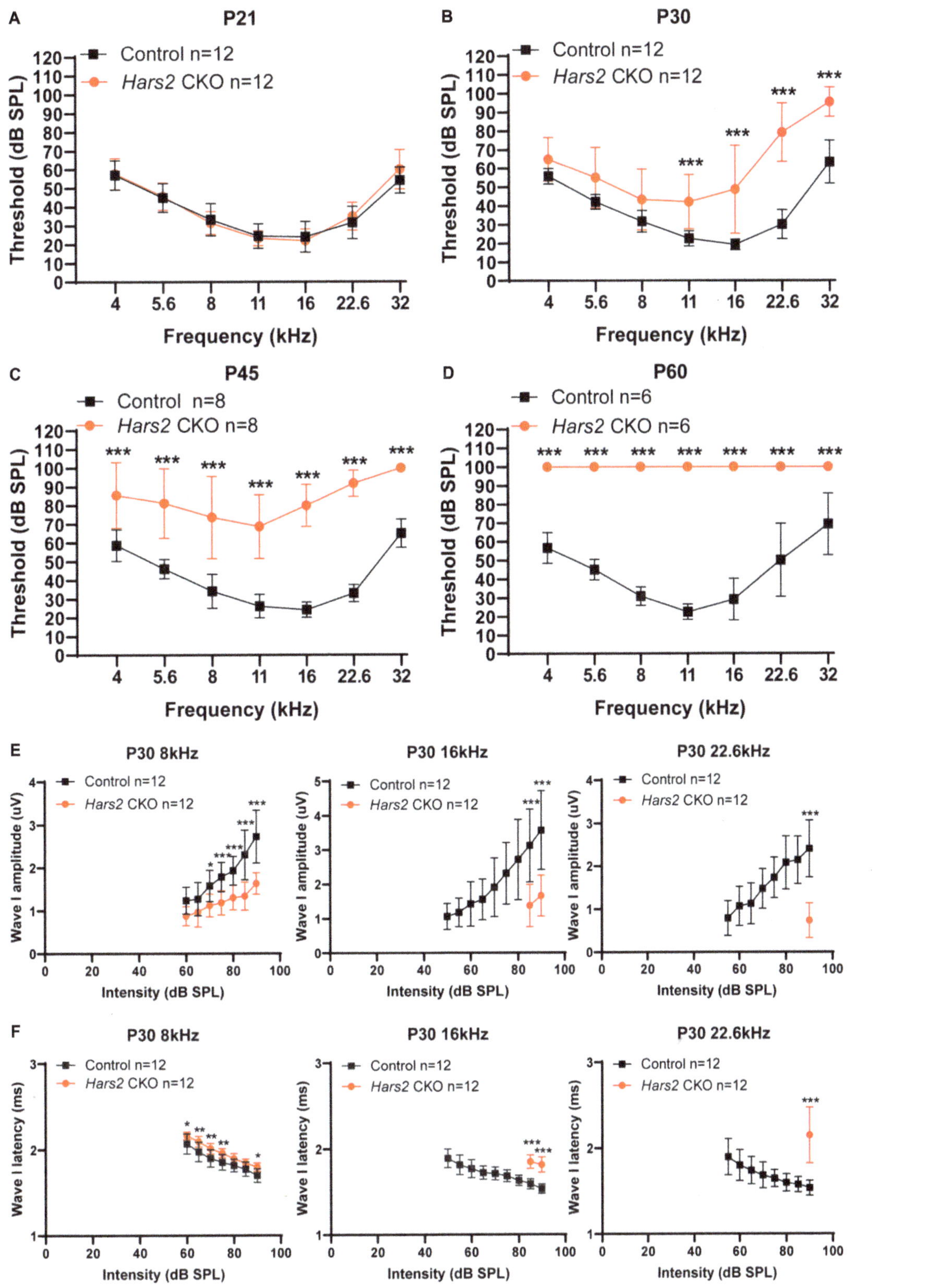

FIGURE 2 | Auditory brainstem response threshold and Wave-I analysis of the *Hars2* CKO mice. **(A)** Indistinguishable ABR thresholds of the *Hars2* CKO and control mice at P21. **(B)** Significantly elevated ABR thresholds at frequencies of 11–32 kHz at P30. **(C)** Further elevated ABR thresholds at all frequencies at P45. **(D)** Profound hearing loss at P60. **(E)** Significantly reduced ABR suprathreshold wave-I amplitudes at frequencies of 8, 16, and 22.6 kHz at P30. **(F)** Significantly prolonged ABR suprathreshold wave-I latencies at frequencies of 8, 16, and 22.6 kHz at P30. * represents $P < 0.05$, ** represents $P < 0.01$, *** represents $P < 0.001$.

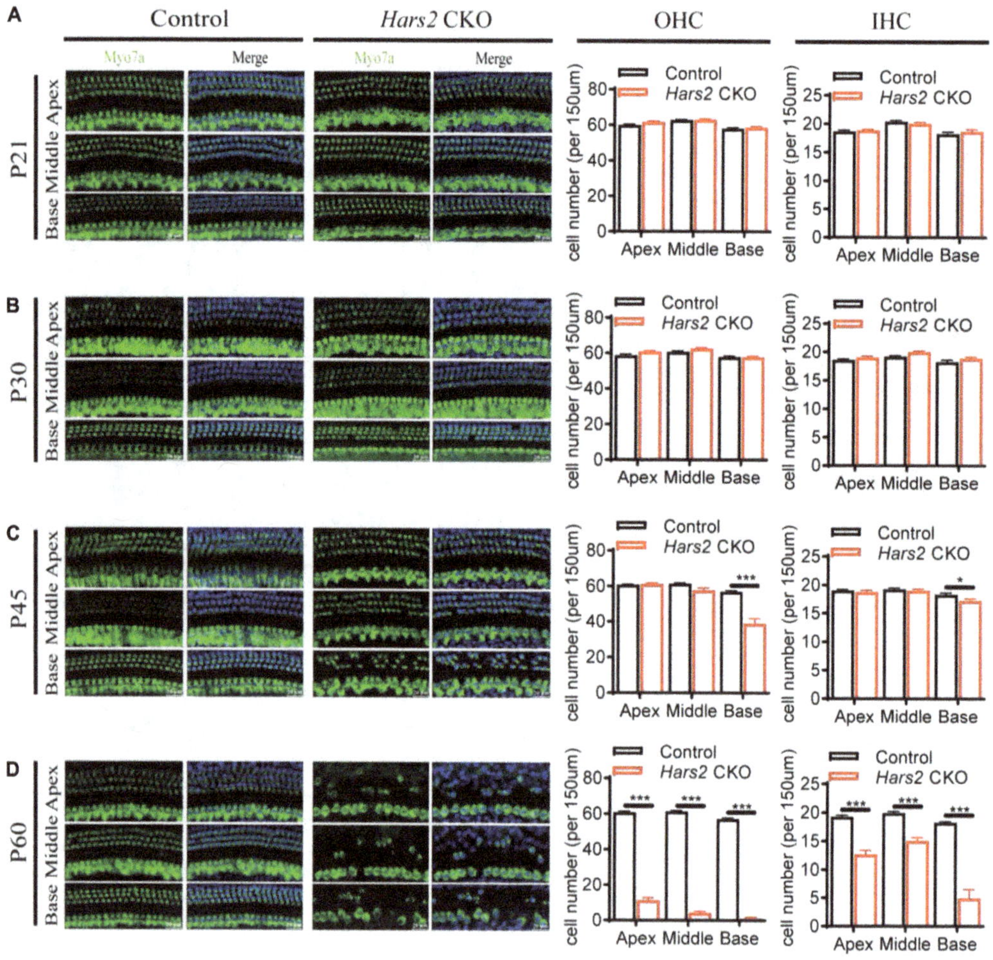

FIGURE 3 | Hair cell loss in the *Hars2* CKO mice. **(A,B)** No significant hair cell loss at P21 and P30. **(C)** Partial loss of hair cells at the basal turn at P45. **(D)** Severe hair cell loss in all turns at P60. Left panels: Whole-mount cochleae were immunostained with anti-Myo7a antibody (green) and DAPI (blue). Right panels: Quantification of the numbers of OHCs (left) and IHCs (right). control: $n = 5$; *Hars2* CKO: $n = 5$. Scale bars = 20 μm. * represents $P < 0.05$, *** represents $P < 0.001$.

Hars2 Knockout Activates Mitochondrial Apoptosis Pathway in Hair Cells

We next investigated that whether hair cell loss of the *Hars2* CKO mice is due to apoptosis. The TUNEL assay was used to label nuclear DNA fragmentation, a key feature of apoptosis (Majtnerová and Roušar, 2018). At P30, all hair cells remain TUNEL-negative (**Supplementary Figure 2**). At P45, TUNEL-positive OHCs can be observed in all three turns of the *Hars2* CKO cochleae, while TUNEL-positive IHCs are present in the basal turn only (**Figures 4A,B**). Expression of multiple pro-apoptotic proteins caspase-3, caspase-9, and cytochrome C are significantly up-regulated in the *Hars2* CKO cochleae, while the anti-apoptotic protein BCL-2 is down-regulated (**Figures 4C,D**).

Hars2 Knockout Elevates Reactive Oxygen Species in Hair Cells

Since mitochondrial ROS has pivotal role in triggering hair cell apoptosis and hearing loss (Wu et al., 2020; Fu et al., 2021b), we then assessed the level of ROS in the *Hars2* CKO cochleae. Increased immunolabeling of the ROS markers 3-NT and 4-HNE can be observed as early as P30 in most turns of cochleae (**Figures 5A–D**). Quantitative reversed transcribed PCR also showed decreased mRNA expression of several antioxidant enzymes xCT, Nqo1, Sod2, and Gsr, and increased expression of the oxidant enzyme Lpo in the *Hars2* CKO cochleae (**Figure 5E**). These results suggested that increased ROS in cochlear hair cells is likely the initiating cause for hearing loss in the *Hars2* CKO mice.

Hars2 Knockout Disrupts Inner Hair Cell Synaptic Transmission

Since the *Hars2* CKO mice has significant hearing loss at P30 without apparent hair cell loss (**Figures 2B, 3B**), we further investigated the IHC functions of the *Hars2* CKO mice at this age. Whole-mount immunostaining showed that the *Hars2* CKO mice has normal IHC ribbon synapse counts as the controls (**Supplementary Figure 3**). Whole-cell patch-clamp recording in IHCs, however, recorded a significantly smaller Ca^{2+} current

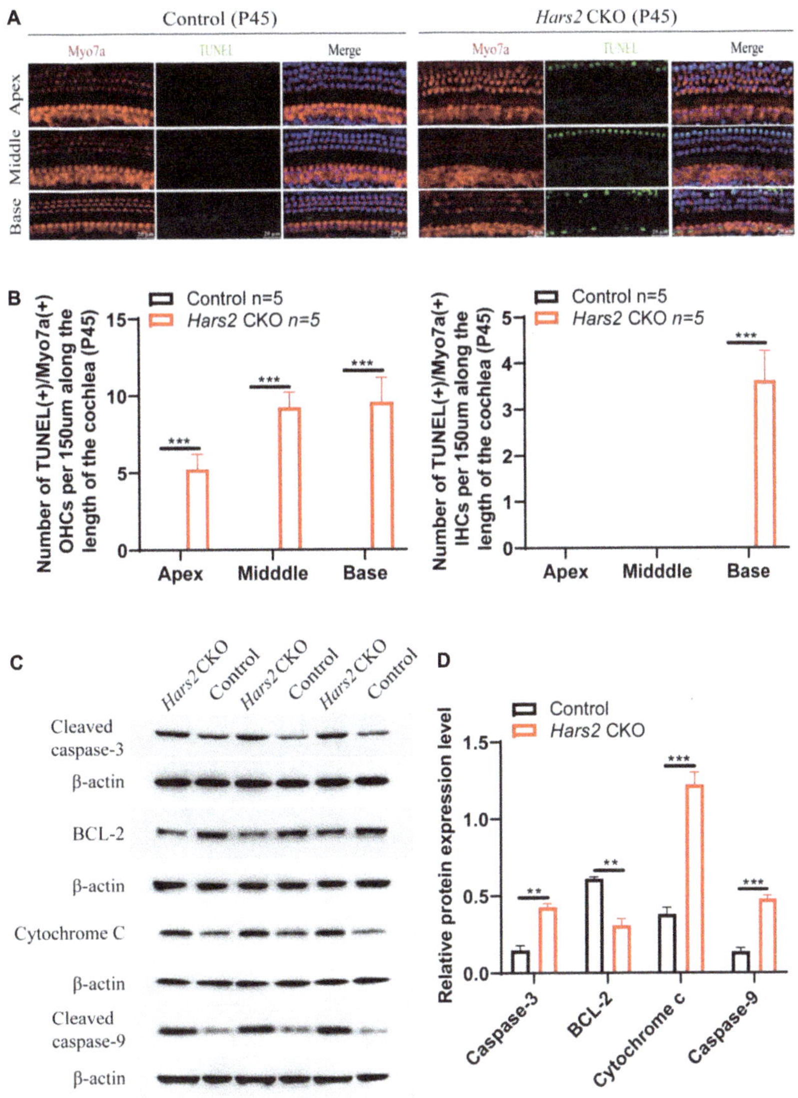

FIGURE 4 | Apoptosis analysis by TUNEL and Western blot in the cochleae of the *Hars2* CKO mice at P45. **(A)** TUNEL (green) and anti-Myo7a (red), DAPI (blue) staining of whole-mount cochlea in the *Hars2* CKO and control mice. Scale bars = 20 μm. **(B)** Quantification of the number of TUNEL positive OHCs and IHCs at the apical, middle, and basal turns of cochlea. **(C)** Protein expression of cleaved caspase-3, BCL-2, cytochrome C, and cleaved caspase-9 detected by Western blotting. **(D)** Relative protein expression levels after normalization against endogenous β-actin. All experiments were replicated in triplets. ** represents $P < 0.01$, *** represents $P < 0.001$.

with lower current amplitude (I_{Ca}), reversal potential (V_{rev}) and half activation potential (V_{half}), and normal steepness of voltage dependence (k_{slope}) for the *Hars2* CKO mice at physiological conditions (**Figures 6A–E**). Membrane capacitance change (ΔC_m), which measures synaptic vesicle release, is normal under short (20 ms) stimulation but significantly reduced under prolonged (200 ms) stimulation (**Figures 6F–J**). The Ca^{2+} efficiency triggering exocytosis, quantified as the ratio of $\Delta C_m/Q_{Ca}$, remain unaltered for both short and prolonged stimulations (**Figures 6H,K**). Taken together, these results suggested that the *Hars2* CKO mice have disrupted IHC synaptic transmission due to reduced calcium influx, which likely contributes to the hearing loss at P30 and is consistent with the decreased supra-threshold amplitude and prolonged latency of the ABR wave I (**Figures 2E,F**).

Hars2 Knockout Causes Accumulation of Morphologically Abnormal Mitochondria in Hair Cells

We finally evaluated the proportion of morphologically abnormal mitochondria, defined by swelling, deformation, loss of cristae, and emergence of large intrinsic vacuoles, in IHCs (**Figure 7**) and OHCs (**Figure 8**) of the *Hars2* CKO mice by Transmission Electron Microscopy (TEM). At P7, the number and distribution of mitochondria in both IHCs and OHCs of the *Hars2* CKO

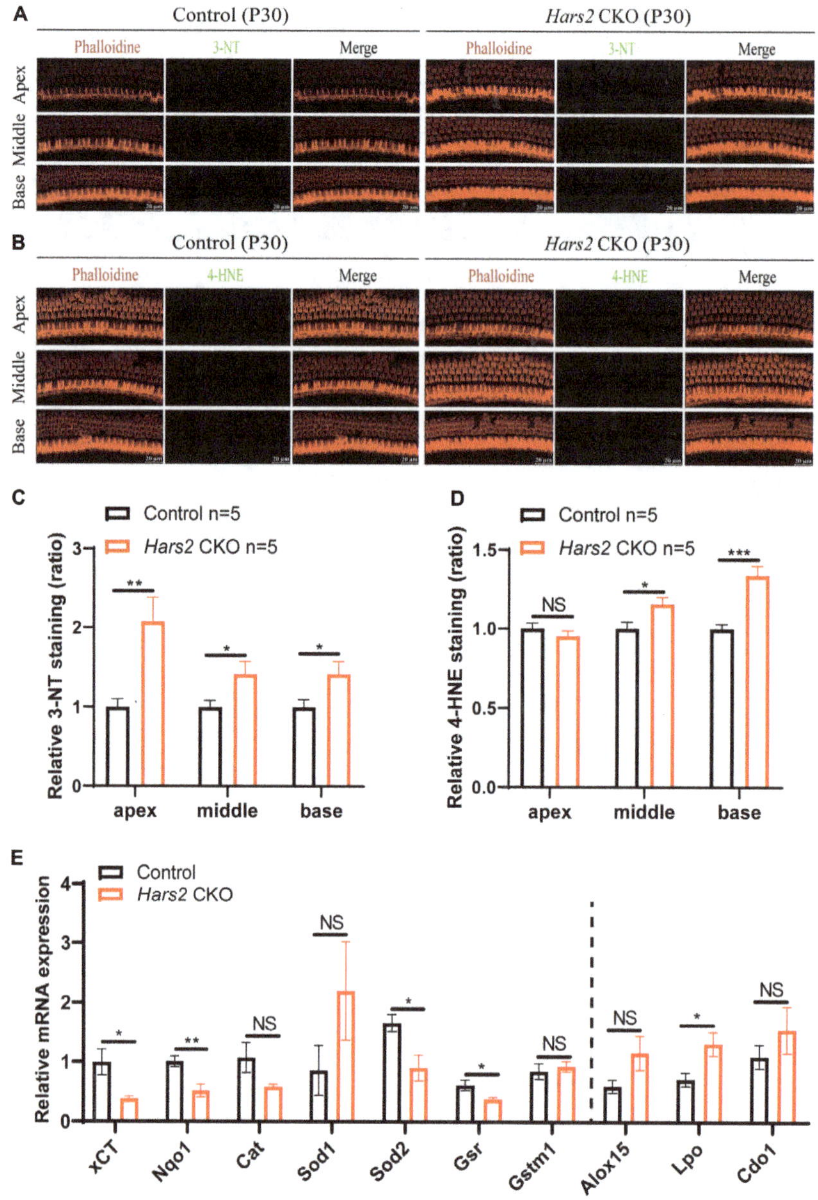

FIGURE 5 | ROS analysis in the cochleae of the *Hars2* CKO mice at P30. **(A,B)** Immunostaining of whole-mount cochleae using anti-3-NT or anti-4-HNE antibodies (green), Phalloidin (red), and DAPI (blue). Scale bars = 20 μm. **(C,D)** Quantification of the 3-NT or 4-HNE immunolabeling in hair cells. **(E)** qPCR analysis of sensory epithelia (without spiral ganglion neurons) showing significantly decreased expression of the antioxidant factors xCT, Nqo1, Sod2, and Gsr and increased expression of pro-oxidant factor Lpo ($n = 6$). NS represents $P > 0.05$, * represents $P < 0.05$, ** represents $P < 0.01$, *** represents $P < 0.001$.

mice are normal, and the ultrastructure of the mitochondria is mostly indistinguishable from the control mice with clearly visible cristae. From P14, a series of abnormal mitochondria can be observed in hair cells of the *Hars2* CKO mice (**Figures 7A, 8A**), which represents reduced inner membrane surface together with low-density mitochondrial mass. The proportion of morphological abnormal mitochondria appears to increase with age and is larger in IHCs than in OHCs (**Figures 7B, 8B**). In addition, cristae surface area, positively correlated with the amount of ATP produced by oxidative phosphorylation (van der Laan et al., 2012; Wollweber et al., 2017), significantly decreases in the *Hars2* CKO mice, again more prominently in IHCs than in OHCs (**Figures 7C, 8C**).

DISCUSSION

The functions of deafness genes play an essential role on the morphology and development of hair cells (Liu et al., 2019d; Qi et al., 2019, 2020; Chen et al., 2021a), synaptic transmission of spiral ganglion neurons (Guo et al., 2020; Guo R. et al., 2021; Hu et al., 2021; Wei et al., 2021), and many other important

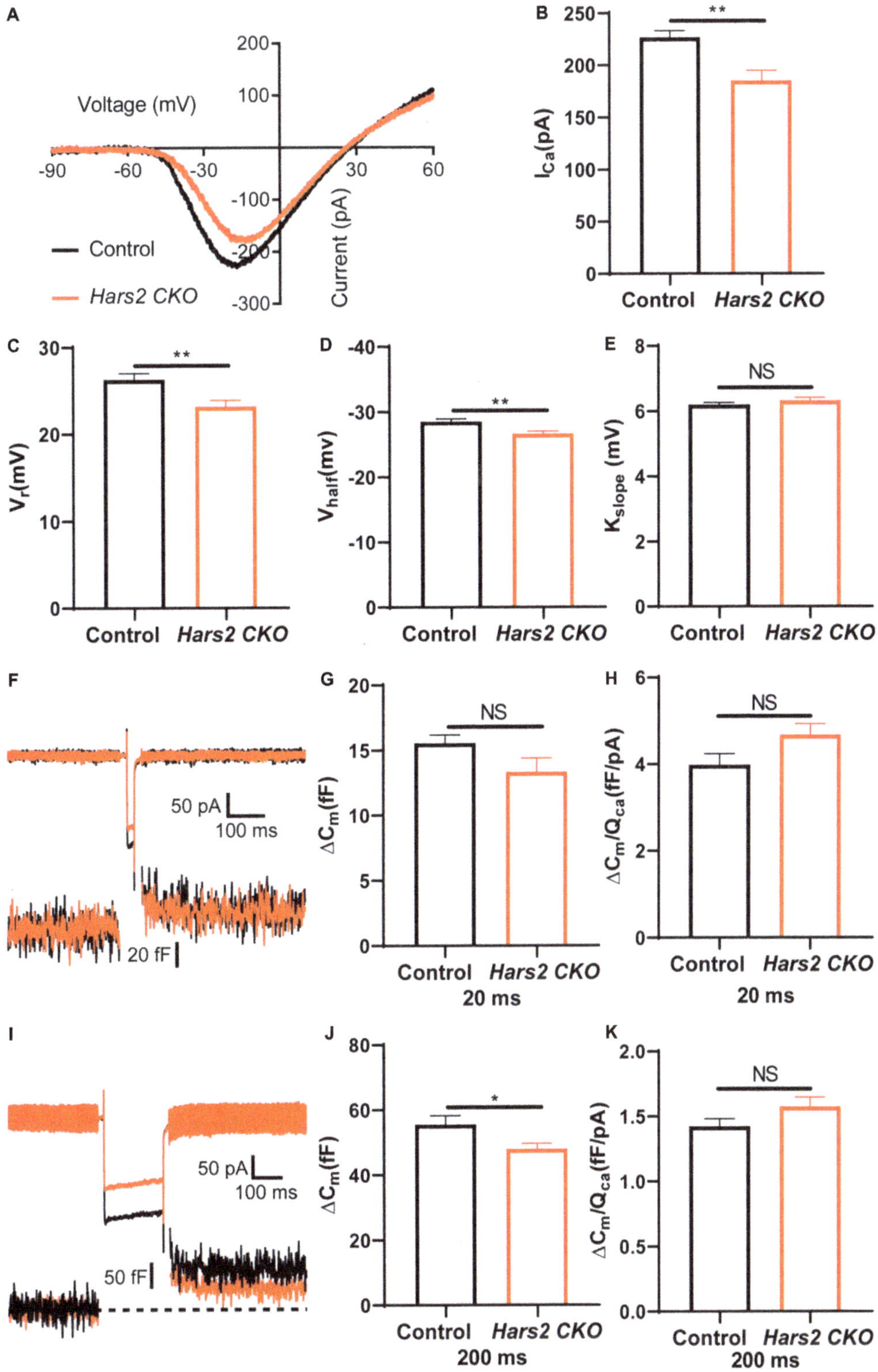

FIGURE 6 | Inner hair cell patch-clamp recording in the *Hars2* CKO mice. **(A)** Representative of the Ca^{2+} current in IHCs of the *Hars2* CKO and control mice. The current response was induced by a voltage ramp from −90 to 60 mV and then leak subtracted. **(B,C)** The Ca^{2+} current amplitude (I_{Ca}) and reversal potential (V_{rev}) are significantly reduced. **(D)** The half activation potential (V_{half}) of calcium current is less negative. **(E)** Slope of activation (k_{slope}) is normal. **(F)** Representative traces of Ca^{2+} current (top) and capacitance (bottom) upon 20 ms step depolarization. **(G)** The membrane capacitance change (ΔC_m) is comparable for stimulations of 20 ms. **(H)** The Ca^{2+} efficiency of exocytosis triggering, quantified as the ratio of $\Delta C_m/Q_{Ca}$, is comparable for stimulation of 20 ms. **(I)** Representative traces of Ca^{2+} current (top) and capacitance (bottom) upon 200 ms step depolarization. **(J)** The ΔC_m is significantly reduced for stimulations of 200 ms. **(K)** The $\Delta C_m/Q_{Ca}$ is comparable for stimulation of 200 ms (control: $n = 5$; *Hars2* CKO: $n = 5$). NS represents $P > 0.05$, * represents $P < 0.05$, ** represents $P < 0.01$.

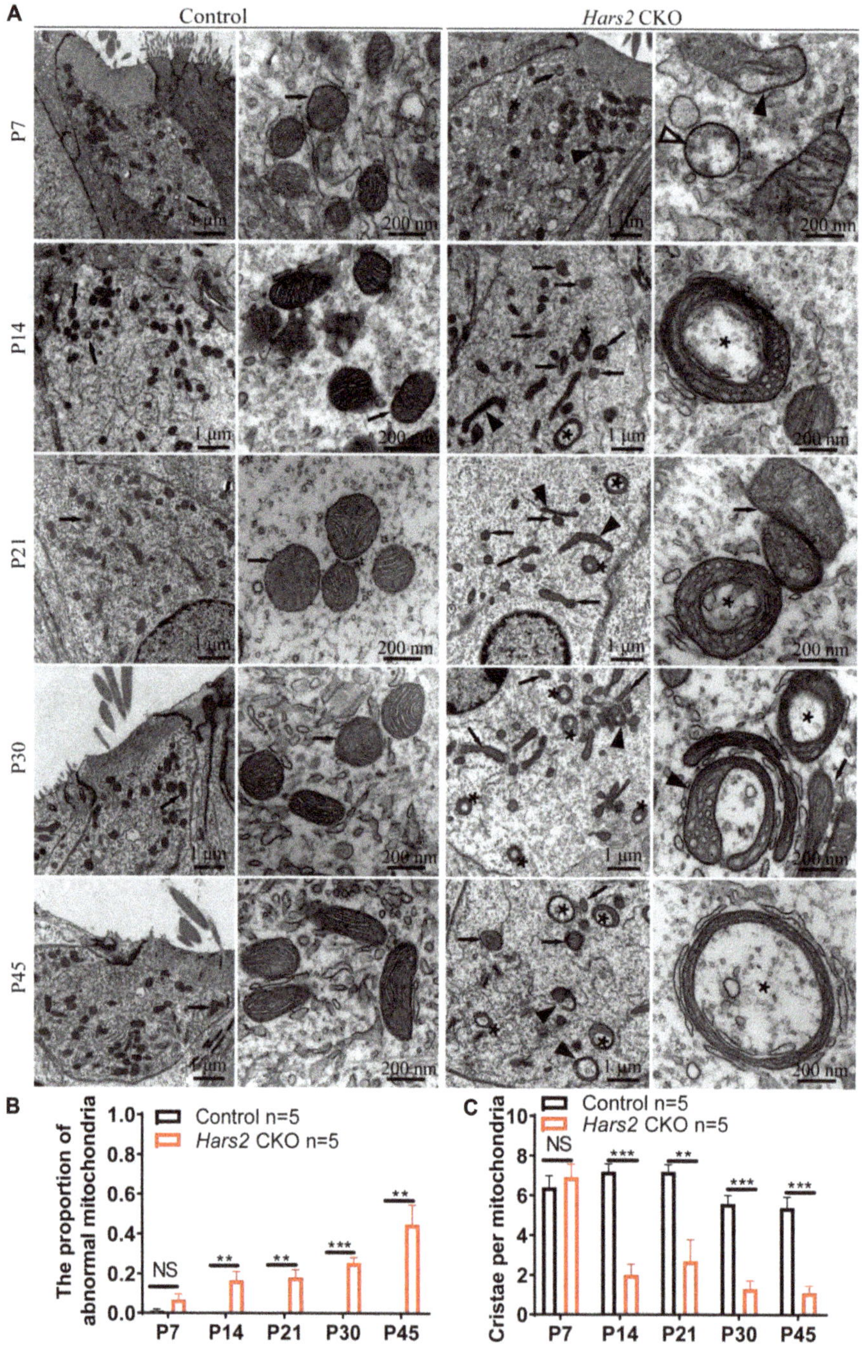

FIGURE 7 | Inner hair cell transmission electron microscopy of the *Hars2* CKO mice between P7 and P45. **(A)** IHCs of the control mice at different ages contains abundant mitochondria with easily-identifiable cristae, whereas various morphologically abnormal mitochondria be observed in IHCs of the *Hars2* CKO mice including swollen (open arrowhead), deformed (black arrowhead) mitochondria, mitochondria with deformed cristae (black arrows), or intrinsic vacuole (black asterisk). **(B)** Quantified proportion of abnormal mitochondria in IHCs. **(C)** Quantified number of mitochondrial cristae per mitochondria in IHCs. NS represents $P > 0.05$, ** represents $P < 0.01$, *** represents $P < 0.001$.

components of the inner ear, including supporting cells, greater epithelial ridge cells and lesser epithelial ridge cells (Ding et al., 2020; Zhang et al., 2020; Chen et al., 2021b). In this study, we generated a *Hars2* conditional knockout mice to investigate the function of HARS2 in hearing and its pathogenic mechanism for deafness. Previous studies have shown that missense mutations in *HARS2*, which account for the majority of reported mutations in humans, lead to significantly decreased protein function (Yu et al., 2020), similar to the loss of function effect in this mouse model. Though HARS2 was found to be widely expressed in

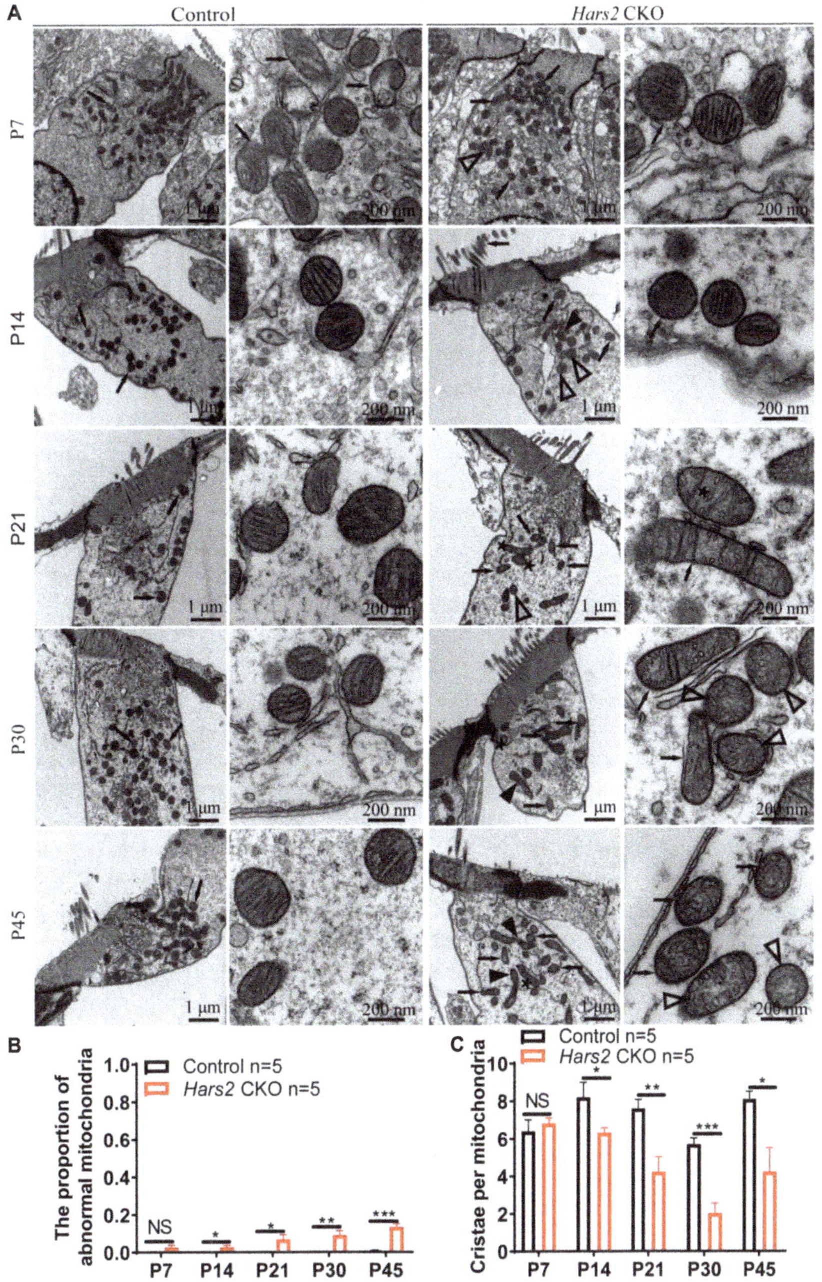

FIGURE 8 | Outer hair cell transmission electron microscopy of the *Hars2* CKO mice between P7-P45. **(A)** OHCs of the control mice at different ages contains abundant mitochondria with easily-identifiable cristae, whereas various morphologically abnormal mitochondria be observed in OHCs of the *Hars2* CKO mice including swollen (open arrowhead), deformed (black arrowhead) mitochondria, mitochondria with deformed cristae (black arrows), or intrinsic vacuole (black asterisk). **(B)** Quantified proportion of abnormal mitochondria in OHCs. **(C)** Quantified number of mitochondrial cristae per mitochondria in OHCs. NS represents $P > 0.05$, * represents $P < 0.05$, ** represents $P < 0.01$, *** represents $P < 0.001$.

many cell types of mouse cochlea (**Figure 1**), the current study chose to focus on cochlear hair cells that have an essential role in converting mechanical sound stimulus into neural electrical signals (Schwander et al., 2010). Notably, our hair cell-specific *Hars2* CKO mice display delayed-onset, rapidly progressive hearing loss (**Figure 2**), which is very similar to the human hearing phenotype associated with the *HARS2* mutations (Yu et al., 2020), supporting our hypothesis that hair cell is among the primary targets for *Hars2*-related pathogenesis in cochlea. At the same time, we acknowledge that the function of HARS2 in other inner ear cell types, such as spiral ganglion neurons and supporting cells, remain to be further studied.

Underlying increasingly elevated ABR hearing thresholds in postnatal *Hars2* CKO mice (**Figure 2**), we observed rapidly progressive hair cell loss due to increased ROS level and activated apoptosis pathway (**Figures 3, 4, 5**). These results are consistent with previous studies on HEK293T cells, which show that the mtARSs are essential in mitochondrial protein synthesis and oxidative phosphorylation (OXPHOS) (Fine et al., 2019; Yu et al., 2020). Reduction of OXPHOS electron transport chain activity may lead to elevated ROS, which in turn can induce opening of mitochondrial permeability transition pore and reduce of mitochondrial membrane potential, triggering mitochondrial apoptotic pathways (Kamogashira et al., 2015).

The hearing loss of the *Hars2* CKO mice, however, cannot be entirely attributed to loss of hair cells, as it already occurs at as early as P30 without apparent hair cell loss (**Figures 2B, 3B**). In hair cells, neurotransmission of the sound signal relies on rapid and sustained vesicle release of the ribbon synapses, which is an energy demanding process relying heavily on mitochondria (Safieddine et al., 2012). Patch-clamp recordings in acute brainstem slices have demonstrated that energy limitations can negatively affect synaptic transmission (Nagase et al., 2014), with similar results also reported in hippocampal slices (Liotta et al., 2012). In this study, by TEM we observed morphological degeneration of mitochondria, which indicate mitochondrial dysfunction in *Hars2* CKO hearing cells at different postnatal periods including P14. In mammalian hair cells, Ca^{2+} influx current triggers both rapid and sustained exocytosis, which releases the readily releasable pool of synaptic vesicles and ensures their efficient recycling (Meyer et al., 2009; Graydon et al., 2011). Besides energy supply, mitochondria also contributes to maintaining of intracellular calcium homeostasis and influx in hair cells (Wang et al., 2019) and is associated with the susceptibility to noise-induced hearing loss (Liu et al., 2020). Although the number of ribbon synapses in IHCs of the *Hars2* CKO mice is unaltered at P30 (**Supplementary Figure 3**), our IHC patch-clamp recording showed that the IHC Ca^{2+} influx current is significantly reduced at physiological conditions (**Figure 6**). Consistently, while the rapid exocytosis and the efficiency of Ca^{2+} triggering exocytosis remains normal, the sustained exocytosis is also reduced in IHCs of the *Hars2* CKO mice. These results are in agreement with previous studies showing that partial block of evoked mitochondria-Ca^{2+} uptake in mature zebrafish hair cells was sufficient to impair presynaptic-Ca^{2+} influx current, especially during sustained stimuli (Castellano-Muñoz and Ricci, 2014; Wong et al., 2019). Overall, our results suggested that *Hars2* deficiency leads to mitochondrial dysfunction, reduced presynaptic Ca^{2+} influx current and compromised sustained exocytosis, which in combination likely contributes to the hearing loss of the *Hars2* CKO mice prior to the hair cell loss.

Our TEM study revealed the progressive morphological abnormalities of mitochondria in hair cells of the *Hars2* CKO mice (**Figures 7, 8**). Mitochondria is a dynamic organelle whose morphology directly reflects its functional status (Friedman and Nunnari, 2014). Here we calculated the proportion of morphologically abnormal mitochondria and the number of mitochondrial cristae per mitochondria to quantify the mitochondrial dysfunction. Interestingly, the distortion and corruption of mitochondria is far more severe in IHCs than in OHCs of the *Hars2* CKO mice. This is in agreement with previous studies on cisplatin-induced hearing loss and noise-induced hearing loss, which showed similar trends for differential mitochondrial damages between IHCs and OHCs (Hill et al., 2016; Chen et al., 2019). However, both previous and our current studies (**Figure 3**) showed that OHCs encounter greater cell loss than IHCs under ROS stress (Choung et al., 2009), suggesting that these two hair cell types perceive the mitochondrial damage differently.

Overall, our study revealed a progressive, rapidly deteriorating course for hair cell mitochondrial damage and hearing loss in the

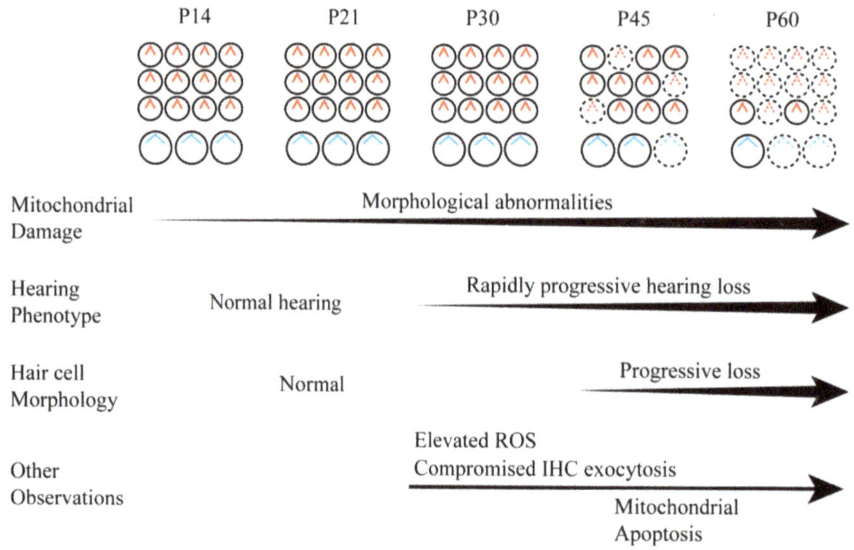

FIGURE 9 | Schematic diagram of the hearing phenotype and hair cell maintenance of the *Hars2* CKO mice between P14 and P60 based on the current morphological and functional studies.

Hars2 CKO mice, accompanied with elevated ROS, compromised IHC sustained exocytosis and eventual hair cell loss (**Figure 9**). As antioxidant drugs targeting mitochondrial ROS pathway have been proven effective to relieve hearing loss associated with noise, ototoxic-drug, and aging (Fetoni et al., 2013; Kamogashira et al., 2015; Kim et al., 2019), HARS2 and other mtARSs may present interesting targets for future therapeutic studies.

CONCLUSION

Our study suggested that *Hars2* is critically required for hair cell survival and maintenance of appropriate function. Mutations in *Hars2* may lead to progressive, rapidly deteriorating hearing loss by hair cell synaptopathy and mitochondrial apoptosis, which are triggered by accumulating mitochondrial damage and elevated ROS stress.

AUTHOR CONTRIBUTIONS

TY and HW designed and supervised the whole project. PX, LW, and XP designed, conducted experiments, and analyzed data. HP helped with confocal imaging and TEM observation. HuL and HoL carried out the IHC patch clamp recordings and analyzed data. QY, YL, and JX assisted in generating *Hars2* CKO mice, performed qPCR and WB analysis. XP, TY, and HW acquired funding. PX, XP, and TY wrote and reviewed the manuscript. All authors contributed to the article and approved the submitted version.

ACKNOWLEDGMENTS

We would like to thank Yu Kong, Xu Wang, Lijun Pan, and Xue Xu (Electron Microscopy Facilities of Center for Excellence in Brain Science and Technology, Chinese Academy of Sciences) for assistance with TEM sample preparation and analysis of TEM images.

REFERENCES

Agnew, T., Goldsworthy, M., Aguilar, C., Morgan, A., Simon, M., Hilton, H., et al. (2018). A Wars2 Mutant Mouse Model Displays OXPHOS Deficiencies and Activation of Tissue-Specific Stress Response Pathways. *Cell Rep.* 25, 3315.e-3328.e. doi: 10.1016/j.celrep.2018.11.080

Akil, O., and Lustig, L. R. (2013). Mouse Cochlear Whole Mount Immunofluorescence. *Bio Protoc.* 3:5. doi: 10.21769/bioprotoc.332

Bock, F. J., and Tait, S. W. G. (2020). Mitochondria as multifaceted regulators of cell death. *Nat. Rev. Mol. Cell Biol.* 21, 85–100. doi: 10.1038/s41580-019-0173-8

Castellano-Muñoz, M., and Ricci, A. J. (2014). Role of intracellular calcium stores in hair-cell ribbon synapse. *Front. Cell Neurosci.* 8:162. doi: 10.3389/fncel.2014.00162

Chen, Y., Gu, J., Liu, J., Tong, L., Shi, F., Wang, X., et al. (2019). Dexamethasone-loaded injectable silk-polyethylene glycol hydrogel alleviates cisplatin-induced ototoxicity. *Int. J. Nanomed.* 14, 4211–4227. doi: 10.2147/IJN.S195336

Chen, Y., Gu, Y., Li, Y., Li, G. L., Chai, R., Li, W., et al. (2021a). Generation of mature and functional hair cells by co-expression of Gfi1, Pou4f3, and Atoh1 in the postnatal mouse cochlea. *Cell Rep.* 35:109016. doi: 10.1016/j.celrep.2021.109016

Chen, Y., Qiang, R., Zhang, Y., Cao, W., Wu, L., Jiang, P., et al. (2021b). The Expression and Roles of the Super Elongation Complex in Mouse Cochlear Lgr5+ Progenitor Cells. *Front. Cell Neurosci.* 15:735723. doi: 10.3389/fncel.2021.735723

Cheng, C., Hou, Y., Zhang, Z., Wang, Y., Lu, L., Zhang, L., et al. (2021). Disruption of the autism-related gene Pak1 causes stereocilia disorganization, hair cell loss, and deafness in mice. *J. Genet. Genomics* 2021:10. doi: 10.1016/j.jgg.2021.03.010

Cheng, C., Wang, Y., Guo, L., Lu, X., Zhu, W., Muhammad, W., et al. (2019). Age-related transcriptome changes in Sox2+ supporting cells in the mouse cochlea. *Stem Cell Res. Ther.* 10:365. doi: 10.1186/s13287-019-1437-0

Choung, Y., Taura, A., Pak, K., Choi, S., Masuda, M., and Ryan, A. (2009). Generation of highly-reactive oxygen species is closely related to hair cell damage in rat organ of Corti treated with gentamicin. *Neuroscience* 161, 214–226. doi: 10.1016/j.neuroscience.2009.02.085

Davis, A. C., and Hoffman, H. J. (2019). Hearing loss: rising prevalence and impact. *Bull World Health Organ.* 97, 646a–646a. doi: 10.2471/blt.19.224683

Dehne, N., Rauen, U., de Groot, H., and Lautermann, J. (2002). Involvement of the mitochondrial permeability transition in gentamicin ototoxicity. *Hear. Res.* 169, 47–55. doi: 10.1016/S0378-5955(02)00338-6

Ding, Y., Meng, W., Kong, W., He, Z., and Chai, R. (2020). The Role of FoxG1 in the Inner Ear. *Front. Cell Dev. Biol.* 8:614954. doi: 10.3389/fcell.2020.614954

Dogan, S. A., Pujol, C., Maiti, P., Kukat, A., Wang, S., Hermans, S., et al. (2014). Tissue-specific loss of DARS2 activates stress responses independently of respiratory chain deficiency in the heart. *Cell Metab.* 19, 458–469. doi: 10.1016/j.cmet.2014.02.004

Du, Z., Yang, Y., Hu, Y., Sun, Y., Zhang, S., Peng, W., et al. (2012). A long-term high-fat diet increases oxidative stress, mitochondrial damage and apoptosis in the inner ear of D-galactose-induced aging rats. *Hear. Res.* 287, 15–24. doi: 10.1016/j.heares.2012.04.012

Fetoni, A. R., De Bartolo, P., Eramo, S. L. M., Rolesi, R., Paciello, F., Bergamini, C., et al. (2013). Noise-Induced Hearing Loss (NIHL) as a Target of Oxidative Stress-Mediated Damage: Cochlear and Cortical Responses after an Increase in Antioxidant Defense. *J. Neurosci.* 33, 4011–4023. doi: 10.1523/jneurosci.2282-12.2013

Figuccia, S., Degiorgi, A., Ceccatelli Berti, C., Baruffini, E., Dallabona, C., and Goffrini, P. (2021). Mitochondrial Aminoacyl-tRNA Synthetase and Disease: The Yeast Contribution for Functional Analysis of Novel Variants. *Int. J. Mol. Sci.* 22:9. doi: 10.3390/ijms22094524

Fine, A. S., Nemeth, C. L., Kaufman, M. L., and Fatemi, A. (2019). Mitochondrial aminoacyl-tRNA synthetase disorders: an emerging group of developmental disorders of myelination. *J. Neurodev. Disord* 11:29. doi: 10.1186/s11689-019-9292-y

Fischel-Ghodsian, N., Kopke, R. D., and Ge, X. (2004). Mitochondrial dysfunction in hearing loss. *Mitochondrion* 4, 675–694. doi: 10.1016/j.mito.2004.07.040

Friedman, J. R., and Nunnari, J. (2014). Mitochondrial form and function. *Nature* 505, 335–343. doi: 10.1038/nature12985

Fu, X., An, Y., Wang, H., Li, P., Lin, J., Yuan, J., et al. (2021a). Deficiency of Klc2 Induces Low-Frequency Sensorineural Hearing Loss in C57BL/6 J Mice and Human. *Mol. Neurobiol.* 2021:2422. doi: 10.1007/s12035-021-02422-w

Fu, X., Wan, P., Li, P., Wang, J., Guo, S., Zhang, Y., et al. (2021b). Mechanism and Prevention of Ototoxicity Induced by Aminoglycosides. *Front. Cell. Neurosci.* 15:692762. doi: 10.3389/fncel.2021.692762

Gong, S. S., Wang, X. Q., Meng, F. L., Cui, L. M., Yi, Q. Z., Zhao, Q., et al. (2020). Overexpression of mitochondrial histidyl-tRNA synthetase restores mitochondrial dysfunction caused by a deafness-associated tRNA(His) mutation. *J. Biol. Chem.* 295, 940–954. doi: 10.1074/jbc.RA119.010998

Graydon, C. W., Cho, S., Li, G. L., Kachar, B., and von Gersdorff, H. (2011). Sharp Ca^{2+} nanodomains beneath the ribbon promote highly synchronous multivesicular release at hair cell synapses. *J. Neurosci.* 31, 16637–16650. doi: 10.1523/jneurosci.1866-11.2011

Guo, L., Cao, W., Niu, Y., He, S., Chai, R., and Yang, J. (2021). Autophagy Regulates the Survival of Hair Cells and Spiral Ganglion Neurons in Cases of Noise, Ototoxic Drug, and Age-Induced Sensorineural Hearing Loss. *Front. Cell Neurosci.* 15:760422. doi: 10.3389/fncel.2021.760422

Guo, R., Li, J., Chen, C., Xiao, M., Liao, M., Hu, Y., et al. (2021). Biomimetic 3D bacterial cellulose-graphene foam hybrid scaffold regulates neural stem cell proliferation and differentiation. *Coll. Surf. B Biointerf.* 200:111590. doi:

10.1016/j.colsurfb.2021.111590

Guo, R., Xiao, M., Zhao, W., Zhou, S., Hu, Y., Liao, M., et al. (2020). 2D Ti(3)C(2)T(x)MXene couples electrical stimulation to promote proliferation and neural differentiation of neural stem cells. *Acta Biomater* 2020:35. doi: 10.1016/j.actbio.2020.12.035

Han, S., Xu, Y., Sun, J., Liu, Y., Zhao, Y., Tao, W., et al. (2020). Isolation and analysis of extracellular vesicles in a Morpho butterfly wing-integrated microvortex biochip. *Biosens Bioelect.* 154:112073. doi: 10.1016/j.bios.2020.112073

He, Z., Fang, Q., Li, H., Shao, B., Zhang, Y., Zhang, Y., et al. (2019). The role of FOXG1 in the postnatal development and survival of mouse cochlear hair cells. *Neuropharmacology* 144, 43–57. doi: 10.1016/j.neuropharm.2018.10.021

He, Z., Guo, L., Shu, Y., Fang, Q., Zhou, H., Liu, Y., et al. (2017). Autophagy protects auditory hair cells against neomycin-induced damage. *Autophagy* 13, 1884–1904. doi: 10.1080/15548627.2017.1359449

He, Z. H., Li, M., Fang, Q. J., Liao, F. L., Zou, S. Y., Wu, X., et al. (2021). FOXG1 promotes aging inner ear hair cell survival through activation of the autophagy pathway. *Autophagy* 2021, 1–22. doi: 10.1080/15548627.2021.1916194

He, Z. H., Zou, S. Y., Li, M., Liao, F. L., Wu, X., Sun, H. Y., et al. (2020). The nuclear transcription factor FoxG1 affects the sensitivity of mimetic aging hair cells to inflammation by regulating autophagy pathways. *Redox Biol.* 28:101364. doi: 10.1016/j.redox.2019.101364

Hill, K., Yuan, H., Wang, X., and Sha, S. (2016). Noise-Induced Loss of Hair Cells and Cochlear Synaptopathy Are Mediated by the Activation of AMPK. *J. Neurosci.* 36, 7497–7510. doi: 10.1523/jneurosci.0782-16.2016

Hu, Y., Li, D., Wei, H., Zhou, S., Chen, W., Yan, X., et al. (2021). Neurite Extension and Orientation of Spiral Ganglion Neurons Can Be Directed by Superparamagnetic Iron Oxide Nanoparticles in a Magnetic Field. *Int. J. Nanomed.* 16, 4515–4526. doi: 10.2147/ijn.S313673

Kamogashira, T., Fujimoto, C., and Yamasoba, T. (2015). Reactive oxygen species, apoptosis, and mitochondrial dysfunction in hearing loss. *BioMed. Res. Internat.* 2015:617207. doi: 10.1155/2015/617207

Kim, Y. R., Baek, J. I., Kim, S. H., Kim, M. A., Lee, B., Ryu, N., et al. (2019). Therapeutic potential of the mitochondria-targeted antioxidant MitoQ in mitochondrial-ROS induced sensorineural hearing loss caused by Idh2 deficiency. *Redox Biol.* 20, 544–555. doi: 10.1016/j.redox.2018.11.013

Konovalova, S., and Tyynismaa, H. (2013). Mitochondrial aminoacyl-tRNA synthetases in human disease. *Mol. Genet. Metab.* 108, 206–211. doi: 10.1016/j.ymgme.2013.01.010

Li, A., You, D., Li, W., Cui, Y., He, Y., Li, W., et al. (2018). Novel compounds protect auditory hair cells against gentamycin-induced apoptosis by maintaining the expression level of H3K4me2. *Drug Deliv.* 25, 1033–1043. doi: 10.1080/10717544.2018.1461277

Lin, X., Li, G., Zhang, Y., Zhao, J., Lu, J., Gao, Y., et al. (2019). Hearing consequences in Gjb2 knock-in mice: implications for human p.V37I mutation. *Aging* 11, 7416–7441. doi: 10.18632/aging.102246

Liotta, A., Rösner, J., Huchzermeyer, C., Wojtowicz, A., Kann, O., Schmitz, D., et al. (2012). Energy demand of synaptic transmission at the hippocampal Schaffer-collateral synapse. *J. Cereb. Blood Flow Metab.* 32, 2076–2083. doi: 10.1038/jcbfm.2012.116

Liu, H., Li, G., Lu, J., Gao, Y. G., Song, L., Li, G. L., et al. (2019a). Cellular Differences in the Cochlea of CBA and B6 Mice May Underlie Their Difference in Susceptibility to Hearing Loss. *Front. Cell Neurosci.* 13:60. doi: 10.3389/fncel.2019.00060

Liu, H., Lu, J., Wang, Z., Song, L., Wang, X., Li, G. L., et al. (2019b). Functional alteration of ribbon synapses in inner hair cells by noise exposure causing hidden hearing loss. *Neurosci. Lett.* 707:134268. doi: 10.1016/j.neulet.2019.05.022

Liu, H., Peng, H., Wang, L., Xu, P., Wang, Z., Liu, H., et al. (2020). Differences in Calcium Clearance at Inner Hair Cell Active Zones May Underlie the Difference in Susceptibility to Noise-Induced Cochlea Synaptopathy of C57BL/6J and CBA/CaJ Mice. *Front. Cell Dev. Biol.* 8:635201. doi: 10.3389/fcell.2020.635201

Liu, W., Xu, L., Wang, X., Zhang, D., Sun, G., Wang, M., et al. (2021). PRDX1 activates autophagy via the PTEN-AKT signaling pathway to protect against cisplatin-induced spiral ganglion neuron damage. *Autophagy* 2021, 1–23. doi: 10.1080/15548627.2021.1905466

Liu, W., Xu, X., Fan, Z., Sun, G., Han, Y., Zhang, D., et al. (2019c). Wnt Signaling Activates TP53-Induced Glycolysis and Apoptosis Regulator and Protects Against Cisplatin-Induced Spiral Ganglion Neuron Damage in the Mouse Cochlea. *Antioxid Redox Signal* 30, 1389–1410. doi: 10.1089/ars.2017.7288

Liu, Y., Qi, J., Chen, X., Tang, M., Chu, C., Zhu, W., et al. (2019d). Critical role of spectrin in hearing development and deafness. *Sci. Adv.* 5:eaav7803. doi: 10.1126/sciadv.aav7803

Lv, J., Fu, X., Li, Y., Hong, G., Li, P., Lin, J., et al. (2021). Deletion of Kcnj16 in Mice Does Not Alter Auditory Function. *Front. Cell Dev. Biol.* 9:630361. doi: 10.3389/fcell.2021.630361

Majtnerová, P., and Roušar, T. (2018). An overview of apoptosis assays detecting DNA fragmentation. *Mol. Biol. Rep.* 45, 1469–1478. doi: 10.1007/s11033-018-4258-9

Matern, M., Vijayakumar, S., Margulies, Z., Milon, B., Song, Y., Elkon, R., et al. (2017). Gfi1(Cre) mice have early onset progressive hearing loss and induce recombination in numerous inner ear non-hair cells. *Sci. Rep.* 7:42079. doi: 10.1038/srep42079

McKay, S. E., Yan, W., Nouws, J., Thormann, M. J., Raimundo, N., Khan, A., et al. (2015). Auditory Pathology in a Transgenic mtTFB1 Mouse Model of Mitochondrial Deafness. *Am. J. Pathol.* 185, 3132–3140. doi: 10.1016/j.ajpath.2015.08.014

Meyer, A. C., Frank, T., Khimich, D., Hoch, G., Riedel, D., Chapochnikov, N. M., et al. (2009). Tuning of synapse number, structure and function in the cochlea. *Nat. Neurosci.* 12, 444–453. doi: 10.1038/nn.2293

Nagase, M., Takahashi, Y., Watabe, A. M., Kubo, Y., and Kato, F. (2014). On-site energy supply at synapses through monocarboxylate transporters maintains excitatory synaptic transmission. *J. Neurosci.* 34, 2605–2617. doi: 10.1523/jneurosci.4687-12.2014

Natarajan, V., Chawla, R., Mah, T., Vivekanandan, R., Tan, S. Y., Sato, P. Y., et al. (2020). Mitochondrial Dysfunction in Age-Related Metabolic Disorders. *Proteomics* 20:e1800404. doi: 10.1002/pmic.201800404

Nemeth, C. L., Tomlinson, S. N., Rosen, M., O'Brien, B. M., Larraza, O., Jain, M., et al. (2020). Neuronal ablation of mt-AspRS in mice induces immune pathway activation prior to severe and progressive cortical and behavioral disruption. *Exp. Neurol.* 326:113164. doi: 10.1016/j.expneurol.2019.113164

Oprescu, S. N., Griffin, L. B., Beg, A. A., and Antonellis, A. (2017). Predicting the pathogenicity of aminoacyl-tRNA synthetase mutations. *Methods* 113, 139–151. doi: 10.1016/j.ymeth.2016.11.013

Pierce, S. B., Chisholm, K. M., Lynch, E. D., Lee, M. K., Walsh, T., Opitz, J. M., et al. (2011). Mutations in mitochondrial histidyl tRNA synthetase HARS2 cause ovarian dysgenesis and sensorineural hearing loss of Perrault syndrome. *Proc. Natl. Acad. Sci. U S A* 108, 6543–6548. doi: 10.1073/pnas.1103471108

Qi, J., Liu, Y., Chu, C., Chen, X., Zhu, W., Shu, Y., et al. (2019). A cytoskeleton structure revealed by super-resolution fluorescence imaging in inner ear hair cells. *Cell Discov.* 5:12. doi: 10.1038/s41421-018-0076-4

Qi, J., Zhang, L., Tan, F., Liu, Y., Chu, C., Zhu, W., et al. (2020). Espin distribution as revealed by super-resolution microscopy of stereocilia. *Am. J. Transl. Res.* 12, 130–141.

Qian, F., Wang, X., Yin, Z., Xie, G., Yuan, H., Liu, D., et al. (2020). The slc4a2b gene is required for hair cell development in zebrafish. *Aging*12, 18804–18821. doi: 10.18632/aging.103840

Safieddine, S., El-Amraoui, A., and Petit, C. (2012). The auditory hair cell ribbon synapse: from assembly to function. *Ann. Rev. Neurosci.* 35, 509–528. doi: 10.1146/annurev-neuro-061010-113705

Schmittgen, T. D., and Livak, K. J. (2008). Analyzing real-time PCR data by the comparative C(T) method. *Nat. Protoc.* 3, 1101–1108. doi: 10.1038/nprot.2008.73

Schwander, M., Kachar, B., and Müller, U. (2010). Review series: The cell biology of hearing. *J Cell Biol.* 190, 9–20. doi: 10.1083/jcb.201001138

Scimemi, P., Santarelli, R., Selmo, A., and Mammano, F. (2014). Auditory brainstem responses to clicks and tone bursts in C57 BL/6J mice. *Acta Otorhinolaryngol. Ital.* 34, 264–271.

Sheffield, A. M., and Smith, R. J. H. (2019). The Epidemiology of Deafness. *Cold Spr. Harb. Perspect. Med.* 9:33258. doi: 10.1101/cshperspect.a033258

Spoendlin, H. (1971). Primary structural changes in the organ of Corti after acoustic overstimulation. *Acta Otolaryngol.* 71, 166–176. doi: 10.3109/00016487109125346

van der Laan, M., Bohnert, M., Wiedemann, N., and Pfanner, N. (2012). Role of

MINOS in mitochondrial membrane architecture and biogenesis. *Trends Cell Biol.* 22, 185–192. doi: 10.1016/j.tcb.2012.01.004

Vikhe Patil, K., Canlon, B., and Cederroth, C. R. (2015). High quality RNA extraction of the mammalian cochlea for qRT-PCR and transcriptome analyses. *Hear Res* 325, 42–48. doi: 10.1016/j.heares.2015.03.008

Wang, M., Sips, P., Khin, E., Rotival, M., Sun, X., Ahmed, R., et al. (2016). Wars2 is a determinant of angiogenesis. *Nat. Commun.* 7:12061. doi: 10.1038/ncomms12061

Wang, X., Zhu, Y., Long, H., Pan, S., Xiong, H., Fang, Q., et al. (2019). Mitochondrial Calcium Transporters Mediate Sensitivity to Noise-Induced Losses of Hair Cells and Cochlear Synapses. *Front. Mole. Neurosci.* 11:469. doi: 10.3389/fnmol.2018.00469

Wang, Y., Zhou, J. B., Zeng, Q. Y., Wu, S., Xue, M. Q., Fang, P., et al. (2020). Hearing impairment-associated KARS mutations lead to defects in aminoacylation of both cytoplasmic and mitochondrial tRNA(Lys). *Sci. China Life Sci.* 2020:1619. doi: 10.1007/s11427-019-1619-x

Wei, H., Chen, Z., Hu, Y., Cao, W., Ma, X., Zhang, C., et al. (2021). Topographically Conductive Butterfly Wing Substrates for Directed Spiral Ganglion Neuron Growth. *Small* 17:e2102062. doi: 10.1002/smll.202102062

Wollweber, F., von der Malsburg, K., and van der Laan, M. (2017). Mitochondrial contact site and cristae organizing system: A central player in membrane shaping and crosstalk. *Biochim. Biophys. Acta Mol. Cell Res.* 1864, 1481–1489. doi: 10.1016/j.bbamcr.2017.05.004

Wong, H. C., Zhang, Q., Beirl, A. J., Petralia, R. S., Wang, Y. X., and Kindt, K. (2019). Synaptic mitochondria regulate hair-cell synapse size and function. *Elife* 8:48914. doi: 10.7554/eLife.48914

Wu, F., Xiong, H., and Sha, S. (2020). Noise-induced loss of sensory hair cells is mediated by ROS/AMPKα pathway. *Redox Biol.* 29:101406. doi: 10.1016/j.redox.2019.101406

Yang, H., Gan, J., Xie, X., Deng, M., Feng, L., Chen, X., et al. (2010). Gfi1-Cre knock-in mouse line: A tool for inner ear hair cell-specific gene deletion. *Genesis* 48, 400–406. doi: 10.1002/dvg.20632

Yu, J., Jiang, W., Cao, L., Na, X., and Yang, J. (2020). Two novel likely pathogenic variants of HARS2 identified in a Chinese family with sensorineural hearing loss. *Hereditas* 157:47. doi: 10.1186/s41065-020-00157-7

Yu, J., Wang, Y., Liu, P., Li, Q., Sun, Y., and Kong, W. (2014). Mitochondrial DNA common deletion increases susceptibility to noise-induced hearing loss in a mimetic aging rat model. *Biochem. Biophys. Res. Commun.* 453, 515–520. doi: 10.1016/j.bbrc.2014.09.118

Zhang, L., Du, Z., and Gong, S. (2021). Mitochondrial Dysfunction and Sirtuins: Important Targets in Hearing Loss. *Neural. Plasticity* 2021:5520794. doi: 10.1155/2021/5520794

Zhang, S., Dong, Y., Qiang, R., Zhang, Y., Zhang, X., Chen, Y., et al. (2021). Characterization of Strip1 Expression in Mouse Cochlear Hair Cells. *Front. Genet.* 12:625867. doi: 10.3389/fgene.2021.625867

Zhang, S., Zhang, Y., Dong, Y., Guo, L., Zhang, Z., Shao, B., et al. (2020). Knockdown of Foxg1 in supporting cells increases the trans-differentiation of supporting cells into hair cells in the neonatal mouse cochlea. *Cell Mol. Life Sci.* 77, 1401–1419. doi: 10.1007/s00018-019-03291-2

Zhang, Y., Li, Y., Fu, X., Wang, P., Wang, Q., Meng, W., et al. (2021). The Detrimental and Beneficial Functions of Macrophages After Cochlear Injury. *Front. Cell Dev. Biol.* 9:631904. doi: 10.3389/fcell.2021.631904

Zhao, J., Li, G., Zhao, X., Lin, X., Gao, Y., Raimundo, N., et al. (2020). Down-regulation of AMPK signaling pathway rescues hearing loss in TFB1 transgenic mice and delays age-related hearing loss. *Aging* 12, 5590–5611. doi: 10.18632/aging.102977

Zheng, Q. Y., Johnson, K. R., and Erway, L. C. (1999). Assessment of hearing in 80 inbred strains of mice by ABR threshold analyses. *Hear. Res.* 130, 94–107. doi: 10.1016/s0378-5955(99)00003-9

Zhong, Z., Fu, X., Li, H., Chen, J., Wang, M., Gao, S., et al. (2020). Citicoline Protects Auditory Hair Cells Against Neomycin-Induced Damage. *Front. Cell Dev. Biol.* 8:712. doi: 10.3389/fcell.2020.00712

Zhou, H., Qian, X., Xu, N., Zhang, S., Zhu, G., Zhang, Y., et al. (2020). Disruption of Atg7-dependent autophagy causes electromotility disturbances, outer hair cell loss, and deafness in mice. *Cell Death Dis.* 11:913. doi: 10.1038/s41419-020-03110-8

16

Chronic Unilateral Hearing Loss Disrupts Neural Tuning to Sound-Source Azimuth in the Rat Primary Auditory Cortex

*Xiuwen Wang, Jing Liu and Jiping Zhang**

Key Laboratory of Brain Functional Genomics, Ministry of Education, NYU-ECNU Institute of Brain and Cognitive Science at NYU Shanghai, School of Life Sciences, East China Normal University, Shanghai, China

Correspondence:
Jiping Zhang
jpzhang@bio.ecnu.edu.cn

Accurate sound localization requires normal binaural input and precise auditory neuronal representation of sound spatial locations. Previous studies showed that unilateral hearing loss profoundly impaired the sound localization abilities. However, the underlying neural mechanism is not fully understood. Here, we investigated how chronic unilateral conductive hearing loss (UCHL) affected the neural tuning to sound source azimuth in the primary auditory cortex (AI). The UCHL was manipulated by the removal of tympanic membrane and malleus in the right ear of young (P14) rats and adult (P57) rats. We recorded the azimuth tuning of neurons in the left AI contralateral to the operated ear in the two groups of rats that experienced 2 months of UCHL, and in the left AI of age-matched control rats. We found that AI neurons in control rats showed predominant preference to sound from contralateral azimuths. However, UCHL weakened the cortical neuronal representation of contralateral azimuths on the operated ear side and strengthened the cortical neuronal representation of ipsilateral azimuths on the intact ear side. This effect was stronger in rats with UCHL at young age than in rats with UCHL in adulthood. Moreover, UCHL degraded the azimuth selectivity and azimuth sensitivity of AI neurons, and this effect was stronger in rats with UCHL in adulthood than in rats with UCHL at young age. These findings highlight a remarkable age-related experience-dependent plasticity of neural tuning to sound source azimuth in AI, and imply a neural mechanism for the impacts of chronic UCHL on sound localization abilities.

Keywords: hearing loss, auditory cortex, azimuth tuning, sound localization, plasticity

INTRODUCTION

The ability to accurately localize and segregate different sound sources is a fundamental acoustical process for human and animals in analyzing signal sounds, monitoring acoustical environment, and guiding subsequent behavioral responses. To localize a sound source, the auditory system relies on the processing of sound spectral, temporal, and level information reaching to the two ears. Unilateral hearing impairments profoundly affect the sound localization ability of human subjects

Abbreviations: ABR, auditory brainstem response; ACon, adult control; AI, primary auditory cortex; AUCHL, adult unilateral conductive hearing loss; CF, characteristic frequency; MT, minimum threshold; PAR75, the preferred azimuth range over which the normalized response strengths are ≥ 0.75; UCHL, unilateral conductive hearing loss; YCon, young control; YUCHL, young unilateral conductive hearing loss.

with hearing loss compared to normal hearing counterparts (Humes et al., 1980; Wilmington et al., 1994). Therefore, normal binaural hearing is necessary for accurate sound localization.

The neural mechanism for processing sound spatial information has been investigated in many previous studies. Behavioral studies by focal lesion or deactivation in the auditory cortex have shown that the AI is necessary for sound localization (Jenkins and Merzenich, 1984; King et al., 2007; Malhotra and Lomber, 2007), and that AI in each hemisphere mainly contributes to localizing sounds in the contralateral auditory space (Jenkins and Merzenich, 1984; Malhotra and Lomber, 2007). Studies in normal hearing animals have demonstrated that many neurons in AI were sensitive to sound source azimuth, i.e., they responded strongly to sound stimuli at some azimuths but poorly at others. Most of the neurons in AI preferred sound stimuli from the contralateral field, and only a small proportion of neurons preferred the sound stimuli from midline or ipsilateral field. This has been demonstrated in cats (Imig et al., 1990; Rajan et al., 1990; Barone et al., 1996; Eggermont and Mossop, 1998), rats (Yao et al., 2013; Gao et al., 2018), and monkeys (Woods et al., 2006). Studies also showed that many azimuth-sensitive neurons in the AI of adult cats determined in binaural conditions immediately became insensitive to sound source azimuth when determined with one ear plugged (Samson et al., 1994), demonstrating the importance of normal binaural input in the spatial sensitivity of AI neurons.

Abnormal binaural hearing is often found in patients with unilateral hearing loss, especially in very young children. During postnatal hearing development, a population of young children experience short-term or chronic UCHL associated with otitis media with effusion. The UCHL attenuates sound transmission to the inner ear with the cochlea remaining largely intact, and produces an imbalance in inputs between the two ears. The UCHL distorts the binaural information for localizing sound source, i.e., the interaural time differences and interaural level differences. Thus, understanding how the neurons in the auditory cortex respond to chronic UCHL at various postnatal ages can provide insights into the impacts of chronic otitis media with effusion and other disorders that affect sound transmission through the external or middle ear. In animal studies, UCHL can be induced by unilateral earplugging (Moore et al., 1989), monaural ear canal ligation (Popescu and Polley, 2010), and monaural disruption of tympanic membrane and ossicles (Tucci et al., 1999; Sumner et al., 2005). These manipulations have become important tools for studying the experience-dependent plasticity in the auditory system. Unilateral ear canal ligation in young rats caused distorted tonotopic maps and a reorganized aural dominance in AI. The representation of the ligated ear in AI was weakened and the representation of the ear with normal hearing was strengthened (Popescu and Polley, 2010). UCHL in young gerbils significantly decreases the metabolic activity in the major ascending projections of the manipulated ear in the central auditory system (Tucci et al., 1999). The most extreme condition of abnormal binaural input is unilateral deafness, e.g., congenital single-sided deafness, bilateral deafness equipped only with one cochlear implant, and unilateral cochlear ablation. The unilateral deafness completely eliminates the input from one of the two ears. Previous studies, by recording local field potentials from the cortical surface of cats, showed that single-sided deafness within an early sensitive period led to unilateral aural preference in favor to the hearing ear (Kral et al., 2013b), and that the plastic reorganizations exhibited hemispheric specificity (Kral et al., 2013a). Further studies by multi-unit recording demonstrated that unilateral hearing prevented non-specific reduction in cortical responsiveness in cat AI, but extensively reorganized aural dominance and binaural responses (Tillein et al., 2016). In addition, previous studies showed that postnatal unilateral cochlea ablation rewired the projection from the non-operated ear to the brainstem (Kitzes et al., 1995; Gabriele et al., 2000), disrupted the maintenance of the banded projections of the dorsal nucleus of the lateral lemniscus in the inferior colliculus ipsilateral to the ablation (Franklin et al., 2006), and led to a dramatic increase in the proportion of neurons in the inferior colliculus ipsilateral to the intact ear (McAlpine et al., 1997). These findings demonstrate a developmental and experience-dependent plasticity in the auditory system.

Accurate sound localization also relies on normal binaural hearing and precise processing of auditory spatial information in the auditory system during postnatal hearing development. In human subjects with congenital UCHL, the performance of sound localization was still below the control level after corrected congenital UCHL (Wilmington et al., 1994). It is possible that abnormal binaural input profoundly affects the neural representation of auditory space in the central auditory system and consequently impairs sound localization performance. However, at present we still have a poor understanding of how chronic UCHL at various postnatal ages affects the neural representation of auditory space in the auditory cortex. In the present study, we investigated whether identical UCHL manipulation carried out in young rats and adult rats produces the same outcome in the neural representation of spatial azimuth in the rat AI. Because previous studies have demonstrated a dominant preference of AI neurons to stimuli from the contralateral auditory space (Imig et al., 1990; Rajan et al., 1990; Barone et al., 1996; Eggermont and Mossop, 1998; Woods et al., 2006; Gao et al., 2018; Yao and Sanes, 2018), we here focused on studying the impacts of postnatal UCHL on the neural tuning to sound source azimuth in the AI contralateral the operated ear. We found that chronic UCHL carried out at both young and adult ages altered the azimuth preference, degraded the azimuth selectivity and sensitivity of AI neurons. Importantly, we found age-related impacts of UCHL on the azimuth tuning of AI neurons exhibited by azimuth preference as well as the azimuth sensitivity and azimuth selectivity of AI neurons.

MATERIALS AND METHODS

Animals and Animal Groups

The Sprague Dawley rats of both sexes were obtained from an in-housing breed stock that originated from the breeding pairs purchased from Shanghai Jie Shi Jie Laboratory Animal Co., Ltd. (Shanghai, China). Four groups of rats were used: (1) Young unilateral conductive hearing loss group (YUCHL group): the rats were operated with UCHL surgery by removing the tympanic membrane and malleus in the right ear at postnatal (P) day 14 (P14), and were reared till the age of P74–P87. (2) Young control group (YCon group): the rats with no UCHL surgery at young age were reared till the age of P74–P87. (3) Adult unilateral conductive hearing loss group (AUCHL group): the rats were operated with UCHL surgery in the right ear at P57, and were reared till the age of P117–P130. (4) Adult control group (ACon group): rats with no UCHL surgery were reared till the age of P117–P130. All rats had free access to food and water, and were reared in the housing environments on 12 h light-dark cycles. The housing temperature was maintained at 20–24°C. The age of rats used for neurophysiological recording was P74–P87 for both the YUCHL group and the YCon group, and was P117–P130 for both the AUCHL group and the ACon group. The purpose of selecting rats within these age ranges for neurophysiological recording was to ensure that all rats used for data recording were in adulthood, and that the impacts of chronic UCHL on azimuth tuning of AI neurons in both the YUCHL group and the AUCHL group were determined within 2 weeks after the rats had 2 months of UCHL experiences.

In the present study, the neurophysiological data were obtained from a total of 95 rats including 29 rats in the YCon group, 27 rats in the YUCHL group, 20 rats in the ACon group, and 19 rats in the AUCHL group, respectively.

Surgery Procedure for UCHL

Unilateral conductive hearing loss was induced in the right ear using the procedures similar to those described in previous studies (Tucci et al., 1999; Xu et al., 2007). Surgical anesthesia was induced with pentobarbital sodium (40 mg/kg i.p.) and was confirmed by a complete elimination of responses to nociceptive stimuli. In the right ear, both the tympanic membrane and the malleus were removed with jeweler's forceps under microscope. Following the surgery the animals were allowed to fully recover under supervision and then were returned to their cages.

Auditory Brainstem Response Measurement

Before doing single-unit recording in the auditory cortex, we measured the ABR from a subset of rats in each group. The main purpose of the ABR measurement was to evaluate the differences in hearing threshold between the intact left ear and the operated right ear with UCHL surgery in the two groups of rats with UCHL.

Rats were anesthetized with urethane (1.5 g/kg i.p.) and then placed in a stereotaxic frame in a double-walled sound-proof room. The inside walls and ceiling of the sound-proof room were covered by sound-absorbing foams to reduce acoustic reflections. The ABR measurements were obtained in a neurophysiology workstation (TDT3, Tucker-Davis Technologies, United States). The multifunction processor (RX6-A5), speaker amplifier (SA1), and multi-field magnetic speakers (MF1) were used to present closed-field acoustic stimuli. The output of the magnetic speakers was calibrated in a closed-field system from 2.0 to 48.0 kHz (sampling rate, 100 kHz) using a one-quarter inch condenser microphone (model 7016, ACO Pacific Inc.). The acoustic signal was present from the calibrated magnetic speaker coupled to the ear. The subdermal needle electrodes (Rochester Electro-Medical, Inc., United States), headstage (RA4LI), preamplifier (RA4PA), and RA16 medusa base station were used to record ABR signals. The electrodes were placed subcutaneously at the vertex (active), the mastoid ipsilateral to the acoustic signal source (reference), and the tail of the rats (ground). The ABR thresholds were measured independently for both ears with tone bursts (5 ms duration, 0.5 ms cosine ramps, 21 Hz repetition rate). The tone bursts were 4–36 kHz in frequency with 4 kHz increments, and 15 dB SPL to 85 dB SPL in level with 5 dB increments. The ABR signals were bandpass filtered (0.3–3 kHz), averaged from 512 stimulus pairs, and analyzed in BioSigRP software. The ABR Wave I threshold was defined as the lowest sound level that could reliably produce an acoustic stimulus-evoked peak which followed the progressive trend for decreasing amplitude and increasing latency obtained over the range of tested sound levels (Popescu and Polley, 2010). We determined the ABR Wave I threshold by visual inspections of ABR data, and by using a statistical measure, i.e., the lowest sound level that evoked a wave I with the peak-to-peak amplitude greater than two standard deviations of the background activity.

The ABR data demonstrated that UCHL surgery induced a significant hearing loss, and the average differences in hearing threshold between the intact ear and the operated ear were within the range of 38–53 dB across the frequencies tested (**Figures 1A,B**, Wilcoxon Signed Rank Test under each tested frequency condition, right ear vs. left ear, all $p < 0.001$ in both YUCHL group and AUCHL group). The average differences in hearing threshold between the intact left ear and the operated right ear did not show significant group differences between the YUCHL group and the AUCHL group (**Figure 1C**, Mann–Whitney test, YUCHL vs. and AUCHL, all $p > 0.05$ under each of the tested frequency condition). The effect of UCHL surgery on the hearing threshold of rats determined in the present study is comparable to that shown in previous studies in gerbils (Tucci et al., 1999).

Animal Surgery for Single-Unit Recording in AI

Surgical anesthesia was induced with urethane (1.5 g/kg i.p.) and maintained by intraperitoneal infusion of urethane via an automatic microinfusion pump (WZ-50C6, China) during the surgery and neurophysiological recording. Atropine sulfate (0.01 mg/kg, sc) was given to reduce bronchial secretions. Body temperature was continuously monitored by a thermal probe and maintained at 37.5°C using a thermostatically controlled heating blanket. The surgical procedures were similar to that described in our previous studies (Jiang et al., 2015; Lu et al., 2016). Briefly, after the trachea of rats was cannulated, the dorsal and temporal skull were exposed. The temporal bone was exposed by partially removing the temporal muscle. A nail (4 cm long) was attached to the dorsal surface of the skulls with 502 super glue and dental cement. The head of the

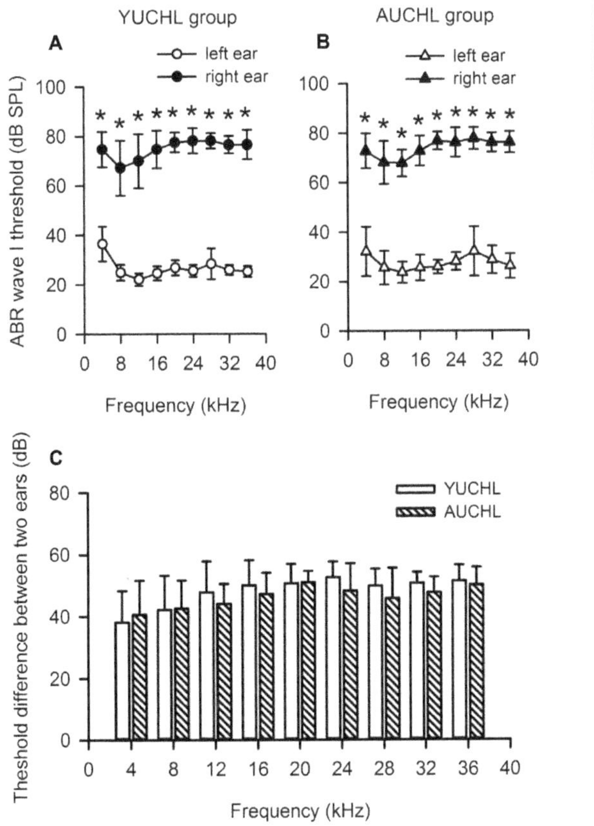

FIGURE 1 | Unilateral conductive hearing loss (UCHL) elevated the auditory brainstem response (ABR) wave I threshold in the operated left ear. YUCHL group: young unilateral conductive hearing loss group; AUCHL group: adult unilateral conductive hearing loss group. Data (shown in mean and standard deviations) were from a subset of rats in the YUCHL group ($n = 15$) and the AUCHL group ($n = 15$). **(A,B)** The ABR wave I thresholds determined independently from the intact left ear and right ear with UCHL in both the YUCHL group **(A)** and the AUCHL group **(B)**. * indicates significantly different in ABR wave I threshold compared to the corresponding data from the left ear (Wilcoxon Signed Rank Test, $p < 0.001$). Note that the ABR thresholds determined in the right ear with UCHL were higher than those in the intact left ear. **(C)** The average differences in ABR wave I thresholds (right ear threshold minus left ear threshold) determined at each frequency. At each frequency, the threshold differences were not significantly different between the two groups (Mann–Whitney test, all $p > 0.05$). See texts in the "Materials and Methods" section for details.

rat was then fixed by the nail to a head holder attached to a stainless steel platform. A craniotomy was performed over the left auditory cortex (contralateral to operated right ear in YUCHL rats and AUCHL rats). The dura was then removed, and the exposed cortex was kept moist by applying warm saline to the cortex.

Systems for Acoustic Stimulus Presentation and Neurophysiological Recording in AI

Acoustic stimulus presentation and single-unit recording were performed through a neurophysiology workstation using TDT System 3 hardware and software (Tucker-Davis Technologies, United States) controlled by a PC. The portion of the workstation for acoustic stimulus presentation includes a multifunction processor (RX6-A5), an electrostatic loudspeaker driver (ED1), and a free field electrostatic loudspeaker (ES1). The acoustic stimuli were delivered through a free-field system. The distance between the loudspeaker and the center of the interaural axis of the rats was constant (20 cm) for all spatial positions tested in the present study. The loudspeaker was able to move freely in the frontal auditory space of the rats by a custom-made motor system. The spatial positions (i.e., azimuths and elevations) of the loudspeaker were monitored by two video cameras. The loudspeaker location directly in front of the rat was assigned to 0° in azimuth, and the loudspeaker elevation aligned to the center of the rat's head was assigned 0° in elevation. In the present study, the loudspeaker elevation was fixed to 0° whereas the loudspeaker azimuth was varied from the left 90° (assigned to −90°) to right 90° (assigned to +90°) in the rat frontal auditory field by a remote control system outside the sound-proof room. The positive azimuths refer to the azimuths contralateral to the cortex (left cortex) being recorded, and the negative azimuths represent the azimuths ipsilateral to the cortex being recorded. The output of the loudspeaker was calibrated from 2.0 to 48.0 kHz (sampling rate, 100 kHz) using a one-quarter inch condenser microphone (model 7016, ACO Pacific Inc.) placed at the center of the interaural axis of rats and faced directly to the loudspeaker. The calibration data were stored in the computer for use in obtaining the desired sound pressure levels in decibel (dB SPLs, re: 20 μPa) within the calibrated frequency range. The acoustic stimuli were tonal stimuli with 50 ms in duration including 2.5 ms rise time and 2.5 ms fall time. The acoustic stimulus frequencies used in the present study did not exceed 46.0 kHz. The interstimulus interval was 1,000 ms.

The recording of neural responses in the auditory cortex to acoustic stimuli was conducted in the sound-proof room. Glass electrodes (1.0–2.0 MΩ impedance, filled with 2M NaCl) were advanced orthogonally to the pial surface of AI by a microdrive (SM-21, Narishige, Japan) that was remotely controlled outside the sound-proof room. Action potentials were recorded, amplified (×1,000), and band pass filtered (0.3–3.0 kHz) by a DAM80 amplifier (WPI, United States), and then fed into a pre-amplifier RA8GA, a RA16 Medusa base station (TDT), and PC for online and offline data processing. The signal was also sent to a digital oscilloscope (TDS 2024, United States) for display and an audio monitor for listening.

Data Collection and Acoustic Stimulus Presentation Paradigm

At the beginning of single-unit recording in the left auditory cortex, the free-field loudspeaker was placed at 30° in azimuth and 0° in elevation in the rat frontal auditory space. The procedure to locate the AI of rats was similar to that described in our previous study (Lu et al., 2016). Preliminary electrode penetrations were made perpendicular to the pial surface of the auditory cortex of each rat to construct a coarse tonotopic map. The positions of the penetrations were within the range of 3.0–5.5 mm posterior to Bregma in anterior–posterior direction, and 3.0–5.0 mm to the Bregma in dorsal–ventral direction. The depth of the penetrations was limited to the range of 300–800 μm below the pial surface. The AI was defined based on electrophysiological properties such as short-latency responses to acoustic stimuli and increasing characteristic frequencies (CFs) of neurons in a caudal to rostral direction (Doron et al., 2002). Once a single unit was well isolated (based on the constancy of amplitude and waveform of evoked action potentials) in AI, the CF of the neuron was determined. We first audio-visually determined the frequency-level ranges that the neuron responded at both 30° and −30° in azimuth. At one of two azimuths which the neuron responded to tonal stimuli at the lowest sound level, we determined the CF of the neuron using a stimulus matrix varied with sound levels (0 to 80 dB SPL in 10-dB steps) and sound frequencies (frequency range: previously audio-visually determined, interval: 1.0 kHz). The CF was the frequency which evoked a response of the neuron at the lowest threshold level. We then determined the rate-level function at the CF and within the level range of 0–80 dB SPL with 10-dB steps. Each stimulus was repeated 20 times. Due to low spontaneous activities in anesthetized rat AI, the MT of the neuron was arbitrarily defined as the sound level that elicited 20% of the maximal spike count in the rate-level function. We used this sound level as the reference level to measure the azimuth tuning curves (or azimuth functions) of the neuron. The azimuth functions of the neuron were determined at the CF, and with an azimuth-level stimulus matrix varied with azimuths (−90°, −70°, −50°, −30°, −10°, 0°, +10°, +30°, +50°, +70°, and +90°) and sound levels (MT+5 dB, MT+10 dB, and MT+20 dB). If the neuron was still available for recording after the three azimuth functions were determined, an additional rate-level function of the studied neuron was obtained to evaluate the stability of the neuron's response. If the neural responses to the same stimuli varied greater than 20%, the data were excluded from further analysis.

The AI neurons tested in the present study all responded transiently to the onset of the sound stimuli. The neural responses to the azimuth-level stimulus matrix were determined based on the total number of spikes per 20 trials of sound stimuli evoked within the sound duration. For each neuron, we plotted the azimuth function at each sound level in both spike counts and normalized response strength (**Figure 2**). We normalized the responses in spike counts by calculating the response strength relative to the maximum spike count in each azimuth function, and the maximum response strength was 1.0 (**Figure 2**, the left *y*-axis indicates spike counts evoked by 20 trials of stimuli, and the right *y*-axis indicates the normalized response strength). For each azimuth function, we determined the preferred azimuth range over which the normalized response strength was ≥0.75 (PAR75). The location of the PAR75 in the horizontal plane was used as a measure of azimuth preference whereas the width of the PAR75 was used as a measure of azimuth selectivity. In each panel of **Figure 2**, the dotted horizontal line indicates the normalized response strength at 0.75, and the horizontal double-headed arrow show the PAR75 determined for each azimuth function. If the dotted line intersects with both sides of the azimuth function, the PAR75 was the azimuth range between the two intersects (**Figure 2A**, horizontal line with double arrowhead). For the unbounded azimuth function, if the dotted line intersects with only one side of the azimuth function, the PAR75 was defined as the azimuth range from the intersect of the dotted line with the azimuth function to the contralateral azimuth limit (i.e., azimuth +90°, **Figure 2B**) or the ipsilateral azimuth limit (i.e., azimuth −90°, **Figure 2C**). If the dotted line did not intersect with either side of the azimuth function, the PAR75 was defined as the azimuth range from −90° to +90° (i.e., PAR75 = 180°, **Figure 2D**). It should be noted that the method to determine PAR75 in the unbounded azimuth functions (**Figures 2B–D**) underestimates the actual extent of PAR75. If an azimuth function has multiple PAR75s, the PAR75 width of the neuron was defined as the sum of the extent of these PAR75s. In addition, the modulation depth of each azimuth function was defined as the difference in normalized response strength between the maximum value and the minimum value (**Figures 2A–D**, vertical lines with double arrowhead). The modulation depth of the azimuth function was used as a measure of azimuth sensitivity.

Statistical analyses were performed in SPSS 13.0, and a criterion of $p < 0.05$ was considered as significantly different between groups.

RESULTS

For each neuron that was available for recording in the rat AI, we determined the azimuth functions at its CF and at the sound levels of MT+5 dB, MT+10 dB, and MT+20 dB, respectively. The data of the azimuth functions from 278 neurons were obtained in the AI of the four groups of rats, including 78 neurons in the YCon group, 73 neurons in the YUCHL group, 61 neurons in the ACon group, and 66 neurons in the AUCHL group. The CF ranges of these AI neurons were 4.0–44.0 kHz in the YCon group, 5.0–41.0 kHz in the YUCHL group, 8.0–41.0 kHz in the ACon group, and 4.2–35.0 kHz in the AUCHL group.

Unilateral conductive hearing loss induced an increase in the MTs of AI neurons contralateral to operated ear in comparison with the MTs of AI neurons in the age-matched control rats. The MTs of AI neurons were significantly higher in the YUCHL group than in the YCon group (YUCHL vs. YCon in mean and standard error, 45.00 ± 1.85 dB SPL vs. 31.46 ± 1.11 dB SPL, Mann–Whitney Test, $z = -5.273$, $p < 0.001$). Similarly, the MTs of AI neurons were significantly higher in the AUCHL group than in the ACon group (AUCHL vs. ACon in mean and standard error, 54.16 ± 2.27 dB SPL vs. 30.77 ± 1.28 dB SPL, Mann–Whitney Test, $z = -5.273$, $p < 0.001$). In the two UCHL groups, the MTs of AI neurons were significantly higher in the AUCHL group than in the YUCHL group (Mann–Whitney Test, $z = -2.942$, $p = 0.003$). No significant differences were found in MTs between the two control groups (YCon vs. ACon, Mann–Whitney Test, $z = -0.577$, $p = 0.564$).

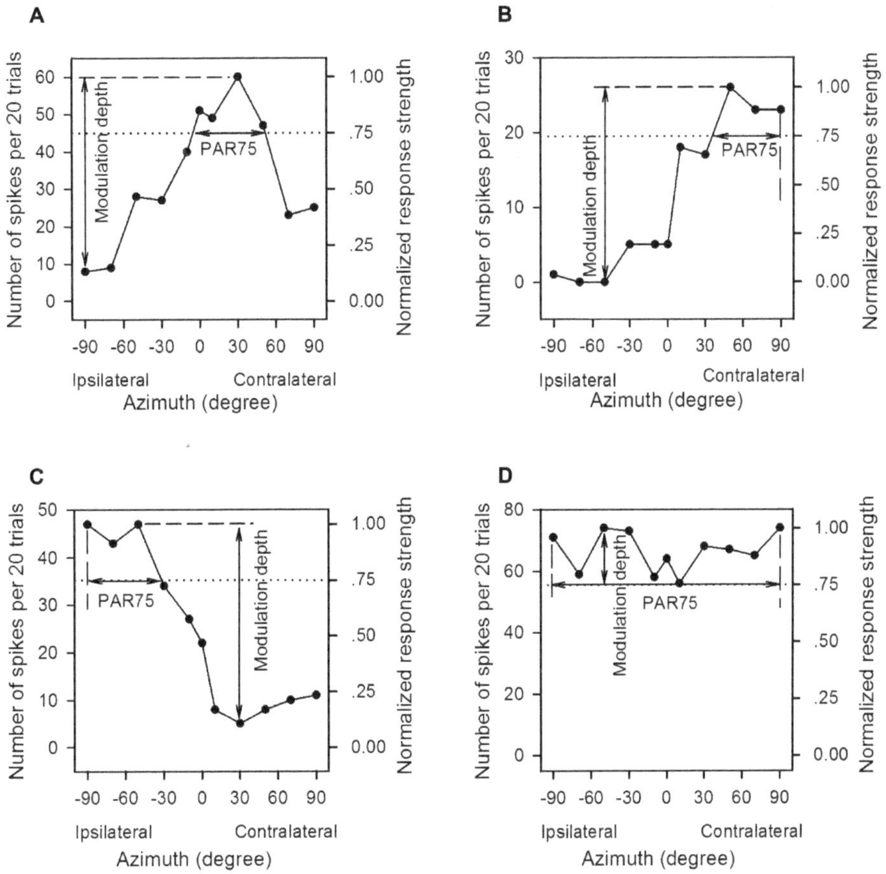

FIGURE 2 | The method to determine the preferred azimuth range and the modulation depth from the azimuth functions of the primary auditory cortex (AI) neurons. **(A–D)** For each panel, the left *y*-axis indicates the number of spikes evoked by per 20 trials of tonal stimuli, and the right *y*-axis indicates the normalized response strength. The spike counts are normalized to the response strengths relative to the maximum spike count in each azimuth function, and the maximum response strength is 1.00. The *x*-axis indicates the speaker location in degree contralateral (positive azimuth) or ipsilateral (negative azimuth) to the cortex (left cortex) being recorded, and 0° is midline azimuth. The dotted line indicates 0.75 in normalized response strength. The range of the horizontal solid line with double arrowhead in each panel is defined as the PAR75, i.e., the preferred azimuth range over which the normalized response strengths are ≥0.75. The range of the vertical solid line with double arrowhead is defined as the modulation depth, i.e., the difference value between the maximum and the minimum normalized response strength in each azimuth function. See texts in the "Materials and Methods" section for details.

Classifications of the Azimuth Functions of Rat AI Neurons

In the frontal auditory space, the azimuths were categorized into contralateral azimuths (from +10° to +90°, not including +10°), central azimuths (from −10° to +10°, including both −10° and +10°), and ipsilateral azimuths (from −10° to −90°, not including −10°) relative to the cortex being recorded. We determined the PAR75 from each azimuth function of an AI neuron measured at a specified sound level, and then categorized the azimuth function at that sound level based on the location and the extent of PAR75. For each azimuth function, it was classified as "contra-field preference" if the PAR75 was restrictively or predominantly distributed within the range of contralateral azimuths (**Figures 3A,B**). The azimuth function was assigned to "ipsi-field preference" if the PAR75 was restrictively or predominantly distributed within the range of ipsilateral azimuths (**Figures 3C,D**). The azimuth function was considered as "central-field preference" if the PRA75 was restrictively or predominantly distributed within the range of central azimuths and with a decline of at least 50% in response on both sides of the maximum response (**Figures 3E,F**). The azimuth function was classified as "omnidirection" if the responses determined at all of the tested azimuths were ≥75% of the maximum response (**Figure 3G**), or if the responses determined at ≥9 of the 11 tested azimuths were ≥75% of the maximum response in the function and the responses at all tested azimuth were ≥50% of the maximum response (**Figure 3H**). The azimuth function was assigned to "multipeak" if there were two or more widely separated peaks in the function, and the PAR75s were distributed within at least two of the three ranges in spatial azimuth, i.e., contralateral azimuths, central azimuths, and ipsilateral azimuths, respectively (**Figure 3I**). If the azimuth function exhibited two peaks and the PAR75s were located within the same lateral-field, the azimuth function was categorized as either contra-field preference or ipsi-field preference.

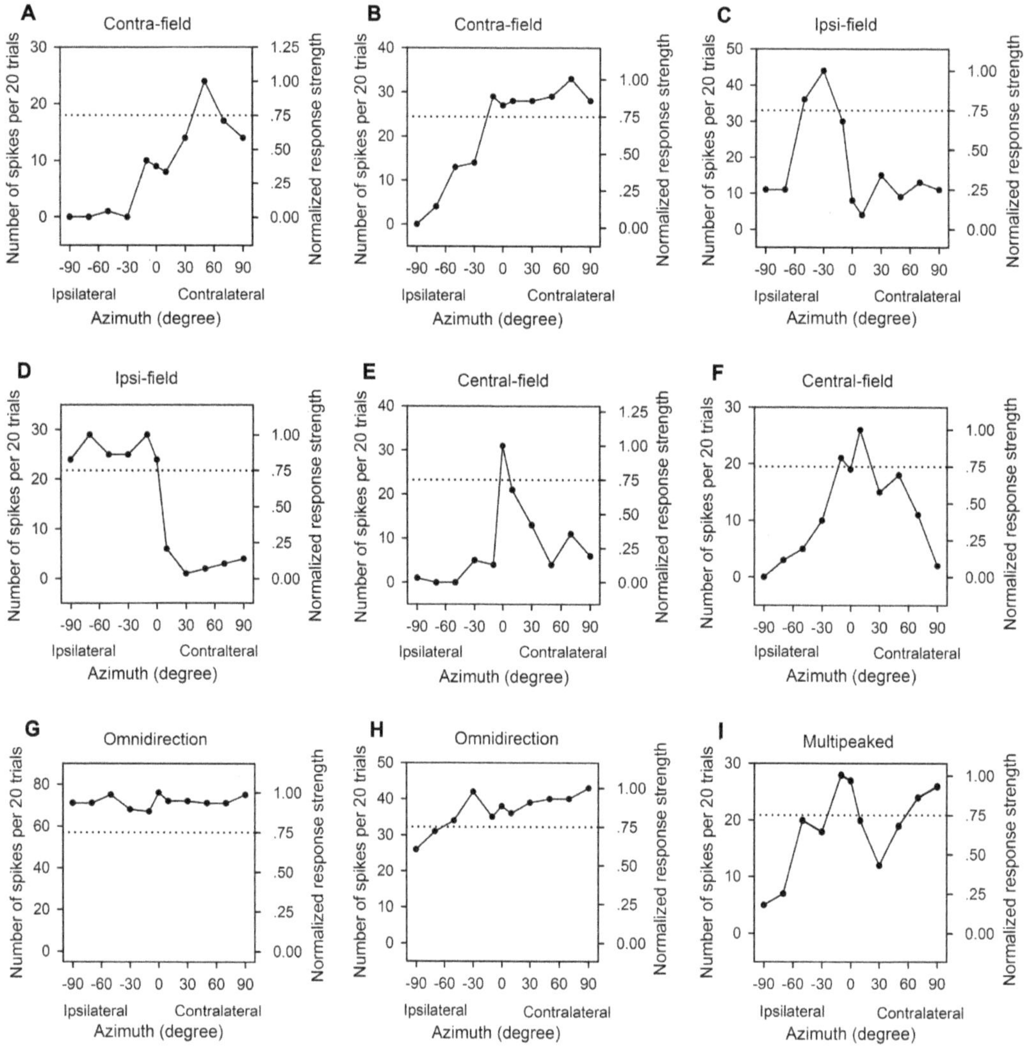

FIGURE 3 | The azimuth functions of nine representative AI neuron with various azimuth preferences. Each panel shows the data from one neuron, the left *y*-axis indicates the number of spikes per 20 trials, and the right *y*-axis indicates the normalized response strength. The *x*-axis indicates the loudspeaker locations in azimuth (degree). The dotted line in each panel indicate 0.75 in normalized response strength. **(A,B)** Contralateral azimuth preference (Contra-field). **(C,D)** Ipsilateral azimuth preference (Ipsi-field). **(E,F)** Central azimuth preference (Central-field). **(G,H)** Omnidirection. **(I)** Multipeak. The frequencies (kHz) and the levels (dB SPL) of sounds used to determine the azimuth functions are as follows: **(A)** 8.0 kHz, 45 dB SPL; **(B)** 9.0 kHz, 60 dB SPL; **(C)** 11.0 kHz, 45 dB SPL; **(D)** 34.0 kHz, 35 dB SPL; **(E)** 14.0 kHz, 30 dB SPL; **(F)** 10.1 kHz, 40 dB SPL, respectively.

The azimuth functions of AI neurons varied with the tested sound levels. **Figure 4** shows the azimuth functions of three AI neurons determined at 5 dB, 10 dB, and 20 dB above the MT of each neuron. It's evident that the azimuth functions varied with neurons, and varied with sound levels for each neuron. The neuron A preferred sound stimuli from contralateral azimuths at MT+5 dB and MT+10 dB conditions, and preferred sound stimuli predominately from contralateral azimuths at MT+20 dB condition (**Figures 4A1,A2**). The preferred azimuth ranges of neuron A increased with increasing sound levels. Neuron B showed clear preference to sound stimuli from ipsilateral azimuths, and the preferred azimuth range of this neuron also varied with sound levels (**Figures 4B1,B2**). Neuron C showed preference to sound stimuli from contralateral azimuths at MT+5 dB, and preference to central azimuths at MT+10 dB (**Figures 4C1,C2**); in contrast, neuron C showed no preference to sound azimuths (i.e., omnidirection) at MT+20 dB condition (**Figures 4C1,C2**).

The Effects of UCHL at Different Postnatal Ages on the Azimuth Functions of AI Neurons

For the population of AI neurons in each group of rats, we determined the average azimuth functions by calculating the means and standard errors of spike counts at each azimuth under various acoustic stimulus conditions (**Figures 5A1–C1**). We then did data analysis (Repeated measure ANOVA with

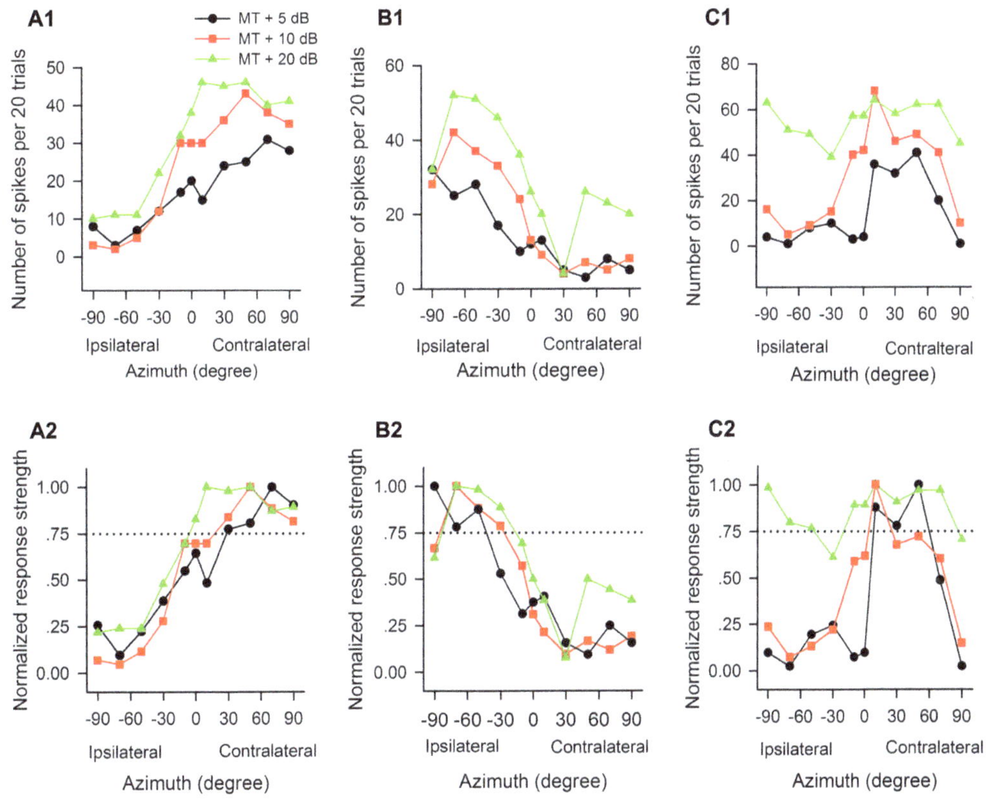

FIGURE 4 | The azimuth functions of three representative AI neurons vary with the change of sound stimulus levels. The data in each column are from one neuron. **(A1–C1)** Azimuth functions shown in number of spikes per 20 trials. **(A2–C2)** Azimuth functions shown in normalized response strength. MT, minimum threshold of the neuron. Curves with different symbols are the azimuth functions determined at the sound levels of MT+5 dB, MT+10 dB, and MT+20 dB, respectively (see the legend in **A1**). The CF (kHz) and MT (dB SPL) of the three neurons are as follows: **(A1,A2)** 13.0 kHz, 35 dB SPL; **(B1,B2)** 34.1 kHz, 30 dB SPL; **(C1,C2)** 35.0 kHz, 20 dB SPL, respectively. Note that the azimuth functions and the azimuth preferences of the three neurons varied with the change of sound levels.

LSD *post hoc* tests) to determine the azimuth preferences of the average azimuth functions shown in spike counts for each group. The data demonstrated a clear preference to sound stimuli from contralateral azimuths for neurons in both the YCon group and the ACon group. For each of the average azimuth functions in the YCon group, the average spike counts at each of the contralateral azimuths (30°, 50°, 70°, and 90°) were greater than those at each of the ipsilateral azimuths (−30°, −50°, −70°, and −90°) (all $p < 0.001$) and at each of the central azimuths (−10°, 0°, and 10°) (all $p \leq 0.01$); similarly, for each average azimuth function in the ACon group, the average spike counts at each of the contralateral azimuths (30°, 50°, 70°, and 90°) were greater than those at each of the ipsilateral azimuths (−30°, −50°, −70°, and −90°) (all $p < 0.001$) and at each of the central azimuths (−10°, 0°, and 10°) (all $p < 0.001$). In contrast, the average azimuth functions in the YUCHL group exhibited ipsilateral azimuth preference under the conditions of MT+5 dB and MT+10 dB (**Figures 5A1,B1**) but showed no azimuth preference under MT+20 dB condition (**Figure 5C1**). Under the conditions of MT+5 dB and MT+10 dB, for each of the average azimuth functions in the YUCHL group, the average spike counts determined at each of the ipsilateral azimuths (−30°, −50°, −70°, and −90°) were greater than those determined at each of the contralateral azimuths (30°, 50°, 70°, and 90°) (all $p < 0.05$); however, no significant differences were found in average spike counts determined at any two tested azimuth pairs in the average azimuth function under MT+20 dB condition (all $p > 0.05$). For the average azimuth functions in the AUCHL group, they exhibited weak preference to the contralateral azimuths: under MT+20 dB condition, the average spikes counts determined at each of the contralateral azimuths (30°, 50°, 70°, and 90°) were greater than those at each of the ipsilateral azimuths (−30°, −50°, −70°, and −90°) (all $p < 0.05$); however, under both MT+5 dB and MT+10 dB conditions, the average spikes counts determined at only a portion of the contralateral azimuths were greater than those at a portion of the ipsilateral azimuths.

We then compared the average azimuth functions (**Figures 5A1–C1**) for population of neurons among the four groups (one-way ANOVA with LSD *post hoc* tests). We found that the average spike counts were not significantly different between the YCon group and the ACon group at each of the azimuths tested (**Figures 5A1–C1**; YCon vs. ACon, all $p > 0.05$). In comparison with the data in both the YCon group and the ACon group, the data in both the YUCHL group and the AUCHL group demonstrated that UCHL consistently

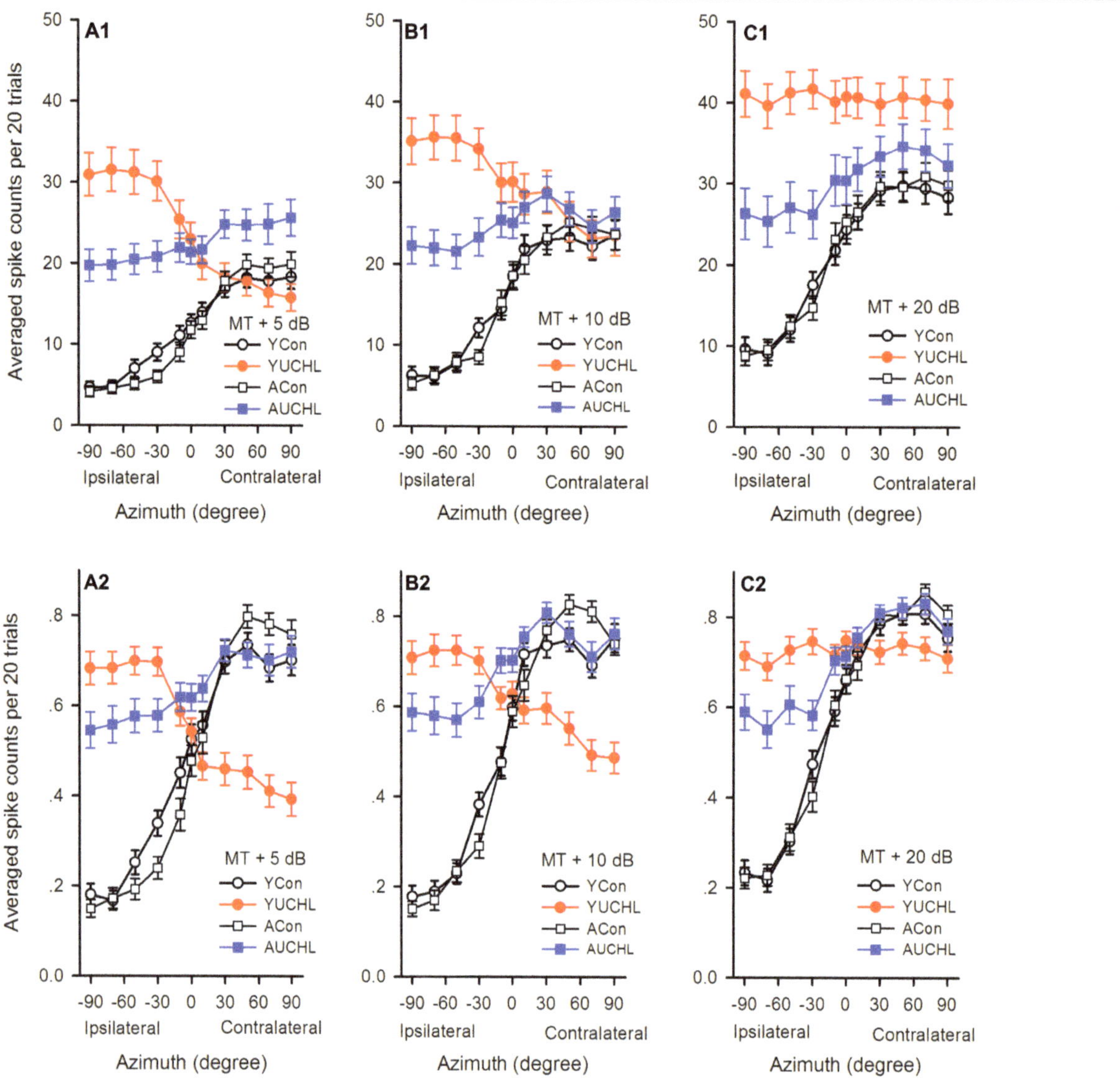

FIGURE 5 | Comparison of the average azimuth functions shown in spikes counts and normalized response strength for the population of AI neurons in the four groups of rats. **(A1–C1)** The average azimuth functions shown in spike counts. **(A2–C2)** The average azimuth functions shown in normalized response strength. The sound levels used to determine the azimuth functions are shown in the legend of each panel. YCon, young control; YUCHL, young unilateral conductive hearing loss; ACon, adult control; AUCHL, adult unilateral conductive hearing loss. The data are shown in mean and standard error.

elevated the responses to stimuli from each of the ipsilateral azimuths (the intact ear side, −30°, −50°, −70°, and −90°) (**Figures 5A1–C1**; at MT+5 dB, all $p < 0.001$, at MT+10 dB, all $p < 0.001$, at MT+20 dB, all $p < 0.01$). Moreover, this elevation of responses to stimuli from the ipsilateral azimuths was more evident in the YUCHL group than in the AUCHL group (**Figures 5A1–C1**; YUCHL vs. AUCHL at each of the ipsilateral azimuths, all $p < 0.001$). For the responses to stimuli from each of the contralateral azimuths (30°, 50°, 70°, and 90°), under MT+5 dB condition, the average spike counts were greater in the AUCHL group than in any one of the other three groups (**Figure 5A1**, all $p < 0.05$) whereas the average spike counts in YUCHL group were not significantly different from the two control groups (**Figure 5A1**, all $p > 0.05$); under MT+10 dB condition, we did not find significant differences in spike counts at each of the contralateral azimuths among the four groups (**Figure 5B1**, all $p > 0.05$); under MT+20 dB condition, at each of the contralateral azimuths, the average spike counts were greater in the YUCHL group than in the two control groups (**Figure 5C1**, all $p < 0.01$) whereas the average spike counts in the AUCHL group were not significantly different from the two control groups (**Figure 5C1**, all $p > 0.05$). In addition, we only found significant differences in the average spike counts between the YUCHL group and the AUCHL group at the azimuth 90° (**Figure 5C1**, YUCHL vs. AUCHL, at the azimuth 90°, $p = 0.04$; at the azimuths 30°, 50°, and 70°, all $p > 0.05$). Therefore, the UCHL at different postnatal periods induced significantly different impacts on the azimuth tuning of AI neurons.

Because the spike counts in the azimuth functions varied with neurons, we compared the mean normalized azimuth functions among the four groups. For each azimuth function, we normalized the spike counts into the response strength relative to the maximum spike count in the azimuth function, and the maximum response strength was 1.0 (**Figures 2–4**). At each of the three sound levels tested (i.e., MT+5 dB, MT+10 dB, and MT+20 dB, respectively), we averaged the normalized response strength in the azimuth functions for the population of AI neurons in each group of rats, and the data were plotted into the mean normalized azimuth functions (**Figures 5A2–C2**). The population data demonstrated that the mean normalized azimuth functions in both the YCon group and the ACon group exhibited clear preferences to sound stimuli from contralateral azimuths (**Figures 5A2–C2**). Statistical analysis (repeated measure ANOVA with LSD *post hoc* tests) showed that, for each normalized mean azimuth function in the YCon group, the average response strength at each of the contralateral azimuths (30°, 50°, 70°, and 90°) was greater than those at each of the central azimuths (−10°, 0°, and 10°; all $p < 0.001$), and was also greater than those at each of the ipsilateral azimuths (−30°, −50°, −70°, and −90°; all $p < 0.001$). Similar findings were shown in the mean azimuth functions in the ACon group. In contrast, the mean normalized azimuth functions for YUCHL group exhibited ipsilateral azimuth preference under the conditions of MT+5 dB and MT+10 dB (**Figures 5A2,B2**), but showed no azimuth preference at MT+20 dB (**Figure 5C2**). Under the conditions of MT+5 dB and MT+10 dB, for each of the mean normalized azimuth functions in the YUCHL group, the average response strength determined at each of the ipsilateral azimuths (−30°, −50°, −70°, and −90°) was greater than those determined at each of the contralateral azimuths (30°, 50°, 70°, and 90°) (all $p < 0.05$); however, no significant differences were found in the average response strengths determined at any two tested azimuth pairs under MT+20 dB condition (all $p > 0.05$). For the AUCHL group, the mean azimuth functions of AI neurons exhibited weak preference to contralateral azimuths. For each of the three mean azimuth functions, the mean response strength determined at each of the contralateral azimuths (30°, 50°, 70°, and 90°) was greater than those determined at each of the ipsilateral azimuths (−30°, −50°, −70°, and −90°) (all $p < 0.05$).

In each of the mean normalized azimuth functions in **Figure 5**, the difference value between the maximum and the minimum average response strength reflect the azimuth sensitivity for population AI neurons. The larger difference value indicates greater azimuth sensitivity. The difference values in each of the mean normalized azimuth functions in the four groups were as follows: at MT+5 dB, 0.57 in YCon group, 0.31 in YUCHL group, 0.65 in ACon group, and 0.19 in AUCHL group (**Figure 5A2**); at MT+10 dB, 0.58 in YCon group, 0.23 in YUCHL group, 0.68 in ACon group, and 0.24 in AUCHL group (**Figure 5B2**); at MT+20 dB, 0.59 in YCon group, 0.04 in AUCHL group, 0.64 in ACon group, and 0.27 in AUCHL group (**Figure 5C2**). These data indicate that the difference values in both the YCon group and the ACon group were larger than those in both the YUCHL group and the AUCHL group. These data suggest that UCHL induced a general decrease of azimuth sensitivity of neurons in the AI contralateral to the operated ear.

The Effect of UCHL at Different Postnatal Ages on the Azimuth Preferences of AI Neurons

For each AI neuron, we determined the PAR75 from each of the azimuth functions determined under the tested sound levels. As shown in **Figure 2**, based on the location of PAR75 in the horizontal plane, we assigned the azimuth preference of the neuron under each sound level condition into one of the five categories: contra-field preference, ipsi-field preference, central-field preference, omnidirection, and multipeak. **Figure 6** shows the percentage of AI neurons in each category of azimuth preference in the four groups of rats. It's evident that, at the tested sound levels, majority of the neurons in both YCon group and ACon group exhibited contra-field preference whereas a small proportion of neurons showed other types of azimuth preference. However, UCHL decreased the percentage of neurons with contra-field preference and increased the percentage of neurons with ipsi-field preference in both YUCHL group and AUCHL group, and this tendency is more evident in the YUCHL group than in the AUCHL group (**Figures 6A–C**). The data for the percentages of AI neurons with contra-field preference in the four groups were as follows: at MT+5 dB, YCon vs. YUCHL, 73.08% vs. 16.44%; ACon vs. AUCHL, 85.25% vs. 48.49%. At MT+10 dB, YCon vs. YUCHL, 69.23% vs. 20.29%; ACon vs. AUCHL, 81.97% vs. 45.61%. At MT+20 dB, YCon vs. YUCHL, 69.23% vs. 20.90%; ACon vs. AUCHL, 78.69% vs. 52.17%. In addition, the data for the percentages of neurons with ipsi-field preference in the four groups were as follows: at MT+5 dB, YCon vs. YUCHL, 1.28% vs. 67.12%; ACon vs. AUCHL, 0.00% vs. 21.21%. At MT+10 dB, YCon vs. YUCHL, 1.28% vs. 52.17%; ACon vs. AUCHL, 0.00% vs. 17.54%. At MT+20 dB, YCon vs. YUCHL, 1.28% vs. 35.82%; ACon vs. AUCHL, 0.00% vs. 13.04%. Moreover, UCHL increased the proportion of omnidirection neurons in both YUCHL group and AUCHL group at MT+10 dB and MT+20 dB conditions, indicating a loss of azimuth selectivity of some AI neurons (**Figures 6B,C**).

We then classified the azimuth preference of each AI neuron based on the overall azimuth preferences tested at the three sound levels (**Figure 6D**). If the azimuth preference of an AI neuron was consistent in one category under the three tested sound levels, we assigned the azimuth preference of the neuron into that category. For some AI neurons, the azimuth preferences were varied under the three tested sound level conditions, so we classified their azimuth preference as "mixed preference." Based on this classification scheme, the proportions of AI neurons with different azimuth preference in the four group of rats were shown in **Figure 6D**. These data demonstrated that most of the AI neurons in the two control groups preferred stimuli from contralateral azimuth. In contrast, UCHL at young age decreased the proportion of neurons with contra-field preference but largely increased the proportion of neurons with ipsi-field preference in YUCHL group; UCHL at adult age also decreased proportion of

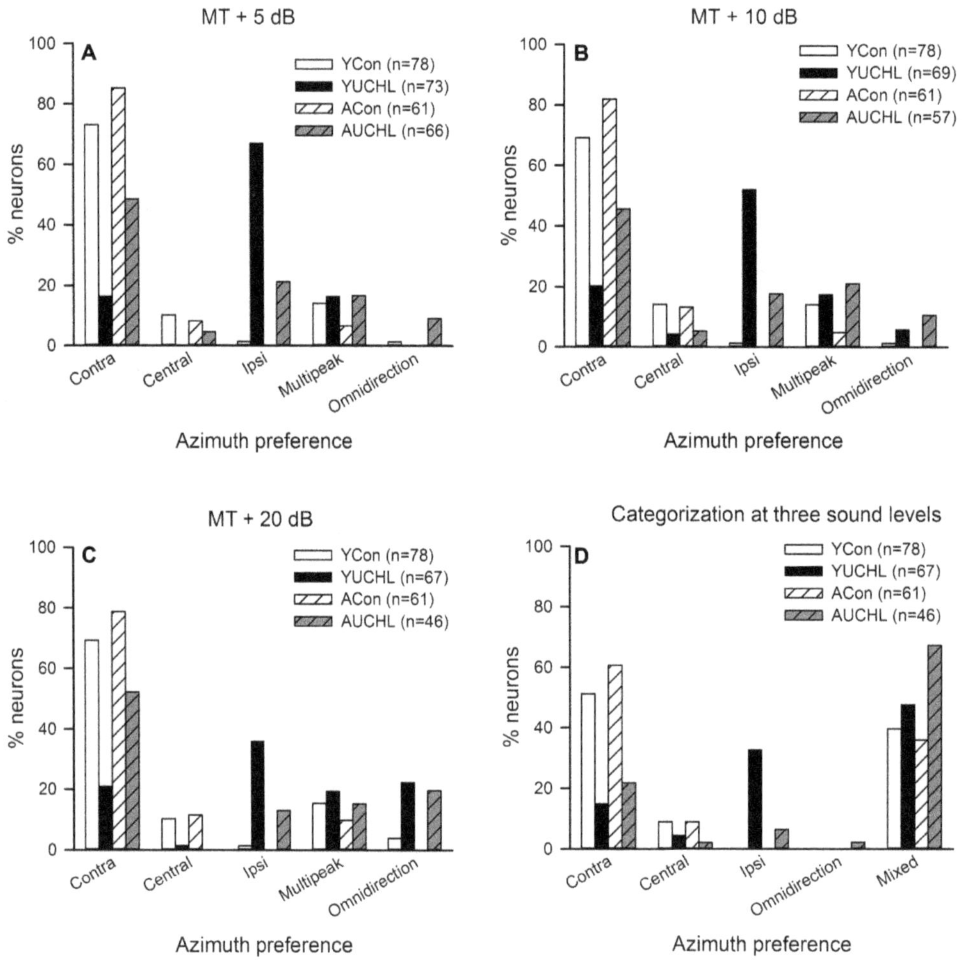

FIGURE 6 | Comparison of the azimuth preference of AI neurons in the four groups of rats. Contra, contra-field preference; Central, central-field preference; Ipsi, ipsi-field preference. Panels **(A–C)** show the percentage of AI neurons with different azimuth preferences determined at each of the three sound levels, i.e., MT+5 dB, MT+10 dB, and MT+20 dB, respectively. Panel **(D)** shows the comparison of the overall azimuth preferences of AI neurons categorized from the azimuth functions determined at all the three sound levels in the four groups. The azimuth preference of an AI neuron was categorized as "mixed" when the azimuth preferences determined at the three sound levels are inconsistent. The 'n' in the legend of each panel show the number of neurons included in the data analysis.

neurons with contra-field preference, but largely increased the proportion of neurons with mixed preference in the AUCHL group (**Figure 6D**).

The Effect of UCHL at Different Postnatal Ages on the Azimuth Selectivity of AI Neurons

The PAR75 width is an index to evaluate the azimuth selectivity of AI neurons. The greater the PAR75 width, the weaker the azimuth selectivity. The distributions of the PAR75 width determined from the four groups of AI neurons are shown in **Figure 7**. The data shown in bar histograms indicated that, under MT+5 dB and MT+10 dB conditions, the PAR75 widths for the majority of the neurons in both the YCon group and the ACon group were $\leq 60°$. In contrast, UCHL decreased the proportion of AI neurons with PAR75 width $\leq 60°$ in both the YUCHL group and the AUCHL group. The proportions of neurons with PAR75 width $\leq 60°$ in the four groups were as follows: at MT+5 dB condition, YCon vs. YUCHL, 70.51% vs. 53.43%, ACon vs. AUCHL, 70.49% vs. 34.85%; at MT+10 dB condition, YCon vs. YUCHL, 58.97% vs. 40.58%, ACon vs. AUCHL, 59.02% vs. 22.81%; at MT+20 dB condition, YCon vs. YUCHL, 33.33% vs. 16.42%, ACon vs. AUCHL, 45.90% vs. 21.74%.

We performed statistical analysis on the PAR75 width of AI neurons in the four groups by Mann–Whitney test (**Figure 7**, panels in the fifth column). The results indicated that no significant differences in the PAR75 width were found between the two control groups (YCon vs. ACon: at MT+5 dB, $Z = -0.121$, $p = 0.904$; at MT+10 dB, $Z = -0.707$, $p = 0.480$; at MT+20 dB, $Z = -1.244$, $p = 0.214$). In comparison with the PAR75 width of AI neurons in the YCon group, UCHL at young age significantly increased the PAR75 width of AI neurons in the YUCHL group (YCon vs. YUCHL, at MT+5 dB, $Z = -3.02$, $p = 0.003$; at MT+10 dB, $Z = -3.276$, $p = 0.001$; at MT+20 dB, $Z = -3.916$, $p < 0.001$). Similarly, in comparison

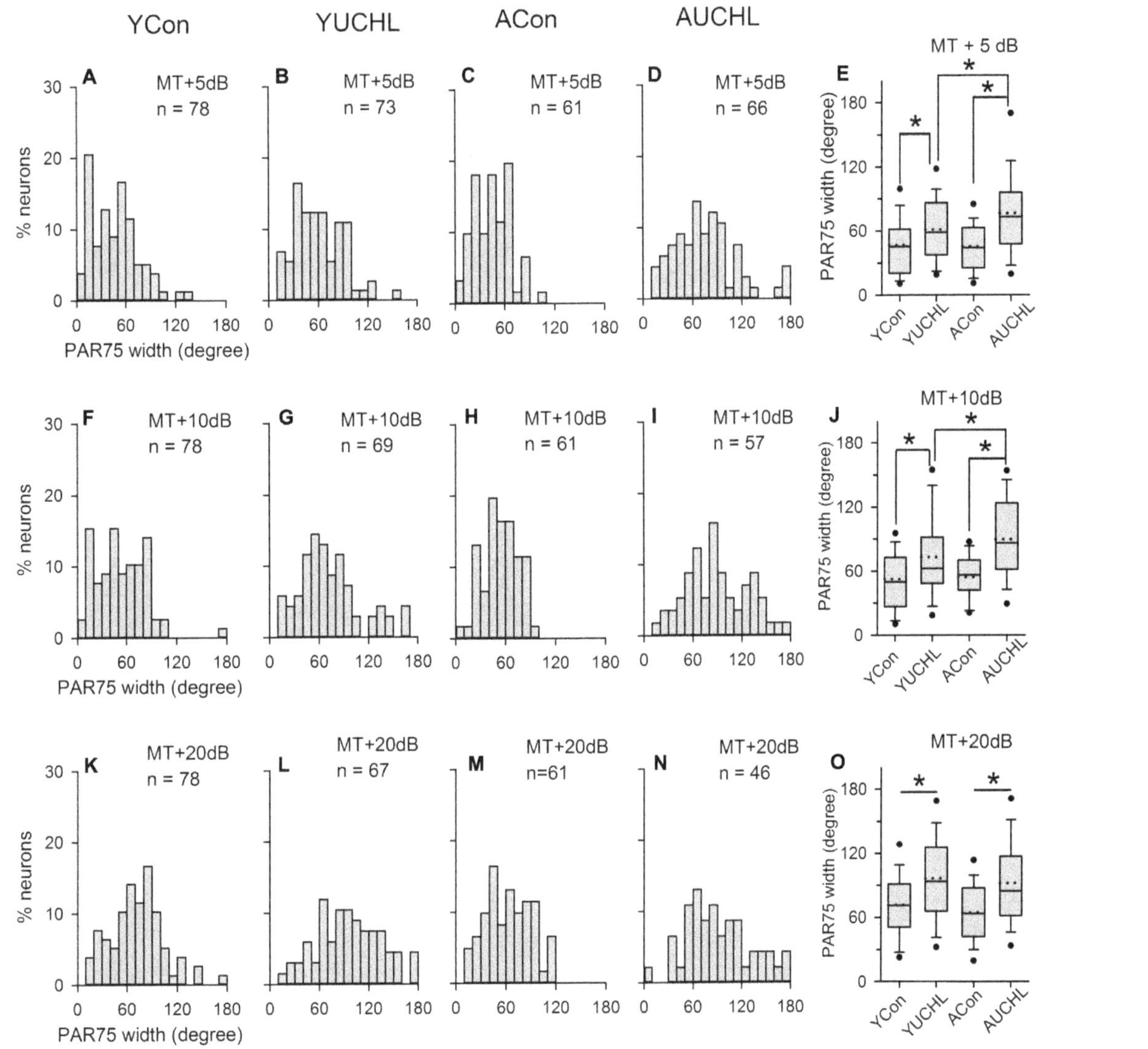

FIGURE 7 | Comparison of the PAR75 width among population of AI neuron from the four groups of rats. The data shown in the panels of the top, middle, and bottom rows are determined at MT+5 dB **(A–D)**, MT+10 dB **(F–I)**, and MT+20 dB **(K–N)** conditions, respectively. Bar histograms show the distributions of PAR75 width of the azimuth functions of A1 neurons from the YCon group (the first column), the YUCHL group (the second column), the ACon group (the third column), and the AUCHL group (the fourth column). **(E,J,O)** The fifth column box plots of the PAR75 width of A1 neurons in the four groups of rats determined at different sound levels. Each box plot shows the median (solid line in the boxes), mean (dotted line in the boxes), quartiles (box extremities), 10th/90th percentiles (error bars), 5th/95th percentiles (filled circles). * indicates significant difference between the two groups (Mann–Whitney test, $p < 0.01$).

with the PAR75 width of AI neurons in the ACon group, UCHL in adulthood significantly increased the PAR75 width of AI neurons in the AUCHL group (ACon vs. AUCHL: at MT+5 dB, $Z = -4.949$, $p < 0.001$; at MT+10 dB, $Z = -5.270$, $p < 0.001$; at MT+20 dB, $Z = -3.565$, $p < 0.001$). Moreover, the effect of UCHL on increasing the PAR75 width was greater in the AUCHL group than in the YUCHL group under both MT+5 dB and MT+10 dB conditions (YUCHL vs. AUCHL: at MT+5 dB, $Z = -2.375$, $p < 0.001$; at MT+10 dB, $Z = -2.605$, $p < 0.009$). However, we did not find significant differences in the PAR75 width of AI neurons between the YUCHL group and the AUCHL group under MT+20 dB condition (YUCHL vs. AUCHL: $Z = -0.777$, $p = 0.43$).

The Effect of UCHL at Different Postnatal Ages on the Azimuth Sensitivity of AI Neurons

The modulation depth of the azimuth function indicates the azimuth sensitivity of an AI neuron. The higher the modulation depth, the greater the sensitivity to sound source azimuth. The data of the modulation depth from the four groups of AI neurons indicate that the ranges of modulation depth were larger in the two groups with UCHL than in the two control groups (**Figures 8A1–C1**). The proportions of AI neurons with high modulation depth (arbitrary ranges: 0.9–1.0) were as follows: at MT+5 dB, YCon vs. YUCHL, 70.51% vs. 53.43%,

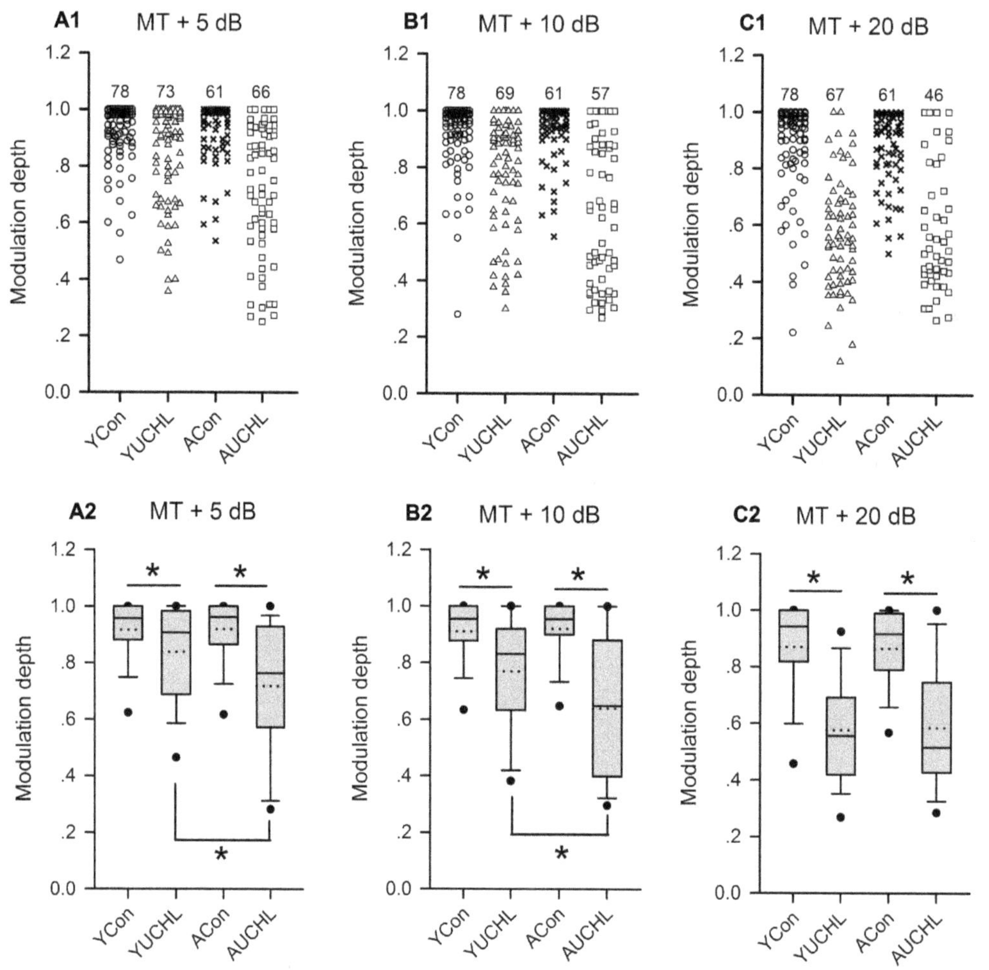

FIGURE 8 | Comparison of the modulation depth of the azimuth functions of AI neurons among the four groups of rats. For each panel, the *x*-axis indicates four different groups of rats, and the *y*-axis represents the value of the modulation depth. MT+5 dB, MT+10 dB, and MT+20 dB are the sound levels used to determine the azimuth functions of AI neurons. **(A1–C1)** The data of modulation depth for each group determined at the tested sound levels, and the number on the top of the symbols for each group is the number of neurons included. **(A2–C2)** The box plots showing the comparison of the modulation depth for the population AI neurons in the four groups of rats. The plots show the median (solid line in each box), mean (dotted line in each box), quartiles (box extremities), 10th/90th percentiles (error bars), and 5th/95th percentiles (filled circles). * indicates significant difference in modulation depth between the two groups (Mann–Whitney test, $p < 0.05$).

ACon vs. AUCHL, 65.57% vs. 31.82%; at MT+10 dB, YCon vs. YUCHL, 69.23% vs. 34.78%, ACon vs. AUCHL, 77.05% vs. 21.05%; at MT+20 dB, YCon vs. YUCHL, 62.82% vs. 7.46%, ACon vs. AUCHL, 50.82% vs. 15.22%. The data indicated that the modulation depth for most of the AI neuron in the two control groups was distributed within the range of 0.9–1.0. In contrast, UCHL decreased the proportion of AI neurons with high modulation depth in both the YUCHL group and the AUCHL group.

The statistical comparison for the modulation depth among the four groups of AI neurons were performed by box plots and by Mann–Whitney test (**Figure 8**). We found no significant differences in modulation depth between the two control groups (YCon vs. ACon: at MT+5 dB, $Z = -0.201$, $p = 0.841$; at MT + 10 dB, $Z = -0.250$, $p = 0.803$; at MT+20 dB, $Z = -0.893$, $p = 0.372$). In comparison with the modulation depth in the YCon group, UCHL significantly decreased the modulation depth of AI neurons in the YUCHL group (YCon vs. YUCHL: at MT+5 dB, $Z = -3.306$, $p = 0.002$; at MT+10 dB, $Z = -5.177$, $p < 0.001$, MT+20 dB, $Z = 7.665$, $p < 0.001$). Similarly, in comparison with the modulation depth in the ACon group, UCHL significantly decreased the modulation depth of AI neurons in the AUCHL group (ACon vs. AUCHL: at MT+5 dB, $Z = -5.742$, $p < 0.001$; at MT+10 dB, $Z = -6.108$, $p < 0.001$; at MT+20 dB, $Z = -5.954$, $p < 0.001$). Moreover, under the conditions of both MT+5 dB and MT+10 dB, the modulation depth of AI neurons was greater in YUCHL group than in AUCHL group (YUCHL vs. AUCHL: at MT+5 dB, $Z = -3.353$, $p = 0.001$; at MT+10 dB, $Z = -2.830$, $p = 0.005$). However, under MT+20 dB condition, we did not find significant differences in the modulation depth between the YUCHL group and the AUCHL group ($Z = -0.207$, $p = 0.836$). These data demonstrated that UCHL decreased the azimuth sensitivity of AI neurons, and this effect was greater in the AUCHL group than in the YUCHL group.

DISCUSSION

Conductive hearing loss produces a partial attenuation of acoustic input to the affected ear (Moore et al., 1989), and UCHL is quite common in human infants with otitis media (Gravel and Wallace, 2000). In animal studies, the disruption of the normal acoustic conduction in the middle-ear has been a common manipulation of conductive hearing loss. The effects of UCHL on the structure and function of the auditory system have been evaluated in the cochlea (Liberman et al., 2015), as well as in the brainstem and auditory cortex (Moore et al., 1989; Tucci et al., 1999; Hutson et al., 2008; Popescu and Polley, 2010; Polley et al., 2013; Yao and Sanes, 2018).

In the present study, we determined the azimuth functions of rat AI neurons and assessed the neural tuning to sound source azimuth by the azimuth preference, the PAR75 width, and the tuning depth of the azimuth functions. We did not find significant differences in the azimuth tuning of AI neurons evaluated by these measurements between the two control groups. The results implied that the age difference between the two control groups did not induce significant changes in the azimuth tuning of rat AI neurons. In comparison with the data in age-matched control groups, the data in both YUCHL group and AUCHL group showed that chronic UCHL induced a lower proportion of contra-field preference neurons in AI, and increased the PAR75 width but decreased the tuning depth of the azimuth functions of AI neurons contralateral to the operated ear. Moreover, UCHL induced a larger percentage of ipsi-field preference neurons in the AI contralateral to the operated ear in the YUCHL group than in the AUCHL group. These results demonstrated that chronic UCHL significantly disrupted the azimuth tuning of AI neurons contralateral to the operated ear, and the effects of UCHL on the azimuth tuning of AI neurons was age-related. The different effects of UCHL on the azimuth tuning of AI neurons shown in developing rats and in adult rats indicated that the timing of UCHL played a critical role in mediating its effects. To our knowledge, the present study is the first demonstration of how chronic UCHL at different postnatal ages affects the azimuth tuning of AI neurons in free-field acoustic stimulus conditions.

In the present study, the responses of AI neurons to stimuli from the azimuths ipsilateral to the operated ear in the average azimuth functions were greater in the two UCHL groups than in the two control groups (**Figure 5**). Interestingly, the responses to stimuli from ipsilateral azimuths were greater in the YUCHL group than in the AUCHL group. Consistent with these changes found in the auditory cortex of UCHL rats, previous studies in the inferior colliculus of ferrets showed that unilateral cochlear removal in adults ferrets led to a rapid and dramatic increase in the proportion of neurons ipsilateral to the intact ear, and unilateral cochlear removal in infancy led to a further increase in responsiveness of individual neurons ipsilateral to the intact ear (McAlpine et al., 1997). We speculate that the changes in responses induced by UCHL in the present study were probably due to both a decrease of inhibition to the ipsilateral input and an increase of ipsilateral input. Because UCHL or unilateral deafness at young age induced an aural preference to the ipsilateral normal hearing ear (Popescu and Polley, 2010; Kral et al., 2013b; Tillein et al., 2016), the greater responses in the YUCHL group than in the AUCHL group at each of the ipsilateral azimuths (**Figure 5**) were possibly due to a greater increase of ipsilateral input in the YUCHL group than in the AUCHL group.

Previous studies in cats related to the present study demonstrated that congenital monaural and binaural deafness resulted in a decrease in sensitivity of AI neurons to interaural time differences (Tillein et al., 2010, 2016). This reduced sensitivity in the AI contralateral to the deaf ear was more pronounced in congenitally monaural deaf cats than in congenitally binaural deaf cats (Tillein et al., 2016). Therefore, both UCHL and unilateral deafness at young age exert significant impacts on the spatial tuning of AI neurons in adulthood.

Neural Tuning to Sound-Source Azimuth in the Auditory Cortex of Normal Hearing Animals

In the present study, the azimuth functions of AI neurons obtained from two control groups demonstrated that more than half of the neurons in the rat AI preferred sound stimuli from the contralateral azimuth in the horizontal plane. This is consistent with the findings shown in previous studies regarding the spatial representation of rat AI neurons measured by spike counts (Yao et al., 2013; Gao et al., 2018) and excitatory postsynaptic potentials (Chadderton et al., 2009). Studies using interaural level differences to mimic the changes of spatial azimuth also demonstrated that most tested neurons in the rat AI preferred acoustic stimuli from contralateral horizontal positions (Kelly and Sally, 1988). Although the criteria used to define the azimuth preference were varied among these studies, the results reached the similar conclusion that most neurons in the rat AI favored the acoustic stimuli in contralateral frontal auditory space. Studies in other species such as cats showed that most neurons in the AI of anesthetized cats responded best to sound stimuli from contralateral azimuths, and a small proportion of neurons preferred sound stimuli from the midline or ipsilateral azimuths (Imig et al., 1990; Rajan et al., 1990; Clarey et al., 1995; Eggermont and Mossop, 1998). These findings obtained in free-field studies were also demonstrated from close-field studies in anesthetized cats by manipulating the interaural level differences (Zhang et al., 2004). Moreover, the overrepresentation to the contralateral field in horizontal plane in AI was further shown in awake cats (Mickey and Middlebrooks, 2003) and alert macaque monkeys (Woods et al., 2006).

Taken together, the overrepresentation of contralateral azimuth is a common feature of neural spatial tuning in AI. This feature has been demonstrated in different animal species, and in both awake and anesthetized conditions. Therefore, any manipulations that induce a change of this feature would imply its consequences of abnormal auditory spatial tuning in AI.

The Effect of UCHL at Young Age on the Azimuth Tuning of AI Neurons

In contrast to the common feature of the overrepresentation of contralateral azimuth in the AI of normal hearing rats, here we show that chronic UCHL in P14 rats induced a significant decrease in the proportion of contra-field preference neurons and a significant increase in the proportion of ipsi-field preference neurons in the AI contralateral to the operated ear (**Figure 6**). The mean normalized azimuth functions for the population AI neurons in the YUCHL group showed a clear preference for the stimuli from the ipsilateral azimuths under MT+5 dB and MT+10 dB conditions (**Figure 5**). These changes in azimuth functions in YUCHL group implied an augment of the responsiveness of AI neurons to acoustic input from the ipsilateral non-operated ear due to UCHL at early postnatal age. The results also showed that the PAR75 width for the azimuth functions of AI neurons was significantly greater in the YUCHL group than in the age-matched YCon group (**Figure 7**), indicating a down regulation of azimuth selectivity by UCHL at early postnatal age. Moreover, UCHL induced a reduction in modulation depth of azimuth functions in the YUCHL group (**Figure 8**), indicating a degraded sensitivity to the change of sound source azimuth. Taken together, UCHL at early postnatal age disrupts the normal spatial tuning of AI neurons to sound source azimuth in adulthood. Related studies in deaf cats showed that both monaural and binaural congenital deafness decreased the sensitivity to interaural time differences in the auditory cortex. The modulation depth in the functions of interaural time differences in the auditory cortex was smaller in congenitally monaural and binaural deaf cats than in hearing control cats (Tillein et al., 2010, 2016). Thus, it is quite clear that postnatal abnormal binaural input results in degraded representations of sound source location in the auditory cortex.

Previous closed-field studies in rodents have demonstrated an experience-dependent plasticity in frequency tuning in AI during postnatal hearing development (Popescu and Polley, 2010; Polley et al., 2013). In normal binaural hearing rats, the AI displayed poor-organized tonotopic maps and low-quality frequency receptive fields in responding to tonal stimuli from the ipsilateral ear. However, chronic UCHL by ear canal ligation in P14 or P28 rats weakened the representation of the contralateral ligated ear in AI and strengthened the representation of the ipsilateral open ear in AI. This was exhibited in adulthood by well-organized ipsilateral tonotopic maps and good quality ipsilateral tonal receptive fields in the AI contralateral to the ligated ear (Popescu and Polley, 2010). Further studies showed that short-term reversible UCHL during the critical periods of mouse hearing development was associated with enhanced sensitivity of AI neurons to the ipsilateral non-operated ear in adulthood (Polley et al., 2013). Studies in cats with unilateral deafness also showed that a massive reorganization of aural preference in favor of the hearing ear was found if the onset of unilateral hearing was before or around the peak of functional synaptogenesis (Kral et al., 2013b), and that unilateral hearing experience led to a functionally asymmetric AI with different neuronal reorganizations and different sensitive periods involved (Kral et al., 2013a). These studies in rodents and cats demonstrated a developmental experience-dependent plasticity in AI from the perspective of frequency tuning and binaural selectivity. The results in the present study provide new evidences for the developmental experience-dependent plasticity in AI from the perspective of azimuth tuning.

At present, we have no direct evidences on the mechanism underlying the effects of chronic UCHL at young age on the azimuth tuning of rat AI neurons. Previous studies showed that chronic UCHL in neonatal ferrets and rhesus monkey did not significantly change the neuronal size of brainstem auditory neurons or the volume of the cochlear nuclei (Moore et al., 1989; Doyle and Webster, 1991). Whereas UCHL in neonatal ferrets in the right ear did not lead to degeneration of the cochlear nucleus on the right side, it led to a significant rearrangement of brainstem connectivity, i.e., a significant increase of projections in the left inferior colliculus from left cochlear nucleus (Moore et al., 1989). Even transient UCHL in developing animals could induce dramatic changes in the structure and function of auditory system. For example, cochlear nucleus neurons innervated by auditory nerve redistributed synaptic AMPA and glycine receptor in response to transient UCHL in P30 rats induced by earplugging (Whiting et al., 2009). Short-term monaural earplugging in P30 rats altered the synthesis and subsequent composition of specific glutamate and glycine receptors and the synapses in the ipsilateral cochlear nucleus (Wang et al., 2011), and led to long-lasting structure and molecular alterations at the endbulb of the Held synapse (Clarkson et al., 2016). In addition, the short-term earplugging in P30 rats induced an increase in postsynaptic density thickness and the upregulation of the postsynaptic GluA3 AMPAR subunit (Clarkson et al., 2016). Early developmental UCHL also resulted in a weakening of neurophysiological representation in the auditory system corresponding to the affected ear. Studies using 2-deoxyglucose uptake as a measure of metabolic activity have shown that, 3 weeks of UCHL induced by malleus removal in P21 gerbils resulted in a marked decrease in glucose uptake in the major ascending projections in the brainstem of the operated ear (Tucci et al., 1999), and in both the inferior colliculus and auditory cortex contralateral to the operated ear (Hutson et al., 2008). These results suggest that neural circuits responsible for integrating input from the two ears may be particularly susceptible early in development, and the abnormal binaural input during early postnatal age could induce plasticity in both structural and functional changes in the central auditory system. In the present study, we found dramatic changes in azimuth tuning of AI neurons induced by UCHL in developing rats, we postulate that these changes in azimuth tuning might be caused by the developmental experience-dependent plasticity in the structure and function of the central auditory system beginning from the cochlear nucleus all the way to the auditory cortex.

The Effect of UCHL in Adulthood on the Azimuth Tuning of AI Neurons

Compared to the data in ACon group, the data in AUCHL group indicated that chronic UCHL in adult rats induced a complex effect on azimuth tuning of AI neurons contralateral to the operated ear: (1) a reduction in the proportion of contra-field preference neurons and an increase in the proportion of mixed preference neurons; (2) an increase in the proportion of ipsi-field preference neurons; (3) an increase in the PAR75 width and a decrease in the modulation depth of azimuth functions. Interestingly, chronic UCHL in adult rats induced a larger increase in the percentage of mixed preference neurons than chronic UCHL in young rats did. In contrast, chronic UCHL in young rats induced a larger increase in the percentage of ipsi-field preference neurons than chronic UCHL in adult rats did. These results suggest that UCHL in developing rats results in a greater weakening of neurophysiological representation associated with the affected ear. These age-dependent effects of UCHL on the azimuth tuning of AI neurons was probably due to the differences in the UCHL-induced plasticity of central auditory system of rats between the YUCHL group and the AUCHL group.

Unilateral conductive hearing loss attenuates the input to the inner ear and alters the normal binaural integration in the central auditory system. Previous studies in adult cats showed that many AI neurons that were sensitive to sound source azimuth in normal binaural hearing conditions immediately became insensitive to azimuth (i.e., either responded well to all azimuths or responded poorly at any azimuth) when one ear was plugged (Samson et al., 1994). Thus, the acute UCHL by earplugging disrupted the normal binaural interaction, and immediately changed the azimuth tuning of cat AI neurons. In contrast to acute UCHL that operated for a few minutes, chronic UCHL that lasts for weeks or months could induce plasticity in the adult central auditory system due to the attenuation of auditory input. Previous studies have shown that, in the fully developed ears of adult mice, the chronic UCHL induced a significant plasticity of the cochlea's afferent and efferent innervations. Chronic UCHL induced by removal of tympanic membrane increased the cochlear-nerve synaptopathy in the ipsilateral ear, and reduced the density of olivocochlear bundle (Liberman et al., 2015). Moreover, chronic UCHL in adult gerbils by malleus removal caused a decrease in metabolic activity measured by 2-deoxyglucose uptake in the cochlear nucleus, lateral lemniscus, and inferior colliculus that primarily receive excitatory inputs from the operated ear (Tucci et al., 1999). UCHL in adult rats also caused a shift in aural dominance in the auditory cortex (but not in the inferior colliculus) contralateral to the operated ear (Popescu and Polley, 2010). These studies demonstrated that chronic UCHL induced a significant plasticity in the adult central auditory system. In the present study, the chronic UCHL in adult rats induced more complex effects on azimuth tuning of AI neurons than the acute UCHL in adult cats did, which suggests that the spatial hearing remains plastic in adulthood. We speculate that the effects of chronic UCHL in adult rats on the azimuth tuning of AI neurons may be attributed to the consequences of UCHL on both the abnormal binaural acoustic input and the experience-dependent plasticity in the adult central auditory system. In the present study, we did not investigate the impacts of acute UCHL on the azimuth tuning of rat AI neurons. Therefore, whether the effects of chronic UCHL in adult rats on the azimuth tuning of AI neurons were indeed caused by the plasticity in AI needs to be further investigated.

Methodology Considerations

In the present study, we focused on investigating the effects of UCHL on the azimuth tuning of AI neurons contralateral to the operated ear because the excitatory drive from the contralateral ear is predominant in the auditory cortex in normal binaural hearing conditions. Previous studies in ferrets showed that unilateral cochlear removal in infancy led to an increase in responsiveness of individual neurons in the ipsilateral inferior colliculus, but had no significant impacts on the responses in the inferior colliculus contralateral to the intact ear (McAlpine et al., 1997). In unilateral deaf cats, the cortex ipsilateral to the hearing ear showed responses to stimulation from both the hearing as well as the deaf ear (Kral et al., 2013b) whereas the cortex contralateral to the hearing ear showed good responsiveness to the hearing ear but weak responses to stimulation of the deaf ear (Kral et al., 2013a). Moreover, congenital unilateral deafness in cats induced a stronger reduction in the sensitivity to interaural time differences in the auditory cortex ipsilateral to hearing ear than in the auditory cortex contralateral to the hearing ear (Tillein et al., 2016). These studies demonstrated a hemispheric specificity of the impacts of single-sided deafness. In the present study, we did not measure the azimuth functions of AI neurons ipsilateral to the operated ear. It's possible that the UCHL also affects the azimuth tuning of AI neurons ipsilateral to the operated ear (or contralateral to the intact ear) due to the attenuation of inhibitory drive or excitatory drive from the operated ear. The AI neurons ipsilateral to the operated ear receive excitatory drive predominantly from the contralateral intact ear, therefore we postulate that the impacts of UCHL on the azimuth tuning of the AI neurons ipsilateral to the operated ear could be weaker than the impacts shown in the present study.

In the single-sided congenital deaf cats, sensitivity of AI neurons to the interaural time differences was reduced, particularly at the AI ipsilateral to the hearing ear (Tillein et al., 2016). In the present study, we used rats as the experimental animals and the CFs of the rat AI neurons included in the data analysis were $\geq$4 kHz. Therefore, the impacts of UCHL on the azimuth functions of the rat AI neurons primarily reflected the impacts on the sensitivity and selectivity of interaural level differences, and the impacts of UCHL on the sensitivity of the interaural time differences of AI neurons are not known in the present study.

In the present study, the number of neurons in each group were within the range of 61–78. Due to the limited time that a well-isolated neuron was available for recording in this acute experiment, we only got few neurons for data analysis in each rat. If more neurons were recorded in each rat, the power for the statistical analysis would be higher than the present situation.

CONCLUSION

In summary, the present study demonstrated that postnatal chronic UCHL at both young age and adult age disrupts the normal neuronal tuning to sound source azimuth in the AI contralateral to the operated ear. Chronic UCHL altered the azimuth preference, degraded the azimuth sensitivity and azimuth selectivity of AI neurons. In addition, UCHL at early postnatal age induced a greater weakening of cortical neurophysiological representation associated with the affected ear than UCHL in adulthood did, indicating age-related effects of UCHL on cortical spatial tuning. The disruption of the azimuth tuning of AI neurons induced by chronic UCHL may be one of the neural mechanisms underlying the poor sound localization abilities shown in chronic UCHL subjects.

AUTHOR CONTRIBUTIONS

JZ and XW designed this study, analyzed the data, and drafted the manuscript. XW and JL engaged in data collection. All authors contributed to the final version of the manuscript and approved its contents.

ACKNOWLEDGMENTS

We acknowledge the support of the NYU-ECNU Institute of Brain and Cognitive Science at NYU Shanghai, and the support by the open project of Key Laboratory of Brain Functional Genomics, Ministry of Education. We thank Xiafei Zhang for his contributions on the manuscript in language editing.

REFERENCES

Barone, P., Clarey, J. C., Irons, W. A., and Imig, T. J. (1996). Cortical synthesis of azimuth-sensitive single-unit responses with nonmonotonic level tuning: a thalamocortical comparison in the cat. *J. Neurophysiol.* 75, 1206–1220.

Chadderton, P., Agapiou, J. P., McAlpine, D., and Margrie, T. W. (2009). The synaptic representation of sound source location in auditory cortex. *J. Neurosci.* 29, 14127–14135. doi: 10.1523/JNEUROSCI.2061-09.2009

Clarey, J. C., Barone, P., Irons, W. A., Samson, F. K., and Imig, T. J. (1995). Comparison of noise and tone azimuth tuning of neurons in cat primary auditory cortex and medical geniculate body. *J. Neurophysiol.* 74, 961–980.

Clarkson, C., Antunes, F. M., and Rubio, M. E. (2016). Conductive hearing loss has long-lasting structural and molecular effects on presynaptic and postsynaptic structures of auditory nerve synapses in the cochlear nucleus. *J. Neurosci.* 36, 10214–10227. doi: 10.1523/JNEUROSCI.0226-16.2016

Doron, N. N., Ledoux, J. E., and Semple, M. N. (2002). Redefining the tonotopic core of rat auditory cortex: physiological evidence for a posterior field. *J. Comp. Neurol.* 453, 345–360.

Doyle, W. J., and Webster, D. B. (1991). Neonatal conductive hearing loss does not compromise brainstem auditory function and structure in rhesus monkeys. *Hear. Res.* 54, 145–151.

Eggermont, J. J., and Mossop, J. E. (1998). Azimuth coding in primary auditory cortex of the cat. I. spike synchrony versus spike count representations. *J. Neurophysiol.* 80, 2133–2150.

Franklin, S. R., Brunso-Bechtold, J. K., and Henkel, C. K. (2006). Unilateral cochlear ablation before hearing onset disrupts the maintenance of dorsal nucleus of the lateral lemniscus projection patterns in the rat inferior colliculus. *Neuroscience* 143, 105–115.

Gabriele, M. L., Brunso-Bechtold, J. K., and Henkel, C. K. (2000). Plasticity in the development of afferent patterns in the inferior colliculus of the rat after unilateral cochlear ablation. *J. Neurosci.* 20, 6939–6949.

Gao, F., Chen, L., and Zhang, J. (2018). Nonuniform impacts of forward suppression on neural responses to preferred stimuli and nonpreferred stimuli in the rat auditory cortex. *Eur. J. Neurosci.* 47, 1320–1338. doi: 10.1111/ejn.13943

Gravel, J. S., and Wallace, I. F. (2000). Effects of otitis media with effusion on hearing in the first 3 years of life. *J. Speech Lang. Hear. Res.* 43, 631–644.

Humes, L. E., Allen, S. K., and Bess, F. H. (1980). Horizontal sound localization skills of unilaterally hearing-impaired children. *Audiology* 19, 508–518.

Hutson, K. A., Durham, D., Imig, T., and Tucci, D. L. (2008). Consequences of unilateral hearing loss: cortical adjustment to unilateral deprivation. *Hear. Res.* 237, 19–31. doi: 10.1016/j.heares.2007.12.007

Imig, T. J., Irons, W. A., and Samson, F. R. (1990). Single-unit selectivity to azimuthal direction and sound pressure level of noise bursts in cat high-frequency primary auditory cortex. *J. Neurophysiol.* 63, 1448–1466.

Jenkins, W. M., and Merzenich, M. M. (1984). Role of cat primary auditory cortex for sound-localization behavior. *J. Neurophysiol.* 52, 819–847.

Jiang, C., Xu, X., Yu, L., Xu, J., and Zhang, J. (2015). Environmental enrichment rescues the degraded auditory temporal resolution of cortical neurons induced by early noise exposure. *Eur. J. Neurosci.* 42, 2144–2154. doi: 10.1111/ejn.12975

Kelly, J. B., and Sally, S. L. (1988). Organization of auditory cortex in the albino rat: binaural response properties. *J. Neurophysiol.* 59, 1756–1769.

King, A. J., Bajo, V. M., Bizley, J. K., Campbell, R. A., Nodal, F. R., Schulz, A. L., et al. (2007). Physiological and behavioral studies of spatial coding in the auditory cortex. *Hear. Res.* 229, 106–115.

Kitzes, L. M., Kageyama, G. H., Semple, M. N., and Kil, J. (1995). Development of ectopic projections from the ventral cochlear nucleus to the superior olivary complex induced by neonatal ablation of the contralateral cochlea. *J. Comp. Neurol.* 353, 341–363.

Kral, A., Heid, S., Hubka, P., and Tillein, J. (2013a). Unilateral hearing during development: hemispheric specificity in plastic reorganizations. *Front. Syst. Neurosci.* 7:93. doi: 10.3389/fnsys.2013.00093

Kral, A., Hubka, P., Heid, S., and Tillein, J. (2013b). Single-sided deafness leads to unilateral aural preference within an early sensitive period. *Brain* 136(Pt 1), 180–193. doi: 10.1093/brain/aws305

Liberman, M. C., Liberman, L. D., and Maison, S. F. (2015). Chronic conductive hearing loss leads to cochlear degeneration. *PLoS One* 10:e0142341. doi: 10.1371/journal.pone.0142341

Lu, Q., Jiang, C., and Zhang, J. (2016). Encoding of sound envelope transients in the auditory cortex of juvenile rats and adult rats. *Int. J. Dev. Neurosci.* 48, 50–57. doi: 10.1016/j.ijdevneu.2015.11.004

Malhotra, S., and Lomber, S. G. (2007). Sound localization during homotopic and heterotopic bilateral cooling deactivation of primary and nonprimary auditory cortical areas in the cat. *J. Neurophysiol.* 97, 26–43.

McAlpine, D., Martin, R. L., Mossop, J. E., and Moore, D. R. (1997). Response properties of neurons in the inferior colliculus of the monaurally deafened ferret to acoustic stimulation of the intact ear. *J. Neurophysiol.* 78, 767–779.

Mickey, B. J., and Middlebrooks, J. C. (2003). Representation of auditory space by cortical neurons in awake cats. *J. Neurosci.* 23, 8649–8663.

Moore, D. R., Hutchings, M. E., King, A. J., and Kowalchuk, N. E. (1989). Auditory brain stem of the ferret: some effects of rearing with a unilateral ear plug on the cochlea, cochlear nucleus, and projections to the inferior colliculus. *J. Neurosci.* 9, 1213–1222.

Polley, D. B., Thompson, J. H., and Guo, W. (2013). Brief hearing loss disrupts binaural integration during two early critical periods of auditory cortex development. *Nat. Comm.* 4:2547. doi: 10.1038/ncomms3547

Popescu, M. V., and Polley, D. B. (2010). Monaural deprivation disrupts development of binaural selectivity in auditory midbrain and cortex. *Neuron* 65, 718–731. doi: 10.1016/j.neuron.2010.02.019

Rajan, R., Aitkin, L. M., Irvine, D. R., and McKay, J. (1990). Azimuthal sensitivity of neurons in primary auditory cortex of cats. I. types of sensitivity and the effects of variations in stimulus parameters. *J. Neurophysiol.* 64, 872–887.

Samson, F. K., Barone, P., Clarey, J. C., and Imig, T. J. (1994). Effects of ear plugging on single-unit azimuth sensitivity in cat primary auditory cortex. II. azimuth tuning dependent upon binaural stimulation. *J. Neurophysiol.* 71, 2194–2216.

Sumner, C. J., Tucci, D. L., and Shore, S. E. (2005). Responses of ventral cochlear nucleus neurons to contralateral sound after conductive hearing loss. *J. Neurophysiol.* 94, 4234–4243.

Tillein, J., Hubka, P., and Kral, A. (2016). Monaural congenital deafness affects aural dominance and degrades binaural processing. *Cereb. Cortex* 26, 1762–1777. doi: 10.1093/cercor/bhv351

Tillein, J., Hubka, P., Syed, E., Hartmann, R., Engel, A. K., and Kral, A. (2010). Cortical representation of interaural time difference in congenital deafness. *Cereb. Cortex* 20, 492–506. doi: 10.1093/cercor/bhp222

Tucci, D. L., Cant, N. B., and Durham, D. (1999). Conductive hearing loss results in a decrease in central auditory system activity in the young gerbil. *Laryngoscope* 109, 1359–1371.

Wang, H., Yin, G., Rogers, K., Miralles, C., De Blas, A. L., and Rubio, M. E. (2011). Monaural conductive hearing loss alters the expression of the GluA3 AMPA and glycine receptor alpha1 subunits in bushy and fusiform cells of the cochlear nucleus. *Neuroscience* 199, 438–451. doi: 10.1016/j.neuroscience.2011.10.021

Whiting, B., Moiseff, A., and Rubio, M. E. (2009). Cochlear nucleus neurons redistribute synaptic AMPA and glycine receptors in response to monaural conductive hearing loss. *Neuroscience* 163, 1264–1276. doi: 10.1016/j.neuroscience.2009.07.049

Wilmington, D., Gray, L., and Jahrsdoerfer, R. (1994). Binaural processing after corrected congenital unilateral conductive hearing loss. *Hear. Res.* 74, 99–114.

Woods, T. M., Lopez, S. E., Long, J. H., Rahman, J. E., and Recanzone, G. H. (2006). Effects of stimulus azimuth and intensity on the single-neuron activity in the auditory cortex of the alert macaque monkey. *J. Neurophysiol.* 96, 3323–3337.

Xu, H., Kotak, V. C., and Sanes, D. H. (2007). Conductive hearing loss disrupts synaptic and spike adaptation in developing auditory cortex. *J. Neurosci.* 27, 9417–9426. doi: 10.1523/JNEUROSCI.1992-07.2007

Yao, J. D., Bremen, P., and Middlebrooks, J. C. (2013). Rat primary auditory cortex is tuned exclusively to the contralateral hemifield. *J. Neurophysiol.* 110, 2140–2151. doi: 10.1152/jn.00219.2013

Yao, J. D., and Sanes, D. H. (2018). Developmental deprivation-induced perceptual and cortical processing deficits in awake-behaving animals. *eLife* 7:e33891. doi: 10.7554/eLife.33891

Zhang, J., Nakamoto, K. T., and Kitzes, L. M. (2004). Binaural interaction revisited in the cat primary auditory cortex. *J. Neurophysiol.* 91, 101–117.

17

The Ganglioside Monosialotetrahexosylganglioside Protects Auditory Hair Cells against Neomycin-Induced Cytotoxicity through Mitochondrial Antioxidation: An *in vitro* Study

Yujin Li[1,2†], Ao Li[1,3,4†], Chao Wang[5], Xin Jin[2], Yaoting Zhang[2], Ling Lu[1,3,4], Shou-Lin Wang[5*] and Xia Gao[1,3,4*]*

[1] Department of Otolaryngology-Head and Neck Surgery, Nanjing Drum Tower Clinical College of Nanjing Medical University, Nanjing, China, [2] Department of Otolaryngology-Head and Neck Surgery, The Affiliated Huaian No. 1 People's Hospital of Nanjing Medical University, Huai'an, China, [3] Research Institute of Otolaryngology, Nanjing, China, [4] Jiangsu Provincial Key Medical Discipline (Laboratory), Department of Otolaryngology-Head and Neck Surgery, Affiliated Drum Tower Hospital of Nanjing University Medical School, Nanjing, China, [5] School of Public Health, Nanjing Medical University, Nanjing, China

Correspondence:
Ling Lu
entluling60@126.com
Shou-Lin Wang
wangshl@njmu.edu.cn
Xia Gao
xiagaogao@hotmail.com

† These authors have contributed equally to this work and share first authorship

Neomycin is a common ototoxic aminoglycoside antibiotic that causes sensory hearing disorders worldwide, and monosialotetrahexosylganglioside (GM1) is reported to have antioxidant effects that protect various cells. However, little is known about the effect of GM1 on neomycin-induced hair cell (HC) ototoxic damage and related mechanism. In this study, cochlear HC-like HEI-OC-1 cells along with whole-organ explant cultures were used to establish an *in vitro* neomycin-induced HC damage model, and then the apoptosis rate, the balance of oxidative and antioxidant gene expression, reactive oxygen species (ROS) levels and mitochondrial membrane potential (MMP) were measured. GM1 could maintain the balance of oxidative and antioxidant gene expression, inhibit the accumulation of ROS and proapoptotic gene expression, promoted antioxidant gene expression, and reduce apoptosis after neomycin exposure in HEI-OC-1 cells and cultured cochlear HCs. These results suggested that GM1 could reduce ROS aggregation, maintain mitochondrial function, and improve HC viability in the presence of neomycin, possibly through mitochondrial antioxidation. Hence, GM1 may have potential clinical value in protecting against aminoglycoside-induced HC injury.

Keywords: monosialotetrahexosylganglioside, neomycin, hair cell, cytotoxicity, reactive oxygen species

INTRODUCTION

Sensorineural hearing loss is a common sensory disorder in humans. Many factors, including viral infections, noise, and exposure to ototoxic drugs, can cause hair cell (HC) damage and induce hearing impairment (Sotoudeh, 2021). Adult mammalian HCs cannot regenerate, and once these cells are damaged, the effects are often permanent (Zhang et al., 2020). Aminoglycoside antibiotics are antibacterial drugs commonly used in clinical treatment and are also the most commonly encountered ototoxic drugs. It is estimated that approximately one-quarter of people who are treated with aminoglycoside antibiotics will develop ototoxicity (Lopez-Novoa et al., 2011). However, these drugs still play a crucial role in the treatment of severe gram-negative bacterial infections and multidrug-resistant tuberculosis and are becoming more irreplaceable as microbial resistance to conventional antimicrobial agents increases (Germovsek et al., 2017). Therefore, exploring the mechanism through which they exert ototoxicity and identifying effective treatment measures is of great significance (Guo et al., 2019). The ototoxic mechanism of aminoglycoside drugs has not been fully elucidated. Recent studies have found that it may be related to oxidative stress (Jiang et al., 2016), apoptosis (Jiang et al., 2017), and mitochondrial dysfunction (Jiang et al., 2017). Previous studies have found that aminoglycoside drugs accumulate in mitochondria after entering HCs and that this can lead to disorders of mitochondrial metabolism, imbalanced expression of prooxidants (ALOX15) and antioxidants (GSR, SOD1, NQO1, GLRX), and the production of excessive reactive oxygen species (ROS) such as hydrogen peroxide (H_2O_2) and hydroxyl radicals (•OH) in cells. Aminoglycosides also disrupt the normal synthesis of mitochondrial proteins and reduce the mitochondrial membrane potential (MMP), leading to increased mitochondrial permeability and release of cytochrome C and ultimately to cell apoptosis (He et al., 2020; Yao et al., 2020). It has been reported that some antioxidants exert protective effects against the ototoxicity of aminoglycosides *in vitro* and *in vivo* (Li et al., 2018; Pham et al., 2020). However, no ideal drug that is protective against ototoxicity has been identified for use in clinical practice (Guo et al., 2019).

Gangliosides are sphingolipid cell membrane components containing sialic acid (Magistretti et al., 2019) that are widely present in the cell membranes of vertebrate tissues. Monosialotetrahexosylganglioside (GM1) is the most extensively studied of the gangliosides to date. GM1 plays a protective role in the nervous system by regulating the expression of BCL-2 protein, reducing the damage caused by free radicals (Rao et al., 2019), increasing mitochondrial activity and stabilizing mitochondrial function (Fazzari et al., 2020). GM1 has also been found to have a cytoprotective effect outside of the nervous system. Franco et al. (2016) found that GM1-containing nanoliposomes protect against light chain protein (LC)-induced human microvascular dysfunction by increasing nitric oxide bioavailability and reducing oxidative and nitrative stress mediated by the Nrf-2-dependent antioxidant stress response. Guo et al. (2021) reported that treatment with GM1 ganglioside (40 μM) significantly decreased α-synuclein accumulation, alleviated mitochondrial dysfunction and oxidative stress, and played an anti-PD role in doxycycline-treated PC12α-Syn A53T cells. In addition, GM-1 treatment was found to significantly decrease auditory brainstem response (ABR) threshold shifts and HC loss after acoustic overexposure, and immunostaining for 4-hydroxynonenal (4-HNE) was found to be reduced by GM-1 treatment, suggesting that GM-1 protects the cochlea against acoustic injury by inhibiting lipid peroxidation (Tanaka et al., 2010) and indicating that GM1 has an antioxidant effect on cochlear HCs.

GM1 has been used as a neuroprotective drug in some countries for the treatment of Alzheimer's disease, stroke, peripheral nerve damage, and Parkinson's disease (Magistretti et al., 2019), and some physicians in China are attempting to use GM1 in the clinical treatment of sudden deafness (Diao and Dong, 2012). However, the protective effect of GM1 against cochlear HC damage and the possible mechanism of this effect are still unclear. Therefore, clarification of the protective effect and mechanism of GM1 on cochlear and HC injury is of practical significance.

Neomycin is a representative ototoxic aminoglycoside drug and is often used in ototoxicity studies. We established a mature neomycin HC injury model in previous experiments (Gao et al., 2019). In the present study, we used neomycin to damage cochlear HC-like HEI-OC-1 cells and used whole-organ explant cultures to establish an *in vitro* model of neomycin-induced HC damage with the aim of investigating the potential protective effect of GM1 on ototoxic HC damage and attempting to provide evidence for the potential clinical use of GM1 in protecting against HC injury caused by aminoglycosides.

MATERIALS AND METHODS

Chemicals and Reagents

GM1 (Macklin, Shanghai, China, G873919), penicillin (CSPC, Shijiazhuang, China, h20033291), CCK-8 Kits (Beyotime, Shanghai, China, C0038), BeyoRT^{TM} II First-Strand cDNA Synthesis Kits with gDNA Eraser (Beyotime, D7170 M), TUNEL Apoptosis Assay Kits (Beyotime, C1086), DMSO (Sigma-Aldrich, Saint Louis, MO, United States, D8371), neomycin (Sigma-Aldrich, N6386-5G), paraformaldehyde (Sigma-Aldrich, 158127), TRIzol reagent (Sangon Biotech, Shanghai, China, B610409-0100), SYBR Green (Roche, Basel, Switzerland, 4913914001), MitoSOX Red (Life Technologies, Carlsbad, CA, United States, M36008), TMRE Mitochondrial Membrane Potential Assay Kits (Abcam, Cambridge, United Kingdom, ab113852), Triton X-100 (Solarbio, Beijing, China, T8260), DAPI (Solarbio, C0060), antibodies against cleaved CASPASE-3 (Thermo Fisher Scientific, Carlsbad, CA, United States, Cat# 43-7800, RRID:AB_2533540), antibody against MYOSIN 7a (Santa Cruz Biotechnology, Santa Cruz, United States, Cat# sc-74516, RRID:AB_2148626), Alexa Fluor 488 goat anti-rabbit IgG (Abcam, Cat# ab150077, RRID:AB_2630356), Alexa Fluor 555 donkey anti-rabbit IgG (Abcam, Cat# ab150062, RRID:AB_2801638), Alexa Fluor 555 goat anti-mouse IgG (Abcam, Cat# ab150118, RRID:AB_2714033), and Alexa Fluor 647 donkey anti-rabbit IgG (Abcam, Cat# ab150077, RRID:AB_2630356) were used in this study.

Cell Culture and Treatment

The House Ear Institute Organ of Corti 1 cell line (HEI-OC-1, RRID: CVCL_D899), which is used as an HC-like model system, expresses Atoh1, Prestin, Myosin7a and other cellular markers specific for auditory and sensory HCs. The cells were cultured in DMEM/F12 containing 10% fetal bovine serum (FBS) and 100 IU/mL penicillin at 37°C in a 5% CO_2 atmosphere. In this study, we exposed cells in FBS-free culture medium to 2 mM neomycin for 24 h to establish an HEI-OC-1 cell injury model, as reported previously (Gao et al., 2019). For the establishment of the HEI-OC-1 cell injury protection model, we plated the cells, cultured them for 12 h, replaced the medium with FBS-free culture medium, and treated the cells with 10–100 μM GM1 or with the corresponding volume of DMSO for 12 h. After 24 h treatment with 2 mM neomycin, the medium was replaced with complete culture medium lacking neomycin and GM1, and the cells were cultured for an additional 12 h before subsequent evaluation (**Figure 1A**).

Whole-Organ Explant Culture

On postnatal day 3 (P3), wild-type FVB mice were placed under deep anesthesia and sacrificed, and the animals' heads were removed and placed in 75% alcohol. The temporal bone cochlea was removed using scissors and placed in a sterile culture dish containing precooled HBSS buffer. Under microscopic view, the volute covering was peeled off, and the spiral ganglia and vascular stripes were separated to obtain a complete basilar membrane, which was then placed face up in the center of a sterile cover glass coated with Cell-tak tissue glue. The cover glass was placed in a 4-well plate and cultured in 120 μL of DMEM/F12 medium containing 2% B27, 1% N-2 and 100 IU/mL penicillin at 37°C in a 5% CO_2 atmosphere. The cochlear HC damage condition was 0.5 mM neomycin for 12 h, as reported previously (Gao et al., 2019). The explants in the GM1 group were cultured in medium to which 20 μM GM1 had been added; after 12 h, 0.5 mM neomycin was added, and the explant was cultured for an additional 12 h. The medium containing GM1 and neomycin was then removed, and the explants were cultured in fresh medium for an additional 12 h for recovery. The control group and the neomycin group were treated with the same volume of DMSO. All procedures involving FVB mice were performed in accordance with the procedures approved by the Animal Care and Use Committee of Nanjing Medical University, and all efforts were made to use the minimum number of animals necessary and to minimize their suffering.

Cell Viability and Number Analysis

Cell viability was measured using a CCK-8 kit. HEI-OC-1 cells were seeded in 96-well plates at 2,000 cells/well. After the treatment described above, 10 μL of CCK-8 was added to each well, and the plates were incubated at 37°C for 30 min. The absorbance at 450 nm was measured using a microtiter plate reader (Bio-Rad). In addition, the HCs of explant-cultured cochleae were immunolabeled using antibodies against MYOSIN 7a and counted by fluorescence labeling

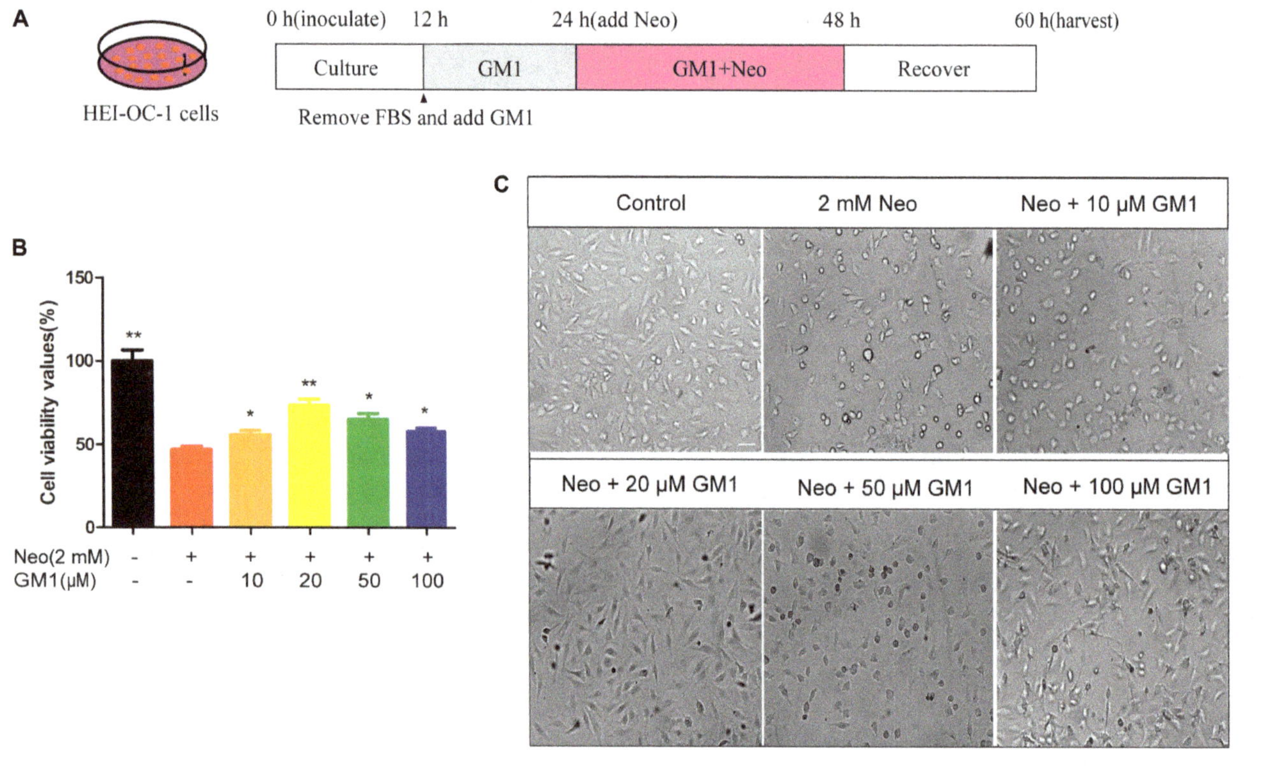

FIGURE 1 | GM1 enhanced HEI-OC-1 cell survival after neomycin exposure. **(A)** Schematic diagram illustrating GM1 and neomycin addition in cell culture. **(B)** Effects of GM1 on the viability of HEI-CO-1 cells after exposure to neomycin. Viability was measured using the CCK-8 assay, and the data are expressed as the mean ± SD of triplicate determinations obtained in three independent experiments. $^{*}p < 0.05$, $^{**}p < 0.01$ compared with neomycin treatment alone. **(C)** Morphology of HC-like HEI-OC-1 cells observed under a live-cell imaging system. Scale bars = 20 μm.

microscopy. The MYOSIN 7a-positive cells in three regions of equal length (160 μm) selected from the apical to the basal turns of the cochlea were viewed under fluorescence microscopy and counted.

Quantitative Real-Time PCR

TRIzol reagent was used to extract total RNA from HEI-OC-1 cells. The concentration and quality of RNA in the samples were measured by NanoDrop spectroscopy (Thermo NanoDrop 2000, United States). A BeyoRT^{TM} II First-Strand cDNA Synthesis Kit with gDNA Eraser was used for reverse transcription according to the instructions supplied by the manufacturer. SYBR Green was used to perform quantitative polymerase chain reaction (qPCR) on a real-time PCR instrument (cfx96, Bio-Rad). *Gapdh* was used as the internal reference gene. The primers were synthesized by Sangon Biotech (Shanghai, China). The primer sequences for the candidate genes are shown in **Table 1**.

Immunofluorescence Assay

An antibody against cleaved CASPASE-3, the TUNEL Apoptosis Assay Kit, MitoSOX Red, the TMRE Mitochondrial Membrane Potential Assay Kit, an antibody against MYOSIN 7a (1:500 dilution), and DAPI (1:1,000 dilution) were used to analyze apoptotic cells, measure ROS, measure MMP, and stain HCs and nuclei. Briefly, after fixation with 4% paraformaldehyde at room temperature for 1 h, the cells and tissues were washed three times with PBST (1 × PBS containing 0.1% Triton X-100) and incubated in blocking medium (PBS containing 10% heat-inactivated donkey serum, 1% Triton X-100, 1% BSA, and 0.02% sodium azide, pH 7.2) at room temperature for 1 h. The samples were then incubated with primary antibodies against cleaved CASPASE-3 or MYOSIN 7a at 4°C for 8 h. After 3 washes with PBST, the samples were labeled with a secondary antibody for 1 h, washed again 3 times with PBST, mounted with a fluorescent blocking agent, and imaged with laser scanning confocal microscopy (Zeiss LSM700, Germany). TUNEL, MitoSox Red, and TMRE signals were measured according to the manufacturer's instructions.

TABLE 1 | Primer sequences for qRT-PCR.

Gene	Sequence (5′ → 3′)	
Gapdh	F:	AGGTCGGTGTGAACGGATTTG
	R:	TGTAGACCATGTAGTTGPAGGTCA
Caspase-3	F:	ATGGAGAACAACAAAACCTCAGT
	R:	TTGCTCCCATGTATGGTCTTTAC
Bax	F:	TGAAGACAGGGGCCTTTTTG
	R:	AATTCGCCGGAGACACTCG
Bcl-2	F:	ATGCTTTGTGGAACTATATGGC
	R:	GGTATGCACCCAGAGTGATGC
Alox15	F:	GGCTCCAACAACGAGGTCTAC
	R:	AGGTATTCTGACACATCCACCTT
Sod1	F:	AACCAGTTGTGTTGTCAGGAC
	R:	CCACCATGTTTCTTAGAGTGAGG
Caspase-9	F:	CCTAGTGAGCGAGCTGCAAG
	R:	ACCGCTTTGCAAGAGTGAAG
Gsr	F:	TGCACTTCCCGGTAGGAAAC
	R:	GATCGCAACTGGGGTGAGAA
Sirt1	F:	TGTGGTGAAGATCTATGGAGGC
	R:	TGTACTTGCTGCAGACGTGGTA

F, forward; R, reverse.

Flow Cytometry Assay

We used DAPI and propidium iodide (PI) to distinguish dead cells from living cells. HEI-OC-1 cells were treated with neomycin in the presence or absence of GM1 and were then treated with trypsin and collected. The cells were washed twice, resuspended in PBS, and diluted to a concentration of 1×10^6 cells/mL in PBS. DAPI and PI were added; the cells were then incubated in the dark at room temperature for 10–20 min and analyzed by flow cytometry (FACSCanto, BD) within 1 h. In addition, MitoSOX Red was used to determine the level of mitochondrial ROS.

Statistical Analysis

All data are expressed as mean ± SD. All statistical analyses were performed using GraphPad Prism 7 software. Two-tailed and unpaired Student's *t*-tests were used to assess the statistical significance of differences between the two groups. One-way ANOVA and Dunnett's multiple comparison tests were used to compare multiple groups. $P < 0.05$ indicated a significant difference.

RESULTS

Monosialotetrahexosylganglioside Protects HEI-OC-1 Cells From Neomycin-Induced Cytotoxicity

As shown in **Figure 1**, exposure to 2 mM neomycin decreased cell viability by approximately half in comparison with the control cells, and GM1 at 10–100 μM exhibited a certain degree of protection; 20 μM GM1 gave the strongest protection. At GM1 concentrations higher than 20 μM, the viability of HEI-OC-1 cells began to decrease (**Figure 1B**). To confirm this finding, we used a live-cell imaging system to observe HEI-OC-1 cells and found that the morphology of living cells in the 20 μM GM1 group was most similar to that of the cells in the control group (**Figure 1C**). Therefore, 20 μM GM1 was used as the treatment concentration in the follow-up experiments in this study.

Monosialotetrahexosylganglioside Decreased Neomycin-Induced Apoptosis in HEI-OC-1 Cells

To confirm the protective effect of GM1 against apoptosis of HEI-OC-1 cells, HEI-OC-1 cells were stained using TUNEL and antibodies against cleaved CASPASE-3. The percentages of TUNEL-positive and cleaved CASPASE-3-positive cells in the neomycin group were significantly higher than those in the control group, and pretreatment with 20 μM GM1 significantly reduced the percentages of TUNEL-positive and

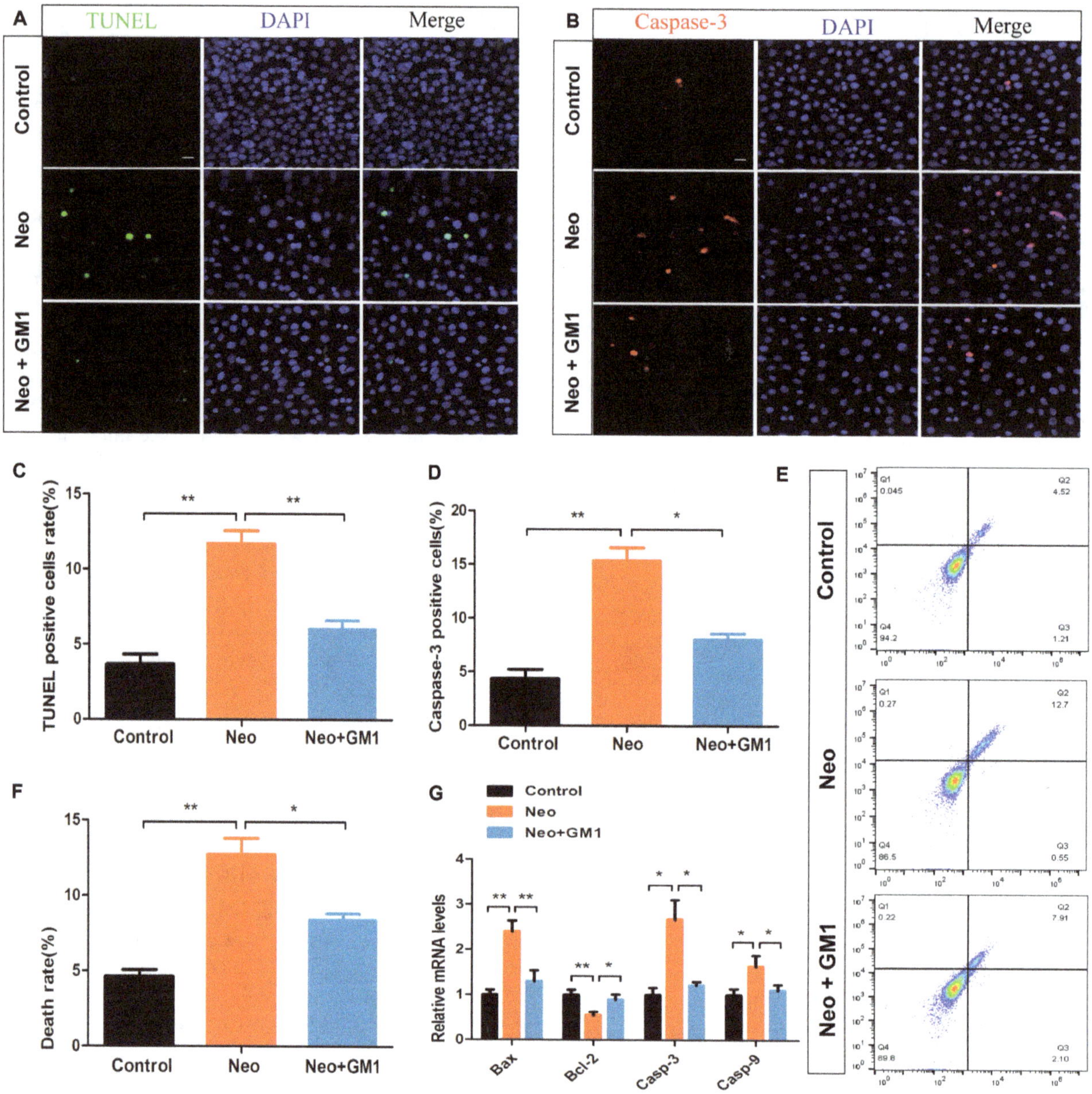

FIGURE 2 | GM1 reduced neomycin-induced apoptosis in HEI-OC-1 cells. **(A)** Immunofluorescence images of apoptotic HEI-OC-1 cells with TUNEL and DAPI double staining. **(B)** Immunofluorescence images of apoptotic HEI-OC-1 cells with cleaved CASPASE-3 and DAPI double staining. **(C,D)** Quantification of the number of apoptotic cells in **(A,B)**. **(E,F)** Survival and percentage of HEI-OC-1 cells determined by DAPI/PI staining flow cytometry. **(G)** Expression of proapoptotic and antiapoptotic genes in HEI-OC-1 cells treated with neomycin and/or GM1 determined by qRT-PCR; the values were normalized to *Gapdh* as an internal control. The data are expressed as the mean ± SD of triplicate samples. $^{*}p < 0.05$, $^{**}p < 0.01$. Scale bars = 20 μm.

cleaved CASPASE-3-positive cells after neomycin exposure (**Figures 2A–D**). Similarly, flow cytometry showed that 20 μM GM1 significantly reduced the death of HEI-OC-1 cells induced by neomycin (**Figures 2E,F**). The qRT-PCR results also showed that the mRNA expression of *Caspase-3, Bax,* and *Caspase-9* decreased significantly, while *Bcl-2* expression increased significantly, in the GM1 group compared with the neomycin group (**Figure 2G**). Taken together, our results suggest that GM1 protects HEI-OC-1 cells from neomycin-induced apoptosis.

Monosialotetrahexosylganglioside Reduced Neomycin-Induced Apoptosis of Hair Cells in Explant-Cultured Cochleae

To explore the protective effect of GM1 on explant-cultured cochleae, TUNEL and antibody staining for cleaved CASPASE-3 were used to measure apoptosis of the cells in the explants after treatment. We found that the percentages of TUNEL-positive

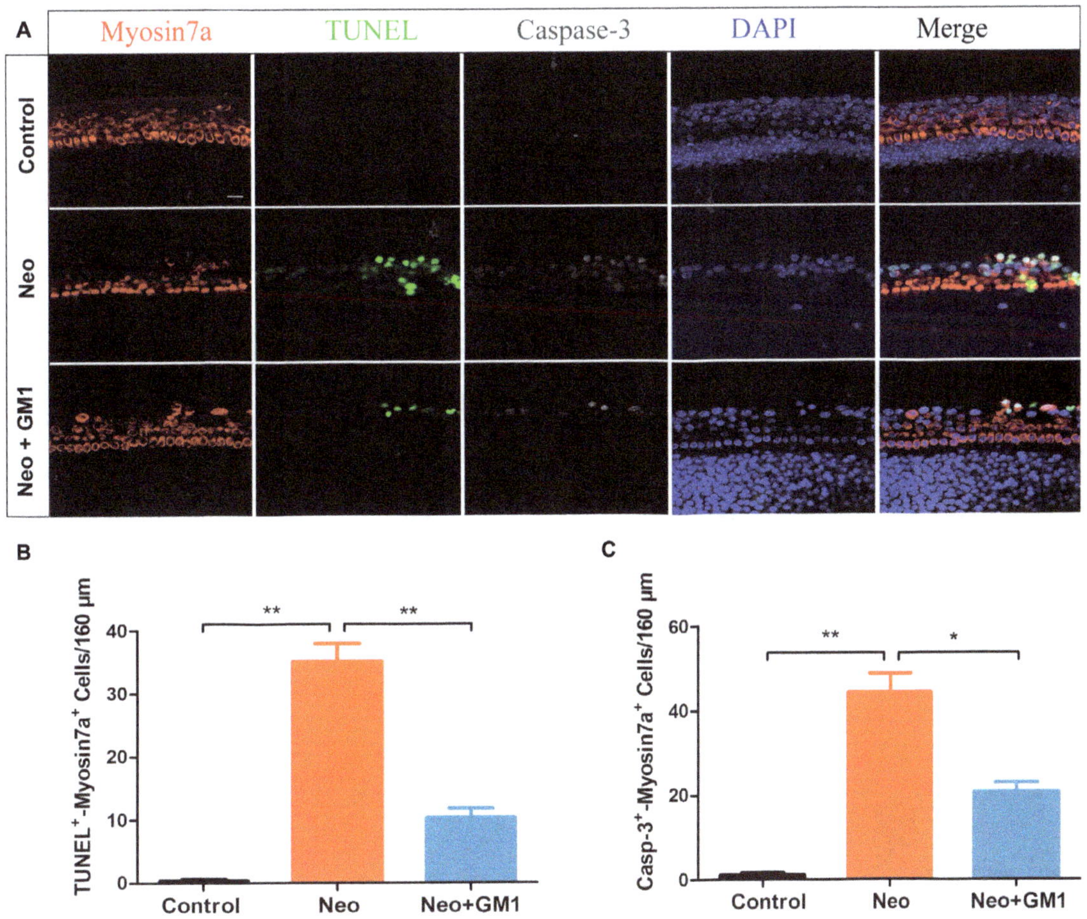

FIGURE 3 | GM1 decreased neomycin-induced HC apoptosis in cochleae. **(A)** Immunofluorescence staining for TUNEL, cleaved CASPASE-3, and MYOSIN 7a in the basal turn of the cochlea in different treatment groups. **(B,C)** Quantification of the number of TUNEL/MYOSIN 7a and cleaved CASPASE-3/MYOSIN 7a double-positive cells per 160 μm of cochlea in **(A)**. The data are expressed as the mean ± SD of triplicate samples. $^{**}p < 0.01$. Scale bars = 16 μm.

and cleaved CASPASE-3-positive cells in the neomycin group were significantly higher than those in the control group and that pretreatment with 20 μM GM1 significantly reduced the percentage of TUNEL-positive and cleaved CASPASE-3-positive cells after neomycin exposure (**Figures 3A–C**), consistent with the results obtained for HEI-OC-1 cells.

Monosialotetrahexosylganglioside Protects Against Neomycin-Induced Hair Cell Loss in Explant-Cultured Cochleae

The procedures used to process the samples in the explant-cultured cochlea experiment are described in **Figure 4A**. MYOSIN 7a and DAPI staining were used to observe the changes in the number of HCs in the apical, middle and basal turns of the cochlea. We found that the number of HCs in the apical turn did not change significantly after neomycin exposure (**Figure 4B**). In contrast, the number of HCs in the middle and basal turns of the cochlea decreased significantly, and GM1 treatment successfully reduced HC loss in the middle and basal turns after neomycin exposure (**Figures 4C–E**).

Monosialotetrahexosylganglioside Attenuates Oxidative Stress in Explant-Cultured Cochleae and HEI-OC-1 Cells After Neomycin Treatment

In this study, MitoSox Red immunofluorescence staining showed that the levels of ROS were significantly increased in the neomycin group compared with the control group and that pretreatment with 20 μM GM1 significantly reduced ROS levels compared with the neomycin group both in explant-cultured cochleae (**Figures 5A,B**) and in HEI-OC-1 cells (**Figures 6A,B**). MitoSOX flow cytometry of HEI-OC-1 cells yielded similar results (**Figure 6C**). qRT-PCR showed that the mRNA expression of *Gsr, Sod1,* and *Sirt1* was significantly upregulated in the GM1 pretreatment group compared with the neomycin group (**Figure 6D**). This suggests that GM1 alleviates the neomycin-induced imbalance in antioxidant-prooxidant gene expression. However, the mRNA expression of *Alox15* did not change significantly after GM pretreatment. We also found that the MMP decreased in the neomycin group but significantly increased

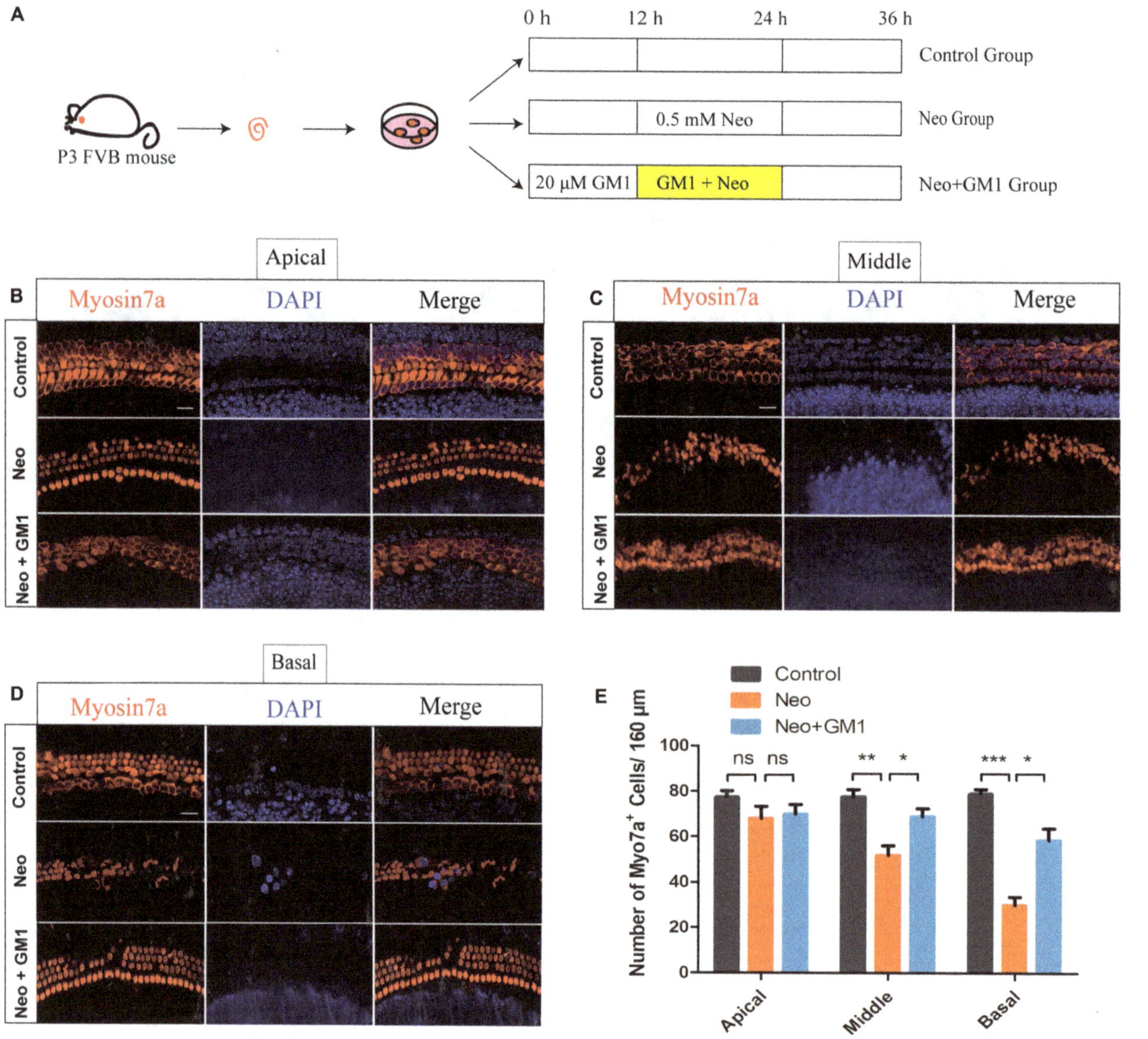

FIGURE 4 | GM1 promoted the survival of cochlear HCs in explant cultures after neomycin exposure. **(A)** Schematic diagram illustrating GM1 and neomycin addition to explant-cultured cochleae. **(B,D)** Immunofluorescence staining of MYOSIN 7a/DAPI in the apical turns **(B)**, middle turns **(C)**, and basal turns **(D)** of explant-cultured cochleae in the different treatment groups. **(E)** Quantification of the number of MYOSIN 7a-positive cells per 160 μm of cochlea in **(B–D)**. The data are expressed as the mean ± SD of triplicate samples $^{*}p < 0.05$, $^{**}p < 0.01$, $^{***}p < 0.001$. Scale bars = 16 μm.

in the GM1 group compared to that in the neomycin group, indicating that 20 μM GM1 treatment can prevent the MMP decrease induced by neomycin exposure in HEI-OC-1 cells (**Figures 7A,B**).

DISCUSSION

Gangliosides are mainly composed of hydrophobic ceramide and hydrophilic oligosaccharide chains containing sialic acid, which are fat-soluble and water-soluble, respectively. Ceramide is composed of long basic hydrophobic chains attached to fatty acids that are embedded in the lipid bilayer of the cell membrane and enhance the stability of the cell membrane structure. Oligosaccharides are linked to the serine residue of ceramide, and the sialic acid in oligosaccharides binds to peripheral calcium ions to maintain normal cellular physiological functions (Schnaar, 2016; Ledeen and Wu, 2018). Recent studies have reported that GM1 exerts antioxidant effects through its regulation of intracellular calcium levels in the hippocampus (She et al., 2009) and its activation of tyrosine kinase Trk receptors (Vlasova Iu et al., 2009) and that it has a protective effect on a variety of cells when applied as an intervention (Nikolaeva et al., 2015; Zhao et al., 2015). In this study, we used the HEI-OC-1 cell line and whole-organ explant cultures to investigate the protective effect of GM1 on neomycin-induced

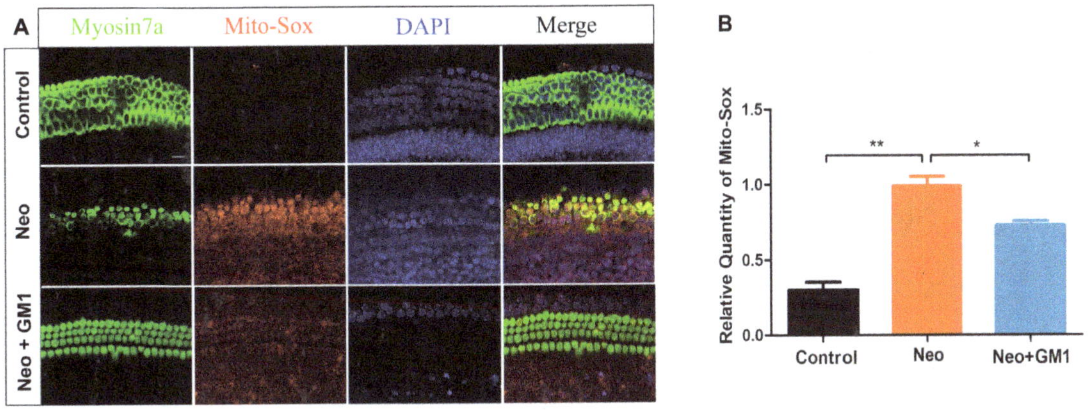

FIGURE 5 | GM1 decreased ROS levels in explant-cultured cochlear HCs after neomycin exposure. **(A)** Immunofluorescence due to MitoSox, MYOSIN 7a and DAPI in the middle turns of explant-cultured cochleae in the different treatment groups. **(B)** Relative MitoSox immunofluorescence intensity. The data are expressed as the mean ± SD of triplicate samples. $^{*}p < 0.05$, $^{**}p < 0.01$. Scale bars = 16 μm.

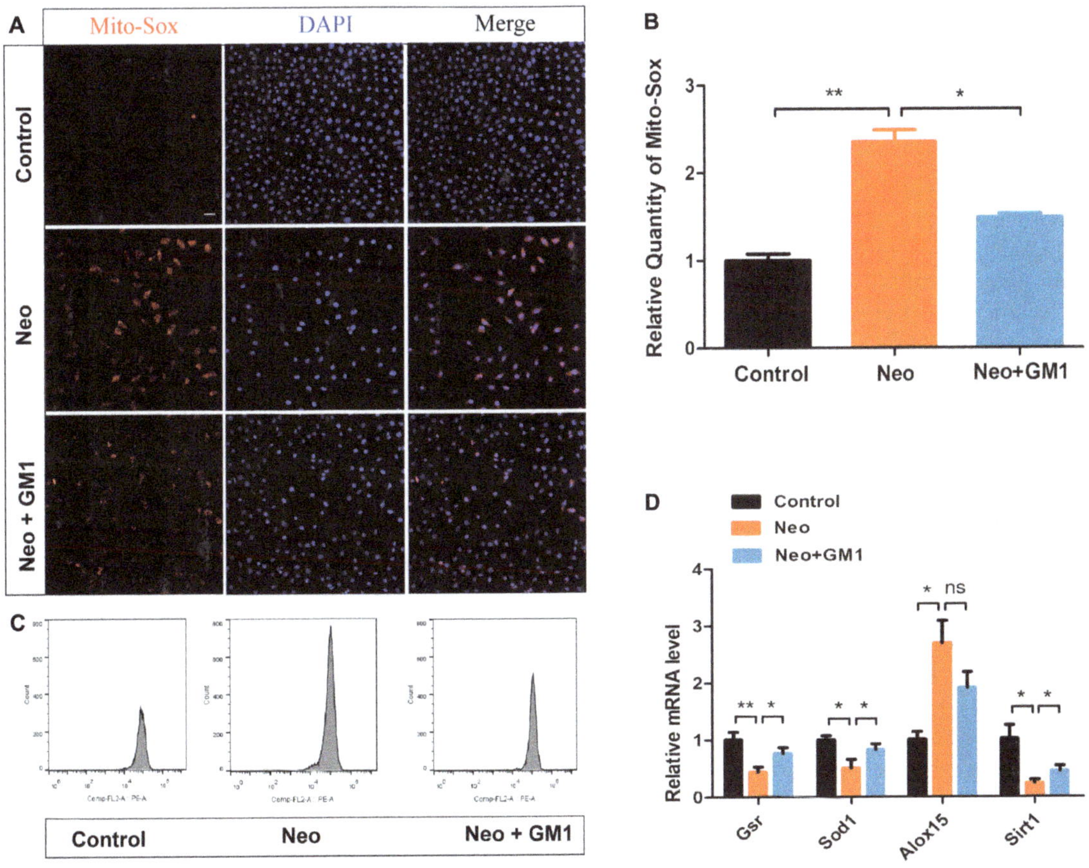

FIGURE 6 | GM1 decreased ROS levels in HEI-OC-1 cells after neomycin exposure. **(A,B)** Immunofluorescence of MitoSox/DAPI in different treatment groups. **(C)** MitoSox levels of HEI-OC-1 cells in different treatment groups determined by flow cytometry. **(D)** mRNA expression levels of redox-related genes in HEI-OC-1 cells determined by qRT-PCR and normalized to *Gapdh*. The data are expressed as the mean ± SD of triplicate samples. $^{*}p < 0.05$, $^{**}p < 0.01$. Scale bars = 20 μm.

HC injury *in vitro*. Our results showed that a protective effect of GM1 on HEI-OC-1 cells is observed when GM1 is applied at concentrations between 10 and 100 μM and that 20 μM is the optimal concentration; beyond this, the protective effect begins to decline, suggesting that GM1 can protect HCs when applied at an appropriate concentration.

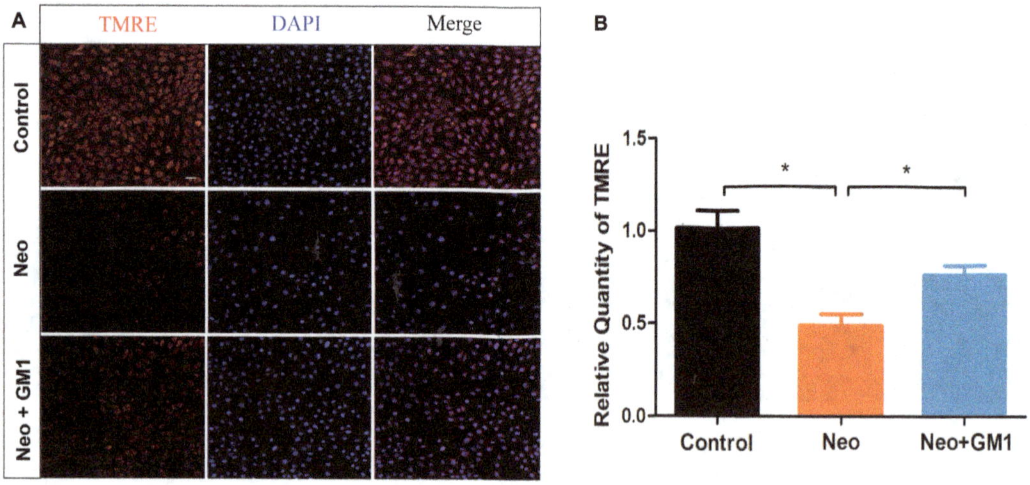

FIGURE 7 | GM1 increases the mitochondrial membrane potential (MMP) after neomycin exposure. **(A)** Immunofluorescence of HEI-OC-1 cells in different treatment groups after labeling using a TMRE staining kit and DAPI. **(B)** Relative immunofluorescence intensities of the cells in **(A)**. The data are expressed as the mean ± SD of triplicate samples. $^{*}p < 0.05$. Scale bars = 20 μm.

Previous studies have suggested that aminoglycoside drugs induce HEI-OC-1 cell apoptosis by promoting the release of proapoptotic factors (Leis et al., 2015). Our previous research also showed that after exposure of HEI-OC-1 cells to neomycin, the expression of proapoptotic genes such as *Caspase 3* and *Bax* increased significantly, while that of the antiapoptotic genes *Bcl-2* and *Nf-kb* decreased significantly (Gao et al., 2019). In the current study, we found that treatment with GM1 decreases the death and apoptosis induced by neomycin. Moreover, our results also showed that exposure of cochlear explant cultures to GM1 protected HC cells in the middle and basal turns of the cochlea from damage; since the damage caused by aminoglycoside drugs shows a decreasing trend from the basal turn to the apical turn of the cochlea (Zhang et al., 2019) and high-frequency hearing loss is the first and most severe impairment in patients with ototoxic hearing loss (Guo et al., 2019), the protective effect of GM1 on high-frequency hearing may have potential clinical significance.

BCL-2 family proteins play a key role in the apoptosis process. Proapoptotic proteins such as BAX change their molecular conformations when they encounter apoptosis signals; they then translocate and insert into the outer mitochondrial membrane, eventually leading to increased permeability of the outer mitochondrial membrane, the release of cytochrome c (Cyt C), and the activation of multiple caspases. BCL-2 can prevent this process (Verma and Syed Mohammed, 2019; Tian et al., 2020; Zeng et al., 2020). Our study found that the mRNA expression of *Bcl-2* was upregulated and that that of *Bax* was downregulated, indicating that GM1 can relieve neomycin-induced HC damage by regulating the mRNA expression of *Bax* and *Bcl-2*. This is consistent with the report by Chen et al. (2019) that GM1 increases *Bcl-2* expression and reduces *Bax* expression, thereby protecting against lead-induced neurological damage in developing rats.

Many studies have found that aminoglycoside antibiotics aggregate in inner ear HCs, where they affect normal metabolism and produce a large number of highly toxic ROS (Han et al., 2020). ROS include hydroxyl radicals (OH•), hydrogen peroxide, superoxide and other free radicals, all of which exhibit great oxygen toxicity. ROS can affect various signaling pathways and physiological activities of cells, including cell growth, division, differentiation and apoptosis. Excessive ROS levels can lead to a variety of diseases (Zhang et al., 2016). Studies have found that aminoglycosides bind to calreticulin, which is highly expressed in cochlear marginal cells and HCs. and disrupt chaperone activity. This binding in turn elevates mitochondrial Ca^{2+} levels, and this leads to elevated levels of both mitochondrial oxidation and cytoplasmic ROS and to an imbalance in the redox state (Jiang et al., 2017). The high reactivity of oxygen free radicals can damage cell components and structures such as nucleic acids and cell membranes. ROS accumulation can also cause mitochondrial depolarization and change mitochondrial membrane permeability. The resulting impairment of mitochondrial function leads to the further accumulation of oxygen free radicals and eventually to apoptosis (He et al., 2020; Zhong et al., 2020). In this study, we found that GM1 significantly decreased ROS levels in HEI-OC-1 cells and explant-cultured cochlear HCs, suggesting that GM1 can alleviate mitochondrial dysfunction after exposure to neomycin. Redox balance plays an important role in the generation and elimination of ROS. In this study, the mRNA expression levels of *Gsr, Sod1,* and *Sirt1* decreased and that of *Alox15* increased significantly after neomycin exposure, and GM1 pretreatment significantly improved the imbalance in the mRNA expression of *Gsr, Sod1,* and *Sirt1* induced by neomycin. These results suggest that exposure of cells to GM1 can correct the imbalance in the expression of prooxidant and antioxidant genes observed after neomycin exposure, thereby reducing the ROS level and preventing HC mitochondrial dysfunction and apoptosis. However, it must be noted that the use of high GM1 concentrations will reduce the protective effect and may cause additional damage to HCs. Drug dosage must be considered in future animal and clinical studies.

In conclusion, our results suggest that GM1 can maintain the normal balance between oxidative and antioxidant gene expression, reduce the accumulation of ROS, and reduce apoptosis after exposure of HEI-OC-1 cells and cultured cochlear HCs to neomycin. These results indicate that GM1 may have potential clinical value in protecting against hearing impairment in individuals treated with aminoglycoside drugs.

AUTHOR CONTRIBUTIONS

YL, AL, and CW performed the experiments, analyzed the data, and wrote the manuscript. LL, S-LW, and XG designed the experiments and provided critical revision. XJ and YZ reviewed the experimental data and conducted the statistical analysis. All authors contributed to the article and approved the submitted version.

ACKNOWLEDGMENTS

We would like to express our sincere appreciation to the Project of Invigorating Health Care through Science, Technology and Education ZDXKB2016015.

REFERENCES

Chen, C., Wang, S., and Liu, P. (2019). Deferoxamine enhanced mitochondrial iron accumulation and promoted cell migration in triple-negative MDA-MB-231 breast cancer cells via a ROS-dependent mechanism. *Int. J. Mol. Sci.* 20:4952. doi: 10.3390/ijms20194952

Diao, Y., and Dong, M. (2012). The observation on curative effect of 90 cases of sudden hearing loss. *Lin chuang er bi yan hou tou jing wai ke za zhi* 36, 306–308.

Fazzari, M., Audano, M., Lunghi, G., Di Biase, E., Loberto, N., Mauri, L., et al. (2020). The oligosaccharide portion of ganglioside GM1 regulates mitochondrial function in neuroblastoma cells. *Glycoconj J.* 37, 293–306. doi: 10.1007/s10719-020-09920-4

Franco, D. A., Truran, S., Weissig, V., Guzman-Villanueva, D., Karamanova, N., Senapati, S., et al. (2016). Monosialoganglioside-containing nanoliposomes restore endothelial function impaired by AL amyloidosis light chain proteins. *J. Am. Heart Assoc.* 5:e003318. doi: 10.1161/JAHA.116.003318

Gao, S., Cheng, C., Wang, M., Jiang, P., Zhang, L., Wang, Y., et al. (2019). Blebbistatin inhibits neomycin-induced apoptosis in hair cell-like HEI-OC-1 cells and in cochlear hair cells. *Front. Cell. Neurosci.* 13:590. doi: 10.3389/fncel.2019.00590

Germovsek, E., Barker, C. I., and Sharland, M. (2017). What do I need to know about aminoglycoside antibiotics? *Arch. Dis. Child Educ. Pract. Ed.* 102, 89–93. doi: 10.1136/archdischild-2015-309069

Guo, J., Chai, R., Li, H., and Sun, S. (2019). Protection of hair cells from ototoxic drug-induced hearing loss. *Adv. Exp. Med. Biol.* 1130, 17–36. doi: 10.1007/978-981-13-6123-4_2

Guo, Y. L., Duan, W. J., Lu, D. H., Ma, X. H., Li, X. X., Li, Z., et al. (2021). Autophagy-dependent removal of α-synuclein: a novel mechanism of GM1 ganglioside neuroprotection against Parkinson's disease. *Acta Pharmacol. Sin.* 42, 518–528. doi: 10.1038/s41401-020-0454-y

Han, H., Dong, Y., and Ma, X. (2020). Dihydromyricetin protects against gentamicin-induced ototoxicity via PGC-1α/SIRT3 Signaling in vitro. *Front. Cell. Dev. Biol.* 8:702. doi: 10.3389/fcell.2020.00702

He, Y., Li, W., Zheng, Z., Zhao, L., Li, W., Wang, Y., et al. (2020). Inhibition of Protein arginine methyltransferase 6 reduces reactive oxygen species production and attenuates aminoglycoside- and cisplatin-induced hair cell death. *Theranostics* 10, 133–150. doi: 10.7150/thno.37362

Jiang, M., Karasawa, T., and Steyger, P. S. (2017). Aminoglycoside-Induced cochleotoxicity: A review. *Front. Cell Neurosci.* 11:308. doi: 10.3389/fncel.2017.00308

Jiang, P., Ray, A., Rybak, L. P., and Brenner, M. J. (2016). Role of STAT1 and oxidative stress in gentamicin-induced hair cell death in organ of corti. *Otol. Neurotol.* 37, 1449–1456. doi: 10.1097/MAO.0000000000001192

Ledeen, R., and Wu, G. (2018). Gangliosides of the nervous system. *Methods Mol. Biol.* 1804, 19–55. doi: 10.1007/978-1-4939-8552-4_2

Leis, J. A., Rutka, J. A., and Gold, W. L. (2015). Aminoglycoside-induced ototoxicity. *Curr. Pharm. Des.* 187:E52. doi: 10.1503/cmaj.140339

Li, A., You, D., Li, W., Cui, Y., He, Y., Li, W., et al. (2018). Novel compounds protect auditory hair cells against gentamycin-induced apoptosis by maintaining the expression level of H3K4me2. *Drug Deliv.* 25, 1033–1043. doi: 10.1080/10717544.2018.1461277

Lopez-Novoa, J. M., Quiros, Y., Vicente, L., Morales, A. I., and Lopez-Hernandez, F. J. (2011). New insights into the mechanism of aminoglycoside nephrotoxicity: an integrative point of view. *Kidney Int.* 79, 33–45. doi: 10.1038/ki.2010.337

Magistretti, P. J., Geisler, F. H., Schneider, J. S., Li, P. A., Fiumelli, H., and Sipione, S. (2019). Gangliosides: treatment avenues in neurodegenerative disease. *Front. Neurol.* 10:859. doi: 10.3389/fneur.2019.00859

Nikolaeva, S., Bayunova, L., Sokolova, T., Vlasova, Y., Bachteeva, V., Avrova, N., et al. (2015). GM1 and GD1a gangliosides modulate toxic and inflammatory effects of E. coli lipopolysaccharide by preventing TLR4 translocation into lipid rafts. *Biochim. Biophys. Acta* 1851, 239–247.

Pham, T. N. M., Jeong, S. Y., Kim, D. H., Park, Y. H., Lee, J. S., Lee, K. W., et al. (2020). Protective mechanisms of avocado oil extract against ototoxicity. *Nutrients* 12:947.

Rao, S., Lin, Y., Du, Y., He, L., Huang, G., Chen, B., et al. (2019). Designing multifunctionalized selenium nanoparticles to reverse oxidative stress-induced spinal cord injury by attenuating ROS overproduction and mitochondria dysfunction. *J. Mater Chem. B* 7, 2648–2656. doi: 10.1039/c8tb02520g

Schnaar, R. L. (2016). Gangliosides of the vertebrate nervous system. *J. Mol. Biol.* 428, 3325–3336. doi: 10.1016/j.jmb.2016.05.020

She, J. Q., Wang, M., Zhu, D. M., Tang, M., Chen, J. T., Wang, L., et al. (2009). Monosialoanglioside (GM1) prevents lead-induced neurotoxicity on long-term potentiation, SOD activity, MDA levels, and intracellular calcium levels of hippocampus in rats. *Naunyn Schmiedebergs Arch. Pharmacol.* 379, 517–524. doi: 10.1007/s00210-008-0379-3

Sotoudeh, H. (2021). Hearing loss prevalence and years lived with disability, 1990–2019: findings from the Global Burden of Disease Study 2019. *Lancet* 397, 996–1009.

Tanaka, S., Tabuchi, K., Hoshino, T., Murashita, H., Tsuji, S., and Hara, A. (2010). Protective effects of exogenous GM-1 ganglioside on acoustic injury of the mouse cochlea. *Neurosci. Lett.* 473, 237–241. doi: 10.1016/j.neulet.2010.02.057

Tian, J., Mo, J., Xu, L., Zhang, R., Qiao, Y., Liu, B., et al. (2020). Scoulerine promotes cell viability reduction and apoptosis by activating ROS-dependent endoplasmic reticulum stress in colorectal cancer cells. *Chem. Biol. Interact* 327:109184.

Verma, J., and Syed Mohammed, T. (2019). Evaluating hearing loss in patients undergoing second line anti tubercular treatment. *Indian J. Otolaryngol. Head Neck Surg.* 71, 1202–1206. doi: 10.1007/s12070-018-1266-y

Vlasova Iu, A., Zakharova, I. O., Sokolova, T. V., Furaev, V. V., Rychkova, M. P., and Avrova, N. F. (2009). Role of tyrosine kinase of Trk-receptors in realization of antioxidant effect of ganglioside GM1 in PC12 cells. *Zh. Evol. Biokhim. Fiziol.* 45, 465–471.

Yao, L., Zhang, J. W., Chen, B., Cai, M. M., Feng, D., Wang, Q. Z., et al. (2020). Mechanisms and pharmacokinetic/pharmacodynamic profiles underlying the low nephrotoxicity and ototoxicity of etimicin. *Acta Pharmacol. Sin.* 41, 866–878.

Zeng, H., Kong, X., Zhang, H., Chen, Y., Cai, S., Luo, H., et al. (2020). Inhibiting DNA methylation alleviates cigarette smoke extract-induced dysregulation of Bcl-2 and endothelial apoptosis. *Tob. Induc. Dis.* 18:51. doi: 10.18332/tid/119163

Zhang, J., Wang, X., Vikash, V., Ye, Q., Wu, D., Liu, Y., et al. (2016). ROS and ROS-mediated cellular signaling. *Oxid Med. Cell Longev.* 2016:4350965. doi: 10.1155/2016/4350965

Zhang, S., Qiang, R., Dong, Y., Zhang, Y., Chen, Y., Zhou, H., et al. (2020). Hair cell regeneration from inner ear progenitors in the mammalian cochlea. *Am. J. Stem Cells* 9, 25–35.

Zhang, Y., Li, W., He, Z., Wang, Y., Shao, B., Cheng, C., et al. (2019). Pre-treatment with fasudil prevents neomycin-induced hair cell damage by reducing the accumulation of reactive oxygen species. *Front. Mol. Neurosci.* 12:264. doi: 10.3389/fnmol.2019.00264

Zhao, H., Li, X., Li, G., Sun, B. O., Ren, L., and Zhao, C. (2015). Protective effects of monosialotetrahexosylganglioside sodium on H2O2-induced human vascular endothelial cells. *Exp. Ther. Med.* 10, 947–953. doi: 10.3892/etm.2015.2603

Zhong, Z., Fu, X., Li, H., Chen, J., Wang, M., Gao, S., et al. (2020). Citicoline protects auditory hair cells against neomycin-induced damage. *Front. Cell. Dev. Biol.* 8:712. doi: 10.3389/fcell.2020.00712

18

Salubrinal Protects against Cisplatin-Induced Cochlear Hair Cell Endoplasmic Reticulum Stress by Regulating Eukaryotic Translation Initiation Factor 2α Signalling

Wen Lu[1†], Kun Ni[1,2†], Zhuangzhuang Li[1†], Lili Xiao[1], Yini Li[1], Yumeng Jiang[1], Jincheng Zhang[3] and Haibo Shi[1*]*

[1] Department of Otolaryngology-Head and Neck Surgery, Shanghai Jiao Tong University Affiliated Sixth People's Hospital, Shanghai, China, [2] Department of Otolaryngology-Head and Neck Surgery, Shanghai Children's Hospital, Shanghai Jiao Tong University, Shanghai, China, [3] Department of Critical Care Medicine, Zhongshan Hospital, Fudan University, Shanghai, China

***Correspondence:**
Jincheng Zhang
pipijincheng@sohu.com
Haibo Shi
hbshi@sjtu.edu.cn

[†] These authors have contributed equally to this work

Objective: Cisplatin is a broad-spectrum anti-tumour drug commonly used in clinical practice. However, its ototoxicity greatly limits its clinical application, and no effective method is available to prevent this effect. Endoplasmic reticulum stress (ERS) is reportedly involved in cisplatin ototoxicity, but the exact mechanism remains unclear. Therefore, this study aimed to investigate the role of eukaryotic translation initiation factor 2α (eIF2α) signalling and its dephosphorylation inhibitor salubrinal in cisplatin ototoxicity.

Methods: We evaluated whether salubrinal could protect against cisplatin-induced damage in House Ear Institute-Organ of Corti 1 (HEI-OC1) cells and mouse cochlear explants. By knocking down eIF2α, we elucidated the vital role of eIF2α in cisplatin-induced damage in HEI-OC1 cells. Whole-mount immunofluorescent staining and confocal microscopy of mouse cochlear explants and HEI-OC1 cells were performed to analyse cisplatin-induced damage in cochlear hair cells and the auditory cell line.

Results: Data suggested salubrinal attenuated cisplatin-induced hair cell injury by inhibiting apoptosis. In addition, salubrinal significantly reduced ERS levels in hair cells *via* eIF2α signalling, while eIF2α knockdown inhibited the protective effect of salubrinal.

Significance: Salubrinal and eIF2α signalling play a role in protecting against cisplatin-induced ototoxicity, and pharmacological inhibition of eIF2α-mediated ERS is a potential treatment for cisplatin-induced damage in the cochlea and HEI-OC1 cells.

Keywords: cisplatin, endoplasmic reticulum stress, salubrinal, apoptosis, hearing loss, ototoxicity

INTRODUCTION

Drug-induced hearing loss is one of the most common types of sensorineural hearing loss (Cunningham and Tucci, 2017). Cisplatin is a broad-spectrum anti-tumour drug commonly used in clinical practice, but its extensive and severe adverse effects on normal tissues greatly limit its clinical application (Wilson et al., 2017). Ototoxicity and nephrotoxicity are the main side effects of cisplatin (Gentilin et al., 2019). Diuretic hydration and other methods may prevent cisplatin nephrotoxic injury (Duan et al., 2020; Bégin et al., 2021). However, the FDA has not yet approved any drug that can effectively prevent cisplatin-induced hearing loss. According to the latest World Hearing Report, 23–50% of adults and up to 60% of children treated with cisplatin suffer from significant hearing loss (Chadha et al., 2021). Hearing loss has a negative effect on a person's quality of life and creates a heavy healthcare burden (Knight et al., 2005; Frisina et al., 2016; Brock et al., 2018). To date, no proven strategy has been established for preventing and treating cisplatin-induced hearing damage, mainly because the mechanism of cisplatin-induced cochlear damage is not fully understood. It is acknowledged that cochlear hair cell (HC) and spiral ganglion cell death is a main pathology contributing to cisplatin-induced hearing loss (Kros and Steyger, 2019). However, an in-depth mechanism of cisplatin damage to cochlea is not well understood, highlighting the importance of further investigation.

The endoplasmic reticulum is found in eukaryotic cells, and it is directly associated with cholesterol metabolism, membrane/secreted proteins, phospholipids, calcium ion signals, and aminoglycosides (Luongo et al., 2017). When the body is subjected to unfavourable stimulation, such as ischemia-reperfusion injury, the endoplasmic reticulum lumen environment is destroyed due to a disorder in Ca^{2+} metabolism (Luongo et al., 2017). As a result, the newly synthesised protein cannot fold normally, resulting in an excessive protein load, which eventually triggers endoplasmic reticulum stress (ERS) (Oyadomari and Mori, 2004; Delaunay-Moisan and Appenzeller-Herzog, 2015; Hetz et al., 2020). An increasing number of studies found that ERS was involved in drug-induced hearing loss and played an important role in the development of ototoxicity, but the precise molecular mechanism was still unclear (Jia et al., 2018; Wen et al., 2021).

Salubrinal (Sal) is a selective protein phosphatase I complex inhibitor, which dephosphorylates eIF2α (Boyce et al., 2005; Binet and Sapieha, 2015). EIF2α phosphorylation reduces the expression of reaction initiators, resulting in reduced synthesis of unfolded proteins and the preservation of the ability to synthesise proteins, which is beneficial for ERS reduction (Hetz, 2012). Therefore, Sal can reduce ERS overexpression and block the initiation of the apoptotic program by selectively inhibiting the dephosphorylation of the PERK-eIF2α phosphate complex (Boyce et al., 2005). Sal plays a cytoprotective role during ERS in various diseases (López-Hernández et al., 2015; Matsuoka and Komoike, 2015; Font-Belmonte et al., 2019). Our previous studies revealed (Zhang et al., 2015, 2020) that Sal treatment improved neurological dysfunction through the inhibition of ER stress after postresuscitation brain injury. This finding suggests that ERS inhibition with Sal could be a neuroprotective strategy. However, whether activating eIF2α phosphorylation with Sal in cochlear HCs could inhibit ERS and thus protect against cisplatin-induced hearing loss is unknown.

In this study, we aimed to investigate the role of eIF2α signalling in cisplatin-induced cochlear damage and establish an effective therapy against cisplatin induced-hearing loss. We hypothesised that Sal could attenuate cisplatin-induced auditory HC apoptosis by inhibiting ERS and this effect was dependent on the eIF2α phosphorylation.

MATERIALS AND METHODS

Animals

All animals were purchased from Shanghai Jie Si Jie Laboratory Animal Co., Ltd. (Shanghai, China). C57BL/6 mice were used in this study for the cochlear explant experiments. Total 28 mice aged P3 was used in our experiments. All experiments were conducted in accordance with the recommendations of the Constitution of the Animal Ethical and Welfare Committee. The study protocol was approved by the Animal Research Committee of the Shanghai Jiao Tong University Affiliated Sixth People's Hospital. Efforts were made to minimise animal pain and the number used as much as possible.

Materials

We used the following reagents and antibodies: Sal (HY-15486; MedChemExpress, Monmouth Junction, NJ, United States), cisplatin (P4394; Sigma-Aldrich, St. Louis, MO, United States), anti-BIP/GRP78 (5,174; Cell Signaling Technology, Danvers, MA, United States), anti-eIF2α (5,324; Cell Signaling Technology), anti-phospho-eIF2α-S51 (AP0692; ABclonal China, Wuhan, China), anti-cleaved caspase 3 (9,661; Cell Signaling Technology), anti-C/EBP homologous protein (CHOP) (2,895; Cell Signaling Technology), anti-cleaved PARP (9,544; Cell Signaling Technology), a rabbit anti-myosin-VIIa antibody (25-6,790; Proteus Bioscience, Ramona, CA, United States), DAPI (ab104139; Abcam, Cambridge, United Kingdom), anti-GAPDH (5,174; Cell Signalling Technology), anti-β-tubulin (2,128; Cell Signalling Technology), and Phalloidin-iFluor 488, 555 (ab176753, ab176756; Abcam), [anti-β-Actin(AC026; ABclonal China, Wuhan, China)].

Cell Culture and Drug Administration

House Ear Institute-Organ of Corti 1 (HEI-OC1) cells provided by Dr. Iris Heredia were cultured according to the guidelines (Kalinec et al., 2016). Before use, the cell line was verified by performing an immunohistochemical analysis of myosin-VIIa, a marker of cochlear hair cells. HEI-OC1 cells were cultured in six-well plates and proliferated under non-permissive conditions (10% CO_2, 33°C) in high-glucose Dulbecco's Modified Eagle's Medium (DMEM) containing 10% foetal bovine serum (Gibco; Thermo Fisher Scientific, Waltham, MA, United States) without antibiotics. When cells reached 80% confluence, subculture was performed using 0.25% trypsin/EDTA (Gibco). Cisplatin (P4394; Sigma-Aldrich) at a final concentration of 20 μM was added and incubated for 24 h to induce HEI-OC1 cell damage.

Cochlear Explants and Drug Administration

The cochlear tissues of C57BL/6J mice on postnatal day 3 (P3) were quickly dissected and cleaned in cold phosphate-buffered saline (PBS) (Sangon Biotech Co., Ltd., Shanghai, China). Next, the cochlea was cultured on glass coverslips coated with Cell-Tak in four-well plates (BD Biosciences, Franklin Lakes, NJ,

United States) with DMEM/F12 growth medium (11330-032; Gibco) containing B-27 supplement (17504-44; Gibco), N-2 supplement (17502-048; Gibco), and ampicillin (50 g/mL, A5354-10ML; Sangon Biotech Co., Ltd.) at 37°C in an incubator environment of 5% CO_2 and 95% O_2. After incubation for a day, we pretreated cochlear explants with or without Sal (10 μM) and then co-treated them with 20 μM cisplatin for 24 h. Cisplatin at a concentration of 20 μM was selected based on our previous study (Li et al., 2022). After removing the cisplatin-containing medium, the cochlear explants were recovered in normal medium for 36 h.

Measurement of Cell Viability

Cell viability analyses were performed using a cell counting kit-8 assay (CCK-8; HY-K0301; MedChemExpress). We trypsinised cells with 0.25% trypsin/EDTA, centrifuged them at 1,000 rpm for 3 min, and resuspended them in medium. Thereafter, HEI-OC1 cells were seeded at a density of 4,000 cells/well in 96-well plates. After 24 h of incubation, the medium was replaced with medium containing cisplatin (20 μM) and different doses of Sal. After 24 h of incubation, CCK8 solution was added per well and incubated with the cells at 37°C for 1 h. Finally, we used a microplate reader to determine the absorbance at 450 nm. The above experiment was repeated thrice.

Immunofluorescence

Immunofluorescence experiments were performed to determine the different apoptosis and ERS markers. After different treatments, the HEI-OC1 cells or cochlear explants were washed with PBS thrice for 15 min. Afterward, we fixed HEI-OC1 cells or cochlear explants with 4% paraformaldehyde (Sangon Biotech Co., Ltd.) for 1 h at 25°C and then washed them thrice with 0.01 M PBS (Sangon Biotech Co., Ltd.). After permeabilisation with 1% Triton X-100 (Solarbio Life Sciences, Beijing, China) for 30 min, non-specific sample binding sites were blocked with 5% bovine serum albumin in PBS (Sigma-Aldrich) at 25°C for 1 h and then incubated with primary antibodies at 4°C overnight (dilution: 1:200–1:500). Subsequently, the samples were washed thrice with PBS and incubated with secondary antibodies (A32723, A32731, A32727, and A32732; Thermo Fisher Scientific) at room temperature for 1 h. Thereafter, the auditory HCs were labelled with FITC-labelled phalloidin (P5282; Sigma-Aldrich), and cell nuclei were labelled with DAPI (Sigma-Aldrich). Finally, we washed the cells thrice with PBS, mounted them with DAPI, and imaged them using an LSM 710 confocal microscope (Zeiss, Oberkochen, Germany). The fluorescence intensity of CHOP was measured using Image J software (NIH, Bethesda, MD, United States).

Western Blotting

HEI-OC1 cells were lysed and prepared in RIPA buffer (Sangon Biotech Co., Ltd.) containing protease and phosphatase inhibitor cocktail (Sangon Biotech Co., Ltd.) on ice for 30 min. Thereafter, cell lysates were centrifuged at 12,000 rpm for 20 min, and the supernatants were collected for protein quantification. Protein concentrations were quantified using a BCA protein assay kit (Sangon Biotech). Equal amounts of proteins were loaded on 10% sodium dodecyl sulphate-polyacrylamide gel for separation *via* electrophoresis and then transferred onto nitrocellulose membranes, which were then blocked with 5% skim milk powder in Tris-buffered saline containing 0.1% Tween 20 (TBST) (Sangon Biotech) for 1 h at room temperature. Subsequently, the membranes were incubated with anti-BIP (5,174; Cell Signaling Technology), anti-eIF2α (5,324; Cell Signaling Technology), anti-phospho-eIF2α-S51 (AP0692; ABclonal), anti-cleaved caspase 3 (9,661; Cell Signaling Technology), anti-CHOP (2,895; Cell Signaling Technology), anti-cleaved PARP (9,544; Cell Signaling Technology), anti-GAPDH (5,174; Cell Signaling Technology), and anti-β-tubulin (2,128; Cell Signaling Technology). The antibodies used ranged from 1:500 to 1:1,000. After incubation with the primary antibodies overnight at 4°C, the membranes were washed thrice for 30 min with 1 × TBST and then incubated with the corresponding secondary antibodies (AS014 and AS003; ABclonal) at room temperature for 2 h. The cell membranes were examined using an Omni-ECL Femto Light Chemiluminescence Kit (SQ201; Epizyme, Cambridge, MA, United States) and imaged using a ChemiDocXRS imaging system (Bio-Rad Laboratories, Hercules, CA, United States). ImageJ software was used to measure band intensities. Each experiment was repeated more than thrice.

Small Interference RNA Transfection

We designed three eIF2α-specific mouse Small Interference RNA (siRNAs) (RiboBio, Guangzhou, China) to knock down eIF2α expression in HEI-OC1 cells. A siRNA encoding a nonsense sequence was designed as the negative control. HEI-OC1 cells were transfected with eIF2α-siRNA or negative-siRNA according to the manufacturer's instructions. HEI-OC1 cells were plated in six-well culture plates at a density of 3×10^5 and transfected with siRNA using Lipofectamine 3000 (L3000001; Invitrogen, Waltham, MA, United States) for 24 h. The transfection efficiency was measured using western blotting. The following siRNAs were used to knock down eIF2α expression: 5′-TCCAAGAGCTTGAAGATTT-3′, 5′-CCTTCTCCAAGAGCTTGAA-3′, and 5′-CTCCAAGAGCT TGAAGATT-3′.

Cell Counts

For HC quantification, cells labelled with myosin7a and showing normal nuclei were considered surviving HCs. To quantify HCs, we imaged the entire cochlea using a Zeiss microscope with a 40 × lens and used ImageJ software to quantify immunopositive cells. The average number of HCs per 130 μm in the apical, middle, and basal turns of the cochlea was calculated for each group. For quantification of apoptotic HCs, we selected only the middle portion of each explant.

Statistical Analysis

Data were analysed using GraphPad Prism statistical software (version 8, GraphPad Software, Inc., San Diego, CA, United States). Normally distributed measures are expressed as mean ± Standard Error of Mean (SEM). Independent sample *t*-tests were performed for comparisons between two groups.

One-way ANOVA was used for comparisons between multiple groups. *P*-values < 0.05 were considered statistically significant.

RESULTS

Sal Reduced the Cytotoxicity of Cisplatin-Induced House Ear Institute-Organ of Corti 1 Cells

Our previous study determined that cisplatin damaged HEI-OC1 cells appropriately at a concentration of 20 μm for 24 h (Li et al., 2022). HEI-OC1 cells were treated with different Sal concentrations (0–100 μM) for 24 h to determine its toxicity. The CCK-8 results showed that Sal did not decrease the viability of HEI-OC1 cells (**Figure 1A**). Therefore, HEI-OC1 cells were treated with or without Sal to determine whether Sal could protect against cisplatin-induced damage. The CCK-8 results showed that viability increased gradually with increasing doses of Sal (0–100 μM) (**Figure 1B**). Since the viability of 50 μM Sal-treated HEI-OC1 cells did not significantly differ from that of 100 μM Sal-treated cells following cisplatin exposure, 50 μM Sal was selected as the treatment condition for 24 h in the rest of this study. Moreover, dead cells on the top of the monolayer are more numerous in the cisplatin-treated group, while 50 μM Sal significantly alleviated this damage (**Figure 1C**). These findings suggest that Sal could effectively reverse cisplatin-induced ototoxicity at an appropriate dose.

Sal Alleviated Cisplatin-Induced Apoptosis in House Ear Institute-Organ of Corti 1 Cells

To determine the protective effect of Sal in HEI-OC1 cells, we measured the percentage of apoptotic cells in the control, Sal, cisplatin, and cisplatin + Sal groups. Immunofluorescence analysis of cleaved caspase 3 showed that the number of cisplatin-induced apoptotic cells was reduced after Sal treatment (**Figures 2A,B**). Consistent with the immunofluorescence results, western blotting showed that the expression of cleaved caspase 3 and cleaved-PARP was significantly reduced after Sal treatment (**Figures 2C–E**). These findings suggested that Sal attenuated cisplatin-induced apoptosis in HEI-OC1 cells.

Sal Decreased Cisplatin-Induced Apoptosis in Cochlear Hair Cells

To determine the effect of Sal in protecting cochlear HCs after cisplatin damage, we used cochlear organ explant cultures. The cochleae of C57BL/6 mice were dissected at P3, and the surrounding tissue and bone were removed using PBS. Cochlear

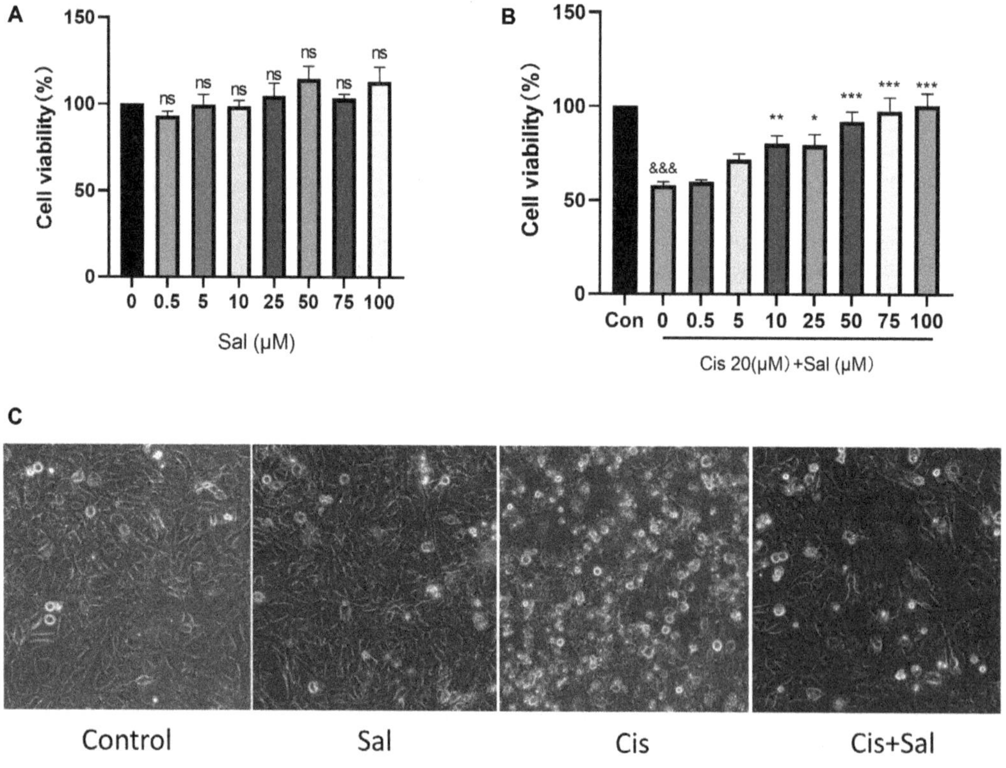

FIGURE 1 | Sal enhances the viability of HEI-OC1 cells after cisplatin damage. **(A)** HEI-OC1 cells were treated with different Sal concentrations for 24 h. **(B)** HEI-OC1 cells were pretreated with or without different Sal concentrations (0–100 μM) for 4 h, followed by 20 μM co-treatment for 24 h except for those in the control group. **(C)** Image of HEI-OC1 cells cultured with different Sal or cisplatin concentrations. Scale bars = 100 μm. Cell viability was measured using the CCK-8 assay. Values are presented as mean ± SEM from independent experiments. *$P < 0.05$, **$P < 0.01$, and ***$P < 0.001$ vs. the control group; $^{\&\&\&}P < 0.001$ vs. the cisplatin group. ns, no statistical difference; Sal, salubrinal; Cis, cisplatin; con, control.

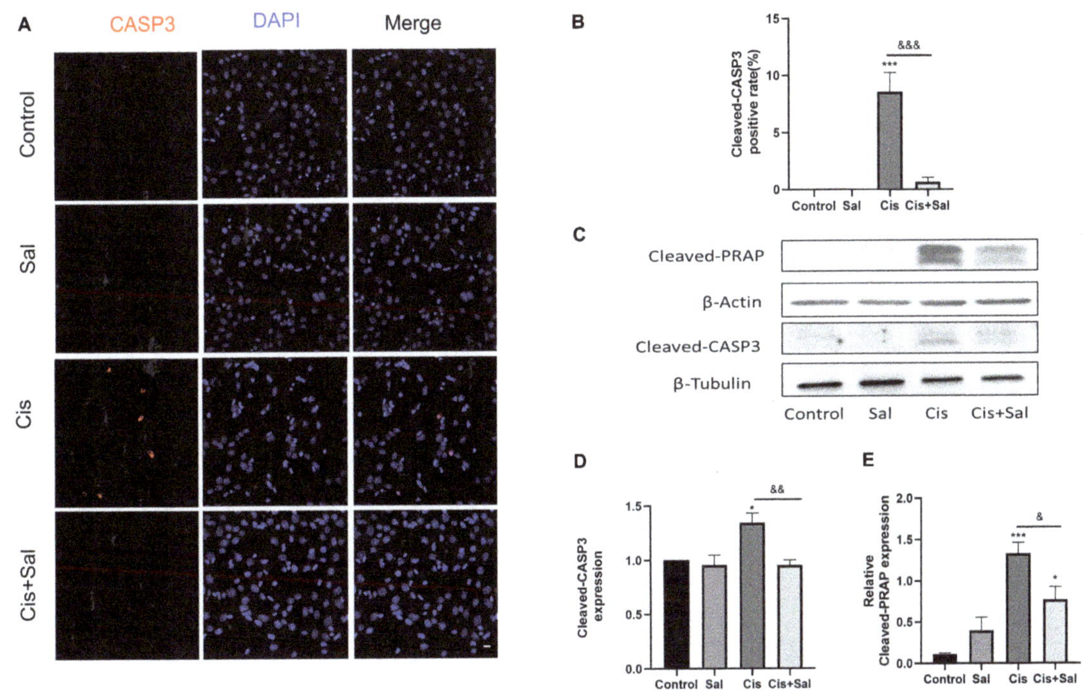

FIGURE 2 | Sal reduces cisplatin-induced apoptosis in HEI-OC1 cells. **(A)** Cleaved caspase 3 (red) and DAPI (blue) double staining showing apoptotic cells after the different treatments (n = 3). **(B)** Quantitative analysis of apoptotic cells in **(A)**. **(C)** Western blotting results showing cleaved PARP (n = 3) and cleaved caspase 3 (n = 3) in the different groups. **(D,E)** Quantitative analysis of the western blotting results in **(C)**. Values are presented as mean ± SEM from independent experiments. $^*P < 0.05$ and $^{***}P < 0.001$ vs. the control group; $^{\&}P < 0.05$, $^{\&\&}P < 0.01$, and $^{\&\&\&}P < 0.001$ vs. the cisplatin group. Sal, salubrinal; Cis, cisplatin. Scale bars = 20 μm.

explants were glued to glass cover slides coated with Cell-Tak (BD Biosciences) and divided into the following groups: control, Sal alone, cisplatin, and Sal + cisplatin (10 μM Sal pretreated for 4 h and 20 μM cisplatin co-treated for 24 h) (**Figure 3A**). To better characterise cochlear HCs, we performed immunofluorescence staining using antibodies against myosin-VIIa. Consistent with the results for HEI-OC1 cells, the number of HCs was significantly reduced in the cisplatin alone group, whereas Sal treatment significantly increased the number of HCs after cisplatin exposure (**Figures 3B–E**). Furthermore, no significant difference was found between the Sal alone and control groups, suggesting that Sal at 10 μM did not affect the survival of HCs. To further validate these results, immunofluorescence staining of cleaved caspase 3 was performed to analyse apoptotic HCs in different groups. Consistent with the number of HCs, the number of cleaved caspase 3-positive HCs was significantly increased in the cisplatin group, when10 μM Sal significantly reduced the cleaved caspase 3-positive HCs in the Sal + cisplatin group (**Figure 4**).

Sal Attenuated Cisplatin-Induced Endoplasmic Reticulum Stress in Hair Cells and House Ear Institute-Organ of Corti 1 Cells

To determine whether Sal protects against cisplatin-induced damage by inhibiting ERS, the expression of CHOP and GRP78/BIP ERS markers was measured in HEI-OC1 cells in the different groups (**Figure 5**). Immunofluorescence staining showed that cisplatin treatment induced nuclear CHOP accumulation compared with the untreated controls (**Figures 5A,B**), whereas Sal and cisplatin co-treatment reduced CHOP expression and increased BIP expression. To further verify that Sal alleviated HC damage, we used immunofluorescence staining of CHOP in the cochlear explants. Similar to the results in HEI-OC1 cells, cisplatin treatment significantly increased CHOP expression, whereas Sal and cisplatin co-treatment significantly decreased CHOP expression (**Figures 5C,D**). Consistent with the immunofluorescence staining results, western blotting results showed that CHOP expression increased in the cisplatin group but decreased in the Sal group (**Figures 5E–H**). These data suggest that cisplatin caused significant ERS in cochlear HCs, and Sal could effectively reverse this damage.

Sal Protected House Ear Institute-Organ of Corti 1 Cells Against Cisplatin-Induced Apoptosis by Eukaryotic Translation Initiation Factor 2α Regulation

Sal selectively attenuates the dephosphorylation of phosphorylated eIF2α and protects cells from ERS-induced apoptosis (Zhang et al., 2015). p-eIF2α expression increased with increasing Sal concentration (**Figures 6A,B**). To investigate

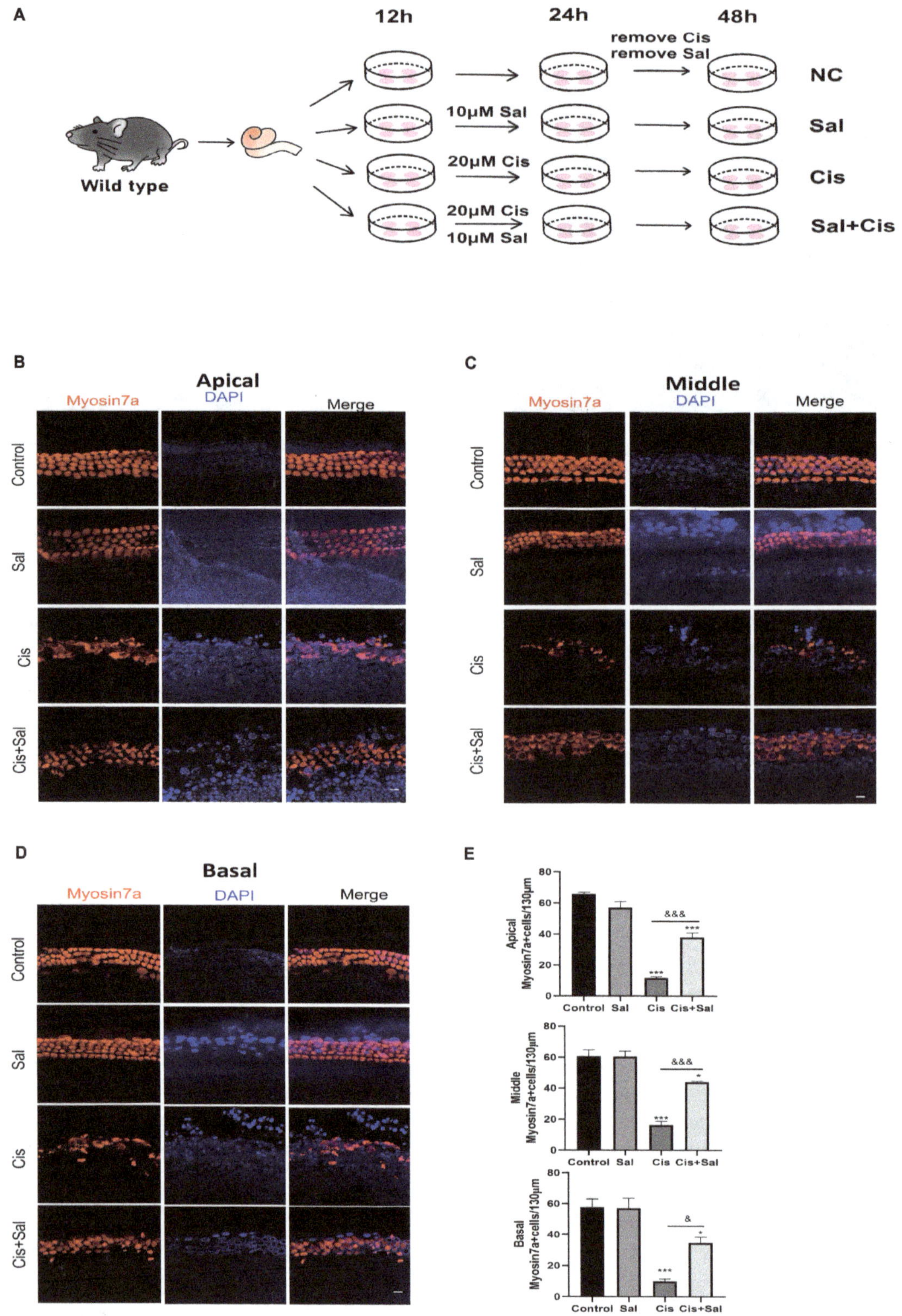

FIGURE 3 | Sal promotes hair cell (HC) survival in the cochlea after cisplatin exposure. **(A)** Schematic diagram of drug addiction in tissue culture. **(B,D)** HCs in the apical **(B)**, middle **(C)**, and basal turns **(D)** of the cochlea were stained with anti-myosin-VIIa antibody and DAPI in the control, 10 μM Sal, 20 μM cisplatin, and 20 μM cisplatin + 10 μM Sal groups. **(E)** Quantification of the number of myosin VIIa-positive cells in the apical, middle, and basal turns of the cochlea. Values are presented as mean ± SEM from independent experiments. **P* < 0.05 and ****P* < 0.001 vs. the control group; &*P* < 0.05 and &&&*P* < 0.001 vs. the cisplatin group. Scale bars = 10 μm.

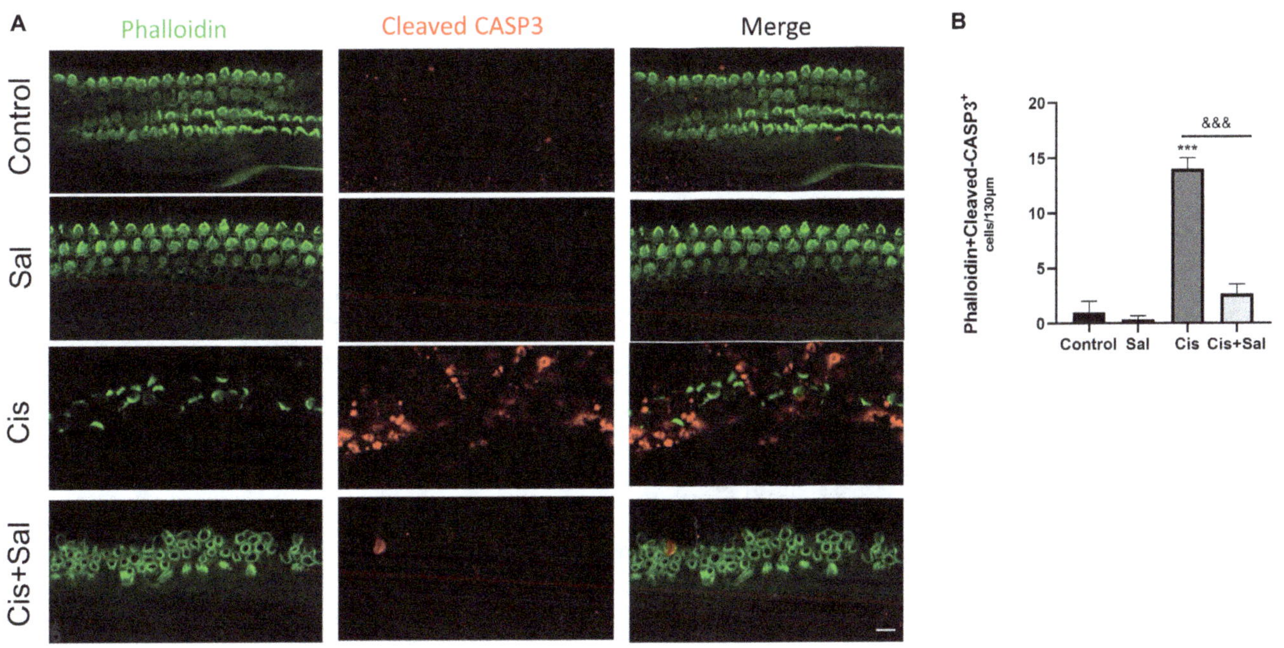

FIGURE 4 | Cisplatin-induced hair cell apoptosis decreases after treatment with Sal. **(A)** Number of cleaved caspase-3-positive cells (red) decreased in the 20 μM cisplatin + 10 μM Sal group compared with that in the cisplatin group (middle turns). **(B)** Quantification of the number of phalloidin + cleaved caspase-3 double-positive cells in **(A)**. Values are presented as mean ± SEM from independent experiments. ***$P < 0.001$ vs. the control group; &&&$P < 0.001$ vs. the cisplatin group. Scale bars = 10 μm.

the role of p-eIF2α in cisplatin-induced cytotoxicity, we further analysed p-eIF2α expression after Sal treatment. Western blotting results showed that p-eIF2α expression significantly decreased in the cisplatin group but increased after Sal treatment (**Figures 6C,D**). Furthermore, Sal treatment did not affect the total amount of eIF2α expression (**Figures 6E,F**). These findings suggest that Sal protected HCs from cisplatin-induced apoptosis by activating the eIF2α pathway.

Silencing Eukaryotic Translation Initiation Factor 2α Enhanced Cisplatin-Induced Hair Cell Death

We transfected HEI-OC1 cells with eIF2α-specific or control siRNA to determine whether eIF2α plays a direct role in the Sal-mediated protective effects against cisplatin-induced cell death. The best knockdown effect was observed in HEI-OC1 cells with a Si-eIF2α mixture (**Figure 7A**). After 36-h transfection, cell viability was analysed using the CCK-8 assay, and results showed that Sal significantly enhanced HEI-OC1 cell viability in the presence of cisplatin. However, cell viability was significantly reduced after eIF2α-specific siRNA treatment compared with that in the control siRNA-treated cells (**Figure 7B**). Furthermore, consistent with the CCK-8 results, western blotting results showed that the expression of cleaved caspase-3 was significantly increased in cells treated with eIF2α-specific siRNA (**Figures 7C,D**). These results suggest that eIF2α was responsible for the protective effects of Sal against cisplatin-induced apoptosis in HCs.

The results for both HEI-OC1 cells and cochlear explants showed that the PERK/ATF4/CHOP signalling branch plays an important role in cisplatin-induced ototoxicity (**Figure 8**).

DISCUSSION

Sal attenuated cisplatin-induced HC damage by inhibiting apoptosis. Furthermore, the effect of Sal was attributed to ERS inhibition, which was dependent on p-eIF2α activity. Knockdown of eIF2α reversed the protective effect of Sal against cisplatin-induced injury in HEI-OC1 cells, leading to cisplatin-induced apoptosis. These results demonstrate that cisplatin-induced HC apoptosis was associated with eIF2α signalling, one of the three major pathways of the unfolded protein response (UPR), while Sal could protect against cisplatin-induced ototoxicity in cochlear HC ERS.

Ototoxic chemicals including cisplatin, acetaminophen, and aminoglycoside disrupt the correct folding of protein or induce mistranslation, leading to the aggregation of unfolding or misfolding proteins in the ER of cochleae (Kalinec et al., 2014; Oishi et al., 2015; Qu et al., 2022). Once the excessive accumulation of unfolding or misfolding proteins occurs in the ER, severe ERS results in an inability to maintain ER homeostasis, leading to cell apoptosis and death (Hetz and Papa, 2018). ERS, evoked by misfolding and unfolding proteins in the ER, can activate the UPR to reduce ER workload by increasing the protein folding capacity, removing misfolded/unfolded proteins from the ER, and inhibiting translation to block new protein

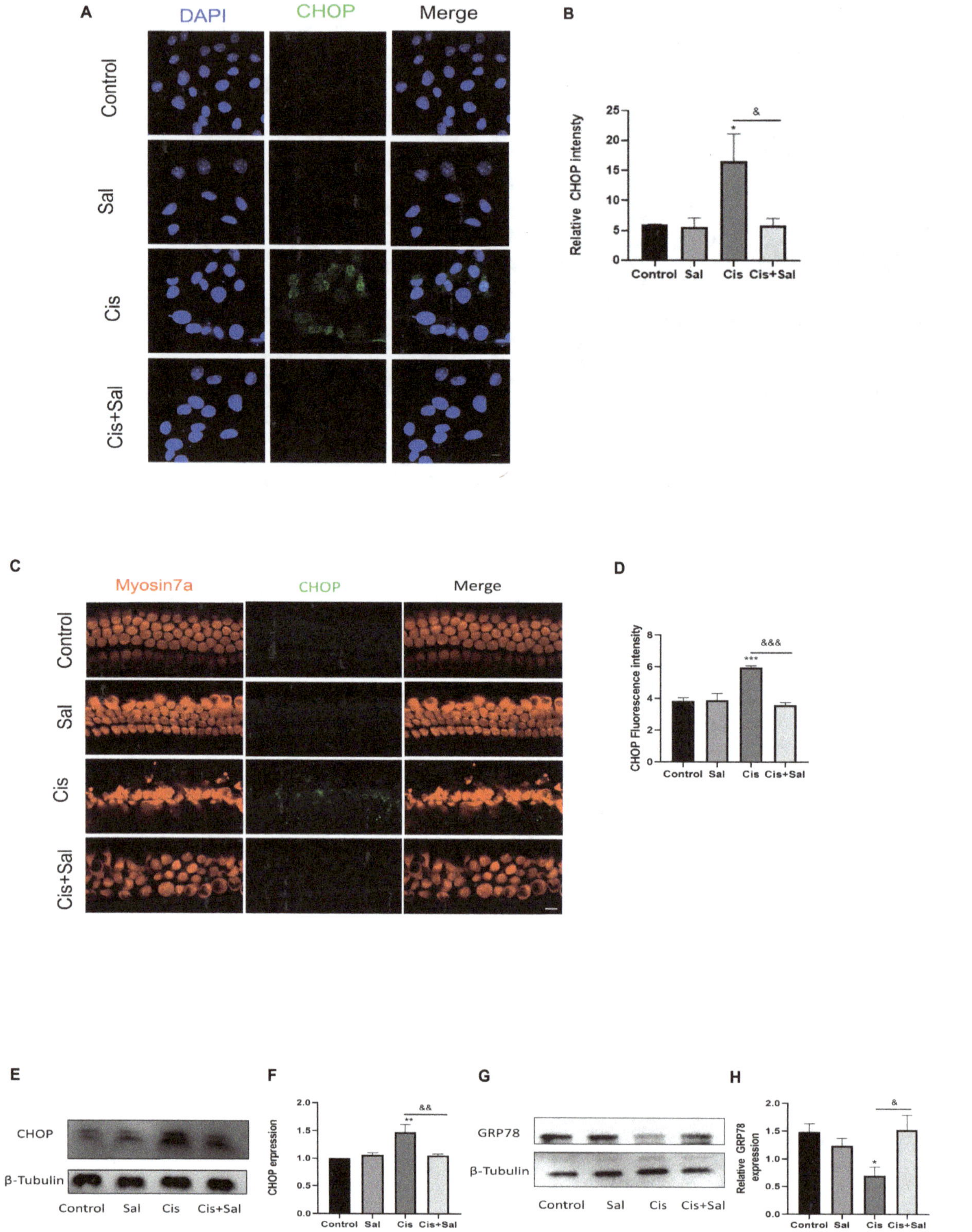

FIGURE 5 | Sal attenuates cisplatin-induced endoplasmic reticulum stress in HEI-OC1 cells. **(A)** HEI-OC1 cells in the different groups were labelled with CHOP ($n = 3$). **(B)** Quantitative analysis of the data shown in **(A)**. **(C)** Cochlear basilar membranes in the different groups were labelled with CHOP ($n = 3$). **(D)** Quantitative analysis of the fluorescence intensity shown in **(C)**. **(E)** Western blotting results showing CHOP expression in HEI-OC1 cells after different treatments ($n = 3$). **(F)** Quantitative analysis of the data shown in **(E)**. **(G)** Western blotting results showing BIP expression in HEI-OC1 cells after different treatments ($n = 3$). **(H)** Quantitative analysis of the data shown in **(G)**. Values are presented as mean ± SEM from independent experiments. $^{*}P < 0.05$, $^{**}P < 0.01$, and $^{***}P < 0.001$ vs. the control group; $^{\&}P < 0.05$, $^{\&\&}P < 0.01$, and $^{\&\&\&}P < 0.001$ vs. the cisplatin group. Scale bars = 10 μm.

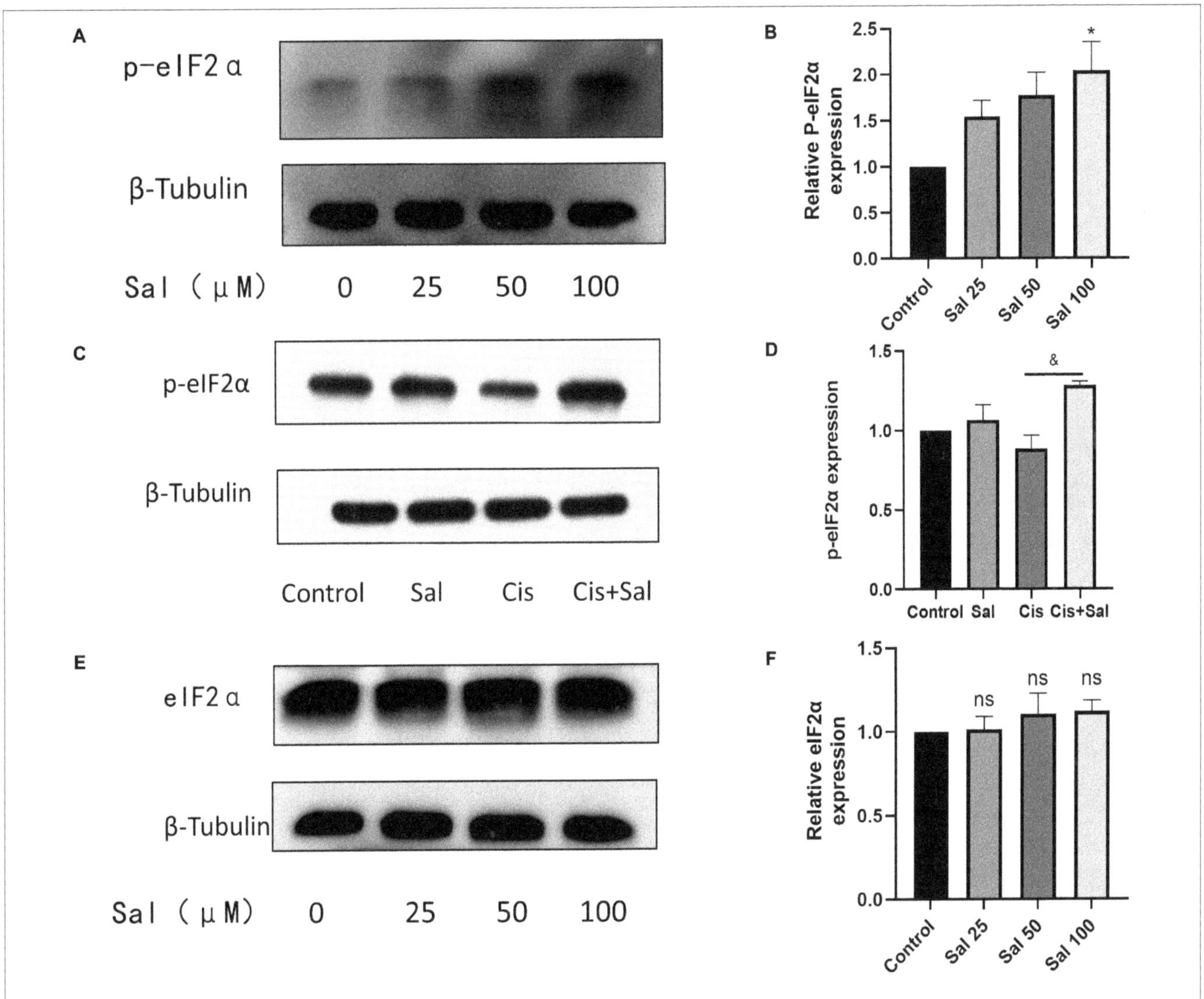

FIGURE 6 | Sal inhibits cisplatin-induced hair cell endoplasmic reticulum stress by inhibiting the dephosphorylation of p-eIF2α. **(A)** As the concentration of Sal increases, p-eIF2α expression increases. **(B)** Quantitative analysis of the data shown in **(A)**. **(C)** Sal increases p-eIF2α expression in hair cell injury after cisplatin exposure. **(D)** Quantitative analysis of the data shown in **(C)**. **(E)** Western blotting results showing the expression of eIF2α after Sal treatment. **(F)** Quantitative analysis of the data shown in **(E)**. Values are presented as mean ± SEM from independent experiments. $^{*}P < 0.05$ vs. the control group; $^{\&}P < 0.05$ vs. the cisplatin group; ns, no statistical difference.

synthesis (Wang et al., 2020). A previous study showed that by inhibiting the accumulation of misfolded/unfolded proteins, upstream of ERS, could effectively attenuate cisplatin-induced damage in auditory HCs (Wen et al., 2021). However, the role of UPR downstream signalling has not been elucidated in HCs. Therefore, whether activating UPR could prevent cisplatin-induced ototoxicity should be further investigated.

UPR mainly consists of three distinct signalling pathways, namely protein kinase R-like endoplasmic reticulum kinase (PERK), activating transcription factor 6 (ATF6), and inositol-requiring kinase 1 (IRE1) (Nakka et al., 2016; Ren et al., 2021). Dysfunction and sustained changes in endoplasmic reticulum function lead to the release of GRP78 PERK, ATF6, and IRE1, which in turn activate associated downstream signalling molecules such as the ERS marker CHOP, ultimately leading to cell death through processes such as apoptosis (Hetz, 2012; Hu et al., 2018). In the current study, we focused on PERK-eIF2α signalling and further investigated the role of eIF2α in cisplatin-induced ototoxicity. The PERK-eIF2α signalling pathway is one of the most critical pathways for the survival of cells exposed to various stressors such as toxic environments, malnutrition, and oxidative stress (Rozpedek et al., 2016). Under ERS, GRP78 is dissociated, and then PERK is activated, which further promotes eIF2α phosphorylation. Phosphorylated eIF2α inhibits general translation, thereby reducing the protein burden of the endoplasmic reticulum and protecting cells from ERS (Godin et al., 2016). Sal has been identified as an inhibitor of eIF2α dephosphorylation (Boyce et al., 2005). Similar to these studies, our results showed that increasing concentrations of Sal increased p-eIF2α expression in HEI-OC1 cells, suggesting

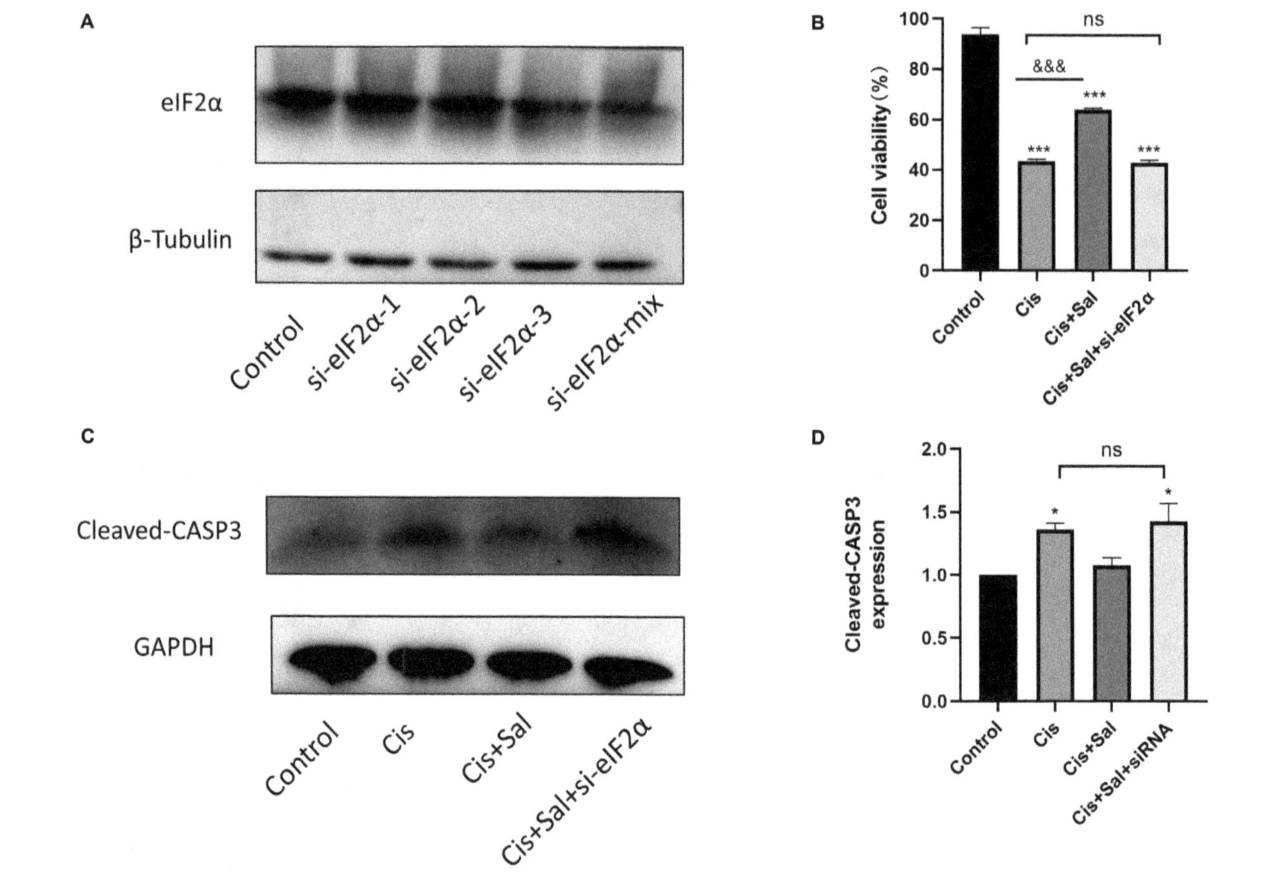

FIGURE 7 | The protective effect of Sal was attributed to eIF2α in HEI-OC1 cells. **(A)** Western blotting results showing the expression of eIF2α transfected with eIF2α-siRNA. **(B)** Effect after eIF2α silencing on cisplatin-induced injury with or without Sal viability in HEI-OC1 cells. **(C,D)** Effects of knocking down eIF2α on cisplatin-induced apoptosis. Western blotting results showing the expression of cleaved caspase in the presence of cisplatin or Sal treatment after eIF2α silencing (n = 3). Values are presented as mean ± SEM from three independent experiments. $^{*}P < 0.05$ and $^{***}P < 0.001$ vs. the control group; $^{\&\&\&}P < 0.001$ vs. the cisplatin group. ns, no statistical difference; Sal, salubrinal; Cis, cisplatin.

that Sal inhibited eIF2α dephosphorylation in a dose-dependent manner in auditory HCs. Furthermore, p-eIF2α decreased after cisplatin treatment, but this reduction was inhibited by Sal treatment, suggesting that p-eIF2α is crucial in cisplatin-induced ERS and apoptosis. However, the role of eIF2α is controversial. Although numerous studies support the notion that phosphorylated eIF2α is beneficial in ERS-induced cell death, eIF2α dephosphorylation has also been shown to contribute to cell survival (Novoa et al., 2003; Duan et al., 2014). Our data demonstrated that cisplatin-induced apoptotic cell death was attenuated if eIF2α could be selectively activated, whereas eIF2α knockdown enhanced cisplatin-induced apoptosis. These results further verified our view that the PERK-eIF2α pathway has a protective role in cisplatin-induced ERS in cochlear cells.

ATF4, which is downstream of eIF2α, has dual effects in ERS, including promoting the transcription of ER chaperones such as GRP78 to help ER recovery and increasing CHOP expression to induce apoptosis. CHOP, also known as growth arrest and DNA damage-inducible gene 153, is commonly expressed at very low levels in normal cells (Oyadomari and Mori, 2004). In response to various ERS stimuli, CHOP expression is upregulated and helps regulate cellular redox and cell death. Thus, CHOP upregulation is also a good biomarker of ERS and is a major downstream effector of the PERK pathway, which functions as a pro-apoptotic factor (Hu et al., 2018; Zhao et al., 2021). BIP plays a crucial role in regulating the dynamic homeostasis of the ER and is a sensor of ERS (Elfiky et al., 2020). BIP dissociates from PERK, IRE1, and ATF6 in response to ERS and triggers UPR, which possesses anti-apoptotic and cytoprotective effects (Hetz, 2012). In the current study, BIP expression decreased in the cisplatin-treated group but increased after Sal treatment. Contrastingly, CHOP was upregulated after cisplatin exposure when Sal strongly decreased the expression. Notably, upregulation of BIP/GRP78 is protective against ischemic injury and also against cisplatin-induced damage in HEI-OC1 cells (Ouyang et al., 2011; López-Hernández et al., 2015; Yi et al., 2020). Our results supported this point and further showed that pharmacological activation of eIF2α-BIP could alleviate cisplatin-induced ERS and apoptosis. Moreover, Sal significantly reduced CHOP expression in cisplatin-induced injury in HEI-OC1 cells and cochleae, suggesting that Sal could also regulate the eIF2α-CHOP pathway to inhibit cisplatin-induced ERS in HCs.

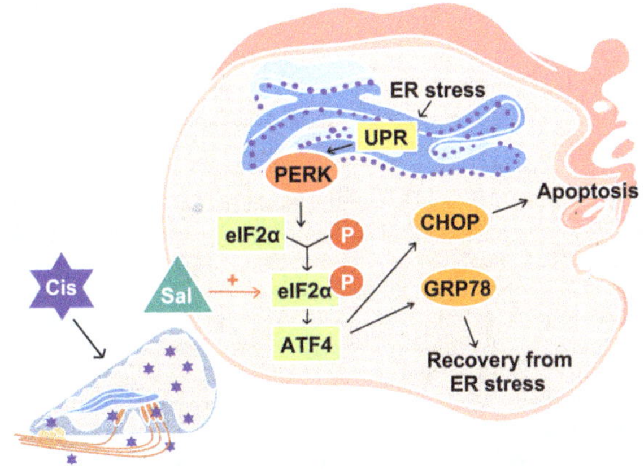

FIGURE 8 | Schematic diagram showing the specific regulatory role of endoplasmic reticulum stress in cisplatin-induced ototoxicity and the main signalling branch exerting a pro-apoptotic effect. PERK and its related PERK/eIF2α/CHOP signalling branch are speculated to play a major role in cisplatin-induced ototoxicity. Sal increases the anti-apoptotic effect of GRP78 by inhibiting the dephosphorylation of eIF2α.

Apoptosis is a positively regulated form of cell death that is mainly involved in cisplatin-induced ototoxicity (Ruhl et al., 2019; Tang et al., 2021). Accumulating evidence indicates that inhibiting apoptosis could effectively protect against cisplatin-induced damage (Wang et al., 2004; Ruhl et al., 2019; Wu et al., 2020). Sal treatment has been proposed to prevent apoptosis in various disease models (López-Hernández et al., 2015; Li et al., 2019, 2020). Consistent with these studies, Sal significantly alleviated cisplatin-induced apoptosis in HEI-OC1 cells and HCs, as evidenced by PARP and caspase-3 levels. In addition, ERS has also been proposed as a potential mechanism for cisplatin-induced ototoxicity. An increasing number of studies have found that ERS plays an important role in drug-induced hearing loss (Gentilin et al., 2019). A previous study found that ERS is involved in spiral ganglion neuron apoptosis after chronic kanamycin-induced deafness (Tu et al., 2019). Moreover, taurine deoxycholic acid attenuates gentamicin-induced cochlear HC death *in vitro* by inhibiting ERS (Hu et al., 2018). In kidney and cancer cell tissues, ERS-induced apoptosis is one of the mechanisms of cisplatin-induced cytotoxicity (Huang et al., 2020; Tham et al., 2020). Our findings are consistent with previous studies showing that Sal effectively inhibits ERS levels, thereby preventing cisplatin-induced apoptosis in HEI-OC1 cells and cochlear HCs. Our results suggest that ERS was hyperactivated in HEI-OC1 cells and HCs after cisplatin exposure, which led to HC apoptosis, and inhibition of ERS could be a promising approach to reduce cisplatin-induced apoptosis. Taken together, our findings suggest that Sal reduces cisplatin-induced apoptosis in HEI-OC1 cells and HCs by attenuating ERS.

This study has several limitations. First, although Sal demonstrates effects associated with preventing cisplatin-induced ototoxicity, it has not been approved by the FDA for clinical application. Second, we demonstrated a protective effect of Sal in cochlear explants and HEI-OC1 cells *in vitro*, but its role *in vivo* was not further explored. Therefore, the role of Sal in protecting against cochlear cisplatin damage and the mechanism involved need to be further investigated and validated in animal models.

CONCLUSION

In conclusion, our findings provide *in vitro* evidence that Sal significantly attenuates ERS in HEI-OC1 and cochlear HCs, subsequently suppressing cisplatin-induced apoptosis. In addition, eIF2α may be an important target for preventing and treating cisplatin ototoxicity. Furthermore, eIF2α plays a crucial role in ERS in HCs, and pharmacological enhancement of eIF2α phosphorylation is a potential therapeutic strategy for cisplatin-induced hearing loss.

AUTHOR CONTRIBUTIONS

WL, KN, and ZL performed all the experiments, analysed the data, and wrote the manuscript. JZ and HS conceived and designed all the experiments. WL and ZL acquired and analysed some of the data. LX, YL, and YJ helped with the experimental design and data interpretation. All authors contributed to the article and approved the submitted version.

ACKNOWLEDGMENTS

We thank Zhen Zhang, Qiang Ma, Qingxiu Yao, Jia Fang, and Chengqi Liu for their help during the experiment.

REFERENCES

Bégin, A. M., Monfette, M. L., Boudrias-Dalle, É, Lavallée, E., Samouelian, V., Soulières, D., et al. (2021). Effect of mannitol on acute kidney injury induced by cisplatin. *Support Care Cancer* 29, 2083–2091. doi: 10.1007/s00520-020-05703-7

Binet, F., and Sapieha, P. (2015). ER stress and angiogenesis. *Cell Metab.* 22, 560–575. doi: 10.1016/j.cmet.2015.07.010

Boyce, M., Bryant, K. F., Jousse, C., Long, K., Harding, H. P., Scheuner, D., et al. (2005). A selective inhibitor of eIF2alpha dephosphorylation protects cells from ER stress. *Science* 307, 935–939. doi: 10.1126/science.1101902

Brock, P. R., Maibach, R., Childs, M., Rajput, K., Roebuck, D., Sullivan, M. J., et al. (2018). Sodium thiosulfate for protection from cisplatin-induced hearing loss. *N. Engl. J. Med.* 378, 2376–2385. doi: 10.1056/NEJMoa1801109

Chadha, S., Kamenov, K., and Cieza, A. (2021). The world report on hearing. *Bull. World Health Organ.* 99, 242A–242A.

Cunningham, L. L., and Tucci, D. L. (2017). Hearing loss in adults. *N. Engl. J. Med.* 377, 2465–2473. doi: 10.1056/NEJMra1616601

Delaunay-Moisan, A., and Appenzeller-Herzog, C. (2015). The antioxidant machinery of the endoplasmic reticulum: protection and signaling. *Free Radic. Biol. Med.* 83, 341–351. doi: 10.1016/j.freeradbiomed.2015.02.019

Duan, Z., Cai, G., Li, J., and Chen, X. (2020). Cisplatin-induced renal toxicity in elderly people. *Ther. Adv. Med. Oncol.* 12:1758835920923430. doi: 10.1177/1758835920923430

Duan, Z., Zhao, J., Fan, X., Tang, C., Liang, L., Nie, X., et al. (2014). The PERK-eIF2α signaling pathway is involved in TCDD-induced ER stress in PC12 cells. *Neurotoxicology* 44, 149–159. doi: 10.1016/j.neuro.2014.06.005

Elfiky, A. A., Baghdady, A. M., Ali, S. A., and Ahmed, M. I. (2020). GRP78 targeting: hitting two birds with a stone. *Life Sci.* 260:118317. doi: 10.1016/j.lfs.2020.118317

Font-Belmonte, E., Ugidos, I. F., Santos-Galdiano, M., González-Rodríguez, P., Anuncibay-Soto, B., Pérez-Rodríguez, D., et al. (2019). Post-ischemic salubrinal administration reduces necroptosis in a rat model of global cerebral ischemia. *J. Neurochem.* 151, 777–794. doi: 10.1111/jnc.14789

Frisina, R. D., Wheeler, H. E., Fossa, S. D., Kerns, S. L., Fung, C., Sesso, H. D., et al. (2016). Comprehensive audiometric analysis of hearing impairment and tinnitus after cisplatin-based chemotherapy in survivors of adult-onset cancer. *J. Clin. Oncol.* 34, 2712–2720. doi: 10.1200/JCO.2016.66.8822

Gentilin, E., Simoni, E., Candito, M., Cazzador, D., and Astolfi, L. (2019). Cisplatin-induced ototoxicity: updates on molecular targets. *Trends Mol. Med.* 25, 1123–1132. doi: 10.1016/j.molmed.2019.08.002

Godin, J. D., Creppe, C., Laguesse, S., and Nguyen, L. (2016). Emerging roles for the unfolded protein response in the developing nervous system. *Trends Neurosci.* 39, 394–404. doi: 10.1016/j.tins.2016.04.002

Hetz, C. (2012). The unfolded protein response: controlling cell fate decisions under ER stress and beyond. *Nat. Rev. Mol. Cell Biol.* 13, 89–102. doi: 10.1038/nrm3270

Hetz, C., and Papa, F. R. (2018). The unfolded protein response and cell fate control. *Mol. Cell* 69, 169–181. doi: 10.1016/j.molcel.2017.06.017

Hetz, C., Zhang, K., and Kaufman, R. J. (2020). Mechanisms, regulation and functions of the unfolded protein response. *Nat. Rev. Mol. Cell Biol.* 21, 421–438. doi: 10.1038/s41580-020-0250-z

Hu, H., Tian, M., Ding, C., and Yu, S. (2018). The C/EBP Homologous Protein (CHOP) transcription factor functions in endoplasmic reticulum stress-induced apoptosis and microbial infection. *Front. Immunol.* 9:3083. doi: 10.3389/fimmu.2018.03083

Huang, Z., Guo, F., Xia, Z., Liang, Y., Lei, S., Tan, Z., et al. (2020). Activation of GPR120 by TUG891 ameliorated cisplatin-induced acute kidney injury via repressing ER stress and apoptosis. *Biomed. Pharmacother.* 126:110056. doi: 10.1016/j.biopha.2020.110056

Jia, Z., He, Q., Shan, C., and Li, F. (2018). Tauroursodeoxycholic acid attenuates gentamicin-induced cochlear hair cell death in vitro. *Toxicol. Lett.* 294, 20–26. doi: 10.1016/j.toxlet.2018.05.007

Kalinec, G. M., Park, C., Thein, P., and Kalinec, F. (2016). Working with Auditory HEI-OC1 cells. *J. Vis. Exp.* 115:54425. doi: 10.3791/54425

Kalinec, G. M., Thein, P., Parsa, A., Yorgason, J., Luxford, W., Urrutia, R., et al. (2014). Acetaminophen and NAPQI are toxic to auditory cells via oxidative and endoplasmic reticulum stress-dependent pathways. *Hear Res.* 313, 26–37. doi: 10.1016/j.heares.2014.04.007

Knight, K. R., Kraemer, D. F., and Neuwelt, E. A. (2005). Ototoxicity in children receiving platinum chemotherapy: underestimating a commonly occurring toxicity that may influence academic and social development. *J. Clin. Oncol.* 23, 8588–8596. doi: 10.1200/JCO.2004.00.5355

Kros, C., and Steyger, P. S. (2019). Aminoglycoside- and cisplatin-induced ototoxicity: mechanisms and otoprotective strategies. *Cold Spring Harb. Perspect. Med.* 9:a033548. doi: 10.1101/cshperspect.a033548

Li, J., Li, X., Liu, D., Hamamura, K., Wan, Q., Na, S., et al. (2019). eIF2α signaling regulates autophagy of osteoblasts and the development of osteoclasts in OVX mice. *Cell Death Dis.* 10:921. doi: 10.1038/s41419-019-2159-z

Li, J., Zhuo, J. Y., Zhou, W., Hong, J. W., Chen, R. G., Xie, H. Y., et al. (2020). Endoplasmic reticulum stress triggers delanzomib-induced apoptosis in HCC cells through the PERK/eIF2α/ATF4/CHOP pathway. *Am. J. Transl. Res.* 12, 2875–2889.

Li, Z., Yao, Q., Tian, Y., Jiang, Y., Xu, M., Wang, H., et al. (2022). Trehalose protects against cisplatin-induced cochlear hair cell damage by activating TFEB-mediated autophagy. *Biochem. Pharmacol.* 197:114904. doi: 10.1016/j.bcp.2021.114904

López-Hernández, B., Ceña, V., and Posadas, I. (2015). The endoplasmic reticulum stress and the HIF-1 signalling pathways are involved in the neuronal damage caused by chemical hypoxia. *Br. J. Pharmacol.* 172, 2838–2851. doi: 10.1111/bph.13095

Luongo, T. S., Lambert, J. P., Gross, P., Nwokedi, M., Lombardi, A. A., Shanmughapriya, S., et al. (2017). The mitochondrial Na(+)/Ca(2+) exchanger is essential for Ca(2+) homeostasis and viability. *Nature* 545, 93–97. doi: 10.1038/nature22082

Matsuoka, M., and Komoike, Y. (2015). Experimental evidence shows salubrinal, an eIF2α dephosphorylation inhibitor, reduces xenotoxicant-induced cellular damage. *Int. J. Mol. Sci.* 16, 16275–16287. doi: 10.3390/ijms160716275

Nakka, V. P., Prakash-Babu, P., and Vemuganti, R. (2016). Crosstalk between endoplasmic reticulum stress, oxidative stress, and autophagy: potential therapeutic targets for acute CNS injuries. *Mol. Neurobiol.* 53, 532–544. doi: 10.1007/s12035-014-9029-6

Novoa, I., Zhang, Y., Zeng, H., Jungreis, R., Harding, H. P., and Ron, D. (2003). Stress-induced gene expression requires programmed recovery from translational repression. *Embo J.* 22, 1180–1187. doi: 10.1093/emboj/cdg112

Oishi, N., Duscha, S., Boukari, H., Meyer, M., Xie, J., Wei, G., et al. (2015). XBP1 mitigates aminoglycoside-induced endoplasmic reticulum stress and neuronal cell death. *Cell Death Dis.* 6:e1763. doi: 10.1038/cddis.2015.108

Ouyang, Y. B., Xu, L. J., Emery, J. F., Lee, A. S., and Giffard, R. G. (2011). Overexpressing GRP78 influences Ca2+ handling and function of mitochondria in astrocytes after ischemia-like stress. *Mitochondrion* 11, 279–286. doi: 10.1016/j.mito.2010.10.007

Oyadomari, S., and Mori, M. (2004). Roles of CHOP/GADD153 in endoplasmic reticulum stress. *Cell Death Differ.* 11, 381–389. doi: 10.1038/sj.cdd.4401373

Qu, Y., Zong, S., Wang, Z., Du, P., Wen, Y., Li, H., et al. (2022). The PERK/ATF4/CHOP signaling branch of the unfolded protein response mediates cisplatin-induced ototoxicity in hair cells. *Drug Chem. Toxicol.* [Online ahead of print] doi: 10.1080/01480545.2022.2039181

Ren, J., Bi, Y., Sowers, J. R., Hetz, C., and Zhang, Y. (2021). Endoplasmic reticulum stress and unfolded protein response in cardiovascular diseases. *Nat. Rev. Cardiol.* 18, 499–521. doi: 10.1038/s41569-021-00511-w

Rozpedek, W., Pytel, D., Mucha, B., Leszczynska, H., Diehl, J. A., and Majsterek, I. J. C. M. M. (2016). The Role of the PERK/eIF2α/ATF4/CHOP signaling pathway in tumor progression during endoplasmic reticulum stress. *Curr. Mol. Med.* 16, 533–544.

Ruhl, D., Du, T. T., Wagner, E. L., Choi, J. H., Li, S., Reed, R., et al. (2019). Necroptosis and apoptosis contribute to cisplatin and aminoglycoside ototoxicity. *J. Neurosci.* 39, 2951–2964. doi: 10.1523/jneurosci.1384-18.2019

Tang, Q., Wang, X., Jin, H., Mi, Y., Liu, L., Dong, M., et al. (2021). Cisplatin-induced ototoxicity: updates on molecular mechanisms and otoprotective strategies. *Eur. J. Pharm. Biopharm.* 163, 60–71. doi: 10.1016/j.ejpb.2021.03.008

Tham, M. J. R., Babak, M. V., and Ang, W. H. (2020). PlatinER: a highly potent anticancer platinum(ii) complex that induces endoplasmic reticulum stress driven immunogenic cell death. *Angew. Chem. Int. Ed. Engl.* 59, 19070–19078. doi: 10.1002/anie.202008604

Tu, Y., Fan, G., Sun, H., Cai, X., and Kong, W. (2019). Endoplasmic reticulum stress is involved in spiral ganglion neuron apoptosis following chronic kanamycin-induced deafness. *Biosci. Rep.* 39:BSR20181749. doi: 10.1042/bsr20181749

Wang, J., Ladrech, S., Pujol, R., Brabet, P., Van De Water, T. R., and Puel, J. L. (2004). Caspase inhibitors, but not c-Jun NH2-terminal kinase inhibitor treatment, prevent cisplatin-induced hearing loss. *Cancer Res.* 64, 9217–9224. doi: 10.1158/0008-5472.Can-04-1581

Wang, Y. C., Li, X., Shen, Y., Lyu, J., Sheng, H., Paschen, W., et al. (2020). PERK (Protein Kinase RNA-Like ER Kinase) branch of the unfolded protein response confers neuroprotection in ischemic stroke by suppressing protein synthesis. *Stroke* 51, 1570–1577. doi: 10.1161/strokeaha.120.029071

Wen, Y., Zong, S., Liu, T., Du, P., Li, H., and Xiao, H. (2021). Tauroursodeoxycholic acid attenuates cisplatin-induced ototoxicity by inhibiting the accumulation and aggregation of unfolded or misfolded proteins in the endoplasmic reticulum. *Toxicology* 453:152736. doi: 10.1016/j.tox.2021.152736

Wilson, B. S., Tucci, D. L., Merson, M. H., and O'Donoghue, G. M. (2017). Global hearing health care: new findings and perspectives. *Lancet* 390, 2503–2515. doi: 10.1016/S0140-6736(17)31073-5

Wu, J., Ye, J., Kong, W., Zhang, S., and Zheng, Y. (2020). Programmed cell death pathways in hearing loss: a review of apoptosis, autophagy and programmed necrosis. *Cell Prolif.* 53:e12915. doi: 10.1111/cpr.12915

Yi, J., Kim, T. S., Pak, J. H., and Chung, J. W. (2020). Protective effects of glucose-related protein 78 and 94 on cisplatin-mediated ototoxicity. *Antioxidants* 9:686. doi: 10.3390/antiox9080686

Zhang, J., Wang, Y., Ju, M., Song, J., Zheng, Y., Lin, S., et al. (2020). Neuroprotective effect of the inhibitor salubrinal after cardiac arrest in a rodent model. *Oxid. Med. Cell Longev.* 2020:7468738. doi: 10.1155/2020/7468738

Zhang, J., Xie, X., Pan, H., Wu, Z., Lu, W., and Yang, G. (2015). Role of endoplasmic reticulum stress in brain damage after cardiopulmonary resuscitation in rats. *Shock* 44, 65–71. doi: 10.1097/SHK.0000000000000367

Zhao, C., Yu, D., He, Z., Bao, L., Feng, L., Chen, L., et al. (2021). Endoplasmic reticulum stress-mediated autophagy activation is involved in cadmium-induced ferroptosis of renal tubular epithelial cells. *Free Radic. Biol. Med.* 175, 236–248. doi: 10.1016/j.freeradbiomed.2021.09.008

19

Detection of BDNF-Related Proteins in Human Perilymph in Patients with Hearing Loss

Ines de Vries[1†], *Heike Schmitt*[1,2†], *Thomas Lenarz*[1,2], *Nils Prenzler*[1], *Sameer Alvi*[3], *Hinrich Staecker*[3], *Martin Durisin*[1†] and *Athanasia Warnecke*[1,2*†]

[1] Department of Otolaryngology, Hannover Medical School, Hanover, Germany, [2] Cluster of Excellence Hearing4all, German Research Foundation, Hannover Medical School, Hanover, Germany, [3] Department of Otolaryngology, Head and Neck Surgery, University of Kansas School of Medicine, Kansas City, MO, United States

***Correspondence:**
Athanasia Warnecke
warnecke.athanasia@mh-hannover.de

† These authors have contributed equally to this work

The outcome of cochlear implantation depends on multiple variables including the underlying health of the cochlea. Brain derived neurotrophic factor (BDNF) has been shown to support spiral ganglion neurons and to improve implant function in animal models. Whether endogenous BDNF or BDNF-regulated proteins can be used as biomarkers to predict cochlear health and implant outcome has not been investigated yet. Gene expression of BDNF and downstream signaling molecules were identified in tissue of human cochleae obtained from normal hearing patients (n = 3) during skull base surgeries. Based on the gene expression data, bioinformatic analysis was utilized to predict the regulation of proteins by BDNF. The presence of proteins corresponding to these genes was investigated in perilymph (n = 41) obtained from hearing-impaired patients (n = 38) during cochlear implantation or skull base surgery for removal of vestibular schwannoma by nanoscale liquid chromatography coupled to tandem mass spectrometry (nano LC-MS/MS). Analyzed by mass spectrometry were 41 perilymph samples despite three patients undergoing bilateral cochlear implantation. These particular BDNF regulated proteins were not detectable in any of the perilymph samples. Subsequently, targeted analysis of the perilymph proteome data with Ingenuity Pathway Analysis (IPA) identified further proteins in human perilymph that could be regulated by BDNF. These BDNF regulated proteins were correlated to the presence of residual hearing (RH) prior to implantation and to the performance data with the cochlear implant after 1 year. There was overall a decreased level of expression of BDNF-regulated proteins in profoundly hearing-impaired patients compared to patients with some RH. Phospholipid transfer protein was positively correlated to the preoperative hearing level of the patients. Our data show that combination of gene expression arrays and bioinformatic analysis can aid in the prediction of downstream signaling proteins related to the BDNF pathway. Proteomic analysis of perilymph may help to identify the presence or absence of these molecules in the diseased organ. The impact of such prediction algorithms on diagnosis and treatment needs to be established in further studies.

Keywords: inner ear, perilymph, BDNF, neurotrophin, bioinformatic analysis, proteomics, diagnostics, cochlear implant

INTRODUCTION

One of the challenges in cochlear implantation is to understand the wide variability in performance amongst users. Candidates with similar history and implanted with the same device can demonstrate outcomes on both ends of the spectrum (Carlson et al., 2012). A plethora of factors may contribute to the variance in speech perception including age, duration of deafness, genetics, surgical technique and device characteristics, neuronal survival, electrode position, or central processing abilities (Carlson et al., 2012; Causon et al., 2015; Kral et al., 2016; Shearer et al., 2017). Since human temporal bone studies have recently shown a link between spiral ganglion population and cochlear implant outcomes (Seyyedi et al., 2014), one of the research targets is to maintain the viable population of spiral ganglion neurons for stimulation. Objective measures of cochlear function also suggest that a healthier neuronal population may result in better speech outcomes (Kim et al., 2010). This raises the possibility of modulating spiral ganglion function and health through drug delivery to the inner ear in conjunction with cochlear implantation.

Neurotrophins are the most promising candidates to support the auditory nerve by increasing neuronal survival. Within the murine inner ear, BDNF and NT-3 seem to regulate the connection of hair cells and neurons (Pirvola et al., 1992, 1997; Flores-Otero and Davis, 2011) and to support the survival and synaptic integrity of the auditory nerve (Mellado Lagarde et al., 2013). Damage to the organ of Corti is thought to result in loss of neurotrophin production and secondary degeneration of the spiral ganglion (Lawner et al., 1997; Staecker and Garnham, 2010). In a number of animal models, the delivery of various growth factors to the cochlea has resulted in increased preservation of neurons, re-growth of peripheral processes, and reduction of the threshold of electrical stimulation, suggesting that combining delivery of neurotrophins or neurotrophin mimetics may improve cochlear implant function (Evans et al., 2009; Wan et al., 2014; Budenz et al., 2015; Ramekers et al., 2015; Wise et al., 2016; Pfingst et al., 2017). Pathway analysis suggests that alterations in neurotrophin signaling should result in a broad range of physiologic changes in the cochlea. BDNF in particular appears to play an important role in both the peripheral and central auditory system (Singer et al., 2014). Despite the vast number of preclinical data concerning BDNF and cochlear health, nothing is known hitherto for the human auditory system. Interestingly, prior evaluations to the proteome of human perilymph (Schmitt et al., 2017) did not detect endogenous BDNF. The raw data of all detected proteins in perilymph by mass spectrometry in detail can be perused in the supplementary material of this prior study (Schmitt et al., 2017).

In order to determine whether BDNF and its regulated proteins are expressed in the adult human cochlea, we performed gene array analysis on human cochlear tissue. The results obtained from gene expression analysis were correlated with the previous reported proteome data of human perilymph samples (Schmitt et al., 2017). Based on the neurotrophin hypothesis, we assumed that patients without any RH would demonstrate altered neurotrophin signaling when compared to patients with RH and this would be reflected on the individual proteomic profiles of the perilymph. To evaluate this, we correlated the presence of BDNF-regulated proteins to preoperative hearing levels and postoperative cochlear implant performance data of the patients.

Abbreviations: BDNF, brain derived neurotrophic factor; CDC42, cell division control protein 42 homolog; CID, collision-induced dissociation; CSF, cerebrospinal fluid; GFAP, glial fibrillary acidic protein; GOA, gene ontology annotations; HSP 90, heat shock protein 90; HTA, human transcriptome array; ID, inner diameter; IPA, Ingenuity Pathway Analysis; IRB, Institutional Review Board; LTQ, linear trap quadrupole; NCAM1, neural cell adhesion molecule 1; NELL2, neural tissue-specific epidermal growth factor-like repeat domain-containing protein; LFQ, label free quantification; NH, no hearing; NT-3, neurotrophin 3; p75NTR, p75 neurotrophin receptor; PI3K, phosphoinositide 3-kinase; PTA, pure tone average; RAS, rat sarcoma; RH, residual hearing; TdT, terminal deoxynucleotidyltransferase; Trk, receptor tyrosine kinase.

MATERIALS AND METHODS

Perilymph and Cochlear Tissue Sampling

Collection of human cochlear tissue for gene array analysis was approved by the University of Kansas School of Medicine Institutional Review Board. Cochleae from three patients with normal hearing were obtained during a transcochlear approach to the posterior fossa for removal of meningioma and analyzed for growth factor gene expression.

Human perilymph was collected with a modified micro glass capillary during inner ear surgeries from 38 patients including three patients undergoing a bilateral cochlear implantation (37 perilymph samples during cochlear implantations and 4 during vestibular schwannoma surgeries) as already described in our previous study (Schmitt et al., 2017). The present study is an extension of a previous study (Schmitt et al., 2017). The data were analyzed with regard to pre-implantation hearing thresholds and cochlear implantation outcome. Patients aged 9 months up to 80 years with different etiologies for sensorineural hearing loss (e.g., Menière's disease, connatal cytomegalovirus infection, large vestibular aqueduct, CHARGE syndrome, meningitis, and auditory neuropathy) were included in this study. In addition, included patients were implanted with different cochlear implant devices and electrode arrays. A short version of the demographic data of the 38 patients undergoing cochlear implantation with perilymph sampling is depicted in **Table 1**. Detailed information about the individual patients is presented in the supporting information (**Supplementary Table S1**). The perilymph samples were obtained by puncturing of the round window membrane directly before the insertion of a cochlear implant electrode array. Protocols for collection of specimens were approved by the Ethics Committee of Hannover Medical School for perilymph by cochlear implantation (approval no. 1883-2013) and for perilymph during translabyrinthal vestibular schwannoma surgeries (approval no. 2403-2014).

Written informed consent was obtained from every patient included in this study.

Genomic Evaluation

Tissue of the cochleae from three patients with normal hearing, undergoing a transcochlear approach to the posterior fossa

TABLE 1 | Demographic data of the 41 patients undergoing CI surgery with perilymph sampling.

Demographic data	Age (mean in years)	*n** (%)
Patients	44.4	41 (100)
Male	44.3	23 (56.1)
Female	44.7	18 (43.9)
No hearing (NH)	36.5	27 (65.9)
Residual hearing (RH)	59.8	14 (34.1)
Children (0–18 years)	2.7	12 (29.3)
Adults (19–80)	61.7	29 (70.7)

**Bilateral samples of patients (n = 3) counted as two individual patients.*

for removal of meningioma were analyzed for growth factor gene expression. The lateral wall, basilar membrane and a portion of the modiolus were removed with an alligator forceps and immediately placed in RNAlater (Qiagen, cat #76104). Total RNA was extracted with Trizol reagent (Thermo Fisher Scientific, cat #15596018) and purified by centrifuging with phase lock heavy gel (Tiagen, cat # WMS-2302830). RNA was analyzed using the Agilent RNA6000 Pico kit in an Agilent Bioanalyzer 2100 to identify RNA degradation if present. Using an Affymetrix GeneChip WT Pico labeling kit, 50 ng of total RNA was TdT end labeled with biotin and hybridized on an Affymetrix HTA 2.0 array. After washing and staining, the chip was read with an Affymetrix GeneChip Scanner 3000 7G using a single scan with default normalization. Expression of genes present at 2 logs over baseline was evaluated. Data (genomic and proteomic) were uploaded into IPA software (Qiagen Bioinformatics) and evaluated based on the effects of varying expression of BDNF. Some proteins were subjected to classification by GOA using *UniProt* (UniProt Consortium, 2015).

Proteomic Analysis

In a prior study, intraoperative perilymph sampling method and analysis by an in depth shot gun proteomics approach were established allowing the analysis of hundreds of proteins simultaneously in very small sample sizes in a microliters range (Schmitt et al., 2017). Perilymph samples were prepared for LC-MS/MS analysis by alkylation and separated using sodium dodecyl sulfate polyacrylamide gel electrophoresis as previously described (Schmitt et al., 2017). Peptide samples were separated with a nano-flow ultra-high pressure liquid chromatography system (RSLC, Thermo Fisher Scientific) equipped with a trapping column (3 μm C18 particle, 2 cm length, 75 μm ID, Acclaim PepMap, Thermo Fisher Scientific) and a 50 cm long separation column (2 μm C18 particle, 75 μm ID, Acclaim PepMap, Thermo Fisher Scientific). The RSLC system was coupled online via a Nano Spray Flex Ion Source II (Thermo Fisher Scientific) to an LTQ-Orbitrap Velos mass spectrometer. Metal-coated fused-silica emitters (SilicaTip, 10 μm i.d., New Objectives) and a voltage of 1.3 kV were used for the electrospray. Overview scans were acquired at a resolution of 60 k in a mass range of m/z 300–1600 in the orbitrap analyzer and stored in profile mode. The top 10 most intensive ions of charges two or three and a minimum intensity of 2000 counts were selected for CID fragmentation with a normalized collision energy of 38.0, an activation time of 10 ms and an activation Q of 0.250 in the LTQ. Fragment ion mass spectra were recorded in the LTQ at normal scan rate and stored as centroid m/z value and intensity pairs. Active exclusion was activated so that ions fragmented once were excluded from further fragmentation for 70 s within a mass window of 10 ppm of the specific m/z value. The relative protein quantification was performed by LFQ and was determined as LFQ intensity (Schmitt et al., 2017, 2018).

Additionally, proteins were subjected to classification by GOA using *UniProt* (UniProt Consortium, 2015). The Gene Ontology (GO) classification allows a mapping of the proteins into the categories *molecular function, biological process,* and *cellular compartment.* Proteins were described using a standardized vocabulary of the *UniProt* Knowledgebase by uploading the UniProt IDs of the proteins to the *UniProt* website http:/www.uniprot.org.

Audiology: Classification of Patients by Audiogram Data

Before surgery and perilymph sampling, pure tone audiometry was performed using a calibrated audiometer according to DIN EN 60318 to detect the acoustic hearing threshold. The test method follows DIN ISO 8253 with headphones for air conduction and headset for bone conduction in both ears. The PTA was analyzed for the frequency region of 500, 1000, and 2000 Hz. This classification was used for a direct correlation of the hearing loss of patients with LFQ intensity of detected proteins.

For the classification of severity of hearing loss in decibels (dB) and percent hearing impairment, a previously described method was used (Shearer et al., 1993). Therefore, the PTA was calculated for the frequency region of 500, 1000, 2000, and 3000 Hz. To obtain an ear-specific level, 25 dB was subtracted from this PTA and multiplied by the factor 1.5. This method includes a broader range of frequency values and allows a more precise classification of severity of hearing loss, especially in our cochlear implant patients with severe hearing loss in the low frequency area. The preoperative audiograms were used to assign patients to one of the two groups:

No hearing: PTA threshold of 91 dB or higher, 100% hearing impairment, *n* = 27 ears.

Residual hearing: PTA threshold of less than 91 dB, some RH, *n* = 14 ears.

Additionally, the postoperative hearing performance with a cochlear implant 1 year after implantation of the 38 patients with perilymph sampling was analyzed. Therefore, data of three audiologic tests (HSM sentence test in quiet and in noise at 10 dB, Freiburg monosyllable word test) 1 year after implantation were included. From the 29 adult patients, the majority of the patients participated in the three tests: HSM sentence test in quiet (*n* = 15), HSM sentence test in noise 10 dB (*n* = 20), Freiburg monosyllable word test (*n* = 22). For children, these types of tests were not applicable.

Statistical Analysis

Mass spectrometric raw data were processed using Max Quant software (version 1.4) and human entries of Swissprot/UniProt database. The threshold for protein identification was set to 0.01 on peptide and protein level.

Data were evaluated with multiple correlation analysis, or generation of heat maps and analysis with Fisher's exact test (Graph Pad Prism V 7). Significance was set at $p < 0.05$.

RESULTS

BDNF and TrkB Are Expressed in the Normal Hearing Human Cochlea

There is only very limited data on neurotrophin signaling in the adult human cochlea. Expression of BDNF mRNA and associated signaling molecules were determined by evaluating cochlear cDNA libraries from patients with normal hearing undergoing surgical removal of rare meningiomas anterior to the brainstem via a transcochlear approach. In these surgeries, hearing was sacrificed to gain better access to the tumor and thus also to the normal hearing cochlea.

Both BDNF and the TrkB receptor were expressed in all three specimens. The array did not differentiate between transcript variants. The low affinity p75NTR was also detectable in all three specimens. To determine the biologically significant pathways regulated by BDNF in the cochlea, we determined which components of neurotrophin signaling were present at a high level in the normal inner ear. As depicted in **Figure 1**, there is a high level of expression of the Ras/ERK pathway members and of CREB. These pathways are not only specific to neurotrophin signaling but may provide targets for pharmacological intervention for experimental or therapeutic purposes.

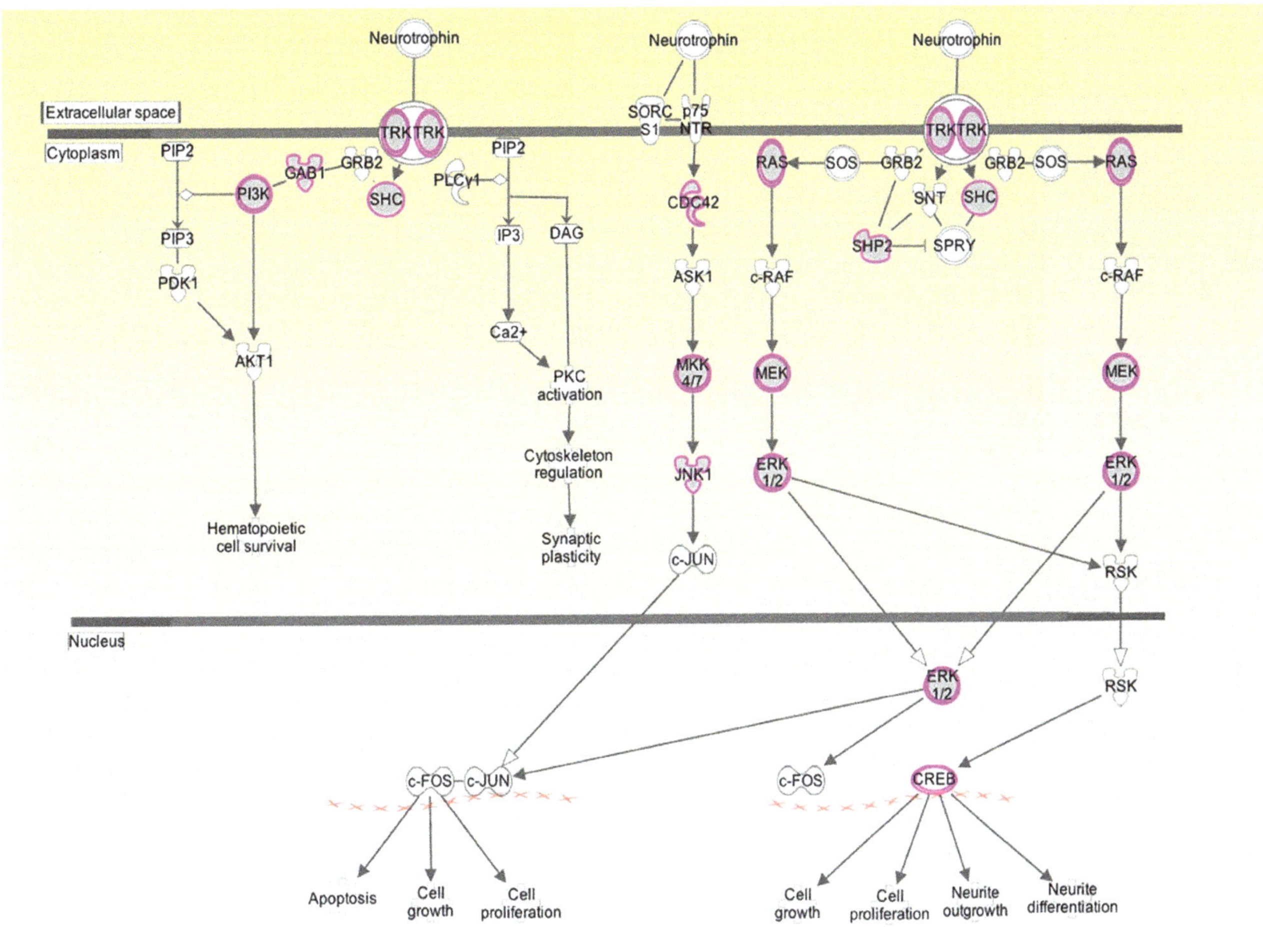

FIGURE 1 | Analysis of human inner ear transcriptome over-layed on a generic human neurotrophin signaling pathway. Purple/gray proteins represent gene products/proteins identified at 10 log folds expression over baseline in the cochlear transcriptome. This suggests that those particular signaling pathways play an active role in the inner ear. Both the high affinity Trk receptor which is found in the spiral ganglion and the low affinity p75NTR which is thought to be in Schwann and glial cells are represented. p75NTR was detectable at 2 log fold expression over baseline expression. The downstream signaling genes were expressed at significantly higher levels.

BDNF Is Predicted to Regulate a Variety of Genes Involved in Neuronal Health in the Human Cochlea

Ingenuity Pathway Analysis software was used to identify pathways related to BDNF signaling that are expressed in all 3 cDNA samples from the normal hearing patients described above at 10-fold higher levels than baseline gene expression levels. In addition, the same software was used to identify the expression of genes in the normal cochlea that are predicted to be regulated by BDNF. A range of proteins, many of which have not been evaluated for their effect on hearing and cochlear biology, have been predicted by the IPA Knowledgebase (**Table 2**). Functions of these genes include microtubule assembly, synaptic vesicle trafficking, protein folding, DNA binding, transcriptional regulation, actin binding, axonogenesis, myelination, ribosomal function, and differentiation. Proteins corresponding to the genes from the cochlear cDNA library (results from mRNA analysis) that were predicted to be regulated by BDNF were not found in the perilymph samples analyzed by mass spectrometry.

BDNF Is Predicted to Regulate a Variety of Proteins That Are Also Present in Human Cochlear Perilymph

The perilymph proteome in 41 perilymph samples of 38 patients undergoing inner ear surgeries with and without RH was evaluated, imported into IPA and queried for predicted relationships between BDNF and the identified proteins. Proteins found in the perilymph at significant concentrations were analyzed by IPA. Some of these proteins correspond to genes that are also predicted to be regulated by BDNF. Using this approach, we were able to indirectly identify genes and proteins relevant to the inner ear and regulated by BDNF. These perilymph proteins and their corresponding genes anticipated to be up and down regulated by reduced BDNF expression and proteins that are predicted to be regulated by reduced BDNF but with no information about the direction of regulation are summarized in **Table 3**. The proteins in **Table 3** are ranked by the occurrence of the protein in perilymph samples of the patients within the three subgroups (downregulated, upregulated, with no information about regulation). Proteins were not detected in every perilymph sample. Proteins listed above in the subgroups have less abundance in the samples of the patients, meaning the proteins are detected in a low number of samples. However, the proteins at the bottom of the subgroup lists are detected in many samples of our patient cohort. Depicted in **Supplementary Figure S1** are the proteins detected in % of the patients. In conclusion, these 41 proteins of the 878 previously determined proteins present in perilymph (Schmitt et al., 2017) were identified in the IPA Knowledgebase as being regulated by BDNF (**Table 3**). There was a wide range of expression profile for the different proteins in different patients with some proteins being expressed in only a few of patients and others being found in every patient, depicted in the supporting information (**Supplementary Figure S1**).

For a more detailed view, GOA analysis was performed with the 41 perilymph proteins. These proteins were classified into the categories *biological process*, *molecular function*, and *cellular component*. The proteins were considered in the GO terms *cellular components*. Most proteins are intracellular proteins located in cell part (mainly intracellular organelle parts), organelle (mainly membrane-bounded organelle), and membrane (especially plasma membrane). But also proteins located in extracellular region part like extracellular exosomes were identified. A table with detailed information about proteins detected in >80% of patients or with direct regulation by BDNF mapped to the category *cellular components* by GOA is exemplarily shown in **Supplementary Table S2**. The main *molecular function* of the considered perilymph proteins depicts besides molecular function regulation and catalytic activity clearly binding with focus

TABLE 2 | Genes predicted to be regulated by BDNF in the normal cochlea.

Symbol	Entrez gene name	Location
ATAT1	Alpha tubulin acetyltransferase 1	Cytoplasm
BDNF	Brain derived neurotrophic factor	Extracellular space
C5orf34	Chromosome 5 open reading frame 34	Other
CADPS2	Calcium dependent secretion activator 2	Plasma membrane
DNAJC21	DnaJ heat shock protein family (Hsp40) member C21	Other
HIST1H2AL	Histone cluster 1H2A family member l	Nucleus
ITIH3	Inter-alpha-trypsin inhibitor heavy chain 3	Extracellular space
MALAT1	Metastasis associated lung adenocarcinoma transcript 1 (non-protein coding)	Nucleus
MYH8	Myosin heavy chain 8	Cytoplasm
OMG	Oligodendrocyte myelin glycoprotein	Plasma membrane
PRSS12	Protease, serine 12	Extracellular space
RPL35A	Ribosomal protein L35a	Cytoplasm
SEMA3E	Semaphorin 3E	Extracellular space
SLC16A7	Solute carrier family 16 member 7	Plasma membrane
TMEM45A	Transmembrane protein 45A	Plasma membrane

TABLE 3 | Perilymph proteins and corresponding abbreviations (gene names) and Uniprot IDs anticipated to be up and down regulated and with no information about regulation by simulation that cochlear BDNF is reduced.

Downregulated	Symbol	Uniprot ID
Neurexin-1 beta	*NRXN1*	F8WB18
Cell division control protein 42 homolog	*CDC42*	P60953
Ubiquitin carboxyl-terminal hydrolase isozyme L1	*UCHL1*	D6RE83
Myelin proteolipid protein	*PLP1*	P60201
Myelin basic protein	*MBP*	E9PMR5
Ryanodine receptor 3	*RYR3*	Q15413
14-3-3 protein gamma	*YWHAG*	P61981
Ryanodine receptor 2	*RYR2*	H7BY35
Osteopontin	*SPP1*	P10451
Protein kinase C-binding protein NELL2	*NELL2*	F8WB6
Heat shock protein HSP 90-alpha	*HSP90AA1*	P07900
Neural cell adhesion molecule 1	*NCAM1*	Q92823
Glial fibrillary acidic protein	*GFAP*	P14136
Upregulated		
Tripeptidyl-peptidase 1	*TPP1*	O14773
Laminin subunit gamma-1	*LAMC1*	P11047
Dihydropyrimidinase-related protein 2	*DPYSL2*	Q16555
Reelin	*RELN*	P78509
Ferritin light chain	*FTL*	P02792
Plexin-B2	*PLXNB2*	O15031
Agrin	*AGRN*	O00468
Annexin A5	*ANXA5*	P08758
Filamin-B	*FLNB*	O75369
Ribonuclease inhibitor	*RNH1*	P13489
Filamin-A	*FLNA*	Q5HY54
78 kDa glucose-regulated protein	*HSPA5*	P11021
Neutrophil gelatinase-associated lipocalin	*LCN2*	P80188
Annexin A2	*ANXA2*	P07355
Phospholipid transfer protein	*PLTP*	P55058
Vimentin	*VIM*	P08670
No information about regulation		
Gamma-secretase C-terminal fragment 59 (Amyloid beta A4 protein)	*APP*	E9PG40
Carboxypeptidase E	*CPE*	P16870
Chromogranin-A	*CHGA*	P10645
Glutamine synthetase	*GLUL*	P15104
Inter-alpha-trypsin inhibitor heavy chain H3	*ITIH3*	Q06033
Vasorin	*VASN*	Q6EMK4
Protein S100-A9	*S100A9*	P06702
Fibrinogen beta chain	*FGB*	P02675
Plasminogen	*PLG*	P00747
Actin, cytoplasmic 1	*ACTB*	P60709
Apolipoprotein E	*APOE*	P02649
Alpha-2-macroglobulin	*A2M*	P01023

on protein and ion binding. The perilymph proteins are involved in manifold *biological processes* with focus on biological regulation. Many proteins are also participated in cellular, developmental and metabolic processes as well as in cellular component regulation, response to stimulus and localization.

Severity of Hearing Loss Correlates to Overall Lower Expression of Perilymph Proteins Predicted to Be Regulated by BDNF

Using IPA software, we identified proteins detected in perilymph with direct or indirect regulation by BDNF and we grouped these regulated perilymph proteins by expected change in expression level when BDNF is decreased. The IPA Knowledgebase predicted that 13 proteins would be down regulated and 16 proteins would be up regulated when BDNF expression diminished (**Table 3**). No predictive information on up or down regulation could be found for the 12 remaining proteins (**Table 3**). Patients were divided into two groups, patients with and without RH based on a cutoff of 90 dB PTA, and correlated to the three groups of proteins regulated by BDNF. These results are shown as a heat map depicting the presence and concentration of the various proteins in patients with and without RH (**Figure 2**). Patients with no preoperative RH had significantly lower levels of the proteins predicted to be down regulated when BDNF decreases (**Figure 2**; left side; $p = 0.007$; Fisher's exact test). For proteins that are predicted to be up regulated, there was also a significant difference between the groups (**Figure 2**; middle; $p = 0.02$; Fisher's exact test). For proteins determined to be regulated by BDNF expression but without predictable change direction, there was no statistically significant difference between RH and non-hearing patients (**Figure 2**; right side).

Preoperative Hearing Loss Correlates to Decreased Perilymph Expression of Phospholipid Transfer Protein

The proteins listed in **Table 3** were correlated to the preoperative hearing level and postoperative performance data with the cochlear implant 1 year after implantation. Comparison of protein levels (LFQ intensity) to the patients' preoperative PTA showed a slightly significant correlation between preoperative PTA and level of phospholipid transfer protein (PLTP) (Pearson $r = -0.3658$; $p = 0.0187$) shown in **Figure 3**. Correlation of the other proteins to the PTA was not significant. PLTP was detectable in the perilymph of the majority of the patients (36/41).

Additionally, the correlation of the relative PLTP concentration (LFQ intensity) in perilymph at the time point during surgery to postoperative hearing performance 1 year after hearing restoration with a cochlear implant was analyzed. Data of audiologic tests (HSM sentence test in quiet and in noise 10 dB, Freiburg monosyllable word test) 1 year after implantation were used for a correlation analysis. Data of the majority of the patients, children excluded, were analyzed: HSM sentence test in quiet ($n = 15$), HSM sentence test in noise 10 dB ($n = 20$), Freiburg monosyllable word test ($n = 22$). There might be a trend toward better understanding in patients with higher PLTP levels in perilymph is shown in **Figure 4**. For confirming these hypotheses further studies are required.

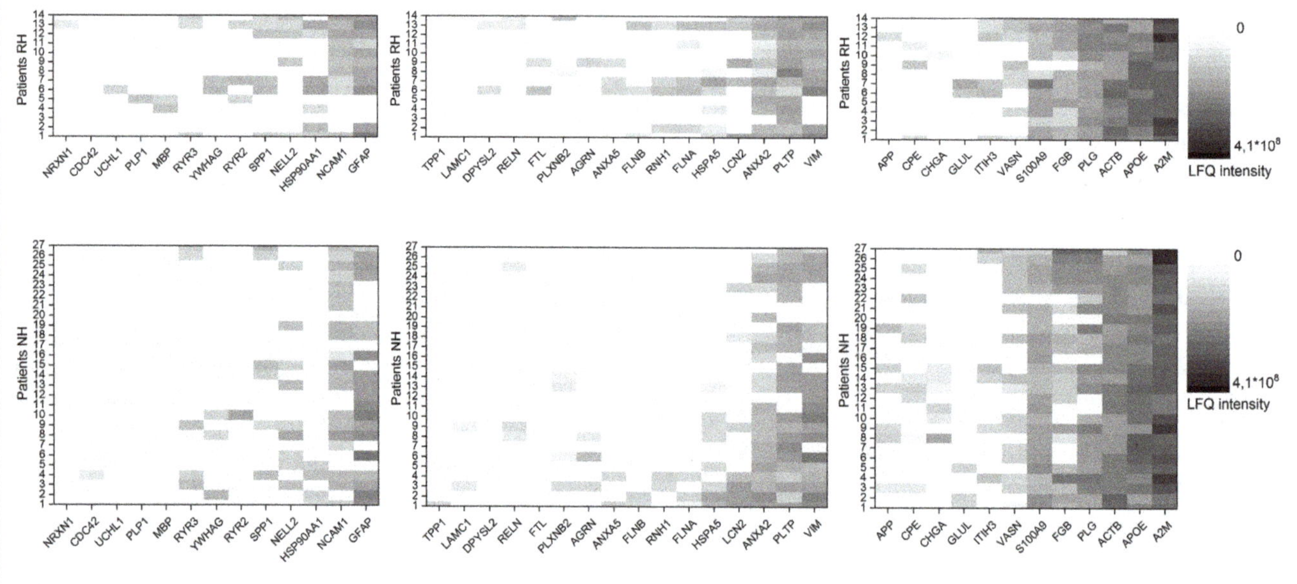

FIGURE 2 | Heat map of proteins predicted to be regulated by BDNF. Shown are proteins anticipated to be downregulated with decrease in BDNF for patients with (RH) and without (NH) residual hearing on the left. Proteins anticipated to be upregulated with decrease in BDNF for patients with (RH) and without (NH) residual hearing in the middle and proteins with no information about the regulation with decrease in BDNF for patients with (RH) and without (NH) residual hearing on the right. Protein values of patients with RH are shown in the upper row, data of patients NH in the lower row. The concentration of the individual proteins was analyzed by label free quantification (LFQ) in human perilymph samples and an increase is shown with deeper shades of violet.

DISCUSSION

The integrity of the spiral ganglion is thought to play a key role in cochlear implant function. Since the studies of Spoendlin demonstrated that aminoglycoside injury of the peripheral auditory system in cats resulted in a secondary degeneration of the spiral ganglion (Spoendlin, 1975), there has been significant interest in understanding the mechanisms that maintain spiral ganglion integrity and function. In humans, the process of spiral ganglion degeneration appears to occur at a different rate than in animal models. There clearly are variations in spiral ganglion populations that occur with different disease processes (Otte et al., 1978). The relationship between spiral ganglion integrity and cochlear implant outcomes in humans has been more difficult to establish. Initial temporal bone studies did not show a clear relationship between spiral ganglion counts and implant outcomes (Fayad et al., 1991). More recent studies with larger numbers, however, do show a relationship between speech outcomes and the quantity of spiral ganglion neurons (Seyyedi et al., 2014). To assess the functionality of the remaining spiral ganglion neurons, animal studies have been used to correlate changes in the electrically evoked compound actual potential of guinea pigs with intact or impaired spiral ganglion neurons (Pfingst et al., 2015b). This potentially correlates to measurable changes in patients undergoing cochlear implantation since an abnormal growth function of the electrically evoked compound action has been correlated to poor cochlear implant speech outcomes (Kim et al., 2010).

An important question that arises is whether neurotrophic factors can influence neuronal survival in humans treated with cochlear implants. Amongst the most studied candidates are

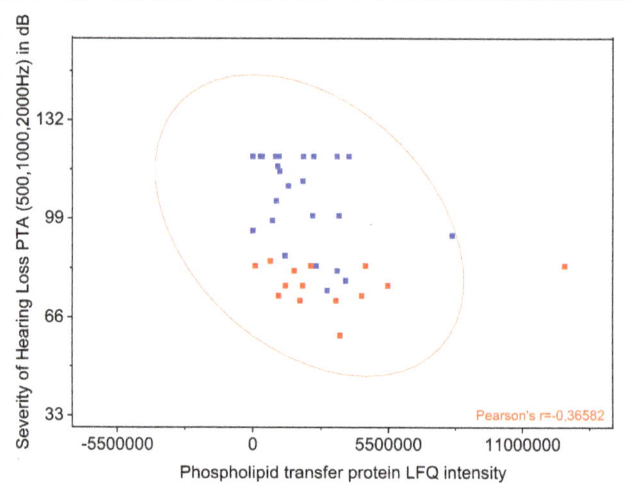

FIGURE 3 | Comparison of PLTP protein levels to the patients' preoperative pure tone average (PTA). Shown is a significant correlation between preoperative PTA (500, 1000, and 2000 Hz) and presence of PLTP. The protein levels were analyzed by label free quantification (LFQ intensity) in human perilymph samples.

the neurotrophins. The function of BDNF in the adult rodent auditory system was recently reviewed (Singer et al., 2014). Diverse studies mainly using knockout and conditional knockout mice suggest that BDNF is initially expressed in auditory hair cells. During maturation of hearing, the pattern of BDNF expression changes to inner phalangeal cells, pillar cells (the cells surrounding the inner hair cell) and spiral ganglion cells

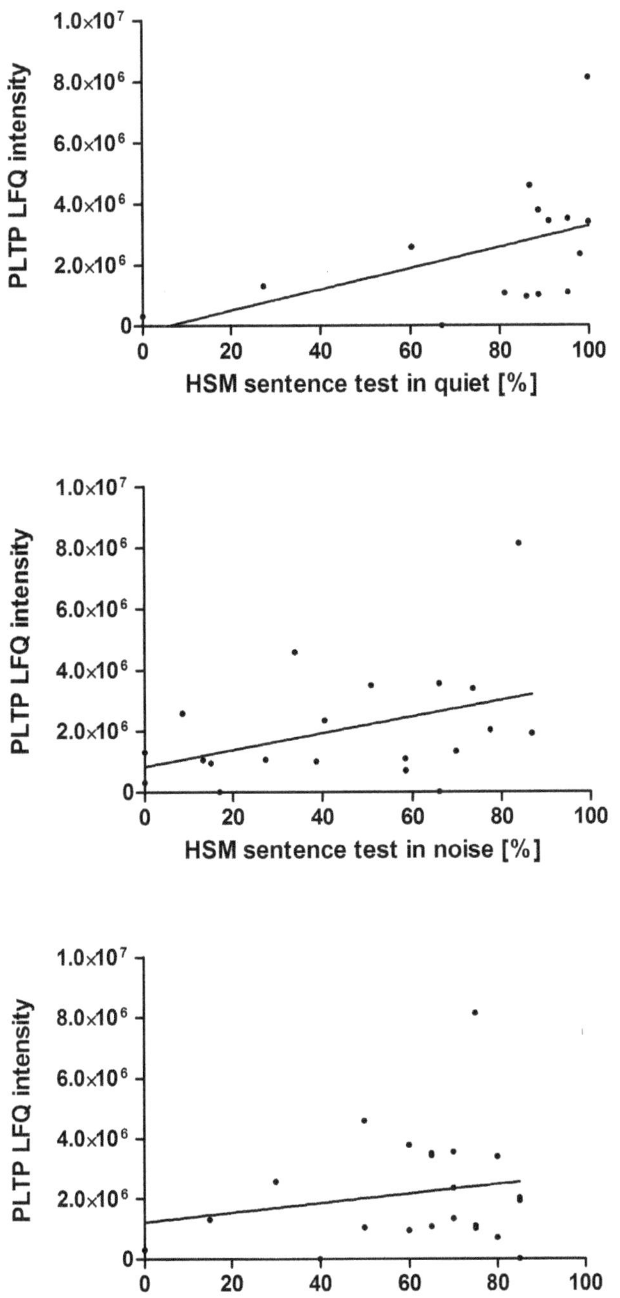

FIGURE 4 | Correlation of the PLTP protein levels to the patients' postoperative hearing performance. Audiologic test data of 29 adult patients of the 41 patients with perilymph sampling 1 year after cochlear implantation are depicted as speech understanding in %. The HSM sentence test in quiet (*n* = 15) is shown on the top, the HSM sentence test in noise at 10 dB (*n* = 20) in the middle and the Freiburg monosyllable word test (*n* = 22) at the bottom. The protein levels were analyzed by label free quantification (LFQ intensity) in human perilymph samples.

(Fritzsch et al., 2004; Kersigo and Fritzsch, 2015; Johnson Chacko et al., 2017). One of the key roles of BDNF in the adult auditory system may include maintenance of ribbon synapse integrity (Zuccotti et al., 2012; Singer et al., 2014). The role of BDNF in the human adult auditory system is less defined. A number of studies have looked at the expression of neurotrophin and their receptors in normal adult human cochlear tissue from cochleae harvested during acoustic neuroma surgery. The TrkB receptor was found to be expressed in the spiral ganglion neurons and in nerve fibers underneath outer hair cells (Liu et al., 2011). BDNF expression was not detectable by immunohistochemistry (Liu et al., 2011). A recent *in situ* hybridization study in adult human inner ear tissue, however, has found BDNF mRNA in auditory hair cells and supporting cells (Johnson Chacko et al., 2017). Expression of the low affinity p75NTR was demonstrated in Schwann cells and glial cells but not in spiral ganglion neurons (Liu et al., 2012). Currently, no human data exists demonstrating what changes in neurotrophin signaling occur as a result of hearing loss. The signaling pathways of BDNF are well understood. Consequently, a potential method of evaluating BDNF effects in the human inner ear is to look at the downstream effects of BDNF signaling.

In the central nervous system, there are clear links to a variety of neurodegenerative pathologies and decreased levels of BDNF expression (Lu et al., 2013). Besides direct degeneration of the tissues producing BDNF, the expression of BDNF can be modulated by inflammatory mediators which may be present as a consequence of cochlear implantation (Calabrese et al., 2014). Additionally, as shown in many studies, BDNF can autoregulate its expression (Zheng et al., 2012). Animal studies have shown that implant function can be improved after cochlear damage by either co-infusing BDNF or inducing production of BDNF through gene therapy (Staecker and Garnham, 2010; Budenz et al., 2012). A key factor in translating these finding into human studies is to identify patients with insufficient endogenous BDNF production or signaling. In addition to electrophysiological measures (Pfingst et al., 2015a), direct or indirect indicators of neurotrophin function in perilymph may be detectable. Unlike in CSF (Calderon-Garciduenas et al., 2016; Li et al., 2016; Martin-de-Pablos et al., 2018), direct detection of BDNF by mass spectrometry have not been demonstrated in perilymph yet (Schmitt et al., 2017).

In the herein presented study, analysis of gene expression in three normal human patients showed the presence of BDNF, TrkB and the p75NTR in the cochlea, supplementing information gained from prior immunohistochemical studies. We compared these data with analysis of proteins in the perilymph of patients undergoing cochlear implantation, therefore having hearing loss, and analyzed their relationship to BDNF signaling. Based on profiling, we show that expression of signaling cascades downstream from neurotrophic tyrosine kinase receptors and the low affinity p75NTR are active in the normal cochlea (**Figure 1**). There is active expression of PI3K, CDC42, and RAS (**Figure 1**) resulting in activation of pathways that maintain cell survival, growth, and neuritogenesis (Sandhya et al., 2013). Using IPA software, we identified a subgroup of the 878 expressed perilymph proteins, identified, and described in a previous study (Schmitt et al., 2017), that may be regulated by BDNF (**Table 3**). The 41 proteins identified based on their relationship to BDNF signaling may be related to the hearing level of the patients since different protein levels between the two patients groups were analyzed (patients with RH and patients with profound hearing loss).

For the proteins that are predicted to be down regulated if BDNF is reduced, patients with no RH prior to implantation expressed lower or absent levels of these proteins. For this group of proteins, ryanodine receptors 2 and 3, and HSP 90 are hair cell specific, so their reduction could be a reflection of loss of hair cells rather than changes in BDNF signaling (Lim et al., 1996; Mammano et al., 2007). Within this group, NELL2 is a spiral ganglion marker (Nelson et al., 2002). GFAP is a marker for spiral ganglion glial cells and supporting cells (Rio et al., 2002) and NCAM1 is associated with the spiral ganglion (Terkelsen et al., 1989). Individually, these proteins did not correlate to preoperative hearing levels. A potential explanation of this is found in the adult rodent data. If BDNF really is only expressed in the higher frequency region of the adult cochlea as suggested by Zuccotti et al. (2012), then our RH and non-hearing patients may not have a significant difference in BDNF expression since most patients undergoing implantation have RH only at lower frequencies. A larger cohort of patients with variable hearing loss will be needed to further refine these outcomes. Interestingly, among these proteins osteopontin is a marker for vestibular hair cells and may also be expressed in lower levels in the marginal cells and in the spiral ganglion (Sakagami, 2000). This protein has a decreased expression in patients without RH, suggesting that there may also be differences in balance function that can be assayed through this approach.

For the proteins that were predicted to be upregulated when BDNF is reduced, filamin A and B are actin binding proteins which can be found in hair cell stereocilia (Ramakrishnan et al., 2012). Plexins are members of a family of transmembrane proteins that control axonal growth and have been demonstrated in the developing spiral ganglion (Lu et al., 2011). Annexin A5 has been described as being present in high concentration in hair cell stereocilia (Krey et al., 2016). Within this group, the patients with profound hearing loss expressed a significantly reduced proteome, when considering proteins regulated by BDNF (**Figure 2**). Again, this may reflect the overall degeneration of the organ of Corti rather than a BDNF regulatory effect. Within this subgroup, however, phospholipid transfer protein showed a statistically significant correlation to preoperative PTA. This protein is generally identified with lipid metabolism but has been identified in the developing inner ear as expressed in cells of a non-hair cell lineage during development (Scheffer et al., 2015). By GOA the molecular, function of this protein is characterized by lipid transporter activity (including phospholipids and ceramides like diacylglycerol, phosphatidic acid, sphingomyelin, phosphatidylcholine, phosphatidylglycerol, cerebroside, and phosphatidyl ethanolamine). Additionally, this protein is involved in different biological processes like ceramide transport, flagellated sperm motility, high-density lipoprotein particle remodeling, lipid metabolic process, lipid transport, phospholipid transport, positive regulation of cholesterol efflux, and vitamin E biosynthetic process. Interestingly, a link between PLTP and the amyloid precursor protein (APP) was discussed suggesting that a deficiency of these proteins accelerates memory dysfunction in mouse models. Additionally, PLTP might play an important role in autophagy modulation (Tong et al., 2015). Its function in the adult inner ear is not defined yet.

When discussing the results obtained from the present study, several limitations need to be considered. The population of the patients included into our analysis is highly heterogenous with different anatomic and molecular pathologies. This can certainly add to the variability in the perilymph proteome that we showed in this study and in prior studies (Schmitt et al., 2017, 2018). In addition, different cochlear implant devices with various electrode arrays have been used for the treatment of the hearing loss, adding more variables to be considered when analyzing the hearing performance with the device. Finally, the low number of patients included and the vast number of proteins identified in the perilymph are limiting the statistical power of the study. The influence of age and gender on gene and protein expression needs also consideration. Thus, future studies need to concentrate on a higher number of homogenous groups of patients.

Despite the limitations, evaluation of the perilymph proteome offers a novel approach for the indirect evaluation of a wide range of biological effects within the cochlea of patients undergoing cochlear implantation. Animal studies have demonstrated that BDNF supplementation can enhance spiral ganglion survival (Evans et al., 2009; Wan et al., 2014; Budenz et al., 2015; Ramekers et al., 2015; Wise et al., 2016; Pfingst et al., 2017). Despite temporal bone pathology and physiological evidence that spiral ganglion survival is variable between disease processes and affects cochlear implant outcomes, we have a very incomplete understanding of the diseased human inner ear. Cochlear "health" is hypothesized to have a significant impact on cochlear implant outcomes (Pfingst et al., 2015b, 2017). The human perilymph proteome in implant patients consists of greater than 800 individual proteins. By focusing on proteins that are regulated by BDNF, we can analyze subgroups that may reflect changes in BDNF signaling or even allow the identification of markers that may reflect BDNF signaling or demonstrate degeneration of hair cells and supporting cells within the organ of Corti.

CONCLUSION

We have demonstrated that BDNF is expressed in cochlear tissue in normal hearing individuals. Patients with profound hearing loss have less BDNF-regulated proteins in their perilymph when compared to patients with some RH. In addition, the expression level of PLTP correlated not only to preoperative hearing but also tend to improved outcome with cochlear implants in individual patients. This initial study identifies a group of proteins that may potentially serve as markers for inner ear health as it relates to cochlear implantation. In order to use this tool for the identification of biomarkers or for the reliable prediction of cochlear implant outcome, large applied studies need to be performed.

AUTHOR CONTRIBUTIONS

IdV acquired and analyzed the data, and wrote the first draft of the manuscript. HS processed and analyzed the perilymph, and wrote the manuscript. TL designed the study, provided financial support, and approved the manuscript. NP collected the perilymph, provided and analyzed the human data, and approved the manuscript. SA performed the bioinformatics analysis of the data, and approved the manuscript. HS designed the study, performed the bioinformatics analysis of the data, and wrote the manuscript. MD collected the perilymph, provided and analyzed the human data, approved the manuscript, and provided financial support. AW designed the study, collected the perilymph, analyzed the data, and wrote the manuscript.

REFERENCES

Budenz, C. L., Pfingst, B. E., and Raphael, Y. (2012). The use of neurotrophin therapy in the inner ear to augment cochlear implantation outcomes. *Anat. Rec.* 295, 1896–1908. doi: 10.1002/ar.22586

Budenz, C. L., Wong, H. T., Swiderski, D. L., Shibata, S. B., Pfingst, B. E., and Raphael, Y. (2015). Differential effects of AAV.BDNF and AAV.Ntf3 in the deafened adult guinea pig ear. *Sci. Rep.* 5:8619. doi: 10.1038/srep08619

Calabrese, F., Rossetti, A. C., Racagni, G., Gass, P., Riva, M. A., and Molteni, R. (2014). Brain-derived neurotrophic factor: a bridge between inflammation and neuroplasticity. *Front. Cell Neurosci.* 8:430. doi: 10.3389/fncel.2014.00430

Calderon-Garciduenas, L., Avila-Ramirez, J., Calderon-Garciduenas, A., Gonzalez-Heredia, T., Acuna-Ayala, H., Chao, C. K., et al. (2016). Cerebrospinal fluid biomarkers in highly exposed pm2.5 urbanites: the risk of alzheimer's and parkinson's diseases in young mexico city residents. *J. Alzh. Dis.* 54, 597–613. doi: 10.3233/JAD-160472

Carlson, M. L., Driscoll, C. L., Gifford, R. H., and McMenomey, S. O. (2012). Cochlear implantation: current and future device options. *Otolaryngol. Clin. North. Am.* 45, 221–248. doi: 10.1016/j.otc.2011.09.002

Causon, A., Verschuur, C., and Newman, T. A. (2015). A Retrospective analysis of the contribution of reported factors in cochlear implantation on hearing preservation outcomes. *Otol. Neurotol.* 36, 1137–1145. doi: 10.1097/MAO.0000000000000753

Evans, A. J., Thompson, B. C., Wallace, G. G., Millard, R., O'Leary, S. J., Clark, G. M., et al. (2009). Promoting neurite outgrowth from spiral ganglion neuron explants using polypyrrole/BDNF-coated electrodes. *J. Biomed. Mater. Res. A* 91, 241–250. doi: 10.1002/jbm.a.32228

Fayad, J., Linthicum, F. H. Jr., Otto, S. R., Galey, F. R., and House, W. F. (1991). Cochlear implants: histopathologic findings related to performance in 16 human temporal bones. *Ann. Otol. Rhinol. Laryngol.* 100, 807–811. doi: 10.1177/000348949110001004

Flores-Otero, J., and Davis, R. L. (2011). Synaptic proteins are tonotopically graded in postnatal and adult type I and type II spiral ganglion neurons. *J. Comp. Neurol.* 519, 1455–1475. doi: 10.1002/cne.22576

Fritzsch, B., Tessarollo, L., Coppola, E., and Reichardt, L. F. (2004). Neurotrophins in the ear: their roles in sensory neuron survival and fiber guidance. *Prog. Brain Res.* 146, 265–278. doi: 10.1016/S0079-6123(03)46017-2

Johnson Chacko, L., Blumer, M. J. F., Pechriggl, E., Rask-Andersen, H., Dietl, W., Haim, A., et al. (2017). Role of BDNF and neurotrophic receptors in human inner ear development. *Cell Tissue Res.* 370, 347–363. doi: 10.1007/s00441-017-2686-9

Kersigo, J., and Fritzsch, B. (2015). Inner ear hair cells deteriorate in mice engineered to have no or diminished innervation. *Front. Aging Neurosci.* 7:33. doi: 10.3389/fnagi.2015.00033

Kim, J. R., Abbas, P. J., Brown, C. J., Etler, C. P., O'Brien, S., and Kim, L. S. (2010). The relationship between electrically evoked compound action potential and speech perception: a study in cochlear implant users with short electrode array. *Otol. Neurotol.* 31, 1041–1048. doi: 10.1097/MAO.0b013e3181ec1d92

Kral, A., Kronenberger, W. G., Pisoni, D. B., and O'Donoghue, G. M. (2016). Neurocognitive factors in sensory restoration of early deafness: a connectome model. *Lancet Neurol.* 15, 610–621. doi: 10.1016/S1474-4422(16)00034-X

Krey, J. F., Drummond, M., Foster, S., Porsov, E., Vijayakumar, S., Choi, D., et al. (2016). Annexin A5 is the most abundant membrane-associated protein in stereocilia but is dispensable for hair-bundle development and function. *Sci. Rep.* 6:27221. doi: 10.1038/srep27221

Lawner, B. E., Harding, G. W., and Bohne, B. A. (1997). Time course of nerve-fiber regeneration in the noise-damaged *mammalian* cochlea. *Int. J. Dev. Neurosci.* 15, 601–617. doi: 10.1016/S0736-5748(96)00115-3

Li, W., Li, X., Xin, X., Kan, P. C., and Yan, Y. (2016). MicroRNA-613 regulates the expression of brain-derived neurotrophic factor in alzheimer's disease. *Biosci. Trends* 10, 372–377. doi: 10.5582/bst.2016.01127

Lim, H. H., Miller, J. M., Dolan, D. F., Raphael, Y., and Altschuler, R. A. (1996). "Noise-induced expression of heat shock proteins in the cochlea," in *Scientific Basis of NoiseInduced Hearing Loss*, eds A. Axelsson, H. Borchgrevink, R. P. Hamernik, P.-A. Hellstrom, and R. J. Salvi (New York,NY: Thieme Medical Publishers), 43–49.

Liu, W., Glueckert, R., Kinnefors, A., Schrott-Fischer, A., Bitsche, M., and Rask-Andersen, H. (2012). Distribution of P75 neurotrophin receptor in adult human cochlea-an immunohistochemical study. *Cell Tissue Res.* 348, 407–415. doi: 10.1007/s00441-012-1395-7

Liu, W., Kinnefors, A., Bostrom, M., and Rask-Andersen, H. (2011). Expression of TrkB and BDNF in human cochlea-an immunohistochemical study. *Cell Tissue Res.* 345, 213–221. doi: 10.1007/s00441-011-1209-1203

Lu, B., Nagappan, G., Guan, X., Nathan, P. J., and Wren, P. (2013). BDNF-based synaptic repair as a disease-modifying strategy for neurodegenerative diseases. *Nat. Rev. Neurosci.* 14, 401–416. doi: 10.1038/nrn3505

Lu, C. C., Appler, J. M., Houseman, E. A., and Goodrich, L. V. (2011). Developmental profiling of spiral ganglion neurons reveals insights into auditory circuit assembly. *J. Neurosci.* 31, 10903–10918. doi: 10.1523/JNEUROSCI.2358-11.2011

Mammano, F., Bortolozzi, M., Ortolano, S., and Anselmi, F. (2007). Ca2+ signaling in the inner ear. *Physiology* 22, 131–144. doi: 10.1152/physiol.00040.2006

Martin-de-Pablos, A., Cordoba-Fernandez, A., and Fernandez-Espejo, E. (2018). Analysis of neurotrophic and antioxidant factors related to midbrain dopamine neuronal loss and brain inflammation in the cerebrospinal fluid of the elderly. *Exp. Gerontol.* 110, 54–60. doi: 10.1016/j.exger.2018.05.009

Mellado Lagarde, M. M., Cox, B. C., Fang, J., Taylor, R., Forge, A., and Zuo, J. (2013). Selective ablation of pillar and deiters' cells severely affects cochlear postnatal development and hearing in mice. *J. Neurosci.* 33, 1564–1576. doi: 10.1523/JNEUROSCI.3088-12.2013

Nelson, B. R., Matsuhashi, S., and Lefcort, F. (2002). Restricted neural epidermal growth factor-like like 2 (NELL2) expression during muscle and neuronal differentiation. *Mech. Dev.* 119(Suppl. 1), S11–S19. doi: 10.1016/S0925-4773(03)00084-4

Otte, J., Schunknecht, H. F., and Kerr, A. G. (1978). Ganglion cell populations in normal and pathological human cochleae. implications for cochlear implantation. *Laryngoscope* 88(8 Pt 1), 1231–1246. doi: 10.1288/00005537-197808000-00004

Pfingst, B. E., Colesa, D. J., Swiderski, D. L., Hughes, A. P., Strahl, S. B., Sinan, M., et al. (2017). Neurotrophin gene therapy in deafened ears with cochlear implants: long-term effects on nerve survival and functional measures. *J. Assoc. Res. Otolaryngol.* 18, 731–750. doi: 10.1007/s10162-017-0633-9

Pfingst, B. E., Hughes, A. P., Colesa, D. J., Watts, M. M., Strahl, S. B., and Raphael, Y. (2015a). Insertion trauma and recovery of function after cochlear implantation: Evidence from objective functional measures. *Hear. Res.* 330(Pt A), 98–105. doi: 10.1016/j.heares.2015.07.010

Pfingst, B. E., Zhou, N., Colesa, D. J., Watts, M. M., Strahl, S. B., Garadat, S. N., et al. (2015b). Importance of cochlear health for implant function. *Hear. Res.* 322, 77–88. doi: 10.1016/j.heares.2014.09.009

Pirvola, U., Hallbook, F., Xing-Qun, L., Virkkala, J., Saarma, M., and Ylikoski, J. (1997). Expression of neurotrophins and Trk receptors in the developing, adult, and regenerating avian cochlea. *J. Neurobiol.* 33, 1019–1033. doi: 10.1002/(SICI)1097-4695(199712)33:7<1019::AID-NEU11>3.0.CO;2-A

Pirvola, U., Ylikoski, J., Palgi, J., Lehtonen, E., Arumae, U., and Saarma, M. (1992). Brain-derived neurotrophic factor and neurotrophin 3 mRNAs in the peripheral target fields of developing inner ear ganglia. *Proc. Natl. Acad. Sci. U.S.A.* 89, 9915–9919. doi: 10.1073/pnas.89.20.9915

Ramakrishnan, N. A., Drescher, M. J., Khan, K. M., Hatfield, J. S., and Drescher, D. G. (2012). HCN1 and HCN2 proteins are expressed in cochlear hair cells: HCN1 can form a ternary complex with protocadherin 15 CD3 and F-actin-binding filamin A or can interact with HCN2. *J. Biol. Chem.* 287, 37628–37646. doi: 10.1074/jbc.M112.375832

Ramekers, D., Versnel, H., Strahl, S. B., Klis, S. F., and Grolman, W. (2015). Temporary neurotrophin treatment prevents deafness-induced auditory nerve degeneration and preserves function. *J. Neurosci.* 35, 12331–12345. doi: 10.1523/JNEUROSCI.0096-15.2015

Rio, C., Dikkes, P., Liberman, M. C., and Corfas, G. (2002). Glial fibrillary acidic protein expression and promoter activity in the inner ear of developing and adult mice. *J. Comp. Neurol.* 442, 156–162. doi: 10.1002/cne.10085

Sakagami, M. (2000). Role of osteopontin in the rodent inner ear as revealed by in situ hybridization. *Med. Electron. Microsci.* 33, 3–10. doi: 10.1007/s007950000001

Sandhya, V. K., Raju, R., Verma, R., Advani, J., Sharma, R., Radhakrishnan, A., et al. (2013). A network map of BDNF/TRKB and BDNF/p75NTR signaling system. *J. Cell Commun. Signal.* 7, 301–307. doi: 10.1007/s12079-013-0200-z

Scheffer, D. I., Shen, J., Corey, D. P., and Chen, Z. Y. (2015). Gene expression by mouse inner ear hair cells during development. *J. Neurosci.* 35, 6366–6380. doi: 10.1523/JNEUROSCI.5126-14.2015

Schmitt, H., Roemer, A., Zeilinger, C., Salcher, R., Durisin, M., Staecker, H., et al. (2018). Heat shock proteins in human perilymph: implications for cochlear implantation. *Otol. Neurotol.* 39, 37–44. doi: 10.1097/MAO.0000000000001625

Schmitt, H. A., Pich, A., Schroder, A., Scheper, V., Lilli, G., Reuter, G., et al. (2017). Proteome analysis of human perilymph using an intraoperative sampling method. *J. Proteome Res.* 16, 1911–1923. doi: 10.1021/acs.jproteome.6b00986

Seyyedi, M., Viana, L. M., and Nadol, J. B. Jr. (2014). Within-subject comparison of word recognition and spiral ganglion cell count in bilateral cochlear implant recipients. *Otol. Neurotol.* 35, 1446–1450. doi: 10.1097/MAO.0000000000000443

Shearer, A. E., Eppsteiner, R. W., Frees, K., Tejani, V., Sloan-Heggen, C. M., Brown, C., et al. (2017).). Genetic variants in the peripheral auditory system significantly affect adult cochlear implant performance. *Hear. Res.* 348, 138–142. doi: 10.1016/j.heares.2017.02.008

Shearer, A. E., Hildebrand, M. S., and Smith, R. J. H. (1993). *Hereditary Hearing Loss and Deafness Overview.* Seattle, WA: University of Washington.

Singer, W., Panford-Walsh, R., and Knipper, M. (2014). The function of BDNF in the adult auditory system. *Neuropharmacology* 76(Pt C), 719–728. doi: 10.1016/j.neuropharm.2013.05.008

Spoendlin, H. (1975). Retrograde degeneration of the cochlear nerve. *Acta Otolaryngol.* 79, 266–275. doi: 10.3109/00016487509124683

Staecker, H., and Garnham, C. (2010). Neurotrophin therapy and cochlear implantation: translating animal models to human therapy. *Exp. Neurol.* 226, 1–5. doi: 10.1016/j.expneurol.2010.07.012

Terkelsen, O. B., Bock, E., and Mollgard, K. (1989). NCAM and Thy-1 in special sense organs of the developing mouse. *Anat. Embryol.* 179, 311–318. doi: 10.1007/BF00305057

Tong, Y., Sun, Y., Tian, X., Zhou, T., Wang, H., Zhang, T., et al. (2015). Phospholipid transfer protein (PLTP) deficiency accelerates memory dysfunction through altering amyloid precursor protein (APP) processing in a mouse model of Alzheimer's disease. *Hum. Mol. Genet.* 24, 5388–5403. doi: 10.1093/hmg/ddv262

UniProt Consortium (2015). UniProt: a hub for protein information. *Nucleic Acids Res.* 43, D204–D212. doi: 10.1093/nar/gku989

Wan, G., Gomez-Casati, M. E., Gigliello, A. R., Liberman, M. C., and Corfas, G. (2014). Neurotrophin-3 regulates ribbon synapse density in the cochlea and induces synapse regeneration after acoustic trauma. *eLife* 3:e03564. doi: 10.7554/eLife.03564

Wise, A. K., Tan, J., Wang, Y., Caruso, F., and Shepherd, R. K. (2016). Improved auditory nerve survival with nanoengineered supraparticles for neurotrophin delivery into the deafened cochlea. *PLoS One* 11:e0164867. doi: 10.1371/journal.pone.0164867

Zheng, F., Zhou, X., Moon, C., and Wang, H. (2012). Regulation of brain-derived neurotrophic factor expression in neurons. *Int. J. Physiol. Pathophysiol. Pharmacol.* 4, 188–200.

Zuccotti, A., Kuhn, S., Johnson, S. L., Franz, C., Singer, W., Hecker, D., et al. (2012). Lack of brain-derived neurotrophic factor hampers inner hair cell synapse physiology, but protects against noise-induced hearing loss. *J. Neurosci.* 32, 8545–8553. doi: 10.1523/JNEUROSCI.1247-12.2012

Correspondence between Cognitive and Audiological Evaluations among the Elderly: A Preliminary Report of an Audiological Screening Model of Subjects at Risk of Cognitive Decline with Slight to Moderate Hearing Loss

Alessandro Castiglione[1,2], Mariella Casa[3], Samanta Gallo[2], Flavia Sorrentino[2], Sonila Dhima[2], Dalila Cilia[1], Elisa Lovo[1], Marta Gambin[1], Maela Previato[1], Simone Colombo[1], Ezio Caserta[2], Flavia Gheller[1], Cristina Giacomelli[1], Silvia Montino[1], Federica Limongi[4], Davide Brotto[2], Carlo Gabelli[3], Patrizia Trevisi[1,2], Roberto Bovo[1,2] and Alessandro Martini[1,2]*

[1] Department of Neurosciences, University of Padua, Padua, Italy, [2] Complex Operative Unit of Otolaryngology, Hospital of Padua, Padua, Italy, [3] Regional Center for the Study and Treatment of the Aging Brain, Department of Internal Medicine, Padua, Italy, [4] Institute of Neuroscience, National Research Council, Padua, Italy

***Correspondence:**
Alessandro Castiglione
alessandro.castiglione@unipd.it

Epidemiological studies show increasing prevalence rates of cognitive decline and hearing loss with age, particularly after the age of 65 years. These conditions are reported to be associated, although conclusive evidence of causality and implications is lacking. Nevertheless, audiological and cognitive assessment among elderly people is a key target for comprehensive and multidisciplinary evaluation of the subject's frailty status. To evaluate the use of tools for identifying older adults at risk of hearing loss and cognitive decline and to compare skills and abilities in terms of hearing and cognitive performances between older adults and young subjects, we performed a prospective cross-sectional study using supraliminal auditory tests. The relationship between cognitive assessment results and audiometric results was investigated, and reference ranges for different ages or stages of disease were determined. Patients older than 65 years with different degrees of hearing function were enrolled. Each subject underwent an extensive audiological assessment, including tonal and speech audiometry, Italian Matrix Sentence Test, and speech audiometry with logatomes in quiet. Cognitive function was screened and then verified by experienced clinicians using the Montreal Cognitive Assessment Score, the Geriatric Depression Scale, and further investigations in some. One hundred twenty-three subjects were finally enrolled during 2016–2019: 103 were >65 years of age and 20 were younger participants (as controls). Cognitive functions showed a correlation with the audiological results in post-lingual hearing-impaired patients, in particular in those affected by slight to moderate hearing loss and aged more than 70 years. Audiological testing can thus be useful in clinical assessment and identification of patients at risk of cognitive impairment. The study was limited by its sample size (CI 95%; CL 10%), strict dependence on language, and hearing threshold. Further investigations should be conducted to confirm the reported results and to verify similar screening models.

Keywords: cognitive decline, hearing loss, Italian Matrix Sentence Test, logatomes, signal-to-noise ratio, slope, speech in noise, screening

INTRODUCTION

Aging is epidemiologically associated with increasing prevalence rates of hearing loss and cognitive decline (Lin et al., 2011a,b; Peracino and Pecorelli, 2016). This association has been widely reported in the literature since a study by Herbst and Humphrey (1980). Even if the rational implications are debated in the literature and a causal relationship remains far from being proven, the audiological and cognitive assessment among elderly still remains a key component of a comprehensive and multidisciplinary approach to determining potential frailty (Panza et al., 2015).

Interest in this topic (Thomson et al., 2017) has grown in the last decade mainly due to demographic and sociocultural changes (Homans et al., 2017; Limongi et al., 2017: Livingston et al., 2017; Rooth, 2017); difficulties in treating neurodegenerative disorders, which has led to increased research into modifiable risk factors (Kostoff et al., 2017; Vos et al., 2017); the potential effects of peripheral hearing loss (Lin et al., 2011b; Lin et al., 2013; Wayne and Johnsrude, 2015; Deal et al., 2017); and rehabilitative as well as economical roles of digital devices (such as hearing aids, cochlear implants, over-the-counter amplification products) (Jorgensen and Messersmith, 2015; Cosetti et al., 2016; Nguyen et al., 2017). Additionally, the growing use of new tests and technologies has globally promoted reassessment of cognitive functions (Shen et al., 2016). The clinical distinction between central and peripheral hearing loss facilitates estimation of different contribution rates (Parham and Kost, 2017), even if, in practice, it is very difficult to quantify the relative portions, especially among older adults. In fact, there are different types of hearing impairment, as well as different types of cognitive decline, and these can be differently correlated or respond differently to treatments.

Defining the specific role of audiology in this context is important, and it is necessary to assess, design tests, and determine range limits in aging populations. To this end, the signal-to-noise ratio (SNR) can be used to define different auditory conditions and it is a good candidate for evaluating the contribution of auditory status to high cognitive functions (Panza et al., 2015; Costa et al., 2016; Livingston et al., 2017; Parham and Kost, 2017; Thomson et al., 2017; Jayakody et al., 2018). The Italian Matrix Sentence Test allows adaptive examination and results in noise (Puglisi et al., 2015). In addition, in selected cases, use of logatomes can elucidate auditory functioning in attention and working memory (Muhler et al., 2009; Moradi et al., 2014; Schubotz et al., 2016).

Thus, we performed a prospective study with cross-sectional measurements to evaluate the use of those tools for identifying older adults affected by hearing impairment and at risk of cognitive decline. In addition, the study aims to contribute in establishing age-appropriate reference intervals of specific tools in different hearing and cognitive impairments.

MATERIALS AND METHODS

One hundred sixty-six subjects were screened for inclusion criteria in this study between 2016 and 2019: adults older than 65 years and native Italian speakers with or without hearing loss or cognitive decline were enrolled as cases. The control group consisted of 20 young students (10 females) (median age 21, range 18–42 years) with normal hearing. Younger adults were also included to normalize reference ranges for different ages and to estimate the statistical power, also by comparing with literature on the same topic.

Exclusion criteria were lack of cooperation, life-threatening diseases, psychotropic therapies, history of disabling cardiovascular diseases, ictus or other potential life-threatening conditions, myocardial infarction, transient ischemic attacks or stroke, familiarity of neurodegenerative processes, or in advanced stages of disease. Patients with a history or family history of neurodegenerative diseases were excluded to avoid the contribution of early-onset diseases, which typically have a genetic etiology (Giau et al., 2019). Additionally, adults with hearing aids or cochlear implants were also excluded to avoid interference of digital devices with the acoustic properties of the auditory stimuli, which could significantly modify the SNR (Gallo and Castiglione, 2019). Patients with hearing impairment of genetic origin and those with severe to profound hearing losses were also excluded. These exclusion criteria were comparable to those of previous reports of investigations of mild cognitive impairment (MCI) among the Italian population to yield homogeneous and comparable data for cutoff settings (Bovo et al., 2007; Conti et al., 2015; Santangelo et al., 2015).

Audiological Assessment

An audiological evaluation was carried out by clinicians and technicians with proven experience in the management of hearing loss. Testing included otoscopy, tonal and speech audiometry in quiet, using disyllabic words, the Italian Matrix Sentence Test (OLSA test), with an adaptive SNR (in dB) at which subjects can recognize 50% of the speech material in noise of 65 dB sound pressure level (SPL) in an open set with a frontal speaker (0 degrees) at 1 m distance and the slope in dB/% for speech discrimination in noise. The audiometric tests were randomly administered in a soundproof booth using the

Noah and Otosuite software with standardized Italian language acoustic materials provided by Otometrics (a division of Natus in Taasrup, Denmark) and HörTech (Oldenburg, Germany).

The following data were obtained in a quiet environment: (1) The pure tone average (PTA) value at 0.5, 1, 2, and 4 kHz, in dB HL (PTA dB HL); (2) the signal/speech recognition threshold (SRT), in dB SPL, at which subjects could identify 50% of disyllabic words; (3) speech audiometry with logatomes. The latter were phonetic units without meaning, which can have the following consonant–vowel construction: CVC, VCVC, CVCV. In the Italian language, these structures can be assimilated to form pseudo-words or words non-words and, in general, presented in the following form: VCV or VCVV. Each list used in the present study consisted of 10 randomly selected logatomes. The choice to use this type of speech audiometry aims to minimize the mnemonic effort of the subjects: the speech intelligibility tends to differ between logatomes and words because they are not supported by semantic and long-term memory (Pisoni, 1996; Chan and Alain, 2018). The average of the intrasubject differences has been estimated between 5 and 20% (in favor of words) of recognized signals, even in the best hearing conditions. To identify different groups and carry out statistical analysis, the difference (hereinafter Log. Diff.) between the maximum intelligibility score, in%, for familiar words and the maximum intelligibility score, in%, for logatomes (i.d. maximum speech score with words - maximum speech score with logatomes) was calculated, and the cutoff was arbitrarily set to 10%, as suggested by a previous report (Moradi et al., 2014) to identify subjects potentially out of reference ranges. This allowed correlation among the Log. Diff. and attention or working memory, particularly if this was difficult among older adults (Santangelo et al., 2015). As mentioned before, the difference in percentage of identification of logatomes and words can be set within 10%, at the maximum comfortable level of acoustic signal in dB SPL for normal-hearing adults without cognitive decline. Thus, the maximum speech discrimination score for disyllabic words in a quiet environment is very close to that for logatomes in quiet, independent of differences in intensity levels. Therefore, the difference in a quiet environment should be less than 10%, even at different dB levels (Moradi et al., 2014).

The OLSA test (HörTech) is a versatile examination that is essentially structured into 20 randomized lists of five-word sentences (Houben et al., 2014), semantically unpredictable and administered after a training session to minimize the learning curve. The test can be useful in evaluating a wide range of conditions and treatments: congenital hearing loss, presbycusis, neuropathies, and auditory rehabilitation with hearing aids or cochlear implants. The test yields three main measurements: (1) the SNR, in dB, at which the subject recognizes 50% of the presented words, even if in different sentences (SNR-SRT); (2) the slope of the discrimination function at SRT (Slope) in percentage (%/dB); and (3) the intelligibility percentage score, in terms of estimated accuracy in understanding whole sentences. The global test in itself is an automated version of the synthetic sentence test, termed the synthetic sentences identification test (SSI) (King-Smith and Rose, 1997; Kaernbach, 2001; Buss et al., 2009; MacPherson and Akeroyd, 2014; Kollmeier, 2015). The novelty and the strength of the test are the speech noise material, with features inspired by ICRA noise, and its simplicity in performing adaptive exams (Dreschler et al., 2001; Wagener et al., 2006; Meister et al., 2013; Akeroyd et al., 2015). Reviewing reference ranges and standard deviations for the Italian language of the OLSA test, published by Puglisi et al. (2015), allowed determination of different levels to identify at-risk patients. The cutoff of the SNR dB (SRT) among the elderly was set to - 0.4 dB based on a reference mean level of −6.7 plus 9 standard deviations (3 SDs include 100% of samples divided by age). Thus, older adults are 6–12 SDs away from normal hearing and hearing in a younger population; the slope cutoff was set to 9.4% (reference level of 13.3% minus 3 SDs) (Puglisi et al., 2015). Audiological tests were conducted blinded to the cognitive status.

Cognitive Assessment

Subjects participated in a screening phase. Cognitive function was screened using the Montreal Cognitive Assessment (MoCA, adjusted for education) score: the presence of mild cognitive dysfunction was suspected when the final score was less than 26. Further clinical investigations were carried out by specialists in the management of dementia and cognitive decline (neuropsychologists and geriatricians). In addition, previous clinical data, including neuroimaging, and history available on digital archives were reviewed by medical doctors for definitive assessment. The evaluation was extended in selected cases to confirm screening results, and it included the forward and backward digit span test, drawing tests (clock, cube, house, pentagons), the trail-making test, the digit symbol substitution test, and the Direct Assessment of Functional Status (DAFS) for measuring Alzheimer's disease severity (Zanetti et al., 1998). The DAFS also helped in defining preservations of daily activities. The Geriatric Depression Scale (GDS) (30 items, long form) was used to screen depressive symptoms.

Mild cognitive decline was confirmed when daily activities were preserved, and cognitive decline was defined when these were compromised based on the diagnostic criteria reported in the literature and the DSM-V. Nevertheless, prior to further investigations and final diagnosis, patients were considered as only being at risk of, or likely to have MCI, because the screening model should be not considered diagnostic.

Participants with good cognitive performance and some degree of hearing loss (if any) in few frequencies, but without disabling hearing impairment, were defined healthy: this group was named the "healthy aging."

The cutoff MoCA score for risk of cognitive impairment has been varied (26, 24, 22) to verify differences in specificity and sensitivity (Davis et al., 2015). In addition, for further analysis, the scores for attention and working memory were set to 4.8 (<5) in the digit span test and MoCA (Moradi et al., 2014; Santangelo et al., 2015), whereas the long-term memory score was set to 2.80 (<3). These scores are the approximate normal/average reference values, reduced by 2 SDs (Moradi et al., 2014; Conti et al., 2015; Davis et al., 2015; Santangelo et al., 2015; Castiglione et al., 2016; Kujawski et al., 2018; Siciliano et al., 2019). Subjects with clinical indications were selected for hearing aid prescription, cochlear implantation surgery, or further cognitive investigations.

Statistical Analysis

Statistical analysis was performed through Microsoft Office Excel 2016 (Redmond, WA, United States) with data analysis plug-ins and MedCalc (Ostend, Belgium). The following tests were used: Student's *t*-test, Mann–Whitney test for independent samples (unpaired), Fisher's exact test and relative risk in 2 × 2 tables, analysis of variance (ANOVA), coefficient of Pearson correlation, and multiple regression analysis. Results were considered significant when $p < 0.01$.

Ethical Issues

This study was carried out in accordance with the recommendations of national and international guidelines. All subjects gave written informed consent in accordance with the Declaration of Helsinki. The protocol was approved by the local ethical committee of the University Hospital of Padua. The research was funded by the University of Padua, the Azienda Ospedaliera di Padova, Cochlear Italia Srl, and Amplifon SpA, as part of the main project PRIHTA-IDECO 2013, approved by the local ethics committee in 2016 (n° AO0379-0059267-CE3361/AO/14).

RESULTS

One hundred sixty-six subjects were included in this study between 2016 and 2019, at the clinic of Otorhinolaryngology of the University Hospital of Padua, as part of the PRIHTA-IDECO 2013 project. Forty-three subjects were excluded because of the degree of hearing loss: severe to profound hearing-impaired patients had a speech recognition score below 50%. The other 123 subjects were then divided into two groups: the cases included 103 subjects (51 females) older than 65 years (median age 71, range 65–93 years). The control group consisted of 20 young students with normal hearing (10 females, median age 21, range 18–42 years). Hearing loss among the cases was classified according to the criteria of the World Health Organization. Among the cases were identified 17 (16.50%) subjects with normal hearing, 21 (20.40%) with slight loss of hearing, and 65 (63.10%) with mild to moderate hearing loss, of which four were with characteristics very close to severe losses. There is also a correlation between hearing loss and age and cognitive decline, so that subjects with better hearing and better cognitive performance are grouped in the age group between 65 and 70 years.

A summary of the characteristics of the cases and controls is given in **Table 1**. Distributions by PTA dB HL, age, and MoCA scores are reported in **Table 2**. No differences were found between the left and the right ear, even if the right ear showed slight advantages in discrimination probably due to interhemispheric dominance ($p > 0.05$). The control group allowed normal range adjustment for testing among the elderly and confirmed the feasibility of the test in different audiological and cognitive conditions.

As expected, significant differences were found between cases and controls in all variables, except for sex. Significant differences were also shown between patients with signs of MCI and those with normal cognitive function in terms of PTA, speech in noise, and the slope of psychometric functions. However, in the present study, GDS results are not significant. Among cases, two subgroups were defined: the healthy aging subgroup with a MoCA score > 26, adjusted for education, without signs of decline in cognitive tests or neuroradiological findings, and the MCI subgroup, identified as individuals at risk of MCI through the MoCA test (**Table 3**), and defined by cognitive scores < 26 adjusted for education (Conti et al., 2015). To give comparable results, *t*-tests and Mann–Whitney tests are reported, as many variables can be considered non-parametric, even when values appear parametric; nevertheless, there were no differences between the groups for either test at $\alpha = 0.01$ (**Table 3**).

Comparison of the three groups revealed significant differences, with increasing *p*-value from CONTROLS to MCI patients. ANOVA revealed significant differences among these two groups ($p < 0.001$), and the results are reported in **Figure 1**.

The study of correlation revealed a moderate to strong coefficient between SNR and MoCA scores. Other correlations and multiple regression analysis are shown in **Table 4**. Age showed the highest negative correlation with cognitive results, but it should be noticed that groups were arbitrarily divided by age and that the MoCA scores were adjusted for years of education. Thus, in higher age groups, the MoCA score could be adjusted for age because after 78 years, participants were unlikely to have been attending educational and recreative programs during childhood, as compared to the new 65-year-old subjects of coming decades (Kujawski et al., 2018). Nevertheless, it should be noticed that the SNR showed the highest negative correlation among the audiological testing results and that the multiple regression analysis reached an R^2 of 0.477. These results suggested a strong correlation with cognitive impairment particularly when the variables were considered together. It could be hypothesized that the cognitive results and the audiological tests, when considered together, can explain approximately 50% of the final score (and its variance) obtained for each subject.

In **Tables 5, 6**, we show the different sensitivity and specificity values for identifying different levels of cognitive impairment. The associated receiver operating characteristic (ROC) curves are illustrated in **Supplementary Figure S1**. The ROC curves show the predictive results of the screening model at various cutoff values. Different ROC curves are shown to compare sensitivity and specificity of different variables for identifying patients with cognitive decline, as represented by a MoCA score < 26 and subsequent confirmed diagnosis of MCI. The SNR reaches highest rates of sensitivity and specificity (**Supplementary Figure S1**). This curve allows intuitive prediction of the sensitivity and specificity of a test for any value obtainable from the test; various tests are also compared to assess which one has the best chance of identifying true positives and true negatives. The audiological evaluation is comparable to those attributed to the MoCA test. Age had suitable characteristics but a lower specificity. These data can only be considered preliminary as a possible screening model that can promote a multidisciplinary approach because the patient often does not know the origin of his own difficulty and may therefore seek help from various specialists. Given that this

TABLE 1 | Major clinical findings in the control group (young adults with normal hearing) and older adults (>65 years, with normal to moderate hearing impairment).

			Controls: 20 (10 F)			*P value*	Cases: 103 (51 F)		
			Mean	**Median**	***SD***	***t*-test**	**Mean**	**Median**	***SD***
		Age (years)	23.20	21	6.22	*<0.001*	72.62	71	7.03
Hearing		PTA dB HL	8.87	10	4.33	***<0.001***	32.77	33.75	15.26
		SRT	13.50	15	5.20	***<0.001***	36.41	35	15.49
		SNR	−6.88	−6.75	0.96	***<0.001***	1.42	−0.3	6.71
		Slope in Noise	15.03	16	4.53	***<0.001***	10.76	10	4.18
		Intelligibility in noise (% of S.I.)	55.48	56	2.9	***<0.001***	50.13	52	7.73
		Logatomes (difference in%)	3.00	2.5	3.35	***<0.001***	11.31	10	12.43
Cognition	MoCA	Tot. MoCA (score)	29.70	30	0.66	***<0.001***	25.15	26	3.89
		Attention and Working Memory	5.80	6	0.41	***<0.001***	4.83	5.00	1.56
		Long-term memory	4.35	4.00	0.67	***<0.001***	2.61	3.00	1.80

F, females; MoCA, Montreal Cognitive Assessment; S.I., Intelligibility (%) of sentences and words in noise around the SNR value; SNR, signal-to-noise ratio; SRT, speech/signal recognition threshold; SD, standard deviation. Bolded values indicate significant results.

TABLE 2 | Age distribution of hearing and cognitive results.

Age (years)	*18–45 (age in years)*	*65–69 (age in years)*	*70–79 (age in years)*	*>79 (age in years)*
n°(of cases)	**20**	**39**	**44**	**20**
MoCA (score)	29.7	27.41	25.15	20.75
Slope (%)	17.3	12.8	10.65	6.95
SNR (dB)	−7	−1.5	1.75	7.89
Intelligibility in Noise (%)	57.9	53	51.25	41.65
PTA (0.5-1-2-4-kHz)	8.62	26.82	33.15	43.5
SRT (%)	9	30.9	36.02	48
Log. Diff. (%)	3	5.5	11.53	22.12
GDS (score)	n.a.	5.48	5.09	5.05
Long Term Memory (score)	4.5	3.8	2.6	2
Attention (score)	5.8	5.8	5.2	3.5
Log Intelligibility (%)	97	77.14	80.6	57.5
MCI (n° of Cases)	0	6	21	17

MoCA, Montreal Cognitive Assessment score (mean); Slope, percentage (mean); SNR, signal-to-noise ratio in dB (mean); S.I., sentence intelligibility in noise, percentage of correct sentences and words (mean); PTA, pure tone average at 500, 1,000, 2,000, and 4,000 Hz (mean in dB HL); SRT, speech/signal recognition threshold, mean in dB SPL of thresholds required to recognize 50% of words in quiet; Log. Diff., difference in% between words intelligibility and logatomes intelligibility (mean); GDS, Geriatric Depression Scale (long form); Memory (long-term), mean of cognitive tests; attention, mean of cognitive tests; MCI, mild cognitive impairment (number of diagnosis for each group); n.a., not applicable. Bolded values indicate significant results.

is proposed as a screening model, high sensitivity is crucial, but subsequent diagnostic confirmation is required.

As mentioned before, the cases were subsequently divided into two subgroups to compare auditory and cognitive functions. In 59 cases, participants were healthy, with good cognitive performance and some degree of hearing loss (if any), but without disabling hearing impairment; this group was named the healthy aging. In contrast, 44 participants were classified as at risk of MCI, showing signs of cognitive impairment. Further cognitive test results and neuroimaging (when possible or indicated) were used to confirm the MoCA results indicative of MCI. Eight of these 44 patients (18.18%) were affected by early-stage vascular cognitive impairment with suggestive neuroradiological findings, 22 (38%) showed memory impairment in multiple domains on cognitive tests, and 14 (38%) were initially classified as having an uncertain or borderline diagnosis (**Table 3**) because of inconclusive diagnostic results or incongruent findings. Eight of the 44 patients (18.18%) were subsequently correctly reevaluated, and MCI in multiple non-amnestic domains was confirmed (**Supplementary Table S1**). The remaining four patients were designated as patients with MCI affecting multiple amnestic domains. Thus, 63.64% (28 of 44) of the screened populations were defined as having amnestic multiple domain MCI, agreeing with reports in the literature. Among the healthy aging group, 9 (of 59) subjects were reevaluated because of inconclusive results probably related to transient anxiety or low attention in performing the test or because they were too fatigued to complete the investigations. Therefore, finally, 23 (of 103) patients required reinterpretation and reanalysis of results.

The relative risk and two-tailed Fisher's exact test for different clinical settings and cutoff values are presented in 2 × 2 tables in **Supplementary Material** (**Supplementary Table S1**).

DISCUSSION

In this preliminary study, we found a significant correlation between cognitive scores and SNR, slope, and logatome intelligibility. Even if the MoCA tests should be considered purely indicative and not diagnostic, the results were verified by clinicians experienced in the management of neurodegenerative processes affecting high cognitive functions. To verify the feasibility of a screening model involving audiological tests, the MoCA score was chosen as representative of real-life cognition. Audiological tests were conducted blinded to the cognitive status, and the results were found to correlate statistically significantly. Using these quantitative and semiquantitative parameters, auditory functioning could be assessed, and the risk

TABLE 3 | Comparisons between the healthy aging group and subjects with or at risk of mild cognitive impairment (MCI).

			103 Cases (51 F)						
			At risk of MCI						
			59 Cases (37 F)				44 Cases (14 F)		
			Healthy aging				MCI* (screened by MoCA)		
			Mean	***Median***	***SD***	***p-value***	***Mean***	***Median***	***SD***
		Age	69.34	68	5.61	***<0.001***	76.95	78	6.44
Hearing		PTA dB HL	27.53	23.75	18.41	***<0.001***	49.52	41.25	19.61
		SRT	25.23	25	10.89	***<0.001***	47.30	45	17.75
		SNR dB (SRT)	−0.83	−3.0	6.07	***<0.001***	4.56	2.9	6.49
		Slope in Noise	12.43	12	3.84	***<0.001***	8.67	8	3.98
		Intelligibility in noise	52.65	54	6.26	***<0.001***	46.51	48.5	8.81
		Logatomes (difference in%)	6.16	0	9.97	***<0.001***	18.78	15	13.23
Cognition	MoCA	Tot. MoCA (score)	27.74	28	1.29	***<0.001***	21.67	22	3.54
		Attention and Working Memory	5.70	6	0.57	***<0.001***	3.44	4	1.59
		Long-term memory	3.3	4	1.48	***=0.001***	1.47	1	1.68
	GDS		5.22	4	3.39	***N.S. (p = 0.8)***	5.28	4	4.34

**F*, females; MCI, mild cognitive impairment as determined by Montreal Cognitive Assessment (MoCA) scores and confirmed with subsequent investigations by specialists; PTA dB HL, The average of pure tone audiometry around the most important frequencies for speech understanding, that is, 500, 1,000, 2,000, and 4,000 Hz. The p-values are obtained by Student's t-test and the Mann–Whitney test in case of non-parametric variables; GDS, 30-item geriatric depression scale; N.S., not significant; SD, standard deviation. Bolded values indicate significant results.*

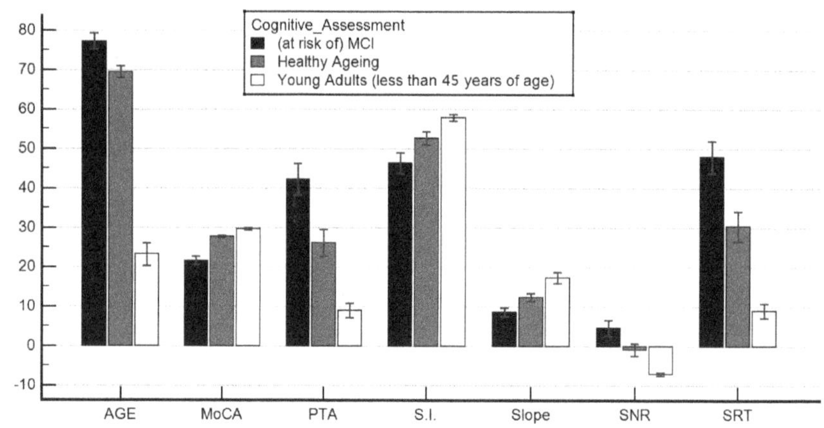

FIGURE 1 | Significant differences among the healthy aging group and the at-risk mild cognitive impairment (MCI) group. This graph shows an analysis of variance for parametric and non-parametric variables. All comparisons were significant; thus, the groups identified through the Montreal Cognitive Assessment (MoCA) test (healthy aging and at risk of MCI) were in fact distinct. They also differed significantly in terms of their audiological profile, although they were not differentiated on the basis of their hearing ability. Healthy aging individuals were also statistically distinct from younger subjects. This suggests cognitive and auditory difficulty/fatigability that physiologically accompanies advancing years. These data, already reported in the literature, were not documented by audiometric comparisons that allow determination of whether loss is paraphysiological. In this way, a healthy aging subject is clearly defined with certain audiometric characteristics: (1) the ability to recognize a signal with a signal-to-noise ratio (SNR) < 0; (2) the pure tone audiometry of less than 30 dB HL; (3) an SRT at rest of less than or equal to 30 dB SPL; (4) a difference between max% words in quiet and logatomes of less than 10; and (5) a slope of psychometric function of greater than 10%. S.I., speech intelligibility in noise. See also **Tables 1–4**.

for cognitive decline can be suspected for further investigations in selected patients. In addition, it is possible to define a reference area or zone, delineated by all of these measures, including individuals with similar characteristics (**Figure 2**). In other words, patients at risk of developing cognitive decline can suffer from a reduced ability to cope with living in a noisy world (auditory frailty). This disadvantage points to the type of rehabilitative action that might reduce the risk of cognitive decline or frailty. The tests might define different contributions to cognitive fatigue by peripheral and central hearing losses, at different ages, thus reflecting a more realistic pattern for longitudinal studies. Even if all tests require cortical efficient functioning, it can be hypothesized that tonal audiometry is one of the simplest tests that a patient can actively perform,

TABLE 4 | Regression analysis and coefficient of correlation of the Montreal Cognitive Assessment (MoCA) score with audiological results.

	Age	*Slope*	*SNR*	*S.I.*	*PTA*	*SRT*	*Log. Diff.*
Coeff. Corr.	−0.670	0.521	−0.544	0.563	−0.469	−0.472	−0.442
R^2	0.449	0.272	0.296	0.317	0.220	0.223	0.195
p_{value}	<0.001	<0.001	<0.001	<0.001	<0.001	<0.001	<0.001
				Multiple Regression (Dependent Y MoCA)			
R^2 adjusted	**Multiple corr. coeff.**	**F-ratio**			**P-value**		
0.477	0.716	14.287			**<0.0001**		

PTA, pure tone average; S.I., sentence intelligibility in noise; SNR, signal-to-noise ratio; SRT, speech/signal recognition threshold; Log. Diff., different discrimination percentages between logatomes and words. Bolded values indicate significant results.

TABLE 5 | Sensitivity and specificity of different audiological results for identifying cognitive impairment.

		MCI			
	TP	**FP**	**TN**	**FN**	**tot**
SNR ≥ -0.4 dB	36	18	41	8	103
Slope ≤ 9.4%	26	9	50	18	103
Logatomes ≥ 10%	38	20	39	6	103
	SNR ≥ -0.4 dB	**≤ 9.4%**	**Log. Diff. ≥ 10%**		
Sens.	0.818	0.743	0.864		
Spec.	0.695	0.735	0.661		

MCI, mild cognitive impairment; Spec, specificity; Sens, sensitivity; SNR, signal-to-noise ratio; tot, total; TP, true positive; FP, false positive; TN, true negative; FN, false negative.

TABLE 6 | Combining Log.Diff.-Slope-SNR (passing two or three criteria for the screening model) increases sensitivity and specificity of audiological screening.

		MCI < 26			
	TP	**FP**	**TN**	**FN**	**tot**
	35	15	44	9	103
	SNR ≥ -0,4 dB AND/OR Slope ≤ 9.4% AND/OR Logatomes Diff. ≥ 10%			***CI 95%***	
Sens.		0.795		0.647–0.902	
Spec.		0.746		0.616–0.850	

Logatomes Diff., the difference in terms of percentage of recognized words/logatomes among the maximum achievable scores in speech audiometry in quiet and the maximum achievable score in logatome audiometry in a quiet environment; MCI, mild cognitive impairment; SNR, signal-to-noise ratio; Sens, sensitivity; Spec, specificity, tot, total; TP, true positive; FP, false positive; TN, true negative; FN, false negative.

and, consequently, it entails poor perceptual involvement of the central neuronal stations. Conversely, progressive involvement of cortical structures is more evident in speech discrimination and in sentence discrimination in noise.

Due to the correlation between hearing loss, aging, and cognitive decline, the results also reflect a pattern of involution, thus the screening model is more congruent for patients with slight to moderate hearing loss among 65–75 years of age (**Table 1**). These results could suggest different contributions of peripheral and central hearing loss to global cognitive functions during aging, and it should suggest range limits for treatments to restore hearing function with hearing aids or cochlear implants.

In the last decade, there has been a great deal of interest in and discussion about the relationship between cognitive decline and hearing loss (Lin et al., 2013; Bernabei et al., 2014; Wayne and Johnsrude, 2015; Hewitt, 2017; Rutherford et al., 2018; Stern and Hilly, 2018; Uchida et al., 2018). Studies on the aging brain have shown that cognitive functions tend to (para-)physiologically decline with advancing years (Ciorba et al., 2011; Ding et al., 2016). In addition, 14.3% of the population over 65 years of age is affected by central auditory processing disorders (CAPD). Older individuals with CAPD seem to be more likely to suffer from dementia than those who are not affected (Martini et al., 2014; Fortunato et al., 2016). The decline can be highlighted in circumstances requiring greater cognitive effort and stressful conditions, such as speech discrimination of words or logatomes in noise or in quiet (Martini et al., 1988; Strauss et al., 2015; Gobara et al., 2016; Taitelbaum-Swead and Fostick, 2016; Bae et al., 2018). Competitive stimuli should be the most sensitive for detecting cognitive efforts or difficulties among elderly people (Pronk et al., 2013). The SNR is a well-known semiquantitative, a parameter, which is useful in the audiological assessment of various conditions of clinical interest, although its role in evaluating cognitive functions is less clear (Pronk et al., 2013; Helfer, 2015; Meister, 2017).

Young subjects have better discrimination than individuals older than 65 years. Furthermore, the use of logatomes can help identify patients with preserved long-term and semantic memory, even though they are at risk of cognitive decline because of impairments in attention and working memory. When semantic content is lacking, speech discrimination requires additional cognitive effort, and subjects with better working memory capacity demonstrate superior performance in the identification of the speech signals (Kim and Oh, 2013). This has been confirmed by neuroimaging studies that show the involvement of both the prefrontal and auditory cortex for the correct identification of ambiguous phonemes (Moradi et al., 2014). In addition, confusion matrices among logatomes (AFA/ATA/ASA, AGIA) can detect some types of cognitive

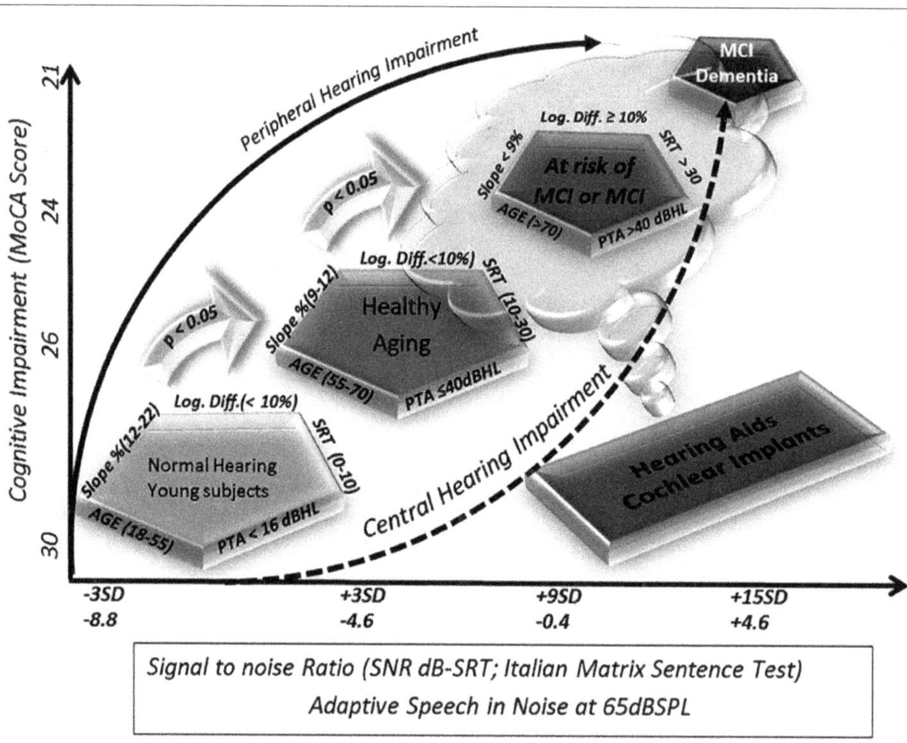

FIGURE 2 | Schematic representation of cognitive decline as defined by different audiological tests. The diagrams summarize the present study. On the *y*-axis, the results of the Montreal Cognitive Assessment (MoCA) score are shown as the average result of the groups shown in the figure as pentagons (ideally defined by five variables, four audiological parameters plus age). On the *x*-axis, there are reference levels for the signal-to-noise ratio (SNR) available in the literature, such as a test for matrices with speech in noise sentences. The test was recently chosen for diffusion in clinical practice in Europe for its easy automatic execution and because it yields easily comparable values regardless of age and language. Starting from the available and official reference levels, and moving in steps of 3 standard deviations, so as to include 100% of the study population, it was possible to identify four different populations, which will by definition be statistically significantly different. The groups used in this study fall exactly within those theoretical values: young subjects, elderly but healthy subjects, and elderly subjects suffering from mild cognitive decline either because they were diagnosed or because they are rated using cognitive tests, and finally, at the opposite extreme, patients suffering from dementia who were so severely affected that they were not able to complete the tests.

disorders among children (Sundstrom et al., 2018), although their role in the audiological and cognitive assessment among older adults is not as clear (Chen and Cowan, 2009). Even if hearing-impaired patients show some disadvantages in speech recognition, the intrasubject differences in identifying words and pseudo-words should be in the 5–20% range (10% $\pm$ 2 standard deviation) at the maximum comfortable level of stimulation in dB SPL (Carrat and Carrat, 1992; Apoux et al., 2001; Moradi et al., 2014; Schubotz et al., 2016). Speech audiometry with logatomes might allow identification of those patients who fall outside of this range (**Tables 5, 6**).

Even if it is not routinely performed, such extensive audiological assessment, including SNR, slope of functions, and logatomes, after 55 years of age might help in identifying patients at risk of cognitive decline prior to 65 years of age in the general population.

Nonetheless, due to the limitations of the present study, this report should be considered a tentative preliminary model of auditory screening in the elderly, which must be confirmed in further studies. To the best of our knowledge, reported results and cutoffs should be considered only among older adults with post-lingual mild to moderate hearing loss, and results are more consistent for people between 65 and 75 years of age. These subjects could take advantages from auditory rehabilitation through hearing aids for moderate hearing losses and cochlear implant for severe to profound hearing losses. Unfortunately, patients with severe to profound hearing loss presented limitations in performing all tests, therefore they required specific settings for subsequent investigations, and they were not comparable to elderly patients with better conditions. Consequently, specific populations, such as severe to profound hearing-impaired patients or subjects with cochlear implants and/or hearing aids, require different range references. Furthermore, protocol testing could be time-consuming especially in untrained centers, or among impaired elderly, thus the screening model might be unsustainable in routine or clinical practice. In addition, the fatigue of older adults might be a bias in the final assessment.

CONCLUSION

In conclusion, our study highlights that, in the elderly, audiological assessment by means of SNR, slope of functions, and logatomes might help in further characterization of selected patients because of their correlation with age, high cognitive functions, and hearing loss. These tests might be helpful not only in the detection of hearing loss but also in early identification of the impairment of high cognitive functions. We also suggest that a stricter relation between audiological and neuropsychological assessment of selected patients should be established, and rehabilitation might benefit from such a comprehensive multidisciplinary approach.

Furthermore, our findings indicate that specific audiological results are representative of cognitive functions during aging, following an irregular progression, in part because they can be assimilated into cognitive tests and involve instructions, training, attention, time, accuracy, and cooperation. A mixed contribution of peripheral and central hearing impairment is involved in real life; nevertheless, these impairments contribute differentially during different stages of life. Irrespective of the causative explanation, hearing impairment presents disadvantages at any stage of life and can affect cognition as well as quality of life, increasing the frailty of subjects. Cognitive assessments should be accompanied by auditory testing.

It is important to remark limitations of the present research, thus there are no conclusive evidences on this topic and further investigations are required.

AUTHOR CONTRIBUTIONS

AC supervised the all tests, collected the data, performed the statistical analysis, wrote the main part of the manuscript, and designed the figures and tables. MC helped in the audiological and cognitive assessment, collected the clinical data, and conducted the cognitive tests. SG and MG conducted the literature review, planned part of the work, and wrote part of the manuscript. EL, DC, FS, FG, EC, SG, SC, MP, and SD performed the audiological tests and collected the data. RB, PT, DB, FL, and CGa provided supervision and consultancy on clinical, audiological, and neuroimaging findings. SM and CGi assessed cognitive-communication deficits. AM is the principal investigator of the PRIHTA-IDECO 2013 project and supervised all of the steps of the research.

ACKNOWLEDGMENTS

We would like to thank all participants, colleagues, and technicians who helped in gathering the information presented in this manuscript. We are particularly grateful to the nurses, the students, and the residents who provided support for the research activities. We also thank Cochlear Italia Srl and Amplifon SpA for technical and logistic assistance. The Italian matrix sentence test was provided by MED-EL Italia and GN Hearing Srl (Natus Medical Srl).

SUPPLEMENTARY MATERIAL

FIGURE S1 | Different receiver operating characteristic curves are shown, to compare sensitivity and specificity of different variables for identifying patients with cognitive decline, as represented by a Montreal Cognitive Assessment (MoCA) score < 26.

TABLE S1 | Twenty-three patients with uncertain results were analyzed through the Fisher Exact Test to estimate the identification rate and relative risk of impairment in attention and working memory using logatomes.

REFERENCES

Akeroyd, M. A., Arlinger, S., Bentler, R. A., Boothroyd, A., Dillier, N., Dreschler, W. A., et al. (2015). International collegium of rehabilitative audiology (ICRA) recommendations for the construction of multilingual speech tests. ICRA working group on multilingual speech tests. *Int. J. Audiol.* 54(Suppl. 2), 17–22. doi: 10.3109/14992027.2015.1030513

Apoux, F., Crouzet, O., and Lorenzi, C. (2001). Temporal envelope expansion of speech in noise for normal-hearing and hearing-impaired listeners: effects on identification performance and response times. *Hear. Res.* 153, 123–131. doi: 10.1016/s0378-5955(00)00265-3

Bae, S., Lee, S., Lee, S., Jung, S., Makino, K., Park, H., et al. (2018). The role of social frailty in explaining the association between hearing problems and mild cognitive impairment in older adults. *Arch. Gerontol. Geriatr.* 78, 45–50. doi: 10.1016/j.archger.2018.05.025

Bernabei, R., Bonuccelli, U., Maggi, S., Marengoni, A., Martini, A., Memo, M., et al. (2014). Hearing loss and cognitive decline in older adults: questions and answers. *Aging Clin. Exp. Res.* 26, 567–573. doi: 10.1007/s40520-014-0266-3

Bovo, R., Ortore, R., Ciorba, A., Berto, A., and Martini, A. (2007). Bilateral sudden profound hearing loss and vertigo as a unique manifestation of bilateral symmetric inferior pontine infarctions. *Ann. Otol. Rhinol. Laryngol.* 116, 407–410. doi: 10.1177/000348940711600603

Buss, E., Hall, J. W., and Grose, J. H. (2009). Psychometric functions for pure tone intensity discrimination: slope differences in school-aged children and adults. *J. Acoust. Soc. Am.* 125, 1050–1058. doi: 10.1121/1.3050273

Carrat, R., and Carrat, X. (1992). [Vocal audiometry: the "phonatome" recognition test. Principle, technique, initial results]. *Rev. Laryngol. Otol Rhinol.* 113, 347–353.

Castiglione, A., Benatti, A., Velardita, C., Favaro, D., Padoan, E., Severi, D., et al. (2016). Aging, cognitive decline and hearing loss: effects of auditory rehabilitation and training with hearing aids and cochlear implants on cognitive function and depression among older adults. *Audiol. Neurootol.* 21(Suppl. 1), 21–28. doi: 10.1159/000448350

Chan, T. M. V., and Alain, C. (2018). Listening back in time: does attention to memory facilitate word-in-noise identification? *Atten. Percept. Psychophys.* 81, 253–269. doi: 10.3758/s13414-018-1586-8

Chen, Z., and Cowan, N. (2009). How verbal memory loads consume attention. *Mem. Cognit.* 37, 829–836. doi: 10.3758/MC.37.6.829

Ciorba, A., Benatti, A., Bianchini, C., Aimoni, C., Volpato, S., Bovo, R., et al. (2011). High frequency hearing loss in the elderly: effect of age and noise exposure in an Italian group. *J. Laryngol. Otol.* 125, 776–780. doi: 10.1017/S0022215111001101

Conti, S., Bonazzi, S., Laiacona, M., Masina, M., and Coralli, M. V. (2015). Montreal cognitive assessment (MoCA)-Italian version: regression based norms and equivalent scores. *Neurol. Sci.* 36, 209–214. doi: 10.1007/s10072-014-1921-3

Cosetti, M. K., Pinkston, J. B., Flores, J. M., Friedmann, D. R., Jones, C. B., Roland, J. T., et al. (2016). Neurocognitive testing and cochlear implantation: insights into performance in older adults. *Clin. Interv. Aging* 11, 603–613. doi: 10.2147/CIA.S100255

Costa, M., Lepore, F., Prevost, F., and Guillemot, J. P. (2016). Effects of aging on peripheral and central auditory processing in rats. *Eur. J. Neurosci.* 44, 2084–2094. doi: 10.1111/ejn.13302

Davis, D. H., Creavin, S. T., Yip, J. L., Noel-Storr, A. H., Brayne, C., and Cullum, S. (2015). Montreal Cognitive Assessment for the diagnosis of Alzheimer's disease and other dementias. *Cochrane Database Syst. Rev.* 10:CD010775. doi: 10.1002/14651858.CD010775.pub2

Deal, J. A., Betz, J., Yaffe, K., Harris, T., Purchase-Helzner, E., Satterfield, S., et al. (2017). Hearing impairment and incident dementia and cognitive decline in older adults: the health ABC study. *J. Gerontol. A Biol. Sci. Med. Sci.* 72, 703–709. doi: 10.1093/gerona/glw069

Ding, X. Q., Maudsley, A. A., Sabati, M., Sheriff, S., Schmitz, B., Schutze, M., et al. (2016). Physiological neuronal decline in healthy aging human brain - An in vivo study with MRI and short echo-time whole-brain (1)H MR spectroscopic imaging. *Neuroimage* 137, 45–51. doi: 10.1016/j.neuroimage.2016.05.014

Dreschler, W. A., Verschuure, H., Ludvigsen, C., and Westermann, S. (2001). ICRA noises: artificial noise signals with speech-like spectral and temporal properties for hearing instrument assessment. International collegium for rehabilitative audiology. *Audiology* 40, 148–157. doi: 10.3109/00206090109073110

Fortunato, S., Forli, F., Guglielmi, V., De Corso, E., Paludetti, G., Berrettini, S., et al. (2016). A review of new insights on the association between hearing loss and cognitive decline in ageing. *Acta Otorhinolaryngol. Ital.* 36, 155–166. doi: 10.14639/0392-100X-993

Gallo, S., and Castiglione, A. (2019). The signal to noise ratio assessment in cochlear implanted patients through the Italian Matrix Sentence Test (Oldenburg Test). *Hearing Balance Commun.* 17, 145–148. doi: 10.1080/21695717.2019.1603949

Giau, V. V., Senanarong, V., Bagyinszky, E., An, S. S. A., and Kim, S. (2019). Analysis of 50 neurodegenerative genes in clinically diagnosed early-onset alzheimer's disease. *Int. J. Mol. Sci.* 20:E1514. doi: 10.3390/ijms20061514

Gobara, A., Yamada, Y., and Miura, K. (2016). Crossmodal modulation of spatial localization by mimetic words. *Iperception* 7:2041669516684244.

Helfer, K. S. (2015). Competing speech perception in middle age. *Am. J. Audiol.* 24, 80–83. doi: 10.1044/2015_AJA-14-0056

Herbst, K. G., and Humphrey, C. (1980). Hearing impairment and mental state in the elderly living at home. *Br. Med. J.* 281, 903–905. doi: 10.1136/bmj.281.6245.903

Hewitt, D. (2017). Age-related hearing loss and cognitive decline: you haven't heard the half of it. *Front. Aging Neurosci.* 9:112. doi: 10.3389/fnagi.2017.00112

Homans, N. C., Metselaar, R. M., Dingemanse, J. G., Van Der Schroeff, M. P., Brocaar, M. P., Wieringa, M. H., et al. (2017). Prevalence of age-related hearing loss, including sex differences, in older adults in a large cohort study. *Laryngoscope* 127, 725–730. doi: 10.1002/lary.26150

Houben, R., Koopman, J., Luts, H., Wagener, K. C., Van Wieringen, A., Verschuure, H., et al. (2014). Development of a Dutch matrix sentence test to assess speech intelligibility in noise. *Int. J. Audiol.* 53, 760–763. doi: 10.3109/14992027.2014.920111

Jayakody, D. M. P., Friedland, P. L., Martins, R. N., and Sohrabi, H. R. (2018). Impact of aging on the auditory system and related cognitive functions: a narrative review. *Front. Neurosci.* 12:125. doi: 10.3389/fnins.2018.00125

Jorgensen, L. E., and Messersmith, J. J. (2015). Impact of aging and cognition on hearing assistive technology use. *Semin. Hear.* 36, 162–174. doi: 10.1055/s-0035-1555119

Kaernbach, C. (2001). Slope bias of psychometric functions derived from adaptive data. *Percept. Psychophys.* 63, 1389–1398. doi: 10.3758/bf03194550

Kim, B. J., and Oh, S. H. (2013). Age-related changes in cognition and speech perception. *Korean J. Audiol.* 17, 54–58. doi: 10.7874/kja.2013.17.2.54

King-Smith, P. E., and Rose, D. (1997). Principles of an adaptive method for measuring the slope of the psychometric function. *Vis. Res.* 37, 1595–1604. doi: 10.1016/s0042-6989(96)00310-0

Kollmeier, B. (2015). Overcoming language barriers: matrix sentence tests with closed speech corpora. *Int. J. Audiol.* 54, 1–2. doi: 10.3109/14992027.2015.1074295

Kostoff, R. N., Zhang, Y., Ma, J., Porter, A. L., and Buchtel, H. A. (2017). *Prevention and Reversal of Alzheimer's Disease.* Atlanta: Georgia Institute of Technology.

Kujawski, S., Kujawska, A., Gajos, M., Topka, W., Perkowski, R., Androsiuk-Perkowska, J., et al. (2018). Cognitive functioning in older people. Results of the first wave of cognition of older people, education, recreational activities, nutrition, comorbidities, functional capacity studies (COPERNICUS). *Front. Aging Neurosci.* 10:421. doi: 10.3389/fnagi.2018.00421

Limongi, F., Siviero, P., Noale, M., Gesmundo, A., Crepaldi, G., Maggi, S., et al. (2017). Prevalence and conversion to dementia of Mild Cognitive Impairment in an elderly Italian population. *Aging Clin. Exp. Res.* 29, 361–370. doi: 10.1007/s40520-017-0748-1

Lin, F. R., Metter, E. J., O'Brien, R. J., Resnick, S. M., Zonderman, A. B., and Ferrucci, L. (2011a). Hearing loss and incident dementia. *Arch. Neurol.* 68, 214–220. doi: 10.1001/archneurol.2010.362

Lin, F. R., Thorpe, R., Gordon-Salant, S., and Ferrucci, L. (2011b). Hearing loss prevalence and risk factors among older adults in the United States. *J. Gerontol. A Biol. Sci. Med. Sci.* 66, 582–590. doi: 10.1093/gerona/glr002

Lin, F. R., Yaffe, K., Xia, J., Xue, Q. L., Harris, T. B., Purchase-Helzner, E., et al. (2013). Hearing loss and cognitive decline in older adults. *JAMA Intern. Med.* 173, 293–299. doi: 10.1001/jamainternmed.2013.1868

Livingston, G., Sommerlad, A., Orgeta, V., Costafreda, S. G., Huntley, J., Ames, D., et al. (2017). Dementia prevention, intervention, and care. *Lancet* 390, 2673–2734. doi: 10.1016/S0140-6736(17)31363-6

MacPherson, A., and Akeroyd, M. A. (2014). Variations in the slope of the psychometric functions for speech intelligibility: a systematic survey. *Trends Hear.* 18:2331216514537722. doi: 10.1177/2331216514537722

Martini, A., Bovo, R., Agnoletto, M., Da Col, M., Drusian, A., Liddeo, M., et al. (1988). Dichotic performance in elderly Italians with Italian stop consonant-vowel stimuli. *Audiology* 27, 1–7. doi: 10.3109/00206098809081568

Martini, A., Castiglione, A., Bovo, R., Vallesi, A., and Gabelli, C. (2014). Aging, cognitive load, dementia and hearing loss. *Audiol. Neurootol.* 19(Suppl. 1), 2–5. doi: 10.1159/000371593

Meister, H. (2017). Speech audiometry, speech perception and cognitive functions. German version. *HNO* 65, 189–194. doi: 10.1007/s00106-016-0229-4

Meister, H., Schreitmuller, S., Grugel, L., Beutner, D., Walger, M., and Meister, I. (2013). Examining speech perception in noise and cognitive functions in the elderly. *Am. J. Audiol.* 22, 310–312. doi: 10.1044/1059-0889(2012/12-0067)

Moradi, S., Lidestam, B., Hallgren, M., and Ronnberg, J. (2014). Gated auditory speech perception in elderly hearing aid users and elderly normal-hearing individuals: effects of hearing impairment and cognitive capacity. *Trends Hear.* 18:2331216514545406. doi: 10.1177/2331216514545406

Muhler, R., Ziese, M., and Rostalski, D. (2009). Development of a speaker discrimination test for cochlear implant users based on the oldenburg logatome corpus. *ORL J. Otorhinolaryngol. Relat. Spec.* 71, 14–20. doi: 10.1159/000165170

Nguyen, M. F., Bonnefoy, M., Adrait, A., Gueugnon, M., Petitot, C., Collet, L., et al. (2017). Efficacy of hearing aids on the cognitive status of patients with alzheimer's disease and hearing loss: a multicenter controlled randomized trial. *J. Alzheimers Dis.* 58, 123–137. doi: 10.3233/JAD-160793

Panza, F., Solfrizzi, V., and Logroscino, G. (2015). Age-related hearing impairment-a risk factor and frailty marker for dementia and AD. *Nat. Rev. Neurol.* 11, 166–175. doi: 10.1038/nrneurol.2015.12

Parham, K., and Kost, K. M. (2017). Presbycusis-peripheral and central. *Ear Nose Throat J.* 96, 462–463. doi: 10.1177/014556131709601206

Peracino, A., and Pecorelli, S. (2016). The epidemiology of cognitive impairment in the aging population: implications for hearing loss. *Audiol. Neurootol.* 21(Suppl. 1), 3–9. doi: 10.1159/000448346

Pisoni, D. B. (1996). Word Identification in Noise. *Lang. Cogn. Process.* 11, 681–687.

Pronk, M., Deeg, D. J., Festen, J. M., Twisk, J. W., Smits, C., Comijs, H. C., et al. (2013). Decline in older persons' ability to recognize speech in noise: the influence of demographic, health-related, environmental, and cognitive factors. *Ear Hear.* 34, 722–732. doi: 10.1097/AUD.0b013e3182994eee

Puglisi, G. E., Warzybok, A., Hochmuth, S., Visentin, C., Astolfi, A., Prodi, N., et al. (2015). An Italian matrix sentence test for the evaluation of speech intelligibility in noise. *Int J. Audiol.* 54(Suppl. 2), 44–50. doi: 10.3109/14992027.2015.1061709

Rooth, M. A. (2017). The prevalence and impact of vision and hearing loss in the elderly. *N. C. Med. J.* 78, 118–120. doi: 10.18043/ncm.78.2.118

Rutherford, B. R., Brewster, K., Golub, J. S., Kim, A. H., and Roose, S. P. (2018). Sensation and psychiatry: linking age-related hearing loss to late-life depression and cognitive decline. *Am. J. Psychiatry* 175, 215–224. doi: 10.1176/appi.ajp.2017.17040423

Santangelo, G., Siciliano, M., Pedone, R., Vitale, C., Falco, F., Bisogno, R., et al. (2015). Normative data for the montreal cognitive assessment in an Italian population sample. *Neurol. Sci.* 36, 585–591. doi: 10.1007/s10072-014-1995-y

Schubotz, W., Brand, T., Kollmeier, B., and Ewert, S. D. (2016). The influence of high-frequency envelope information on low-frequency vowel identification in noise. *PLoS One* 11:e0145610. doi: 10.1371/journal.pone.0145610

Shen, J., Anderson, M. C., Arehart, K. H., and Souza, P. E. (2016). Using cognitive screening tests in audiology. *Am. J. Audiol.* 25, 319–331. doi: 10.1044/2016_AJA-16-0032

Siciliano, M., Chiorri, C., Passaniti, C., Sant'elia, V., Trojano, L., and Santangelo, G. (2019). Comparison of alternate and original forms of the Montreal Cognitive Assessment (MoCA): an Italian normative study. *Neurol. Sci.* 40, 691–702. doi: 10.1007/s10072-019-3700-7

Stern, D., and Hilly, O. (2018). [The relationship between hearing loss and cognitive decline in the elderly and the efficiency of hearing rehabilitation in preventing cognitive decline]. *Harefuah* 157, 374–377.

Strauss, A., Henry, M. J., Scharinger, M., and Obleser, J. (2015). Alpha phase determines successful lexical decision in noise. *J. Neurosci.* 35, 3256–3262. doi: 10.1523/JNEUROSCI.3357-14.2015

Sundstrom, S., Lofkvist, U., Lyxell, B., and Samuelsson, C. (2018). Prosodic and segmental aspects of nonword repetition in 4- to 6-year-old children who are deaf and hard of hearing compared to controls with normal hearing. *Clin. Linguist. Phon.* 32, 950–971. doi: 10.1080/02699206.2018.1469671

Taitelbaum-Swead, R., and Fostick, L. (2016). The effect of age and type of noise on speech perception under conditions of changing context and noise levels. *Folia Phoniatr. Logop.* 68, 16–21. doi: 10.1159/000444749

Thomson, R. S., Auduong, P., Miller, A. T., and Gurgel, R. K. (2017). Hearing loss as a risk factor for dementia: a systematic review. *Laryngoscope Investig. Otolaryngol.* 2, 69–79. doi: 10.1002/lio2.65

Uchida, Y., Sugiura, S., Nishita, Y., Saji, N., Sone, M., and Ueda, H. (2018). Age-related hearing loss and cognitive decline - The potential mechanisms linking the two. *Auris Nasus Larynx* 46, 1–9. doi: 10.1016/j.anl.2018.08.010

Vos, S. J. B., Van Boxtel, M. P. J., Schiepers, O. J. G., Deckers, K., De Vugt, M., Carriere, I., et al. (2017). Modifiable risk factors for prevention of dementia in midlife, late life and the oldest-old: validation of the LIBRA Index. *J. Alzheimers Dis.* 58, 537–547. doi: 10.3233/JAD-161208

Wagener, K. C., Brand, T., and Kollmeier, B. (2006). The role of silent intervals for sentence intelligibility in fluctuating noise in hearing-impaired listeners. *Int. J. Audiol.* 45, 26–33. doi: 10.1080/14992020500243851

Wayne, R. V., and Johnsrude, I. S. (2015). A review of causal mechanisms underlying the link between age-related hearing loss and cognitive decline. *Ageing Res. Rev.* 23, 154–166. doi: 10.1016/j.arr.2015.06.002

Zanetti, O., Frisoni, G. B., Rozzini, L., Bianchetti, A., and Trabucchi, M. (1998). Validity of direct assessment of functional status as a tool for measuring Alzheimer's disease severity. *Age Ageing* 27, 615–622. doi: 10.1093/ageing/27.5.615

Permissions

All chapters in this book were first published by Frontiers; hereby published with permission under the Creative Commons Attribution License or equivalent. Every chapter published in this book has been scrutinized by our experts. Their significance has been extensively debated. The topics covered herein carry significant findings which will fuel the growth of the discipline. They may even be implemented as practical applications or may be referred to as a beginning point for another development.

The contributors of this book come from diverse backgrounds, making this book a truly international effort. This book will bring forth new frontiers with its revolutionizing research information and detailed analysis of the nascent developments around the world.

We would like to thank all the contributing authors for lending their expertise to make the book truly unique. They have played a crucial role in the development of this book. Without their invaluable contributions this book wouldn't have been possible. They have made vital efforts to compile up to date information on the varied aspects of this subject to make this book a valuable addition to the collection of many professionals and students.

This book was conceptualized with the vision of imparting up-to-date information and advanced data in this field. To ensure the same, a matchless editorial board was set up. Every individual on the board went through rigorous rounds of assessment to prove their worth. After which they invested a large part of their time researching and compiling the most relevant data for our readers.

The editorial board has been involved in producing this book since its inception. They have spent rigorous hours researching and exploring the diverse topics which have resulted in the successful publishing of this book. They have passed on their knowledge of decades through this book. To expedite this challenging task, the publisher supported the team at every step. A small team of assistant editors was also appointed to further simplify the editing procedure and attain best results for the readers.

Apart from the editorial board, the designing team has also invested a significant amount of their time in understanding the subject and creating the most relevant covers. They scrutinized every image to scout for the most suitable representation of the subject and create an appropriate cover for the book.

The publishing team has been an ardent support to the editorial, designing and production team. Their endless efforts to recruit the best for this project, has resulted in the accomplishment of this book. They are a veteran in the field of academics and their pool of knowledge is as vast as their experience in printing. Their expertise and guidance has proved useful at every step. Their uncompromising quality standards have made this book an exceptional effort. Their encouragement from time to time has been an inspiration for everyone.

The publisher and the editorial board hope that this book will prove to be a valuable piece of knowledge for researchers, students, practitioners and scholars across the globe.

List of Contributors

Shu-Qi Wang, Jing-Qi Xu and Pei-Dong Dai
Department of Facial Plastic Reconstruction Surgery, Eye and ENT Hospital of Fudan University, Shanghai, China
ENT Institute, Eye and ENT Hospital of Fudan University, Shanghai, China

Chen-Long Li, Li-Li Chen, Liu-Jie Ren, Tian-Yu Zhang and You-Zhou Xie
Department of Facial Plastic Reconstruction Surgery, Eye and ENT Hospital of Fudan University, Shanghai, China
ENT Institute, Eye and ENT Hospital of Fudan University, Shanghai, China
Hearing Medicine Key Laboratory, National Health Commission of China, Shanghai, China

Wen-Juan Yao
School of Mechanics and Engineering Science, Shanghai University, Shanghai, China
Shanghai Institute of Applied Mathematics and Mechanics, Shanghai, China

Lingna Guo
State Key Laboratory of Bioelectronics, School of Life Sciences and Technology, Jiangsu Province High-Tech Key Laboratory for Bio-Medical Research, Southeast University, Nanjing, China
Department of Otolaryngology Head and Neck Surgery, The Second Affiliated Hospital of Anhui Medical University, Hefei, China

Wei Cao
Department of Otolaryngology Head and Neck Surgery, The Second Affiliated Hospital of Anhui Medical University, Hefei, China

Yuguang Niu
Department of Ambulatory Medicine, The First Medical Center of PLA General Hospital, Beijing, China

Shuangba He
Department of Otolaryngology Head and Neck Surgery, Nanjing Tongren Hospital, School of Medicine, Southeast University, Nanjing, China

Renjie Chai
State Key Laboratory of Bioelectronics, School of Life Sciences and Technology, Jiangsu Province High-Tech Key Laboratory for Bio-Medical Research, Southeast University, Nanjing, China
Co-Innovation Center of Neuroregeneration, Nantong University, Nantong, China
Institute for Stem Cell and Regeneration, Chinese Academy of Sciences, Beijing, China
Beijing Key Laboratory of Neural Regeneration and Repair, Capital Medical University, Beijing, China

Jianming Yang
Department of Otolaryngology Head and Neck Surgery, The Second Affiliated Hospital of Anhui Medical University, Hefei, China

Joseph A. Bellairs
Department of Otolaryngology-Head and Neck Surgery, University of Washington, Seattle, WA, United States

Van A. Redila, Ling Tong and Edwin W. Rubel
Department of Otolaryngology-Head and Neck Surgery, University of Washington, Seattle, WA, United States
Virginia Merrill Bloedel Hearing Research Center, University of Washington, Seattle, WA, United States

Patricia Wu
Virginia Merrill Bloedel Hearing Research Center, University of Washington, Seattle, WA, United States
Department of Biological Structure, University of Washington, Seattle, WA, United States

Alyssa Webster and Julian A. Simon
Fred Hutchinson Cancer Research Center, Seattle, WA, United States

David W. Raible
Department of Otolaryngology-Head and Neck Surgery, University of Washington, Seattle, WA, United States
Virginia Merrill Bloedel Hearing Research Center, University of Washington, Seattle, WA, United States,
Department of Biological Structure, University of Washington, Seattle, WA, United States

Dongmei Tang, Xiaoling Lu, Ruonan Huang, Huiqian Yu and Wenyan Li
State Key Laboratory of Medical Neurobiology and MOE Frontiers Center for Brain Science, ENT Institute and Department of Otorhinolaryngology, Eye & ENT Hospital, Fudan University, Shanghai, China
NHC Key Laboratory of Hearing Medicine, Fudan University, Shanghai, China

Dongxin Liu, Ruijuan Dong, Jing Chen and Shuo Wang
Otolaryngology—Head & Neck Surgery, Beijing Tongren Hospital, Beijing Institute of Otolaryngology, Capital Medical University, Beijing, China

Jiong Hu and Gabriella Musacchia
Department of Audiology, University of the Pacific, San Francisco, CA, United States

Xue Wang, Yuechen Han, Fang Chen, Man Wang, Yun Xiao, Haibo Wang, Lei Xu and Wenwen Liu
Department of Otolaryngology-Head and Neck Surgery, Shandong Provincial ENT Hospital, Cheeloo College of Medicine, Shandong University, Jinan, China
Shandong Institute of Otorhinolaryngology, Jinan, China

Jinan Li, Chang Liu, Samuel Kaefer, Mariam Youssef and Bo Zhao
Department of Otolaryngology-Head and Neck Surgery, Indiana University School of Medicine, Indianapolis, IN, United States

Junmin Chen, Penghui Chen, Baihui He, Tianyu Gong, Yue Li, Jifang Zhang, Jingrong Lv, Shule Hou and Jun Yang
Department of Otorhinolaryngology—Head & Neck Surgery, Xinhua Hospital, Shanghai Jiaotong University School of Medicine, Shanghai, China
Ear Institute, Shanghai Jiaotong University School of Medicine, Shanghai, China
Shanghai Key Laboratory of Translational Medicine on Ear and Nose Diseases, Shanghai, China

Fabio Mammano
Department of Physics and Astronomy "G. Galilei", University of Padua, Padua, Italy
Department of Biomedical Sciences, Institute of Cell Biology and Neurobiology, Italian National Research Council, Monterotondo, Italy

Ryan J. Longenecker, Rende Gu, Jennifer Homan and Jonathan Kil
Sound Pharmaceuticals Inc., Seattle, WA, United States

Fuxin Ren, Bin Zhao and Fei Gao
Shandong Medical Imaging Research Institute, Shandong University, Jinan, China

Jianfen Luo
Department of Otolaryngology-Head and Neck Surgery, Shandong Provincial ENT Hospital, Shandong University, Jinan, China
Shandong Provincial Key Laboratory of Otology, Jinan, China

Wen Ma
Department of Otolaryngology, Jinan Central Hospital, Shandong University, Jinan, China

Qian Xin
The Second Hospital of Shandong University, Jinan, China

Lei Xu, Zhaomin Fan, Haibo Wang and Yu Ai
Department of Otolaryngology-Head and Neck Surgery Shandong Provincial ENT Hospital, Shandong University, Jinan, China
Shandong Provincial Key Laboratory of Otology, Jinan, China

Chama Belkhiria, Rodrigo C. Vergara, Simón San Martín, Alexis Leiva and Bruno Marcenaro
Department of Neuroscience, Faculty of Medicine, University of Chile, Santiago, Chile
Biomedical Neuroscience Institute, Faculty of Medicine, University of Chile, Santiago, Chile

Melissa Martinez
Department of Neurology and Neurosurgery, Clinical Hospital of the University of Chile, Santiago, Chile

Carolina Delgado
Department of Neuroscience, Faculty of Medicine, University of Chile, Santiago, Chile
Department of Neurology and Neurosurgery, Clinical Hospital of the University of Chile, Santiago, Chile

Paul H. Delano
Department of Neuroscience, Faculty of Medicine, University of Chile, Santiago, Chile
Biomedical Neuroscience Institute, Faculty of Medicine, University of Chile, Santiago, Chile
Department of Otolaryngology, Clinical Hospital of the University of Chile, Santiago, Chile

Chama Belkhiri, Rodrigo C. Vergara, Simón San Martín, Alexis Leiva and Bruno Marcenaro
Department of Neuroscience, Faculty of Medicine, University of Chile, Santiago, Chile
Biomedical Neuroscience Institute, Faculty of Medicine, University of Chile, Santiago, Chile

Julia Sarant, Peter Busby and Richard Dowell
Department of Audiology and Speech Pathology, The University of Melbourne, Melbourne, VIC, Australia

Robert Briggs
The Royal Victorian Eye and Ear Hospital, Melbourne, VIC, Australia

Shimei Zheng
Department of Otolaryngology-Head and Neck Surgery, Yijishan Hospital of Wannan Medical College, Wuhu, China

Dongmei Tang, Chang Liu and Yingzi He
State Key Laboratory of Medical Neurobiology and MOE Frontiers Center for Brain Science, ENT Institute and Department of Otorhinolaryngology, Eye & ENT Hospital, Fudan University, Shanghai, China
NHC Key Laboratory of Hearing Medicine, Fudan University, Shanghai, China

Xin Wang
Nantong Laboratory of Development and Diseases, School of Life Sciences, Co-innovation Center of Neuroregeneration, Key Laboratory of Neuroregeneration of Jiangsu and MOE, Nantong University, Nantong, China

Na Zuo, Renchun Yan, Cheng Wu, Jun M, Shaofeng Liu and Chuanxi Wang
Department of Otolaryngology-Head and Neck Surgery, Yijishan Hospital of Wannan Medical College, Wuhu, China

Hongfei Xu
Department of Forensic Medicine, Soochow University, Suzhou, China

Dong Liu
Nantong Laboratory of Development and Diseases, School of Life Sciences, Co-innovation Center of Neuroregeneration, Key Laboratory of Neuroregeneration of Jiangsu and MOE, Nantong University, Nantong, China

Dona M. P. Jayakody
Ear Science Institute Australia, Subiaco, WA, Australia
Ear Sciences Centre Faculty of Health and Medical Sciences, The University of Western Australia, Crawley, WA, Australia

Holly K. Menegola and Jack Goodman-Simpson
Ear Science Institute Australia, Subiaco, WA, Australia

Jessica M. Yiannos
Ear Science Institute Australia, Subiaco, WA, Australia
School of Human Sciences, The University of Western Australia, Crawley, WA, Australia

Peter L. Friedland
Department of Otolaryngology Head Neck Skull Base Surgery, Sir Charles Gairdner Hospital, Nedlands, WA, Australia
School of Medicine, University Notre Dame, Fremantle, WA, Australia

Kevin Taddei
School of Medical and Health Sciences, Edith Cowan University, Joondalup, WA, Australia

Simon M. Laws
Collaborative Genomics Group, School of Medical and Health Sciences, Edith Cowan University, Joondalup, WA, Australia
School of Pharmacy and Biomedical Sciences, Faculty of Health Sciences, Curtin Health Innovation Research Institute, Curtin University, Bentley, WA, Australia

Michael Weinborn
School of Medical and Health Sciences, Edith Cowan University, Joondalup, WA, Australia
School of Psychological Science, The University of Western Australia, Nedlands, WA, Australia

Ralph N. Martins
School of Medical and Health Sciences, Edith Cowan University, Joondalup, WA, Australia
Department of Biomedical Sciences, Faculty of Medicine and Health Sciences, Macquarie University, Sydney, NSW, Australia

Hamid R. Sohrabi
School of Medical and Health Sciences, Edith Cowan University, Joondalup, WA, Australia
Department of Biomedical Sciences, Faculty of Medicine and Health Sciences, Macquarie University, Sydney, NSW, Australia
Centre for Healthy Ageing, School of Psychology and Exercise Science, Murdoch University, Murdoch, WA, Australia

Pengcheng Xu, Longhao Wang, Huihui Liu, Hongchao Liu, Yun Lin, Jun Xu, Hao Wu, Tao Yang and Qingyue Yuan
Department of Otolaryngology-Head and Neck Surgery, Shanghai Ninth People's Hospital, Shanghai Jiao Tong University School of Medicine, Shanghai, China
Ear Institute, Shanghai Jiao Tong University School of Medicine, Shanghai, China
Shanghai Key Laboratory of Translational Medicine on Ear and Nose Diseases, Shanghai, China

Hu Peng
Department of Otolaryngology-Head and Neck Surgery, Changzheng Hospital, Second Military Medical University, Shanghai, China

Xiuhong Pang
Department of Otolaryngology-Head and Neck Surgery, Taizhou People's Hospital, The Fifth Affiliated Hospital of Nantong University, Taizhou, China

Xiuwen Wang, Jing Liu and Jiping Zhang
Key Laboratory of Brain Functional Genomics, Ministry of Education, NYU-ECNU Institute of Brain and Cognitive Science at NYU Shanghai, School of Life Sciences, East China Normal University, Shanghai, China

Yujin Li
Department of Otolaryngology-Head and Neck Surgery, Nanjing Drum Tower Clinical College of Nanjing Medical University, Nanjing, China
Department of Otolaryngology-Head and Neck Surgery, The Affiliated Huaian No. 1 People's Hospital of Nanjing Medical University, Huai'an, China

Ao Li, Xia Gao and Ling Lu
Department of Otolaryngology-Head and Neck Surgery, Nanjing Drum Tower Clinical College of Nanjing Medical University, Nanjing, China
Research Institute of Otolaryngology, Nanjing, China
Jiangsu Provincial Key Medical Discipline (Laboratory), Department of Otolaryngology-Head and Neck Surgery, Affiliated Drum Tower Hospital of Nanjing University Medical School, Nanjing, China

Chao Wang
School of Public Health, Nanjing Medical University, Nanjing, China

Xin Jin and Yaoting Zhang
Department of Otolaryngology-Head and Neck Surgery, The Affiliated Huaian No. 1 People's Hospital of Nanjing Medical University, Huai'an, China

Shou-Lin Wang
School of Public Health, Nanjing Medical University, Nanjing, China

Wen Lu, Zhuangzhuang Li, Lili Xiao, Yini Li, Yumeng Jiang and Haibo Shi
Department of Otolaryngology-Head and Neck Surgery, Shanghai Jiao Tong University Affiliated Sixth People's Hospital, Shanghai, China

Kun Ni
Department of Otolaryngology-Head and Neck Surgery, Shanghai Jiao Tong University Affiliated Sixth People's Hospital, Shanghai, China
Department of Otolaryngology-Head and Neck Surgery, Shanghai Children's Hospital, Shanghai Jiao Tong University, Shanghai, China

Jincheng Zhang
Department of Critical Care Medicine, Zhongshan Hospital, Fudan University, Shanghai, China

Ines de Vries, Nils Prenzler and Martin Durisin
Department of Otolaryngology, Hannover Medical School, Hanover, Germany

Heike Schmitt, Thomas Lenarz and Athanasia Warnecke
Department of Otolaryngology, Hannover Medical School, Hanover, Germany
Cluster of Excellence Hearing4all, German Research Foundation, Hannover Medical School, Hanover, Germany

Sameer Alvi and Hinrich Staecker
Department of Otolaryngology, Head and Neck Surgery, University of Kansas School of Medicine, Kansas City, MO, United States

Alessandro Castiglione
Department of Neurosciences, University of Padua, Padua, Italy
Complex Operative Unit of Otolaryngology, Hospital of Padua, Padua, Italy

Mariella Casa and Carlo Gabelli
Regional Center for the Study and Treatment of the Aging Brain, Department of Internal Medicine, Padua, Italy

Samanta Gallo, Flavia Sorrentino, Ezio Caserta, Flavia Gheller, Cristina Giacomelli, Silvia Montino, Davide Brotto and Sonila Dhima
Complex Operative Unit of Otolaryngology, Hospital of Padua, Padua, Italy

Dalila Cilia, Elisa Lovo, Marta Gambin, Maela Previato and Simone Colombo
Department of Neurosciences, University of Padua, Padua, Italy

Federica Limongi
Institute of Neuroscience, National Research Council, Padua, Italy

Patrizia Trevisi, Roberto Bovo and Alessandro Martini
Department of Neurosciences, University of Padua, Padua, Italy
Complex Operative Unit of Otolaryngology, Hospital of Padua, Padua, Italy

Index

N

O

P

R

S

T

V

www.ingramcontent.com/pod-product-compliance
Lightning Source LLC
LaVergne TN
LVHW080954210926
848485LV00004B/834